D. Ba

Principles and Practice of S
Laparoscopy

Advanced Course July 1994
Many thanks for your help, David

James

and Simon.

PRINCIPLES AND PRACTICE OF SURGICAL LAPAROSCOPY

Edited by

Simon Paterson-Brown
Consultant Surgeon, Royal Infirmary, Edinburgh

and

James Garden
Senior Lecturer and Honorary Consultant Surgeon, University Department of Surgery, Royal Infirmary, Edinburgh

W. B. Saunders Company Ltd
London Philadelphia Toronto Sydney Tokyo

W. B. Saunders Company Ltd 24–28 Oval Road
London NW1 7DX

The Curtis Center
Independence Square West
Philadelphia, PA 19106-3399, USA

Harcourt Brace & Company
55 Horner Avenue
Toronto, Ontario M8Z 4X6, Canada

Harcourt Brace & Company, Australia
30–52 Smidmore Street
Marrickville, NSW 2204, Australia

Harcourt Brace & Company, Japan Inc
Ichibancho Central Building, 22-1 Ichibancho
Chiyoda-ku, Tokyo 102, Japan

This book is printed on acid-free paper

A catalogue record for this book is available from the British Library

ISBN 0-7020-1712-4

Typeset by Paston Press Ltd, Loddon, Norfolk

Printed in Great Britain by The University Press, Cambridge

Contents

Bypass surgery – biliary

Colorectal surgery

Benign oesophageal surgery

Antiulcer surgery

Abdominal trauma

Staging of abdominal malignancy

Thoracic sympathectomy

List of Contributors

S. Banting FRACS, P.O. Box 2022, 360 High Street, Kew 3101, Australia.

R. Bendavid MD, Consultant Surgeon, Department of Surgery, Shouldice Hospital, 7750 Bayview Avenue, Box 370, Thornhill, Ontario L3T 4A3, Canada.

D. Burris MD FACS, Assistant Professor of Surgery, Uniformed Services University of the Health Sciences, Bethesda, Maryland; Fellow, Trauma/ Critical Care, Washington Hospital Center, 110 Irving Street NW, Washington DC 20010, USA.

D. Carr-Locke MD FRCP FACG, Director of Endoscopy, Gastroenterology Division, Brigham and Women's Hospital, 75 Francis Street, Boston, Massachusetts 02115, USA.

D. C. Carter MD FRCS FRCP(Edin), Regius Professor of Surgery, Royal Infirmary, Lauriston Place, Edinburgh EH3 9YW.

H. R. Champion FRCS(Edin) FACS, Professor of Surgery, Chief, Division of Surgery for Trauma, Uniformed Services University of the Health Sciences, Bethesda, Maryland; Chief, Trauma and Surgical Critical Care, Washington Hospital Center, 110 Irving Street NW, Washington DC 20010, USA.

B. Dallemagne MD, Consultant Surgeon, Clinique Saint-Joseph, 75 rue de Hesbaye, Liege 4000, Belgium.

A. Darzi MD FRCS(I), Consultant Surgeon, Central Middlesex Hospital, Park Royal, Acton Lane, London NW10 7NS.

A. de Beaux FRCS, Surgical Registrar, Royal Infirmary, Lauriston Place, Edinburgh EH3 9YW.

H. A. F. Dudley CBE ChM FRCS FRACS, Emeritus Professor of Surgery, University of London, Broombrae, Glenbuchat, Strathdon, Aberdeenshire AB3 8UE.

K. C. H. Fearon MD FRCS, Senior Lecturer and Honorary Consultant Surgeon, Royal Infirmary, Lauriston Place, Edinburgh EH3 9YW.

G. A. Fielding FRACS, Consultant Surgeon, Royal Brisbane Hospital, Herston 4029, Queensland, Australia.

O. J. Garden BSc MD FRCS, Senior Lecturer and Honorary Consultant Surgeon, Royal Infirmary, Lauriston Place, Edinburgh EH3 9YW.

J. D. Greig MD FRCS, Senior Registrar, Royal Infirmary, Lauriston Place, Edinburgh, EH3 9YW.

M. Hashmonai MD FACS, Head, Department of Surgery B, Rambam Medical Centre; Associate Professor of Surgery, Technion-Israel Institute of Technology, Haifa, Israel.

T. Hennessy MD MCh FRCS FRCS(I), Regius Professor of Surgery, Trinity College, Dublin, and St. James's Hospital, James Street, Dublin 8, Ireland.

A. Hill MB FRCS(I), Central Middlesex Hospital, Park Royal, Acton Lane, London NW10 7NS.

T. T. Irvin MB PhD ChM FRCS(Edin), Consultant Surgeon, Royal Devon and Exeter Hospital (Wonford), Barrack Road, Exeter, Devon EX2 5DW.

C. Jehaes MD, Department of Surgery, Clinique Saint-Joseph, 75 rue de Hesbaye, Liege 4000, Belgium.

T. G. John FRCS, Lecturer in Surgery, Royal Infirmary, Lauriston Place, Edinburgh EH3 9YW.

N. Katkhouda MD, Associate Professor of Surgery, Chief, Division of Outpatient and Minimally Invasive Surgery, Department of Surgery, University of Southern California, School of Medicine, Los Angeles, CA 90033, USA.

A. Lee FRCA, Consultant Anaesthetist, Royal Infirmary, Lauriston Place, Edinburgh EH3 9YW.

D. Lichtenstein MD, Instructor in Medicine, Harvard Medical School, Associate Physician, Gastroenterology Division, Brigham and Women's Hospital, 75 Francis Street, Boston, Massachusetts 02115, USA.

R. Lombard MD, Department of Surgery, Clinique Saint-Joseph, 75 rue de Hesbaye, Liege 4000, Belgium.

S. Markiewicz MD, Department of Surgery, Clinique Saint-Joseph, 75 rue de Hesbaye, Liege 4000, Belgium.

D. Menzies MS FRCS, Consultant Surgeon, Colchester District General Hospital, Turner Road, Colchester, Essex CO4 5JL.

J. R. T. Monson MD FRCS(I) FRCS FACS, Professor of Surgery, Castle Hill Hospital, Castle Road, Cottingham, North Humberside HU16 5JQ.

M. Morino MD, Associate Professor of Surgery, Department of Surgery, University of Turin, Corso A. M. Dogliotti 14, 10126 Torino, Italy.

R. W. Motson MS FRCS, Consultant Surgeon, Colchester District General Hospital, Turner Road, Colchester, Essex CO4 5JL.

J. Mouiel MD FACS, Professor of Surgery, Hôpital Saint-Roch, 5 rue Pierre Devoluy, BP 319, Nice 06006, France.

A. Nagy MD FRCS(C), Head, Section of Laparoscopic Surgery, Department of Surgery, University of British Columbia, Vancouver, British Columbia V5Z 1H8, Canada.

L. K. Nathanson MB ChB FRACS, Consultant Surgeon/Senior Lecturer, Royal Brisbane Hospital, Herston 4029, Queensland, Australia.

M. G. Ochsner MD FACS, Assistant Professor of Surgery, Uniformed Services University of the Health Sciences, Bethesda, Maryland; Attending Surgeon, Trauma/Critical Care, Washington Hospital Center, 110 Irving Street NW, Washington DC 20010, USA.

M. O'Riordain MD FRCS(I), Senior Registrar, University Department of Surgery, Regional Hospital, Wilton, Cork, Eire.

N. O'Rourke MB BS FRACS, Honorary Consultant, Department of Surgery, North Hampshire Hospital, Aldermaston Road, Basingstoke, Hampshire RG24 9NA.

S. Paterson-Brown MPhil MS FRCS, Consultant Surgeon, Royal Infirmary, Lauriston Place, Edinburgh EH3 9YW.

J. Petelin MD FACS, Clinical Assistant Professor of Surgery, Shawnee Mission Medical Center, 9100 West 74th Street, Shawnee Mission, Kansas 66021, USA.

R. K. S. Phillips MS FRCS, Consultant Surgeon, St Mark's Hospital, City Road, London EC1V 2PS.

G. Plant MBBS FRCR, Consultant Radiologist, North Hampshire Hospital, Aldermaston Road, Basingstoke, Hampshire RG24 9NA.

M. Rees MBBS MS FRCS, Consultant Surgeon, North Hampshire Hospital, Aldermaston Road, Basingstoke, Hampshire RG24 9NA.

J. A. Ross PhD, Non-clinical Lecturer, University Department of Surgery, Royal Infirmary, Lauriston Place, Edinburgh EH3 9YW.

R. C. G. Russell MS FRCS, Consultant Surgeon, The Middlesex Hospital, Mortimer Street, London W1N 8AA.

B. A. Salky MD FACS, Chief, Division of Laparoscopic Surgery, Department of Surgery, Mount Sinai Medical Center, 1 Gustave L. Levy Place, New York 10029, USA.

M. Schein MD FCS(SA), Consultant Surgeon, Bnei Zion Medical Centre, Clinical; Senior Lecturer and Deputy Head, Technion-Israel Institute of Technology, Haifa, Israel.

H. J. Scott, MS FRCS, Senior Registrar, Ashford Hospital, Ashford, Middlesex.

N. J. Standfield MS FRCS, Senior Lecturer, Hammersmith Hospital, Royal Postgraduate Medical School, Du Cane Road, London W12 0NN.

R. W. Stitz MD, Royal Brisbane Hospital, Herston 4029, Queensland, Australia.

M. Sutter MD, Senior Resident, Division of General Surgery, University of British Columbia, 906-750 West Broadway, Vancouver, British Columbia V5Z 1H8, Canada.

T. V. Taylor MD ChM FRCS Eng. FRCS Ed. FACG, Chief, General Surgery, DVA Medical Center Hospital, Associate Professor of Surgery, Baylor College of Medicine, 2002 Holcombe Boulevard, Houston, Texas 77030, USA.

A. Watson MD FRCS FRACS, Consultant Surgeon, The Wellington Hospital, London NW8 9LE.

J. Weerts MD, Consultant Surgeon, Clinique Saint-Joseph, 75 rue de Hesbaye, Liege 4000, Belgium.

Preface

Over the last few years laparoscopy, once the preserve of the practising gynaecologist and occasional surgical enthusiast, has at last become established in general surgery. The surgical revolution which followed the successful introduction of laparoscopic cholecystectomy, has now united all clinicians who operate within the two main body cavities into a common group of minimal access surgeons. However, the very attraction of a swift post-operative recovery and reduced wound pain – the driving force behind the acceptance of minimal access techniques over conventional surgery by patients and surgeons alike – has brought with it new problems, many of which remain unanswered.

The speed of introduction of laparoscopic surgery took many surgeons by surprise, most having to embark upon a rapid re-learning process in order not to be left behind. The understandable desire to search for more procedures which might be performed using minimal access techniques has called into question many of the traditional surgical methods and teachings. Although questioning of surgical dogma must always be encouraged, lessons learnt by meticulous attention to detail, experimental analysis and clinical trials over the last half century of open surgery must not be abandoned too readily just to facilitate the laparoscopic approach.

We are now at a crossroads in the management of most surgical conditions. New technology has rendered the majority of operations possible within the scope of minimal access and laparoscopic techniques, but the data for many are not yet available to guide the surgeon in whether such procedures are appropriate. In this book we have been fortunate to be able to draw upon the enormous experience of surgeons at the fore of clinical practice in the treatment of surgical conditions by both established open and laparoscopic techniques. By presenting the current expectations from open surgical operations with the early results of comparable laparoscopic procedures, along with the operative techniques used, we hope the readers will be able to judge for themselves for which surgical conditions the laparoscopic approach is most suitable.

The very speed of these changes in surgical therapy may render much of the data in this book out of date within a few years, but if the principles behind these surgical decisions are understood, then surgery can proceed with the same objectives for which our predecessors taught us to strive: safe surgery, low morbidity, and maximum chance for cure in cases of malignant disease.

The authors gratefully acknowledge the immense support provided by their long-suffering wives, Sheila and Mandy, during the evenings and weekends sacrificed in the preparation of this book. We are grateful to colleagues for having provided us with such excellent work and hope that those recalcitrant colleagues who required repeated prompting to deliver manuscripts, agree that our efforts were justified. We would also wish to acknowledge the skilled secretarial assistance of Carole Tomlinson and are grateful to Rachael Stock and Seàn Duggan of WB Saunders Company Limited, for their continued support and patience. We are very grateful to David Gardner and Gillian Lee for drawing the illustrations.

Simon Paterson-Brown
O. James Garden

1

Introduction

H. A. F. DUDLEY

Access to body cavities in order to undertake surgical procedures by other means than making a large, if well designed hole through the chest or abdominal wall has been a technique waiting for its time. For many years gynaecologists have practised the art of viewing the pelvic organs through an instrument not very dissimilar from the cystoscope but their expertise was somewhat jealously guarded and their techniques relatively crude. Moreover, they largely confined their expertise to diagnosis though in recent years laparoscopic sterilization has become an application of importance.

Outside the field of gynaecology things began to change about 20 years ago. Some abdominal surgeons felt that they might be able to make a diagnosis of, say, inoperable malignant disease by laparoscopic observation which could be further underpinned by taking a biopsy without resort to formal laparotomy. Most of their colleagues remained conservative – as is usual in the surgical profession until some compelling argument is brought forward – so that the occasional pioneers were largely disregarded. Nevertheless a shift in attitude was underway. On the one hand it was the outcome of a drive towards "minimally invasive surgery" which had been pioneered by urologists and radiologists in relation to the urinary system and which had lead first to transcutaneous techniques of access to the renal pelvis and then to methods of gaining a view of the urinary tract above the bladder.[1] On the other hand it was a combination of increased interest in reducing the morbidity of conventional abdominal surgery, combined with a clearer understanding of the ability to make a diagnosis in acute abdominal pain without resort to opening the abdomen by a formal incision so as to "look and see rather than wait and see".

All these factors have come together in the late 1980s and early 1990s to create a new and rapidly growing movement which not only exploits the skills of those who can look down a monocular telescope – as did the urologists – but can also relate what they see to their knowledge of conventional anatomy in order to carry out complex procedures in three-dimensional space. As is well known, the telescope has now been replaced by the television camera but the two-dimensional problem still persists. Exactly how this movement took off will be a subject for surgical historians to explore many years hence but one of the seminal studies was that of Sugarbaker and his colleagues who first precisely focused attention on the role of laparoscopic examination in the "acute abdomen".[2] They showed, as is considered in more detail elsewhere in this book, that it was possible to avoid unnecessary laparotomy in a significant number of patients and so save them from the discomforts and possible complications of an abdominal exploration as well as reducing expenditure in the health system as a whole.

Nevertheless it has to be admitted that for better or for worse (and I usually take the latter view), what most captures the surgical imagination is *therapy* rather than *diagnosis*. The next development was the realization that it was possible to remove the gall bladder, first with the relatively primitive instruments of the gynaecologists but later, as the technology gained momentum, with more effective tools.[3]

Laparoscopic cholecystectomy was truly a watershed in the development of minimal access surgery in fields other than urology and has resulted – as this book indubitably shows – in an explosion of techniques which are now challenging conventional surgery. It has now certainly become *possible* to carry out extremely complex procedures such as oesophagectomy, hiatus hernia repair and restorative resection of the distal colon and rectum through numerous small ports in the abdominal and/or thoracic wall. The question that remains to be answered is whether the advantages of this type of approach are sufficient to make them a new standard against which conventional open surgery, with its big exposures and precise Halstedian dissection, should be judged. To this I will briefly return.

The great plus point for endoscopic surgery in the chest and abdomen is that it avoids the physiological disturbance which is caused by the incision and the distraction of structures required to gain access. It is reasonably certain that we have underestimated these matters and have tended blindly to ascribe all the diverse features of the response to injury to the operation as a whole rather than to specific aspects such as the extent of the wound required, eventration and the handling of viscera. The objective biological evidence is not yet fully available – though some of it is considered in this volume – but it is striking that patients are often so little disturbed by endoscopic procedures that they are able to leave hospital much earlier than convention would expect. It is reasonable for endoscopic surgeons to assume that they have almost completely removed the 'wound factor' both in relation to its general effects and also, of more importance to the patient, in terms of the subjective disturbance created by pain which is also an important trigger of adaptive events. It is, however, as yet unclear whether endoscopic surgery may not lead to problems of its own. Amongst these are the potential but still insufficiently evaluated, though possibly deleterious, effects of a prolonged pneumoperitoneum which are discussed in more detail elsewhere in this volume.

In the abdomen there is another small but possibly important point. It has always been conventional teaching that every laparotomy is *exploratory* in that, however precise the preoperative diagnosis, other findings are sought so that they can be dealt with if this is perceived necessary. Such an attitude is open to question but with minimal access surgery has largely to be abandoned. The risk of an error of omission is small but should be kept in mind.

The next matter which has to be addressed is whether conventional and endoscopic procedures have comparable outcomes in dealing with disease and disorder. In the short term, do they have the same (and, it is to hoped, minimal) complication rate? In the long term, do they yield the same results, such as for example recurrence of hernia and freedom from residual malignant disease? To assess such matters the discipline of clinical medicine has developed the controlled trial with its formal assignment of a random sample to a group which receives the best conventional treatment and one which is allotted to the new. This is a wonderful scientific apparatus but one which has significant problems in relation to the introduction of a new surgical technique.[4] First it is impossible to set up a sample which is "blind" to the new approach and therefore results may be conditioned by the treatment that has been perceived to have been administered. Second, and more important in the present context, there are the social and surgical preconceptions which drive the patient and the surgeon to think *a priori* that the new is preferable to the old which makes the recruitment to a trial difficult.[5] With minimally invasive procedures this viewpoint is reinforced for the patient by the perceived short term advantages in terms of freedom from pain, little or no time in hospital and a speedy return to normal activities. Surgeons also are particularly susceptible to the tug of the new because they have an intuitive liking for technical change and possible advance which leads them to embrace (sometimes one has to say falsely) anything that is novel and exciting in therapy.

Again, this book is written at a time when the evidence is not available but what is somewhat disturbing is that it may well never be possible to obtain it. Both for the reasons that I have given and the experience of those who work in the field of minimal access surgery, the conventional approach of clinical trials is well nigh impossible and as yet we have not accepted a different analytic apparatus which permits us properly to judge new techniques of which minimal access surgery is but one example. There are of course circumstances where the advantage is so obvious that neither a formal trial nor a subtle statistical analysis is necessary. However, there are situations where comparison with conventional treatment is definitely required; resective treatment for malignant disease is a good example. The use of laparoscopic techniques for resection of gastrointestinal malignancy is clearly an attractive option but there must be *a priori* doubts about the efficacy of clearance, the possibility of seeding in the peritoneal cavity or along the track of insertion of an instrument and the necessary abandonment of such niceties as mediolateral dissection in colon cancer.

In all fields thoughtful and prospective analysis of results is vital so that they can at least be compared with previous best practice but even this is being forgotten in a technical rush to exploit the new equipment which is becoming available and the skills that surgeons are able to deploy. The example of laparoscopic cholecystectomy is familiar to all: rapid conversion of all but a few surgeons;[6] a steep "learning curve" with an initially high incidence of complications which may in some instances, such as bile duct injury, persist above the level found in open surgery; an increased number of operations which may possibly be the outcome of relaxing the established indications for the procedure;[7] and finally, only a retrospective – and therefore partially flawed – analysis of results.

In the same general area as this last matter is the possible effect of the laparoscopic option on surgical decision making. Cutting into the body has always been viewed as something which should be done only after the most careful consideration and if there is no obvious and equally satisfactory alternative. This is of course right but since the turn of the century good indications have been established which justify an open operation and, though surgeons still have to exert their authority and personality to persuade both patients and their internal medicine colleagues that the proposed course of action is correct, surgical judgement is on the whole respected. However, now that there is the possibility of doing the same thing without the most visible (and sometimes the most painful) feature of a surgical procedure – the incision – there is the slight but definite possibility of a retreat from or reluctance to undertake an open procedure when it is unequivocally needed. A recent case in England has highlighted some aspects of such reluctance when a patient who had undergone hysterectomy developed complications suggestive of intestinal obstruction and though open surgery was recommended, a laparoscopic procedure was undertaken. The bowel was perforated and though open surgery was later done, the patient died.[8] It is true that the same sequence of events can follow open surgery but it is, in my view, particularly likely to occur in circumstances where minimal access surgery is available. One anecdote does not make a cogent premise but the possibility should be borne in mind, particularly in that with increasing public experience of and satisfaction with endoscopic techniques, pressure to avoid open surgery will also come from patients.

A further matter which attracts my attention is whether surgical principles and outcomes inherited from our teachers and built into our standards of performance are being too hastily abandoned or falsely challenged. Inguinal hernia is a case in point. Though no one would claim that everything is known about hernia repair, it has in the last half century been possible to get recurrence rates down to very small numbers by the application of such principles as flush ligation of the sac and careful suture repair of the fascia transversalis. Admission to hospital is not often necessary and the well-planned incisions used are virtually invisible after a few months. Yet we are now faced with a drive to use the laparoscope and often prosthetic inserts for repair even though it would seem from first principles that there is nothing much to gain and perhaps something to lose. Of course it is always right to question principles which have perhaps been too long taken for granted but such a challenge should be based on sound premises that are associated with the welfare of the patient rather than the attractions to the surgeon of a new method which he or she wishes to exploit. It may well be that some of my cautious attitude to change that has not been well considered on logical grounds may prove as wrong as the statements of some surgeons at the close of the last century who believed that certain parts of the body would always be beyond the reach of surgery. Nevertheless a note of conservatism is required.

The pages of this book bear witness to the extraordinary wave of activity that has been unleashed by the throwing of the "gestalt switch"[9] of endoscopic surgery. There is little doubt that the next few years will better establish where the balance should be struck between open and minimal access surgery in the chest and abdomen. Where this lies will greatly influence many aspects of clinical surgery: allocation of resources, the training of the next generation and quite possibly the design of operating facilities. There will further be an increasing need for interaction between surgeons on the one hand and scientists and engineers on the other so that what we might loosely term "remote operating" using complicated optics and three-dimensional observation of the operating field becomes ever more possible. We are only on the threshold of the possibilities and in some ways it is remarkable that so much has been achieved, so safely, with what is quite crude apparatus. As in other surgical fields, we can look forward to increasing refinement in instruments and techniques but again we must hope that this will be the subject of scientific endeavour rather than, as has appeared to happen with orthopaedic implants, the outcome of fashion and hard selling by industry.

REFERENCES

1. Fitzpatrick JM, Wickham JEA. Minimally invasive surgery. *Br J Surg* 1990; **77**: 721–2.
2. Sugarbaker PH, Bloom BS, Sanders JH, Wilson RE. Pre-operative laparoscopy in diagnosis of acute abdominal pain. *Lancet* 1975; **1**: 442–5.
3. Dubois F, Icard P, Berthelot G, Levard H. Coelioscopic cholecystectomy. *Ann Surg* 1990; **211**: 60–2.
4. Dudley HAF. The controlled clinical trial and the advance of reliable knowledge: an outsider looks in. *Br Med J* 1983; **287**: 957–60.
5. Neugebauer E, Troidl W, Spangenburger A, Dietrich R, Lefering R and the Cholecystectomy Study Group. Conventional versus laparoscopic cholecystectomy and the randomised controlled trial. *Br J Surg* 1991; **78**: 150–4.
6. Leman F. Laparoscopic cholecystectomy: a cautionary note. *Br J Surg* 1991; **78**: 1400.
7. Orlando R, Russell JC, Lynch J, Mattie A. Laparoscopic cholecystectomy. A statewide experience. *Arch Surg* 1993; **128**: 494–9.
8. Brahms D. 'Keyhole' surgery with fatal complications. *Lancet* 1993; **341**: 170.
9. Kuhn T. *The Structure of Scientific Revolutions*. Chicago, University of Chicago Press, 1962.

2

The Inflammatory and Metabolic Response to Open Surgery and Minimally Invasive Surgery

M. O'RIORDAIN, J. A. ROSS and K. C. H. FEARON

INTRODUCTION

In 1932 Sir David Cuthbertson[1] wrote that following long bone fracture or soft tissue injury, "there is an early and rapid catabolism of the tissues, . . . that the main site of catabolism is skeletal muscle . . . that the time of maximum catabolism is contemporaneous with the first sign of regeneration of the injured part . . . and that in a few cases net catabolism could continue for up to one to two months". He concluded that "The early acceleration of the catabolism of protein is a special effort to meet an urgent need". These observations have formed the basis for most subsequent metabolic research into the response to surgical injury and hence are a suitable starting point for this discussion on how a laparoscopic approach may modify the metabolic and immunological sequelae of open surgery.

Sir David Cuthbertson emphasized that the metabolic changes observed following surgery fulfilled an urgent need that was basic to survival. In the past few years we have come to understand how this process is mediated not only via afferent neurogenic stimuli activating the classical neuroendocrine pathways but also via factors produced in the injured tissue and released into the systemic circulation. The most important group of these locally produced factors are called cytokines. These small polypeptides were first recognized as key intercellular messengers in the immune system but are now known to be produced by a great variety of cells and have the potential for autocrine, paracrine and endocrine effects. The importance of the neuroendocrine and cytokine responses in maintaining/restoring homoeostasis following minor or moderate tissue injury is beyond doubt. However, the metabolic and immunological responses which ensure short term survival are now recognized to bring about much more prolonged metabolic changes which may influence duration of convalescence and delay return to full health. Moreover, in the severely injured or septic patient, if such responses are uncontrolled or markedly prolonged then this may compromise ultimate survival.[2] The introduction of the laparoscopic approach to chest and abdominal surgery now allows us to examine the influence of the wound itself on the physiological response to surgery. This provides a unique chance to unravel further the interplay between neuroendocrine and cytokine pathways and their influence on outcome. This chapter is thus divided into sections that describe the metabolic changes that follow tissue injury, the classic neuroendocrine response, the cytokine response and finally how all these changes are modified by a laparoscopic approach.

THE METABOLIC RESPONSE

It has long been established that the extent and degree of the metabolic changes which follow tissue injury depend on the severity of that injury. Clearly for the majority of surgical procedures which can be performed laparoscopically the degree of injury is of a mild or moderate nature. The following description of the metabolic changes which occur after surgery necessarily reflects this limitation. The metabolic response may also be modified by the preoperative nutritional status of the patient, the use of concurrent nutritional support and by the manipulation of the cytokine or neuroendocrine systems which mediate the response. However, since few patients undergoing elective laparoscopic procedures are grossly malnourished, receive TPN or undergo epidural anaesthesia, these factors will not be considered further.

The Metabolic Response to Starvation

It is important to appreciate that apart from the 24–48 hours surrounding the period of surgery and until spontaneous oral diet returns, the dominant metabolic influence is that of progressive starvation. Anorexia and a reduced food intake occur over a considerable period and the effects can be seen many weeks after discharge from hospital. It is well documented that even after a simple abdominal procedure such as open cholecystectomy, patient habitual energy intake is not reached until approximately the seventh postoperation day, nitrogen losses in the immediate postoperation period are not completely restored until the eighteenth postoperation day, and less than 15% of patients will have regained their preoperation stable weight 30 days after surgery.[3]

During starvation the body rapidly uses up its glycogen reserves and is faced with providing approximately 100 g of glucose per day to satisfy cerebral and red cell energy requirements. The body's main energy reserve is fat but the brain is unable to utilize free fatty acids directly. The problem is overcome by the liver converting free fatty acids to ketone bodies which can then be utilized by the brain. However, the changeover to the brain utilizing ketone bodies requires an

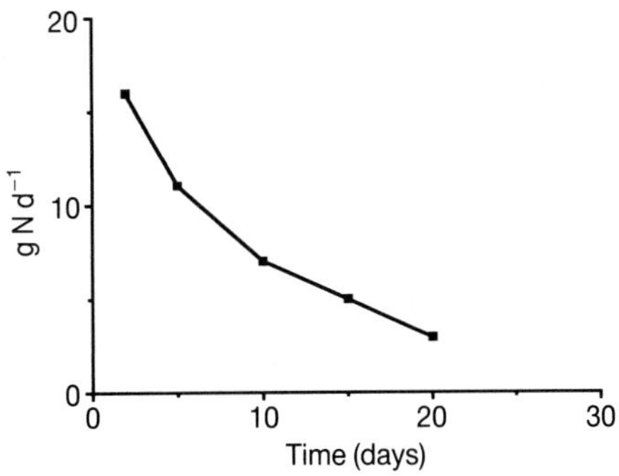

Figure 2.1 Urinary nitrogen loss during total starvation in a 70 kg male.

increase in circulating ketone body levels which occurs progressively over the first 7–10 days of a fast. The gap is filled by mobilizing amino acids from skeletal muscle to support hepatic gluconeogenesis. Hence during early starvation[4] there are substantial urinary nitrogen losses associated with accelerated hepatic gluconeogenesis, followed by a fall once glucose requirements diminish (Fig. 2.1). Conservation of body fuels is further achieved by a fall in the rate of various energy requiring metabolic cycles (for example, protein turnover) and an overall decrease in energy expenditure. This pattern of events is somewhat modified in the "starving" surgical patient since, independent of the influence of surgery *per se*, most of these individuals will receive up to two litres of 5% dextrose per day which in effect will supply at least a proportion of endogenous glucose requirements and may change the hormonal milieu responsible for the switch to hepatic ketogenesis.

The Metabolic Response to Surgery

Following minor or moderate surgical injury the starvation response which allows fuel conservation is modified, particularly in the first 24–72 hours. Patients develop a systemic acute phase response comprising a low grade pyrexia, leucocytosis, complement activation and the production of hepatic acute phase proteins. The acute phase proteins are believed to be important in the host survival response. Some acute phase proteins are opsonins which enhance the phagocytosis of bacteria or damaged host cells and others are antiproteases which limit destruction of host tissues.[5] The acute phase protein response is generally regarded as under the primary control of the cytokine network and is discussed in the next section. The major metabolic changes that accompany the acute phase reaction include a rise in energy expenditure and an increase in the supply of the various substrates required for maintenance of hepatic acute phase protein synthesis, for upregulation of the immune system and for healing and repair in the injured tissue. In order to supply energy substrates, rates of lipolysis and gluconeogenesis are increased and free fatty acid and glucose levels rise in the plasma.[6] Clearly, loss of adipose tissue, at least in the short term, has little functional effect on the patient. Of much greater importance is the loss of protein mass which results from accelerated turnover and use of amino acids for gluconeogenesis and as substrates for new protein synthesis.

Skeletal muscle is the largest organ in humans, comprising 40% of total protein content of the body. It acts as the prime labile amino acid store after injury. Following moderate surgical trauma protein synthesis rates in skeletal muscle fall dramatically (by one third within two hours of the start of surgery)[7] and this is accompanied by a fall in protein degradation rates, the overall effect being a net release of amino acids (particularly branched chain amino acids) into the plasma. It must be emphasized, however, that the maximum rates of nitrogen loss from the body following moderate surgical trauma rarely exceed 8–14 g N d^{-1} (approximately 300–500 g d^{-1} wet weight lean tissue) and that this rate of loss seldom continues for more than a few days. Perhaps of greater interest is that protein synthesis rates and intracellular amino acid levels may remain altered for more than 30 days postoperation and may relate to the postoperative fatigue observed long after the acute protein catabolism has resolved.[3]

THE CONTROL OF THE METABOLIC RESPONSE TO SURGICAL TRAUMA

The principal cause of the increased basal metabolic rate, protein catabolism and nitrogen loss which occur after major surgery appears to be the production of hormones which are "counter-regulatory" to insulin and which include cortisol, adrenaline and glucagon. These hormones rise rapidly during surgery[8] and the infusion of these stress hormones may mimic the effects of surgical trauma or sepsis in healthy volunteers causing lipolysis, proteolysis and an increase in resting energy expenditure.[9,10] The metabolic response to surgery occurs very rapidly and a fall of approximately 30% in skeletal muscle protein synthesis occurs as early as 90 minutes after cholecystectomy.[7] The speed of onset of the response suggests that a neural mechanism is involved. It is likely that during surgery, afferent somatic and visceral neurogenic signals activate the hypothalamo-pituitary-adrenal axis to cause the release of cortisol and adrenaline into the systemic circulation. Indeed, perioperative epidural blockade greatly influences the metabolic response to surgery. Epidural blockade extending from T4 to S5 in patients undergoing lower abdominal surgery prevents the outpouring of adrenaline and cortisol,[11] prevents the normal increase in arterial glucose or free fatty acid concentrations[6] and abrogates the usual increase in urinary nitrogen excretion.[12]

The situation is less clear in upper abdominal or thoracic surgery where such blockade of the neuroendocrine axis fails to prevent the rise in serum cortisol or resting energy expenditure.[6,13] It has been suggested that in the latter situation, although pain relief may be complete and sustained, fast conducting nerve fibres may not be completely blocked, thus allowing the neuroendocrine axis to be activated. It is likely, however, that the failure of epidural anaesthesia in this situation is due also to the production of other mediators by the wound or traumatized tissue.

IMMUNE CONTROL OF METABOLISM

More recently it has become apparent that cells of the immune system may also control metabolism in major trauma or sepsis. Immune cells rapidly invade the surgical wound and become activated, releasing proinflammatory cytokines into the systemic circulation. Gut derived endotoxin may also activate and stimulate cytokine production from these cells.[14] Cytokines are naturally occurring heterogeneous peptides and glycoproteins synthesized principally by the cells of the reticuloendothelial and immune systems. They are mediators of inflammation secreted by one cell which act on another cell. They may act locally or exist in active form in the circulation. The principal proinflammatory cytokines interleukin-1 (IL-1), IL-6 and tumour necrosis factor (TNF) are released primarily by activated macrophages, but also by other cells including neutrophils. Such cytokines appear to operate as a network of interacting signals with both synergistic and antagonistic effects on the release of other cytokines and mediators. IL-1 is known to act on the hypothalamus[15,16] with the release of corticotrophin-releasing factor and the activation of the hypothalamo-pituitary-adrenal axis. The influence of the immune system on the hypothalamo-pituitary-adrenal axis is important as it completes the bidirectional control loop between the immune and the endocrine systems: corticosteroids have been shown to downregulate the immune system and inhibit the production of proinflammatory cytokines by the macrophage. The interaction is likely to be much more complicated than this and shorter feedback loops may also occur: mononuclear leucocytes express adrenergic receptors as well as receptors for ACTH while monocytes produce a substance which directly induces release of cortisol from adrenocortical cells.[17]

It is important to emphasize that the effects of each cytokine may not be compartmentalized or dissected from those of the other cytokines and the synergistic and complementary actions of all are required to generate the full clinical response. Indeed, it is likely that other cytokines, as well as non-cytokine mediators such as the prostaglandins and leukotrienes, heat shock proteins, kinins and endocrine hormones play an important role in a manner which is as yet not fully understood. Of the proinflammatory cytokines, IL-6 has been best studied in the postoperative patient principally because it is readily measurable in serum and is thought to be the main cytokine controlling hepatic acute phase

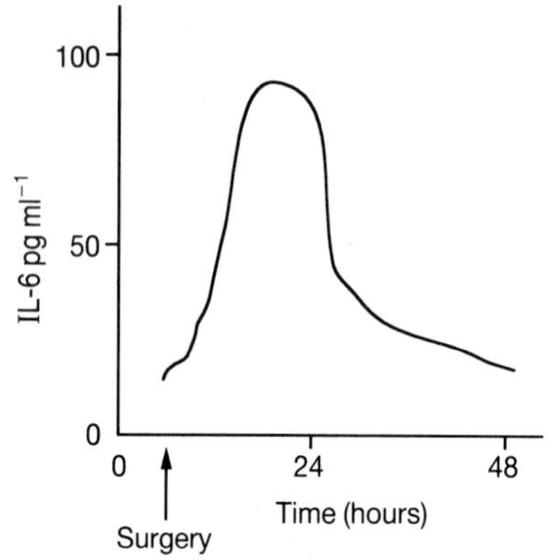

Figure 2.2 Typical IL-6 response following major elective surgery.

response production (Fig. 2.2). Serum IL-6 becomes elevated between 12 and 24 hours after major surgery and this elevation remains for at least 48–72 hours.[18] The serum IL-6 concentration appears to be proportional to the severity of the injury.[19]

Control of the Acute Phase Response

The acute phase protein response appears to be principally under the control of certain proinflammatory cytokines (IL-1, IL-6 and TNF) produced by the cells of the monocyte/macrophage lineage. There is evidence that IL-1 and TNF induce the upregulation of IL-6 production[20] and that IL-6[21] is the cytokine primarily involved in delivering the final signal for an alteration in the regulation of protein synthesis to hepatocytes. Recently, IL-6 induced transcriptional activation[22] of a set of human acute phase proteins and nuclear transcription factors which interact with the C-reactive protein promoter[23] has been described. The full actions of these cytokines are beyond the scope of this chapter and are reviewed elsewhere.[24]

IL-1 was the original proinflammatory cytokine and was initially known as endogenous pyrogen (Fig. 2.3). While it is a principal mediator of inflammation with activation of the immune response, it also induces production of the immunosuppressive prostaglandin E_2 (PGE_2). TNF was originally described as an endogenous mediator of fat loss in chronic parasitic infections which lead to cachexia. More recently it has been ascribed a role in the endogenous response to overwhelming sepsis. TNF has been implicated in protein catabolism,[25] although the evidence for this is not clear. IL-6, in common with other cytokines, displays pleiotropic effects and thereby influences the biology of a number of different cell types (for example, IL-6 plays a major role in the control of antibody production from B cells).

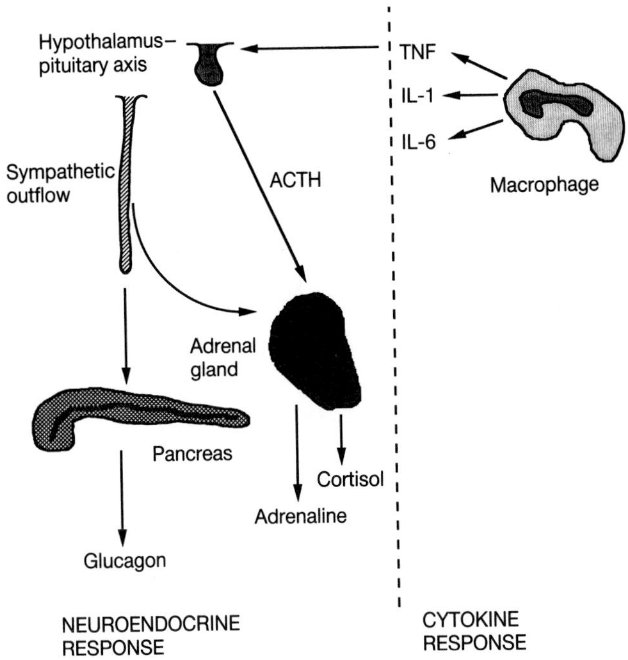

Figure 2.3 Inter-relationships of the classic neuroendocrine response and the inflammatory (cytokine) response.

It has been assumed that the hepatocyte plays a passive role during the acute phase response. Isolated hepatocytes are insensitive to endotoxin, a triggering factor for the release of cytokines (IL-1, TNF and IL-6) from cells of the monocyte lineage, but when cocultured with Kupffer cells, synthesize acute phase proteins.[26] This is analogous to the acute phase protein response identified *in vivo*. Although IL-6 responsive elements have been demonstrated in a number of genes coding for acute phase proteins, other control mechanisms, including those synergistic or antagonistic with IL-6 control, cannot be excluded. The relative importance of locally produced and circulating cytokines in the alteration in hepatic protein synthesis is unclear. Although the addition of crude supernatants from endotoxin stimulated Kupffer cells induces an acute phase protein response with suppression of albumin and transferrin production in isolated hepatocytes, the induction is significantly less than that detected in Kupffer cell/hepatocyte coculture systems. This may indicate that a Kupffer cell membrane bound or secreted protein synergizes with the IL-6 signal to maximize the induction of acute phase protein production. TNF in particular is a shortlived protein with the potential to exist in a transmembrane form[27] and this may be the functionally important form with regard to intercellular signalling in the liver.

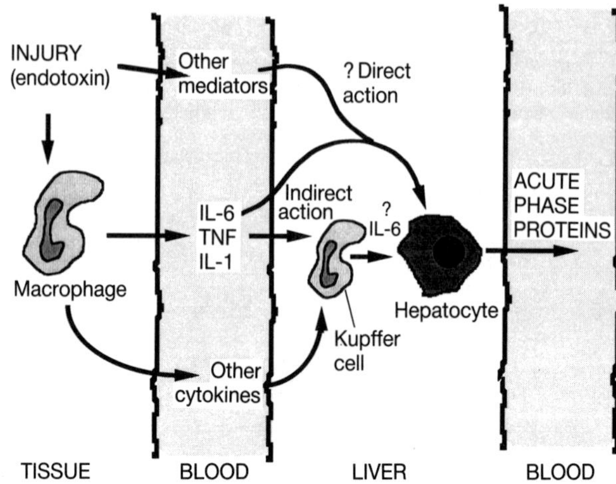

Figure 2.4 Hypothetical scheme for the control of hepatocyte acute phase protein production.

It may be that during the acute phase response Kupffer cells (or related cells such as peripheral blood macrophages) become activated, releasing proinflammatory cytokines such as IL-6, which then act on the hepatocyte to induce production of the acute phase proteins with suppression of normal export proteins (Fig. 2.4). This may be important in multiple organ failure syndrome where overstimulation by the Kupffer cell may well play an important role in the pathogenesis of the hepatic dysfunction seen in this condition.[28]

Other Mediators

A number of other mediators have been implicated in the control of the acute phase response. Nitric oxide, a product of arginine metabolism within many types of cell (including the macrophage), may suppress hepatic protein synthesis.[29] It also causes hypotension and has been implicated in the generation of a systemic acute phase response. While it appears that nitric oxide may well play a significant role in the pathogenesis of sepsis, its role in the metabolic response to surgery is unknown. More information is available on the role of the prostaglandins, but again their contribution is unclear. Prostaglandins are known to be elevated after major trauma or burns[30] and indeed may contribute to the T cell suppression seen in these conditions. In addition, the administration of cyclo-oxygenase inhibitors such as ibuprofen may reduce the production of acute phase response proteins after elective surgery. However, these inhibitors also enhance the production of proinflammatory cytokines *in vitro* and this would be expected to induce an acute phase response. The reduction in acute phase protein production produced by these agents occurs without an alteration in serum cytokines. There is no evidence that the prostaglandins work directly on the hepatocyte and reports regarding the mechanism of action of the cyclo-oxygenase inhibitors are conflicting. It may well be that these drugs work not by their actions on cyclo-oxygenase activity but rather by some other mechanism not as yet defined.

OVERALL BENEFIT OF STRESS RESPONSE TO THE HOST

As previously discussed, the metabolic and acute phase responses to trauma have evolved as complex mechanisms to optimize host survival. Whilst a moderate acute phase response may be beneficial, a response which is prolonged in duration or intensity may be detrimental. A severe stress response occurring in reaction to major trauma leads to the gross catabolism of body protein. The hepatic acute phase proteins are produced at the expense of the normal hepatic export proteins such as albumin, prealbumin or transferrin and production of these is suppressed. Upregulation of the immune system leads to the over-production of the proinflammatory cytokines with signs of systemic sepsis syndrome while T cell regulatory functions appear to be compromised. Neutrophils are activated and contribute to adult respiratory distress syndrome (ARDS). Such a severe stress response may have been appropriate before the development of modern intensive care (where this stress response remained the host's only chance of recovery from injury). However, with today's intensive care and surgical techniques the patient may be artificially provided with many of the beneficial effects of the acute phase response, including the provision of substrates such as glucose and amino acids, the use of potent antibacterial agents, the removal (debridement) of necrotic tissue and the repair of open wounds. In this situation the detrimental effects of the acute phase response outweigh the benefits.

Therapeutic Manipulation of the Acute Phase Response in the Surgical Patient

There are few animal or clinical data indicating whether it is beneficial to attenuate the acute phase response following surgery. Except in extreme circumstances, we do not know whether the combined effects of the stress response are beneficial or detrimental to the host. The typical surgical patient undergoing major abdominal surgery falls somewhere in the middle of a clinical spectrum ranging from the subject with a trivial injury to the patient with major overwhelming sepsis. Most patients undergoing abdominal surgery demonstrate a relatively minor self-limiting acute phase response where none of the major detrimental effects such as major protein catabolism or sepsis syndrome are seen. Nevertheless, the detrimental effects of the acute phase response may be more subtle in these patients and may be manifest as muscle fatigue, loss of grip strength or general weakness persisting for many weeks after the operation.

In a recent study, Schulze and coworkers[31] have attenuated the acute phase response to surgery by means of a combined regimen which included preoperative steroids, perioperative intrathecal neural blockade and postoperative cyclo-oxygenase inhibition. Fatigue scores were improved in the treated group. However, the number of patients in this study was small. Larger trials are required to determine whether blockade of the acute phase response would compromise the natural ability of a patient to respond to a serious or unforeseen complication such as bacterial invasion or anastomotic leak. In addition, the acute phase response plays a role in wound healing and the consequences of its blockade on wound and anastomotic healing need to be elucidated. Clearly the optimal situation would be to limit the trauma which initiated the acute phase response in the first instance. Once the primary insult has occurred, however, it is not clear whether a therapeutic attempt to inhibit the response should be made.

Laparoscopic Surgery and the Minimization of Surgical Trauma

While these dilemmas are being clarified, it would appear that the most logical strategy is to minimize the injury which initiates the acute phase response in the first instance. The stress response associated with a surgical operation may be related to the degree of tissue trauma caused by the surgery. The latter is particularly related to the length of the incision. However, other factors such as extent of bowel handling,[19] stretching of the peritoneum[32] or the amount of internal tissue damage may also play a role. At present, we do not have good methods of estimating the degree of trauma induced by a particular surgical procedure. Until these tools are developed, we can only speculate that laparoscopic surgery may reduce the traumatic challenge. For the meanwhile, perhaps the best method of resolving the issue is to measure the stress response to surgery, examining the metabolic, neuroendocrine, cytokine and acute phase responses.

MODIFICATION OF THE METABOLIC RESPONSE AS A RESULT OF LAPAROSCOPY

Open cholecystectomy has been used frequently as a model of moderate surgical trauma and therefore it is not surprising that with the advent of laparoscopic surgery, most of the information comparing the metabolic response between open and closed techniques concerns this operation. Our own and recent studies[32,33] will be considered with respect to the metabolic, neuroendocrine and cytokine response and also in relation to the patient's clinical course.

Metabolic Response

Very little information is available on the metabolic sequelae of laparotomy versus laparoscopically performed procedures. The principal model used to date has been cholecystectomy. Since at least 45% of patients undergoing the laparoscopic procedure are discharged on their first postoperative day it is difficult to undertake controlled metabolic studies. In the study by Mealy and coworkers[32] no significant difference was demonstrated in urinary urea excretion in the first 24 hours following either the open or closed operation. However, the latter was not a randomized study, total urinary nitrogen was not measured and patients were allowed to eat during the collection period. Since the duration of postoperative fasting is known to be longer in patients undergoing the open procedure,[33] these problems make interpretation of the data difficult.

Neuroendocrine Response

Following cholecystectomy using either an open or laparoscopic technique, there appears to be no significant change in the immediate postoperative period and for the ensuing 48 hours in the pattern of elevated serum cortisol concentrations or urinary cortisol excretion.[32,33] Similarly, the plasma catecholamine response does not appear to differ between the two types of surgery.[33] These findings suggest that there is equivalent activation of the neuroendocrine axis via afferent neurogenic stimuli from a laparotomy wound versus the induction and maintenance of a pneumoperitoneum. Previous studies using epidural morphine administration in patients undergoing open cholecystectomy have suggested that postoperative pain is a factor involved in the stress response following surgery.[34] In the studies comparing laparotomy with laparoscopic cholecystectomy, pain scores were generally higher for longer in the laparotomy group and analgesic consumption was at least doubled.[32,33] If analgesics had not been freely available one might have expected the open operation to have induced a more prolonged stress response.

Cytokine and Acute Phase Response

Much attention has focused on the cytokine and acute phase response observed in open versus laparoscopic surgery. Returning to the cholecystectomy model,

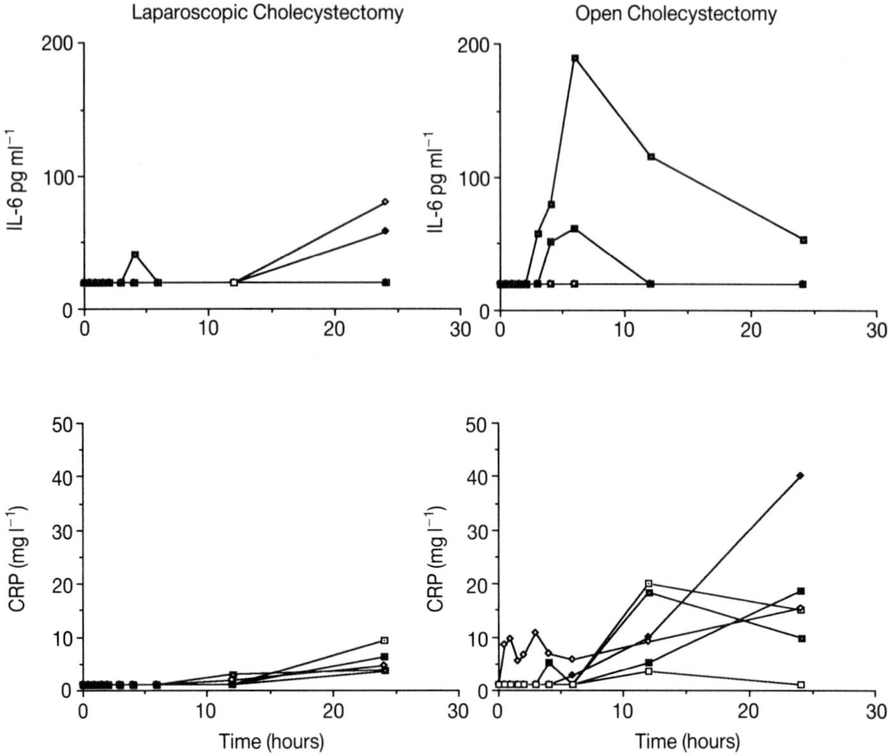

Figure 2.5 Kinetics of interleukin-6 and C-reactive protein in patients who underwent laparoscopic cholecystectomy (n = 5) or conventional cholecystectomy (n = 6). Of those who underwent laparoscopic cholecystectomy, two had detectable IL-6 at 24 hours but all had CRP levels of <10 mg l^{-1}. Those patients who had open cholecystectomy demonstrated a more heterogeneous response in terms of both circulating IL-6 and CRP levels. The minimum limit of detection of the IL-6 ELISA was 20 pg ml^{-1} and of the CRP ELISA was 1 mg l^{-1}.

our own data (Fig. 2.5) and at least three different studies[32,33,35] have confirmed significantly higher circulating C-reactive protein (CRP) concentrations at 24 hours postoperation in patients undergoing the open as opposed to the laparoscopic procedure. Moreover, Joris and coworkers have shown that for up to 48 hours following surgery, plasma interleukin-6 levels are higher in the open cholecystectomy group.[33] In contrast, our own studies would suggest a more heterogeneous serum IL-6 response to open cholecystectomy, some patients having a response similar to that observed with the laparoscopic technique whilst others produce a more dramatic response. Our findings are therefore similar to those of Roumen and coworkers.[36] It has previously been shown that the increase in concentration of circulating interleukin-6 is approximately proportional to the severity of the surgery.[19] Moreover, as stated previously, interleukin-6 appears to be the main regulator of hepatocyte acute phase protein production by human hepatocytes.[22,23] Overall these data tend to suggest greater tissue trauma in the open cholecystectomy group and a consequently greater and more prolonged acute phase response.

Clinical Course of Patients

In these studies of laparoscopic cholecystectomy overall hospital stay was reduced by nearly 50% and the patients' improved recovery was associated with a decreased duration of postoperative fasting, an improvement in simple respiratory function tests and a decrease in analgesic consumption.[32,33] This improved outcome occurred with no obvious difference in activation of the neuroendocrine stress response but with significantly less activation of the cytokine/acute phase response. It is tempting to extrapolate from these findings to suggest that the cytokine/acute phase response might be the dominant factor in determining certain aspects of postoperative recovery. However, more detailed analysis of these responses in a variety of models will be required before any such judgement can be made.

CONCLUSION

Clearly a laparoscopic approach will diminish the amount of tissue damage and the degree of activation of the neuroendocrine and cytokine pathways that follows surgery. The effects of these changes on patient recovery are self-evident. However, this brief survey of the modifications which occur has served to emphasize the lack of detailed metabolic studies comparing patients treated either laparoscopically or by conventional surgery. Much more work is required in order to understand the mechanisms by which the inflammatory response is brought about and how further changes in anaesthesia, analgesia or surgical technique might reduce the catabolic response to surgery and shorten the duration of recovery.

Acknowledgements

The authors would like to thank J. Maingay for assistance with the IL-6 and CRP ELISAs. Work in the authors' laboratory is supported by the Leverhulme Trust. M.G. O'Riordain is supported by a University of Edinburgh Research Fellowship.

REFERENCES

1. Cuthbertson D. Observations on disturbance of metabolism produced by injury to the limbs. *Q J Med* 1932; **25**: 233–46.

2. Dofferholff ASM, Bom VJJ, de Vries-Hospers HG *et al.* Patterns of cytokines, plasma endotoxin, plasminogen activator inhibitor and acute phase proteins during the treatment of severe sepsis in humans. *Crit Care Med* 1992; **20**: 185–92.
3. Petersson B, Wernerman J, Waller SO, von der Decken A, Vinners E. Elective abdominal surgery depresses muscle protein synthesis and increases subjective fatigue: effects lasting more than 30 days. *Br J Surg* 1990; **77**: 796–800.
4. Cahill GF. Starvation: some biological aspects. In: *Nutrition and Metabolism in Patient Care* (eds Kinney JM, Jeebebhoy KN, Hill GL and Owen OE), pp. 193–204. Philadelphia, WB Saunders, 1988.
5. Stahl WM. Acute phase protein response to tissue injury. *Crit Care Med* 1987; **15**: 545–50.
6. Hakenson E, Rutberg H, Jorfeldt L, Mortensson J. Effects of the extradural administration of morphine or bupivacaine on the metabolic response to upper abdominal surgery. *Br J Anaesth* 1985; **57**: 394–9.
7. Essen P, McNurlan MA, Wernerman J, Vinners E, Garlick PJ. Uncomplicated surgery, but not general anaesthesia decreases muscle protein synthesis. *Am J Physiol* 1992; **262**: E253-E260.
8. Alberti KGMM, Batstone GF, Path MRC, Foster KJ, Johnstone DG. Relative role of various hormones in mediating the metabolic response to injury. *J Parent Ent Nutr* 1980; **4**: 141–5.
9. Watters JM, Bessey PQ, Dinarello CA, Wolff SM, Wilmore DW. Both inflammatory and endocrine mediators stimulate host response to sepsis. *Arch Surg* 1986; **121**: 179–90.
10. Bessey PQ, Watters JM, Aoki TT, Wilmore DW. Combined hormonal infusion stimulates the metabolic response to injury. *Ann Surg* 1984; **200**: 264–81.
11. Kehlet H. The modifying effect of general and regional anaesthesia on the endocrine–metabolic response to surgery. *Reg Anaesth* 1982; **7**: 538–44.
12. Carli F, Webster J, Pearson M *et al.* Protein metabolism after abdominal surgery: effect of 24-H extradural block with local anaesthetic. *Br J Anaesth* 1991; **67**: 729–34.
13. Schulze S, Roikjaer O, Hasselstrom L, Jensen NH, Kehlet H. Epidural bupivacaine and morphine plus systemic indomethacin eliminates pain but not the systemic response and convalescence after cholecystectomy. *Surgery* 1988; **103**: 321–7.
14. Deitch EA. The role of intestinal barrier failure and bacterial translocation in the development of systemic infection and multiple organ failure. *Arch Surg* 1990; **125**: 403–4.
15. Besedovsky H, del Rey A, Sorkin E, Dinarello CA. Immunoregulatory feedback between interleukin-1 and glucocorticoid hormones. *Science* 1986; **233**: 652–4.
16. Sapolski R, Rivier C, Yamamoto G, Plotsky P, Vale W. Interleukin-1 stimulates the release of hypothalamic corticotrophin-releasing factor. *Science* 1987; **238**: 522–4.
17. Buzzetti R, McLoughlin L, Scavo D, Rees LH. A critical assessment of the interactions between the immune system and the hypothalamo-pituitary-adrenal axis. *J. Endocrinol* 1989; **120**: 183–7.
18. Parry-Billings M, Baigrie RJ, Lamont PM, Morris PJ, Newsholme EA. Effects of major and minor surgery on plasma glutamine and cytokine levels. *Arch Surg* 1992; **127**: 1237–40.
19. Cruickshank AM, Fraser WD, Burns HJG, van Damme J, Shenkin A. Response of serum interleukin-6 in patients undergoing elective surgery of varying severity. *Clin Sci* 1990; **79**: 161–5.
20. Shimizu H, Mitomo K, Watanabe T *et al.* Involvement of a NF-kB-like transcription factor in the activation of the interleukin-6 gene by inflammatory lymphokines. *Mol Cell Biol* 1990; **10**: 561–8.
21. Heinrich PC. Interleukin-6 and the acute phase protein response. *Biochem J* 1990; **265**: 621–36.

22. Morrone G, Giliberto G, Oliviero S *et al.* Recombinant interleukin-6 regulates the transcriptional activation of a set of human acute phase genes. *J Biol Chem* 1988; **263**: 12554–8.
23. Majello B, Arcone R, Toniatto C, Giliberto G. Constitutive and IL-6 induced nuclear factors that interact with the human C-reactive protein promoter. *EMBO J* 1990; **9**: 457–65.
24. Akira S, Hirano T, Taga T, Kishimoto T. Biology of the multifunctional cytokines: IL-6 and related molecules (IL-1 and TNF). *FASEB J* 1990; **4**: 2860–7.
25. Sherry BA, Gelin J, Fong Y *et al.* Anti-cachectin/tumor necrosis factor antibodies attenuate development of cachexia in tumor models. *FASEB J* 1989; **3**: 1956–62.
26. West MA, Billiar TR, Curran RJ, Cerra FB, Simmons RL. Endotoxin modulation of hepatocyte secretory and cellular protein synthesis is mediated by Kupffer cells. *Arch Surg* 1988; **123**: 1400–5.
27. Leuttig B, Decker T, Lohmann-Matthes M-L. Evidence for the existence of two forms of membrane tumour necrosis factor: an integral protein and a molecule attached to its receptor. *J Immunol* 1989; **143**: 4043–4048.
28. Shiratori Y, Tanaka M, Hai K *et al.* Role of endotoxin-responsive macrophages in hepatic injury. *Hepatology* 1990; **11**: 183–92.
29. Billiar TR, Curran RJ, Stuehr DJ *et al.* An L-arginine-dependent mechanism mediates Kupffer cell inhibition of hepatocyte protein synthesis *in vitro*. *J Exp Med* 1989; **169**: 1467–72.
30. Arturson G. Prostaglandins in human burn wound secretion. *Burns* 1977; **3**: 112–18.
31. Schulze S, Sommer P, Bigler D *et al.* Effect of combined prednisolone, epidural analgesia, and indomethacin on the systemic response after colonic surgery. *Arch Surg* 1992; **127**: 325–31.
32. Mealy K, Gallagher H, Barry M, Lennon F, Traynor O, Hyland J. Physiological and metabolic responses to open and laparoscopic cholecystectomy. *Br J Surg* 1992; **79**: 1061–4.
33. Joris J, Cigarini I, Legrand M *et al.* Metabolic and respiratory changes after cholecystectomy performed via laparotomy or laparoscopy. *Br J Anaesth* 1992; **69**: 341–5.
34. Rutberg H, Hakanson E, Anderberg B, Jorfeldt L, Martensson J, Schildt B. Effect of the extradural administration of morphine or bupivacaine on the endocrine response to upper abdominal surgery. *Br J Anaesth* 1984; **56**: 233–7.
35. Jakeways MSR, Mitchell V, Hashim IA *et al.* Metabolic and inflammatory changes following laparoscopic cholecystectomy. *Proc Nut Soc* 1992; in press.
36. Roumen RMH, van Meurs PA, Kuypers HHC, Kraak WAG, Sauerwein RW. Serum interleukin-6 and C-reactive protein responses in patients after laparoscopic or conventional cholecystectomy. *Eur J Surg* 1992; **158**: 541–4.

3

General Anaesthesia for Laparoscopic Surgery

A. LEE

The dramatic increase in the range of operations performed using minimally invasive surgical techniques is likely to continue and to obtain the maximum benefit for the patient, anaesthetic practice must complement the surgery. Diagnostic laparoscopy and short laparoscopic surgical procedures have been commonplace in gynaecological practice for many years. At first sight, general surgical operations performed laparoscopically present the anaesthetist with a familiar situation, but the anaesthetic techniques used in gynaecology may not be readily transferred to the field of general surgery. The duration of surgery, the age of the patient and the incidence of pre-existing medical problems are often greater with general surgery. Features specific to the laparoscopic technique required for general surgery may affect the cardiorespiratory stability of the patient during the procedure, e.g. the requirement for reverse Trendelenburg position.

In addition to the usual needs of the operative period, namely a sleeping, analgesed and adequately relaxed patient, the aims of anaesthesia for laparoscopic surgery should include a clearheaded, rapid recovery from anaesthesia and the provision of adequate postoperative analgesia allowing early ambulation, resumption of oral intake and short hospital stay.

The surgeon's experience of the reduction in surgical stress and the rapid recovery of patients after laparoscopically performed surgery means that older patients with multiorgan disease, who may otherwise be considered unfit for a conventional procedure, will be presented for assessment. Potential problems should be addressed in advance with the aim being to identify and reverse acute pathology and optimize chronic dysfunction. The procedures themselves are frequently prolonged and the effects of the pneumoperitoneum need to be appreciated and allowed for. The possibility of conversion to open surgery should always be anticipated. Appropriate monitoring and recovery facilities are no less essential than after more conventional forms of surgery.

PHYSIOLOGICAL DISTURBANCES DURING LAPAROSCOPIC SURGERY

Predictable physiological changes occur during laparoscopic surgery. These are caused by the anaesthetic agents and techniques employed, e.g. intermittent positive pressure ventilation, the pneumoperitoneum which produces primary mechanical effects and features secondary to carbon dioxide (CO_2) absorption, the various operative tilting manoeuvres required and the stress of the operation itself. Less commonly, severe physiological disturbances secondary to complications of the technique occur. The anaesthetist needs to understand and manage the patient appropriately in the face of expected physiological derangements and be alert to the early features of a developing complication, e.g. pneumothorax, gas embolism, extraperitoneal CO_2 insufflation. The expected physiological features of the technique will be discussed below. Clinical presentation and management of complications will be considered with the intraoperative course.

Cardiovascular System

Minor cardiovascular disturbances are not uncommon during laparoscopic procedures and occasional catastrophic events have been reported.[1–6]

With modern equipment it is usual to maintain a pneumoperitoneum with a pressure of approximately 2 kPa (15 mmHg) using CO_2 as the insufflating gas. Studies which report on the effects of pneumoperitoneum at pressures up to and in some cases exceeding 5.5 kPa (40 mmHg) have limited relevance to routine clinical practice.[7] Cardiovascular disturbances are predominantly related to the pneumoperitoneum but factors such as the anaesthetic agents, the position of the patient, the structures being stimulated surgically and the insufflating gas used are important.[8,9] The interaction of some of these factors with the cardiovascular effects caused by the pneumoperitoneum can produce more exaggerated disturbances than those that occur when individual factors such as the pneumoperitoneum or Trendelenburg position are examined in isolation.[7,10,11] The cardiovascular effects caused by the pneumoperitoneum will be considered together. Other cardiovascular disturbances will be discussed separately.

Effect of the Pneumoperitoneum

Simple clinical measurements of blood pressure and heart rate may give a misleading impression of cardiovascular stability.[12] Several studies have examined the effect of pneumoperitoneum on cardiac output in animal models and in humans. Implanted aortic flow probes and thermodilution techniques have been used to measure cardiac output in animals. Invasive indocyanine green and non-invasive thoracic impedance methods have been used in humans.[10,12–14]

The use of a flow probe to measure inferior vena caval blood flow allows an understanding of the relationship between central venous pressure measurements and venous return during increasing intra-abdominal pressure.[7,14]

Cardiac output decreases when the intra-abdominal pressure exceeds 2.7 kPa (20 mmHg).[13,14] Insufflation up to pressures of 2.7 kPa may have minimal effect on cardiac output, but this is dependent on other factors, in particular intravascular volume status.[11] Dogs made hypervolaemic can maintain cardiac output even at intra-abdominal pressures of 5.5 kPa.[7] There is also a relationship between the degree of Trendelenburg tilt employed during laparoscopy and the maintenance of cardiac output. In dogs a decrease in cardiac output with increasing intra-abdominal pressure is aggravated by reverse Trendelenburg position and partially alleviated by Trendelenburg position.[10]

Central venous pressure is a misleading measure of venous return to the heart after abdominal insufflation. Animal studies have shown that while central venous pressure consistently increases, the transmural pressure gradient (mean right atrial pressure–mean pleural pressure) decreases because of a marked increase in pleural pressure.[14] This occurs at intra-abdominal pressures as low as 2.7 kPa and there is a concurrent decrease in supradiaphragmatic inferior vena caval blood flow to the heart, leading to a decrease in cardiac output.

A consistent effect of the pneumoperitoneum on the cardiovascular system is an increase in systemic vascular resistance.[14] In conjunction with minimal changes in heart rate this can lead to relatively normal values for heart rate and blood pressure in the presence of significantly reduced cardiac output and oxygen delivery.[8] The increased peripheral vascular resistance is partially accounted for by compression of the abdominal aorta and an increase in splanchnic arteriolar vasoconstriction secondary to the increase in intra-abdominal pressure. This is most marked if there is concurrent hypovolaemia.[7] Venous return is increased by the increase in mean systemic pressure secondary to compression of splanchnic venules; however, this is more than offset by the increase in venous resistance due to vena caval compression with increasing intra-abdominal pressure. Hypervolaemia can maintain the patency of the vena cava, reduce venous resistance and lead to an augmentation of venous return secondary to the increase in mean systemic venous pressure.

Another possible mechanism leading to increased systemic vascular resistance is the increase in plasma arginine vasopressin (AVP) concentration which occurs with the increase in intra-abdominal pressure.[15] A tenfold increase over basal levels has been recorded with increases in intra-abdominal pressure of <1.3 kPa (10 mmHg). An increase in plasma AVP concentration can occur in the absence of blood pressure, heart rate or acid-base disturbances and does not appear to be related to underlying disease or level of anxiety. It is most likely that an increase in plasma AVP concentration occurs secondary to a reduction in left atrial transmural pressure gradient rather than being due to a reduction in thoracic blood volume, a known factor causing release of AVP.[15,16] Changes in thoracic blood volume have not been demonstrated at intra-abdominal pressures of <1.3 kPa, a pressure level at which plasma AVP concentration increases.

Sympathetic stimulation from pain or hypercarbia may also lead to an increase in systemic vascular resistance.[17]

Dysrhythmias

Bradycardia is a common rhythm disturbance during laparoscopy.[4,18] It may occur secondary to pelvic manipulations during gynaecological procedures or follow peritoneal stretching during insufflation. It is presumed to be a vagally mediated problem and responds promptly to vagolytic drugs such as atropine. Modern anaesthetic agents, in particular the newer neuromuscular blocking agents such as atracurium and vecuronium, produce minimal or no vagolytic effects. As a result bradycardia may become a more frequent problem. Opioid drugs (e.g. fentanyl) have been shown to have central effects that may contribute to the incidence of intraoperative bradycardia.

Tachycardia is less frequently observed during laparoscopic surgery, but may occur secondary to inadequate anaesthesia, hypercarbia, blood loss or following the use of vagolytic agents such as atropine.

Hypercarbia in association with the use of halothane leads to a high incidence of intraoperative dysrhythmias, most commonly ventricular ectopics.[5] This complication can frequently be avoided by the use of another volatile agent (e.g. enflurane) which does not sensitize the myocardium to circulating catecholamines, mechanical ventilation to normocarbia or the use of another gas for insufflation. Nitrous oxide supports combustion and is not a suitable alternative to CO_2 as the use of diathermy is contraindicated. Helium is a possible alternative.[19]

Changes in Blood Pressure

Hypotension is not uncommon during laparoscopy and usually indicates a significant decrease in cardiac output. It may be related to technical problems with the anaesthetic, e.g. inappropriate dose of anaesthetic agent, hypoxia or diminished venous return as a consequence of mechanical hyperventilation. It may occur secondary to surgical factors, e.g. vagal stimulation causing bradycardia, or significant haemorrhage. Most commonly, intraoperative hypotension during laparoscopic surgery is a result of the pneumoperitoneum causing diminished venous return to the heart. Rarely, hypotension may be associated with complications such as gas embolism, pneumothorax or serious dysrhythmia.

Hypertension may occur secondary to hypercarbia following carbon dioxide absorption from the peritoneal cavity leading to sympathetic nervous stimulation or may more simply be the result of inadequate analgesia or anaesthesia.[20]

Respiratory System

Conventional abdominal surgery has profound effects on respiratory function demonstrable for many days postoperatively. This is particularly true when an upper abdominal incision is required for procedures such as cholecystectomy. Laparoscopic surgery may have a less detrimental effect on respiratory function, but the effects of prolonged pneumoperitoneum need to be considered.

Several studies have examined the respiratory effects of laparoscopy, some in a purely descriptive fashion, others in a randomized manner compared to open surgery. Parameters evaluated include simple respiratory function tests, other lung volumes, e.g. functional residual capacity and physiological dead space, oxygenation and the degree of hypercarbia and its causes. The time courses of these changes have been investigated with a reasonably consistent pattern emerging from different researchers.

Lung Volumes

Forced expiratory volume in one second (FEV_1) and forced vital capacity (FVC) are markedly reduced after open abdominal procedures and reductions to 50% of normal after upper abdominal surgery are not uncommon 24 hours postoperatively.[21,22] Recovery is slow and reductions of >20% are still frequently present on the third postoperative day. In contrast, the reductions in FEV_1 and FVC after laparoscopic surgery (cholecystectomy), are much less marked at 24 hours (FEV_1 85% and FVC 70% of preoperative values).[23] By day 3, respiratory function tests have almost returned to normal following laparoscopic cholecystectomy with the FEV_1 92% and FVC 91% of preoperative values.

A 30% decrease in functional residual capacity from preoperative values is common 24 hours after open cholecystectomy. This is slow to resolve, being 75% of preoperative values by day 3.[23] Following laparoscopic cholecystectomy, a 10% decrease at 24 hours is more usual with full recovery of FRC by day 3.[23,24] A postoperative reduction in FRC is associated with atelectasis and hypoxaemia and is of clinical relevance. Alterations in lung volumes postoperatively may be related to pain, but the above differences between laparoscopic and conventional surgery can be demonstrated in patients with similar pain scores postoperatively, albeit requiring less analgesic medication after a laparoscopically performed procedure.[23] Significant changes in FRC and the development of atelectasis following laparoscopic surgery can be predicted in patients aged >60 years, current smokers and those with respiratory symptoms preoperatively.[24] There may be a subset of patients who have a greater than average impairment of respiratory function after laparoscopic procedures. These patients have impaired respiratory function to start with and are least able to withstand a further deterioration postoperatively.[25] The patient with significant pulmonary dysfunction who is presented for anaesthetic assessment because of the perceived lack of respiratory problems associated with laparoscopic surgery may still become a significant postoperative problem.

Small but significant decreases in carbon monoxide diffusing capacity occur at 24 hours postoperatively.[24]

Arterial Blood Gas Analysis

Hypoxaemia. Whilst hypoxaemia occurs after both laparoscopic and conventional abdominal surgery, it has been demonstrated to be of shorter duration following laparoscopic procedures.[22–24] Two days after laparoscopic surgery arterial oxygenation has returned to preoperative values, but is still reduced several days after conventional surgery. Impaired oxygenation is the result of ventilation perfusion mismatching secondary to reduced functional residual capacity and atelectasis. The time course is consistent with the changes in lung volumes demonstrated postoperatively. This cause of hypoxaemia is easily corrected with supplemental oxygen administered by facemask.

Hypercarbia. Carbon dioxide pneumoperitoneum is associated with hypercarbia secondary to absorption of gas from the peritoneal cavity.[26] This does not occur when nitrous oxide or helium is the insufflating gas.[5,19,26] The rise in intra-abdominal pressure produces an increase in dead space, but this is insufficient to account for the degree of hypercarbia.[26,27] The rate of CO_2 absorption from the peritoneal cavity has been quantified at 40 ml min^{-1}, i.e. an increase of approximately 30% over a measured basal production of 145 ml min^{-1}.[28] A 20–30% increase in minute ventilation is sufficient to eliminate the increased CO_2 load and maintain normocapnia. This technique helps to avoid dysrhythmias, vasodilatation and excessive respiratory drive which sometimes manifests itself as straining of the abdominal muscles when muscle relaxation is inadequate. This straining to breathe can result in the triggering of the high pressure alarm on the insufflation machine.

An appropriate level of ventilation to excrete the increased CO_2 load can be judged from the end tidal CO_2 tension measured using a capnograph. In fit patients the arterial–alveolar CO_2 gradient is small and increases only slightly following CO_2 absorption from the pneumoperitoneum.[29,30] Some patients have little scope to increase their alveolar ventilation because of severe pre-existing lung disease.[26] These patients may have difficulty in eliminating this moderately increased CO_2 load and develop marked hypercarbia.[31] This may not be reflected in the end-tidal CO_2 tension measured by the capnograph due to a large arterial–alveolar CO_2 gradient.[32] Measurement of arterial blood gases is required intraoperatively in patients with severe lung disease and conversion to open surgery may be necessary if hypercarbia becomes excessive. The use of helium as an insufflating gas would be particularly useful in this group of patients.[19,26]

Postoperatively arterial CO_2 tension is unchanged from preoperative values.[22]

Postoperative Respiratory Complications

Many studies confirm the expectation of reduced impairment of respiratory function after laparoscopic surgery when compared with conventional surgery, but as yet there is little evidence of a reduction in the clinical sequelae such as pneumonia. Larger studies of postoperative complications will be required.

Renal Function

In animal studies an increase in intra-abdominal pressure to 2.7 kPa leads to a reduction in renal blood flow and glomerular filtration rate to less than 25% of baseline. This effect is secondary to renal vein compression rather than a decrease in cardiac output.[33]

Temperature Control

Heat loss from the open abdomen can be considerable and it might be expected that heat loss after laparoscopic surgery would be less. However, decreases in body temperature comparable to or greater than those following conventional surgery have been reported.[34,35] This reflects the duration of surgery and the use of cold insufflating gas and highlights the need to treat all aspects of the intraoperative course carefully. A heated mattress on the operating table, a condenser humidifier in the anaesthetic circuit and warming of fluids will normally be adequate.

ANAESTHETIC MANAGEMENT

Laparoscopy may be performed under local anaesthesia, central nervous system blockade using an epidural or spinal technique, general anaesthesia with the patient breathing spontaneously through a facemask, laryngeal mask or endotracheal tube or general anaesthesia with the patient ventilated. Spontaneously breathing techniques are commonly used for short procedures (less than 30 minutes), but for longer procedures paralysis, intubation and mechanical ventilation will provide better operating conditions.

Preoperative Preparation

The increasing trend towards day case and short stay surgery is given impetus by the use of laparoscopic techniques, but this should not compromise patient care. Patients with coexisting medical problems should have a thorough preoperative assessment. All patients should be in the optimum condition for surgery. In additition to appropriate preoperative investigations, it is advisable to group and save blood for rapid crossmatch if required.

A preoperative visit by the anaesthetist should be standard practice. This will allow for a review of the patient's general fitness for surgery, assessment of the need for premedication and an explanation of procedures relating to the anaesthetic and postoperative analgesia.

Premedication is not essential but a short-acting, orally administered anxiolytic such as temazepam 1–2 hours before surgery is most appropriate if requested. Subcutaneous heparin may be administered at this time for prophylaxis against deep venous thrombosis.

Induction

Reliable intravenous access should be sited preoperatively in preparation for possible major haemorrhage. Monitoring prior to induction will normally consist of continuous electrocardiography, intermittent non-invasive blood pressure measurement and pulse oximetry.

Patients considered at risk of regurgitation should be preoxygenated and then undergo a rapid sequence induction utilizing cricoid pressure to guard against the aspiration of gastric contents.

An induction agent such as propofol which is rapidly cleared from the body may allow a more clearheaded and rapid recovery from anaesthesia. The avoidance of suxamethonium may reduce the incidence of muscle pain postoperatively in patients who are going to mobilize early, but this has not been confirmed after outpatient laparoscopy.[36]

A nasogastric tube placed after induction will allow a distended stomach to be decompressed resulting in improved surgical access to the operative field. Pressure points should be carefully padded. Methods to conserve heat should be employed. The eyes should be protected and the patient positioned appropriately before surgery if an operative cholangiogram is to be performed.

Maintenance

A variety of anaesthetic agents may be used. There are potential differences in the incidence of postoperative sequelae using different techniques, but these are relatively minor distinctions and no one technique has emerged as ideal. Nausea and vomiting may be more likely if an intravenous opioid has been used rather than a volatile anaesthetic alone, but analgesia may then be inadequate for smooth anaesthesia. Nitrous oxide does not cause significant bowel distension or postoperative emetic sequelae after laparoscopic cholecystectomy, as has been reported following other operations, but does have the potential to worsen the haemodynamic effects of venous CO_2 embolism compared to a technique in which 100% oxygen is administered.[37–39] Halothane has the potential to cause dysrhythmias in the presence of hypercarbia, but is not contraindicated in a ventilated patient.[5]

The best anaesthetic is the one with which the anaesthetist is most familiar and can use smoothly. General principles should include the use of short-acting agents to allow rapid recovery. Paralysis and mechanical ventilation to normocapnia is usual. A commonly employed technique would be induction using propofol, muscle paralysis with atracurium or vecuronium, maintenance with nitrous oxide and a volatile agent, e.g. enflurane in oxygen, with or without small increments of fentanyl to ensure intraoperative stability.

Monitoring

Intraoperative monitoring should include continuous ECG, intermittent non-invasive blood pressure and pulse oximetry. Capnography is mandatory to aid ventilatory management in the presence of CO_2 absorption from the peritoneal cavity and is important in the detection of complications. Intraoperative arterial blood gas analysis is appropriate in patients with severe respiratory problems. Airway pressures should be monitored, a nerve stimulator to assess degree of neuromuscular block is usual and monitoring of temperature during long procedures is valuable. A precordial or oesophageal stethoscope is useful in the detection of gas embolism and the oesophageal stethoscope has been used to confirm at an early stage that pneumoperitoneum is developing correctly.[40] Characteristic tympanic sounds are heard with surgical percussion over the right costal margin.

Management of Intraoperative Complications

Gas Embolism

Venous gas embolism is a well-recognized cause of cardiovascular collapse and death during laparoscopy.[41–43] It is most likely to occur with insufflation through a misplaced Veress needle. Whilst air embolism through open venous channels during craniotomy is well recognized, it is unlikely to occur from gas correctly sited in the peritoneal cavity. Air embolism has been reported from the use of a NdYag laser intraoperatively.[44] This instrument employs a constant flow of gas at 0.5 l min^{-1} to cool the tip while in use and care should be taken not to bury the tip in tissues such as the gall bladder bed.

The clinical features of gas embolism include a splashing millwheel murmur, cyanosis, hypotension and a progressive decrease in end-tidal CO_2 tension. This occurs as cardiac output and lung perfusion are compromised, resulting in a higher ventilation to perfusion ratio. The incidence of minor episodes of gas embolism is unknown. Features suggestive of gas embolism were noted using oesophageal or precordial auscultation in 0.6% of patients undergoing laparoscopy in a recent study, but this is not confirmed using precordial Doppler ultrasound detection.[45,46] Massive gas embolism results in cardiovascular collapse. The reduction and then cessation of cardiac output is associated with the sudden loss of expired CO_2.

Management of severe gas embolism is immediate cessation of insufflation followed by positioning of the patient in a steep left lateral Trendelenburg position in an attempt to prevent right ventricular outflow obstruction by gas in the heart. Placement of a central venous line may permit aspiration of gas. Cardiac massage should be instituted if the above position does not promptly result in restoration of cardiac output. 100% oxygen should be administered as soon as the problem is suspected.

Pneumothorax

There are many reports of pneumothorax occurring during laparoscopy, most recently associated with laparoscopic cholecystectomy.[47–50] CO_2 can enter the pleural space through a pleuroperitoneal connection or by an extraperitoneal route if gas escapes from the peritoneal cavity through a puncture hole in the mesentery or falciform ligament.[48,49] Clinical features may include a decrease in arterial oxygen saturation, increased airway pressure, diminished breath sounds, hyper-resonance of the chest, hypotension, tachycardia or bradycardia. Subcutaneous emphysema may be present.[47] The diagnosis can be confirmed by chest X-ray, but this should not delay emergency treatment if required.

Analysis of aspirated gas can confirm that it has originated from peritoneal insufflation as it will be nearly 100% CO_2.[49] This analysis is readily performed in theatre using the capnograph. CO_2 is rapidly absorbed and management can often be conservative even with a large pneumothorax, providing the patient is well oxygenated and haemodynamically stable.[50] Aspiration rather than formal chest drain insertion is acceptable if the gas is CO_2 since pneumothorax should not recur when the pneumoperitoneum is released.[49]

Pneumopericardium and pneumomediastinum have also been reported after laparoscopy.[51,52] Conservative management should be followed if the patient is haemodynamically stable.

Subcutaneous Emphysema

This can result from accidental subcutaneous insufflation of gas or leakage of gas into subcutaneous tissue around a trocar site.[53,54] The initial clinical feature is an increase in end-tidal CO_2.[53–55] This is associated with increased arterial CO_2 tension and respiratory acidosis. An increase in airway pressure may be secondary to the requirement for an increase in ventilation to eliminate the CO_2 load or indicate the development of a pneumothorax.

Accurate placement of the insufflating needle and tightly fitting trocars are important in the prevention of this complication. The patient with subcutaneous emphysema should be carefully examined to ensure that a pneumothorax is not present. An increase in ventilation is required to offset the respiratory acidosis. CO_2 absorption from subcutaneous tissue is very rapid and this complication resolves quickly once the pneumoperitoneum is released.

Bradycardia

This is usually a result of vagal overactivity. Prophylactic atropine is appropriate in the young patient with marked vagal tone prior to surgical stimulation or in the patient on beta blockers in whom vagal stimulation can result in extreme bradycardia, but most anaesthetists do not give atropine as a routine. The management of bradycardia includes a rapid assessment to ensure that there are no anaesthetic problems resulting in hypoxia, requesting the surgeon to cease any stimulating procedures, particularly if involving peritoneum, and the administration of atropine. A freely running intravenous infusion will transport the drug centrally and produce a rapid response. Doses of 0.3–0.6 mg as a bolus are appropriate. Persisting or recurring bradycardia should be preventable by complete vagal blockade; 2.4 mg of atropine may then rarely be required. If bradycardia is severe, the pneumoperitoneum should be released until stability is achieved.

Hypotension

Blood loss should be replaced with intravenous fluids and any dysrhythmias treated appropriately. Anaesthetic administration should be reduced to the minimum commensurate with the prevention of awareness. Hypotension is likely to be associated with decreased venous return to the heart and the administration of fluid to increase preload should help alleviate the problem. In the case of severe hypotension, gas embolism should be considered. The Trendelenburg position can rapidly increase venous return and the pneumoperitoneum should be released until the situation is under control if hypotension is profound and persisting.[6]

Cardiovascular Collapse

Sudden cardiovascular collapse during laparoscopy is a well-recognized complication of the technique and has several possible causes, most notably severe vagal overactivity and gas embolism. The incidence of cardiac arrest during laparoscopy has been reported as one in 2500.[1]

Severe bradycardia may progress to asystole. There may be more than one mechanism by which this can occur. Bradycardia may be the initial presenting feature or hypoxia secondary to intrapulmonary shunting may then lead to bradycardia and cardiac arrest. Gross intrapulmonary shunting with hypoxia has been described in the absence of gas embolism.[2] This may represent an atypical vagal reaction. Rapid surgical incision into the abdominal cavity with release of pneumoperitoneum has been reported to reverse asystole.[1]

POSTOPERATIVE CARE

General Postoperative Management

Arterial oxygen desaturation is less of a problem than after open surgery, but supplemental oxygen should be administered routinely at least until the patient is fully awake and able to maintain an acceptable arterial oxygen saturation breathing air.

Nausea and/or vomiting may be a troublesome postoperative symptom. Opioid drugs are well recognized as a potent cause of nausea and vomiting in the setting of minor to moderate pain and their avoidance in the postoperative period, together with the use of short-acting agents intraoperatively only when required, may be helpful. Antiemetics such as cyclizine or droperidol may be given prophylactically at induction. The introduction of ondansetron, although expensive, is promising in the patient prone to this distressing complication.[56] Gastric decompression before removal of the nasogastric tube at the end of surgery may be useful.

Postoperative hypothermia should not be a significant problem if active measures to prevent heat loss have been taken intraoperatively, but it is a reported complication of laparoscopic surgery and heat loss in the immediate postoperative period should be minimized.

Routine monitoring of heart rate, blood pressure and respiratory rate should be performed postoperatively until it is clear that the patient is stable.

Postoperative Analgesia

Pain is less of a problem than after open surgery, but still needs consideration.[23] Somatic pain from the portal sites can be alleviated with local anaesthetic infiltration. This must be performed carefully and adequate analgesia will require at least 20 ml of 0.5% bupivacaine for four incisions. Additional analgesia may be required to deal with the pain from intra-abdominal structures, most notably after laparoscopic sterilization. Shoulder tip pain may occur from diaphragmatic irritation following the pneumoperitoneum. This can be minimized by ensuring that residual gas is evacuated from the peritoneal cavity at the completion of surgery.[57] A non-steroidal anti-inflammatory agent (NSAID) can provide additional analgesia and avoid or reduce the requirements for opioid drugs. Diclofenac can be administered as a suppository, ketorolac can be given intravenously. Use of NSAIDs should be a positive decision rather than routine practice in view of the known and potentially serious side effects in some individuals, e.g. renal failure and exacerbation of asthma. Intraperitoneal instillation of a local anaesthetic may reduce the incidence of shoulder tip pain postoperatively.[58]

If pain relief is still inadequate a clear plan of action is required. Commonly, additional local anaesthetic infiltration at one of the portals is all that is necessary. This can be performed in the recovery area. Oral medication may be tolerated and sufficient and if not, the administration of an opioid should be considered. In patients after cholecystectomy a small dose of pethidine may be the most suitable agent.

Assessment Before Discharge

Some laparoscopic surgical procedures may be performed on a day case basis, e.g. laparoscopic sterilization. More major procedures such as cholecystectomy usually necessitate an overnight stay and review the following day. Facilities should always be available for more prolonged patient admission, e.g. if the surgeon has had to resort to open surgery.

Various tests have been proposed to assess patient fitness for discharge. In general, the patient should be conscious, able to communicate normally, able to stand and walk steadily, not suffering from severe pain or severe nausea or vomiting. Appropriate oral analgesia should be organized for the immediate period after discharge.

CONCLUSION

Laparoscopic surgical techniques represent a considerable advance in surgical practice with undoubted benefits for patients. It is essential that careful thought is given to the anaesthetic techniques employed to best complement the surgery and maximize the advantages. An understanding of the physiological processes in relation to pneumoperitoneum can improve anaesthetic management. Methods of prevention and treatment of the potentially serious complications which can occur during laparoscopic surgery, as well as the clinical features important for diagnosis, must be understood by anyone anaesthetizing these patients if patient safety is not to be compromised.

REFERENCES

1. Shifren JL, Adlestein L, Finkler NJ. Asystolic cardiac arrest: a rare complication of laparoscopy. *Obstet Gynecol* 1992; **79**: 840–1.
2. Brantley JC, Riley PM. Cardiovascular collapse during laparoscopy: a report of two cases. *Am J Obstet Gynecol* 1988; **159**: 735–7.
3. Motew M, Ivankovich AD, Bieniarz J, Albrecht RF, Zahed B, Scommegna A. Cardiovascular effects and acid-base and blood gas changes during laparoscopy. *Am J Obstet Gynecol* 1973; **115**: 1002–12.
4. Doyle DJ, Mark PWS. Reflex bradycardia during surgery. *Can J Anaesth* 1990; **37**: 219–22.
5. Scott DB, Julian DG. Observations on cardiac arrhythmias during laparoscopy. *Br Med J* 1972; **1**: 411–13.

6. Lee CM. Acute hypotension during laparoscopy: a case report. *Anesth Analg* 1975; **54**: 142–3.
7. Kashtan J, Green JF, Parsons EQ, Holcroft JW. Hemodynamic effects of increased abdominal pressure. *J Surg Res* 1981; **30**: 249–55.
8. Johannsen G, Andersen M, Juhl B. The effect of general anaesthesia on the haemodynamic events during laparoscopy with CO_2-insufflation. *Acta Anaesth Scand* 1989; **33**: 132–6.
9. Bongard FS, Pianim N, Liu SY, Lippmann M, Davis I, Klein S. Using helium for insufflation during laparoscopy. *JAMA* 1991; **266**: 3131.
10. Williams MD, Murr PC. Laparoscopic insufflation of the abdomen depresses cardiopulmonary function. *Surg Endosc* 1993; **7**: 12–16.
11. Diamant M, Benumof JL, Saidman LJ. Hemodynamics of increased intra-abdominal pressure: interaction with hypovolemia and halothane anesthesia. *Anesthesiology* 1978; **48**: 23–7.
12. Lenz RJ, Thomas TA, Wilkins DG. Cardiovascular changes during laparoscopy. Studies of stroke volume and cardiac output using impedance cardiography. *Anaesthesia* 1976; **31**: 4–12.
13. Kelman GR, Swapp GH, Smith I, Benzie RJ, Gordon NLM. Cardiac output and arterial blood–gas tension during laparoscopy. *Br J Anaesth* 1972; **44**: 1155–62.
14. Ivankovich AD, Miletich DJ, Albrecht RF, Heyman HJ, Bonnet RF. Cardiovascular effects of intraperitoneal insufflation with carbon dioxide and nitrous oxide in the dog. *Anesthesiology* 1975; **42**: 281–7.
15. Herruzo JAS, Castellano G, Larrodera L *et al.* Plasma arginine vasopressin concentration during laparoscopy. *Hepato-gastroenterol* 1989; **36**: 499–503.
16. Melville RJ, Frizis HI, Forsling ML, LeQuesne LP. The stimulus for vasopressin release during laparoscopy. *Surg Gyn Obstet* 1985; **161**: 253–6.
17. Reid CW, Martineau RJ, Hull KA, Miller DR. Haemodynamic consequences of abdominal insufflation with CO_2 during laparoscopic cholecystectomy. *Can J Anaesth* (abs.) 1992; **39**: A132.
18. Myles PS. Bradyarrhythmias and laparoscopy: a prospective study of heart rate changes with laparoscopy. *Aust NZ Obstet Gynaecol* 1991; **31**: 171–3.
19. Fitzgerald SD, Andrus CH, Baudendistel LJ, Dahms TE, Kaminski DL. Hypercarbia during carbon dioxide pneumoperitoneum. *Am J Surg* 1992; **163**: 186–90.
20. Monk TG, Weldon BC. Anesthetic considerations for laparoscopic surgery. *J Endourol* 1992; **6**: 89–94.
21. Frazee RC, Roberts JW, Okeson GC *et al.* Open versus laparoscopic cholecystectomy. A comparison of postoperative pulmonary function. *Ann Surg* 1991; **213**: 651–4.
22. Joris J, Cigarini I, Legrand M *et al.* Metabolic and respiratory changes after cholecystectomy performed via laparotomy or laparoscopy. *Br J Anaesth* 1992; **69**: 341–5.
23. Putensen-Himmer G, Putensen C, Lammer H, Lingnau W, Aigner F, Benzer H. Comparison of postoperative respiratory function after laparoscopy or open laparotomy for cholecystectomy. *Anesthesiology* 1992; **77**: 675–80.
24. Johnson D, Litwin D, Osachoff J *et al.* Postoperative respiratory function after laparoscopic cholecystectomy. *Surg Lap Endosc* 1992; **2**: 221–6.
25. Cooney CM, Lyons JB, Hennigan A, Blunnie WP, Moriarty DC. Ventilatory function following laparoscopic cholecystectomy. *Can J Anaesth* (abs.) 1992; **39**: A54.
26. Leighton T, Pianim N, Liu SY, Kono M, Klein S, Bongard F. Effectors of hypercarbia during experimental pneumoperitoneum. *Am Surg* 1992; **58**: 717–21.
27. Puri GD, Singh H. Ventilatory effects of laparoscopy under general anaesthesia. *Br J Anaesth* 1992; **68**: 211–13.
28. Tan PL, Lee TL, Tweed WA. Carbon dioxide absorption and gas exchange during pelvic laparoscopy. *Can J Anaesth* 1992; **39**: 677–81.

29. Brampton WJ, Watson RJ. Arterial to end-tidal carbon dioxide tension difference during laparoscopy. Magnitude and effect of anaesthetic technique. *Anaesthesia* 1990; **45**: 210–14.
30. Brown DR, Fishburne JI, Roberson VO, Hulka JF. Ventilatory and blood gas changes during laparoscopy with local anaesthesia. *Am J Obstet Gynecol* 1976; **124**: 741–5.
31. Ho HS, Gunther RA, Wolfe BM. Intraperitoneal carbon dioxide insufflation and cardiopulmonary functions. Laparoscopic cholecystectomy in pigs. *Arch Surg* 1992; **127**: 928–32.
32. Wittgen CM, Andrus CH, Fitzgerald SD, Baudendistel LJ, Dahms TE, Kaminski DL. Analysis of the hemodynamic and ventilatory effects of laparoscopic cholecystectomy. *Arch Surg* 1991; **126**: 997–1000.
33. Harman PK, Kron IL, McLachlan HD, Freedlender AE, Nolan SP. Elevated intra-abdominal pressure and renal function. *Ann Surg* 1982; **196**: 594–7.
34. Rose DK, Cohen MM, Soutter DI. Laparoscopic cholecystectomy: the anaesthetist's point of view. *Can J Anaesth* 1992; **39**: 809–15.
35. Wallasvaara MT, Paloheimo M. Ventilation and body temperatures during laparoscopic vs. open cholecystectomy. *Anesth Analg* (abs.) 1992; **74**: S340.
36. Zahl K, Apfelbaum JL. Muscle pain occurs after outpatient laparoscopy despite the substitution of vecuronium for succinylcholine. *Anesthesiology* 1989; **70**: 408–11.
37. Hovorka J, Korttila K. Nitrous oxide does not increase nausea and vomiting following gynaecological laparoscopy. *Can J Anaesth* 1989; **36**: 145–8.
38. Taylor E, Feinstein R, White PF, Soper N. Anesthesia for laparoscopic cholecystectomy. Is nitrous oxide contraindicated? *Anesthesiology* 1992; **76**: 541–3.
39. Steffey EP, Johnson BH, Eger EI II. Nitrous oxide intensifies the pulmonary arterial pressure response to venous injection of carbon dioxide in the dog. *Anesthesiology* 1980; **52**: 52–5.
40. Beckmann CRB, Dadabhoy Z, Beckmann CA, Yeko TR. Auscultation with an esophageal stethoscope. A new test for pneumoperitoneum. *J Reprod Med* 1991; **36**: 298–300.
41. Root B, Levy MN, Pollack S, Lubert M, Pathak K. Gas embolism death after laparoscopy delayed by "trapping" in portal circulation. *Anesth Analg* 1978; **57**: 232–7.
42. Yacoub OF, Cardona I, Coveler LA, Dodson MG. Carbon dioxide embolism during laparoscopy. *Anesthesiology* 1982; **57**: 533–5.
43. Clark CC, Weeks DB, Gusdon JP. Venous carbon dioxide embolism during laparoscopy. *Anesth Analg* 1977; **56**: 650–2.
44. Greville AC, Clements EAF, Erwin DC, McMillan DL, Wellwood JM. Pulmonary air embolism during laparoscopic laser cholecystectomy. *Anaesthesia* 1991; **46**: 113–14.
45. Hynes SR, Marshall RL. Venous gas embolism during gynaecological laparoscopy. *Can J Anaesth* 1992; **39**: 748–9.
46. Wadhwa RK, McKenzie R, Wadhwa SR, Katz DL, Byers JF. Gas embolism during laparoscopy. *Anesthesiology* 1978; **48**: 74–6.
47. Doctor NH, Hussain Z. Bilateral pneumothorax associated with laparoscopy. A case report of a rare hazard and review of literature. *Anaesthesia* 1973; **28**: 75–81.
48. Smiler BG, Falick VS. Complication during anaesthesia and laparoscopy. *JAMA* 1973; **226**: 676.
49. Gabbott DA, Dunkley AB, Roberts FL. Carbon dioxide pneumothorax occurring during laparoscopic cholecystectomy. *Anaesthesia* 1992; **47**: 587–8.
50. Heddle RM, Platt AJ. Tension pneumothorax during laparoscopic cholecystectomy. *Br J Surg* 1992; **79**: 374.
51. Nicholson RD, Berman ND. Pneumopericardium following laparoscopy. *Chest* 1979; **76**: 605–7.

52. Pascual JB, Baranda MM, Tarrero MT, Gutierrez MFM, Garrido IM, Errasti CA. Subcutaneous emphysema, pneumomediastinum, bilateral pneumothorax and pneumopericardium after laparoscopy (letter). *Endosc* 1990; **22**: 59.
53. Kent RB III. Subcutaneous emphysema and hypercarbia following laparoscopic cholecystectomy. *Arch Surg* 1991; **126**: 1154–6.
54. Lew JKL, Gin T, Oh TE. Anaesthetic problems during laparoscopic cholecystectomy. *Anaesth Intens Care* 1992; **20**: 91–2.
55. Bard PA, Chen L. Subcutaneous emphysema associated with laparoscopy. *Anesth Analg* 1990; **71**: 101–2.
56. Leeser J, Lip H. Prevention of postoperative nausea and vomiting using ondansetron, a new, selective, 5-HT_3 receptor antagonist. *Anesth Analg* 1991; **72**: 751–5.
57. Shrivastav P, Nadkarni P. Prevention of shoulder pain after laparoscopy. *Lancet* 1992; **339**: 744.
58. Narchi P, Benhamou D, Fernandez H. Intraperitoneal local anaesthetic for shoulder pain after day-case laparoscopy. *Lancet* 1991; **338**: 1569–70.

4

Principles, Technique and Complications of Laparoscopy

S. PATERSON-BROWN

INTRODUCTION

There have been great changes in the instrumentation and techniques for laparoscopy since the concept was first introduced by Kelling in 1902,[1] when he used a cystoscope with air insufflation to examine the peritoneal cavity of a dog. When Kelling went on to use this technique in patients he preferred to approach the peritoneum by direct cutdown through a supraumbilical incision for safety.[2] It was not until much later that carbon dioxide replaced room air for insufflation[3] and Veress reported his springloaded needle for percutaneous puncture.[4] However, in spite of the technological revolution which has occurred in laparoscopic surgery during the last few years the principles of the technique remain the same: safe puncture of the peritoneal cavity, adequate pneumoperitoneum before insertion of trocars and careful inspection of the intra-abdominal viscera using further ports as appropriate, inserted under direct vision.

With the introduction of videophotography and the additional equipment required for laparoscopic surgery, the surgeon has become reliant on many more external factors than is the case for most open surgical procedures. The smooth running of all laparoscopic procedures will therefore depend upon a full understanding of the laparoscopic equipment and technology by the whole operating team. Furthermore, arrangements should be made for additional essential instruments and back-up equipment to be available should they be required.

COMPLICATIONS OF LAPAROSCOPY

The complications associated with diagnostic as opposed to therapeutic laparoscopy are a consequence of the pneumoperitoneum and instrumental injuries. The majority of major complications result from puncture injuries following incorrect insertion of the Veress needle or trocars.[5] These may only be minor lacerations to the omentum, small intestine or mesentery, but major injuries to the colon, abdominal aorta and iliac vessels have all been reported,[6] some with disastrous consequences.[7] Although blind insertion of instruments into the peritoneal cavity will always have an inherent, albeit small risk of major injury, this can and should remain negligible if careful attention is paid to the technique employed. A large multicentre confidential enquiry reported by the Royal College of Obstetrics and Gynaecology[6] reported 1818 complications in 50 247 gynaecological patients undergoing laparoscopy. There were only four deaths and these resulted from gas embolism (1), perforated bowel (1) and cardiac arrests (2). These figures represent a morbidity of 4% and a mortality of eight per 100 000. Of these laparoscopies, 20 586 were for diagnostic purposes only and the remainder for sterilization procedures. There were 127 intra-abdominal injuries associated with diagnostic laparoscopy with an overall complication rate of 30 per 1000 procedures, of which 23 per 1000 were considered serious.

The pneumoperitoneum may result in complications due to the raised intra-abdominal pressure, excessive absorption of the insufflating gas and gas emboli. Both cardiac arrhythmias and acid-base disturbances have been reported following insufflation of carbon dioxide,[8,9] but these complications can be reduced if the patient is paralysed and ventilated rather than performing the procedure using spontaneous breathing.[10] When the abdominal pressure rises above 20 mmHg not only is the ventilatory capacity reduced but so is the central venous pressure, pulse pressure and cardiac output due to reduced venous return.[11] Even at lower pressures these physiological changes may be of significance in patients with severe cardiorespiratory disease. Indeed many surgeons and anaesthetists advocate that severe cardiac and respiratory disease remain a contraindication for laparoscopy. These problems can be reduced in part by lowering the insufflation pressure which can almost be eliminated if the abdominal wall is externally supported, as has been demonstrated by some Japanese surgeons.[12]

Attention has recently been drawn to the possible increased risk of deep vein thrombosis and pulmonary embolism associated with laparoscopic surgery.[13] In an experimental model the insufflation pressures used for laparoscopic procedures produced venous hypertension in the common femoral vein, which resolved upon release of the pneumoperitoneum.[13] As laparoscopic procedures by and large take longer to perform than the open operation, these observations, if substantiated by future studies, may have important consequences on both the indications for laparoscopic procedures and the patient selection.

As surgeons have become more experienced in the techniques of laparoscopy the number of contraindications have been reduced. Suspicions of intra-abdominal adhesions or overt intestinal obstruction are not contraindications providing an open technique for insufflation is used. Similarly, external hernias and hiatal hernias are now treated laparoscopically so no longer constitute a contraindication; however, in the latter care must be taken to keep the insufflation pressures low to prevent cardiorespiratory compromise or pneumomediastinum. Insufflation and insertion of instruments must be carried out with great care when performing laparoscopy in patients with bleeding disorders, and a direct approach for insufflation with careful haemostasis is advisable in severe cases. Severe cardiorespiratory disease remains one of the only absolute contraindications to laparoscopy, though abdominal wall elevation after direct insertion of the laparoscopic ports without any significant pneumoperitoneum[12] may also solve the problems relating to insufflation in these patients.

PATIENT PREPARATION

Laparoscopy may be performed under local or general anaesthesia. If local anaesthesia is attempted, this should be performed in a sterile environment with adequate sedation and facilities available for conversion to immediate general anaesthesia and laparotomy if required. It is advisable to ensure the bladder is not full before commencing the procedure, but routine catheterization is not essential if care is taken to ensure the bladder is not palpable. Prophylactic urinary catheterization before laparoscopy is associated with a significantly higher incidence of urinary tract infection compared with patients who are not catheterized.[14] If pneumoperitoneum is to be produced by direct cutdown the risk of bladder injury is reduced. As for open surgery, catheterization should still be carried out for pelvic surgery, when suprapubic ports are required or a lengthy procedure is contemplated. All patients undergoing laparoscopy and laparoscopic surgery must give full informed consent regarding the possible recourse to laparotomy.

PRODUCTION OF A PNEUMOPERITONEUM

Insufflating Agent

Room air may still be employed for diagnostic laparoscopy and is used routinely in some centres.[15] However, carbon dioxide remains the agent of choice for most procedures. When laparoscopy is performed under local anaesthesia carbon dioxide may still be used for insufflation[16] although some surgeons prefer the additional analgesic properties associated with the use of nitrous oxide.[17] However, if this is used electrocoagulation is contraindicated.

Open Technique

The direct approach to the peritoneum initially advocated by Kelling[2] remains popular amongst many surgeons for one of two reasons: firstly the small but definite risk of visceral injury associated with all blind techniques, irrespective of the experience of the surgeon; and secondly the increasing number of surgeons who are now performing laparoscopy, many for the first time, with little or no

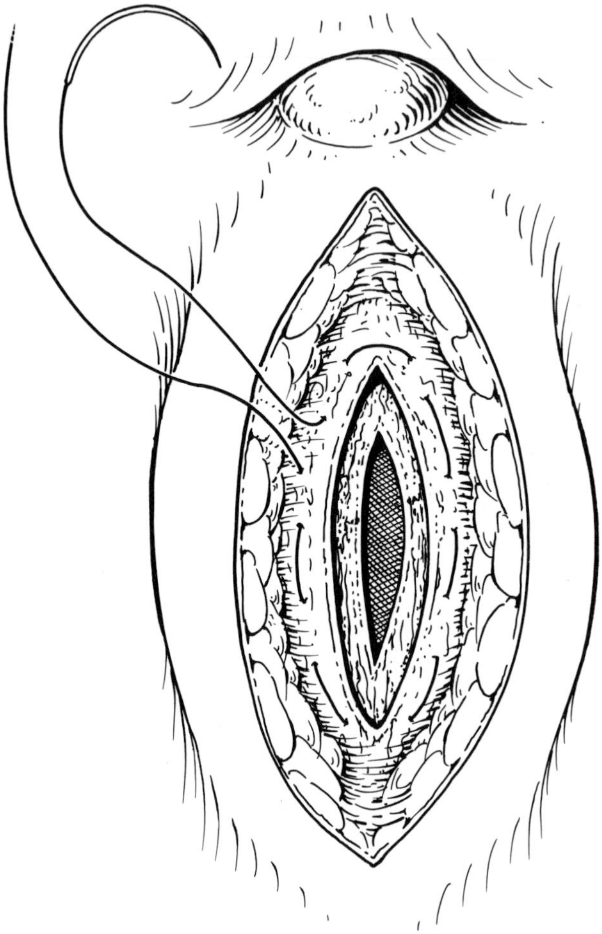

Figure 4.1 Open laparoscopy performed through an infraumbilical incision with a pursestring suture passed through peritoneum and linea alba.

experience in the basic techniques of laparoscopy. This is particularly true for the acute abdomen where many junior surgeons are being encouraged to perform diagnostic laparoscopy, perhaps proceeding to laparoscopic appendicectomy if indicated. As the majority of elective laparoscopic surgery is still performed by the senior surgical staff, compared with the opposite for emergency procedures, the junior staff may receive little or no supervised training in the basic techniques of laparoscopy.

There are two different open techniques. The first involves a direct cutdown onto the peritoneum through a small supraumbilical or infraumbilical incision. A pursestring suture is placed around the fascia of the incised linea alba and peritoneum (Fig. 4.1) in order to prevent excessive gas leak once the laparoscopic port has been inserted. This technique has been greatly facilitated by the

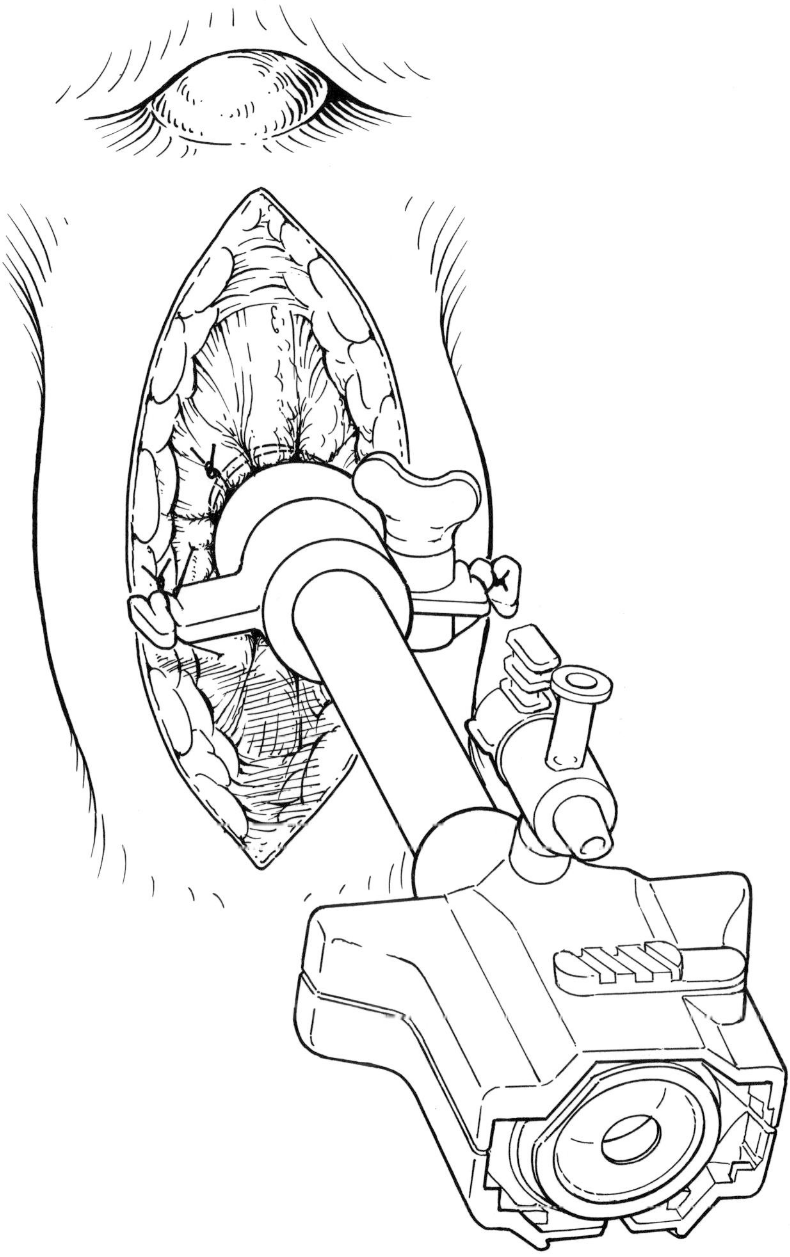

Figure 4.2 Hasson port inserted through an infraumbilical incision with a suture on each side securing it in place.

introduction of a modified trocar and port by Hasson,[18] which has a blunt tip and two wings to which the sutures are attached in order to immobilize the port. If the Hasson type trocar and port are used then two strong nylon sutures should be inserted on each side of the incision rather than a pursestring suture. The edges of both the linea alba and peritoneum are incorporated in the suture, which is pulled up while at the same time inserting the external winged section of the port firmly into the opening in the peritoneal cavity and the sutures locked into place (Fig. 4.2). The inner port can then be advanced through the external device to which it is firmly screwed. Once the laparoscopy has been completed the defect is closed. This technique may be used anywhere on the anterior abdominal wall and is particularly appropriate in patients who have had previous abdominal surgery where underlying adhesions are suspected.

A second and much simpler technique has been developed by Fielding in Australia (G Fielding, 1992, personal communication; see also Chapter 8.2). This technique involves a small incision over the everted umbilicus at a point where the skin and peritoneum are adjacent. Because the umbilicus has been everted (so the angle of insertion of the laparoscopic port becomes oblique) and the incision required is relatively small, a suture is not usually required to prevent gas leakage, although one may be required to stabilize the port. Following good skin preparation of the umbilicus, toothed grasping forceps (the author often uses a towel clip) are inserted into the apex of the umbilicus which is everted. A vertical incision is then made from the apex of the umbilicus in a caudal direction (Fig. 4.3) into which two small retractors are inserted to reveal the cylindrical umbilical tube running from the undersurface of the umbilical skin down to the defect in the linea alba. This tube is incised from its apex (just deep to the skin) downwards towards its junction with the linea alba (Fig. 4.4) and further blunt dissection through this plane permits direct entry into the peritoneum. This is best performed with blunt artery forceps which should be kept as perpendicular as possible to the abdominal wall to prevent entry into the preperitoneal space.

Once the peritoneal cavity has been breached the laparoscopic port (without trocar) can then be inserted directly (Fig. 4.5) and insufflation commenced. A blunt internal trocar facilitates insertion of this port and an external grip which can be attached to the port helps to secure it in position. When employing this technique it is useful to insert a single suture through the defect which can then be used to stabilize the port, prevent any intraoperative gas leak during the procedure and also to close the incision at the end.

A recent study comparing open and closed methods of laparoscopy has demonstrated better safety, quicker insufflation and a financial saving on disposable ports associated with the open method.[19]

Closed Technique Under General Anaesthesia

Following endotracheal intubation and full muscle relaxant anaesthesia, the abdomen is palpated and the suprapubic region examined for evidence of a full

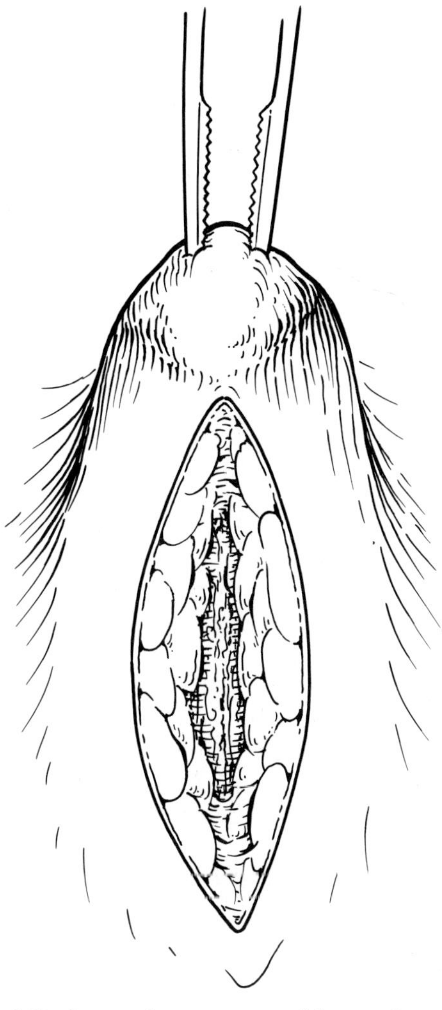

Figure 4.3 Transumbilical open laparoscopy with eversion of the umbilicus using toothed grasping forceps.

bladder. If present, a urinary catheter should be inserted and some surgeons perform this as a routine. It is not necessary to insert a nasogastric tube at this stage, though one may be required to decompress the stomach and duodenum during operations in the upper abdomen. The most common site for insertion of the Veress needle is through a supraumbilical or infraumbilical incision at an angle towards the patient's pelvis over the pelvic brim with the patient in the Trendelenburg position and the anterior abdominal wall raised by the surgeon's left hand. It does not matter whether a transverse or longitudinal incision is made although the latter has been reported to heal better in the subumbilical region.[20] The internal obturator of the springloaded Veress needle will be pushed back as the needle traverses the abdominal wall and will spring forward once the peritoneal cavity has been entered. Confirmation of position should be obtained before high flow insufflation is commenced and can be achieved by a number of methods:

1. There is a negative intraperitoneal pressure compared with atmospheric pressure and therefore air will be drawn into the needle after it enters the peritoneal space. This may produce an audible hiss[21] or alternatively a drop of water placed on the hub of the needle before insertion will be drawn into the needle as it enters the peritoneal cavity.

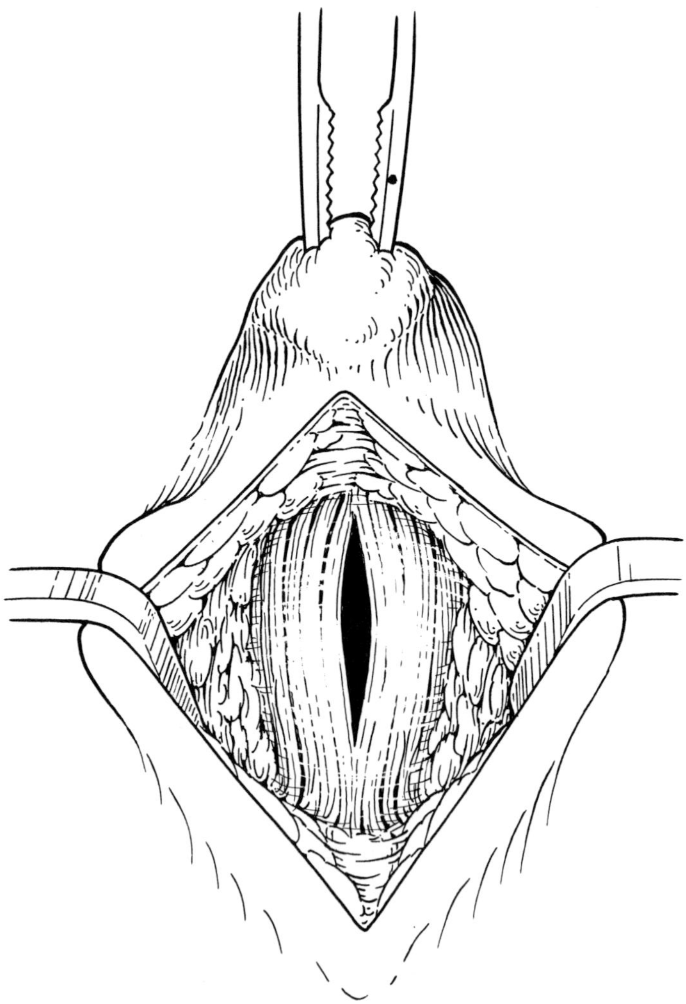

Figure 4.4 Incision through the umbilical tube.

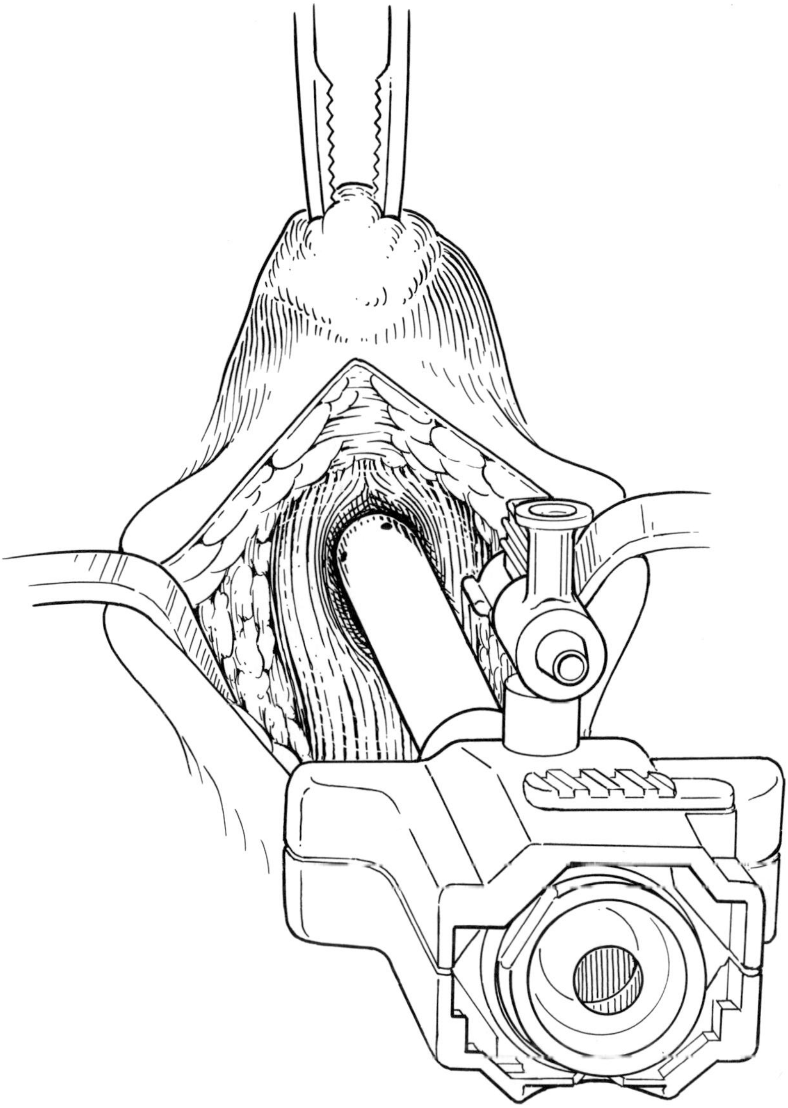

Figure 4.5 Insertion of the port after extending the incision through the umbilical tube down to the peritoneum with blunt dissection using artery forceps.

2. It should not be possible to aspirate fluid which has been injected through the needle if the needle lies within the peritoneal space.
3. The initial insufflation pressure through the needle before insertion should be approximately the same as that after insertion for the same flow rate.
4. The initial insufflation pressure after insertion should not exceed 10 mmHg for a flow rate of 1 l min^{-1}.

The flow rate may be increased after confirmation of position of the Veress needle. With many of the new insufflators the high flow capacity ranges from 3–9 $l\ min^{-1}$. This rate will not be achieved through the small diameter Veress needle, but will be possible if an open approach has been used and insufflation is performed directly through the laparoscopic port.

Before inserting the laparoscopic trocar and cannula it is essential that an adequate pneumoperitoneum has been achieved into which the trocar can be inserted. If the abdominal wall is not suitably distended there is a significant risk that blind insertion of the trocar can injure underlying viscera and therefore it is not the volume of gas insufflated but the pressure reached which is the important factor. The trocar is inserted towards the pelvis with the surgeon's left hand controlling the shaft to prevent a sudden "give" as the peritoneal cavity is entered. The recent introduction of disposable laparoscopic ports and trocars with a springloaded guard has reduced the chance of injury to underlying structures but does not eliminate the potential danger.[22] A gentle twisting action will usually permit a controlled entry of the trocar without excessive force being required.

Production of a pneumoperitoneum in patients who have undergone previous abdominal surgery or who present with intestinal obstruction is not contraindicated but poses additional problems and potential complications. The surgeon has two options: the first, and obviously the safer, is to perform an open technique, either in the umbilical region or through a point distant from the scars, and with overt signs of intestinal obstruction the open approach is mandatory; alternatively a closed approach may be employed with the Veress needle inserted away from the area of possible adhesions. Percutaneous ultrasonography may be used to identify adhesions between the viscera and the anterior abdominal wall,[23] confirmed by demonstrating that during respiration the viscera adjacent to the abdominal wall do not alter position.

A semiopen approach has recently been published whereby a supraumbilical incision is made down to the linea alba which is elevated with skin hooks.[24] The Veress needle is then passed through into the peritoneal cavity.

Closed Technique Under Local Anaesthesia

The patient is prepared and draped as described earlier and intravenous sedation may be useful. The point of insertion of the laparoscope is infiltrated with a local anaesthetic agent such as 0.5% bupivacaine down to and including the peritoneum. Following adequate anaesthesia the Veress needle is inserted as previously described. It is often helpful to ask the patient to cough during insertion of the Veress needle as this contracts the abdominal wall and prevents the needle being pushed into the underlying viscera. When inserting the Veress needle under local anaesthesia the author prefers to use a point midway between the pubic symphysis and the sacral prominence. The needle is inserted slowly perpendicular to the skin until the linea alba is felt. The patient is then asked to cough at the moment the Veress needle is pushed through.

Once correct positioning of the Veress needle has been confirmed insufflation proceeds at $1\ \mathrm{l\ min^{-1}}$ using either carbon dioxide or nitrous oxide (as discussed earlier). It is important not to insufflate too quickly as rapid distension of the parietal peritoneum may be painful. The port and trocar are then inserted, usually through a periumbilical incision, after adequate insufflation, again asking the patient to cough on insertion.

When laparoscopy is performed in patients with ascites, the ascitic fluid should be drained during the preceding 24 hours. The catheter used for drainage is then left in situ and used for insertion of the insufflating agent the following day.

LAPAROSCOPIC INSPECTION AND INSERTION OF ADDITIONAL PORTS

Once the laparoscope has been inserted and connected to the videocamera, if available, detailed inspection of the peritoneal cavity can begin. As for open laparotomy, this is best performed in a routine fashion and as the laparoscope is usually inserted towards the pelvis, these structures are best examined first. Laparoscopic inspection of most viscera requires the insertion of a second port through which a blunt palpating probe can be inserted. Although the tactile sensation of the surgeon's hand cannot be emulated, this probe does permit viscera to be manipulated and both 'fixity' and consistency can often be determined. Examination of the small and large intestine is possible using atraumatic grasping forceps and if necessary a second port can be inserted for additional instruments. Many recesses and structures remain poorly visualized using end-viewing laparoscopes, such as the spleen and superior surface of the liver, and oblique-viewing laparoscopes should be used, of which the 30° is the most popular.

All additional ports should be inserted under direct laparoscopic vision and in all cases the surgeon must use one hand to steady the shaft of the trocar and prevent a sudden plunge of the instrument through the abdominal wall into the underlying viscera.

COMPLETION OF LAPAROSCOPY, CLOSURE AND ANALGESIA

Once the laparoscopy has been completed the ports should all be removed under direct vision to ensure there is no bleeding from the incisions and once the pneumoperitoneum has been released the camera and port may be removed. It is important to remove as much insufflating gas as possible at the end of the procedure to reduce postoperative pain and in particular shoulder tip pain. The mechanism is thought to be due to either stretching of the peritoneum or formation of carbonic acid from the insufflated carbon dioxide and some studies have shown that the insertion of a suction drain for only a few hours reduces the frequency and severity of pain in the early postoperative period.[25] Fascial defects greater than 10 mm should be closed where possible and the skin incisions closed as appropriate. A J-shaped needle with an absorbable suture is useful for the fascial suture.

The use of local anaesthetic wound infiltration greatly reduces the postoperative analgesic requirement and 0.5% bupivacaine is a commonly used agent which has activity for up to 12 hours. Non-steroidal anti-inflammatory suppositories are also used.

REFERENCES

1. Kelling G. Uber oesophagoskopie, gastroskopie und colioskopie. *Munch Med Wochschr* 1902; **49**: 21–4.
2. Kelling G. Zur colioskopie und gastroskopie. *Arch Klin Chir* 1923; **126**: 226–9.
3. Fervers C. Die laparoskopie mit dem cystoskop. *Medsche Klin* 1933; **29**: 1042–5.
4. Veress J. Neues instrument zur ausfuhrung von brust-oder bauchpunktionen und pneumothoraxbehandlung. *Dt Med Wschr* 1938; **64**: 1480–1.
5. Mintz M. Risks and prophylaxis in laparoscopy: a survey of 100 000 cases. *J Reprod Med* 1977; **18**: 269–72.
6. Chamberlain GVP, Carron Brown JA. *Report of the Working Party of the Confidential Enquiry into Gynaecological Laparoscopy*. London, Royal College of Obstetricians and Gynaecologists, 1978.
7. Peterson HB, Greenspan JR, Ory HW. Death following puncture of the aorta during laparoscopic sterilization. *Obstet Gynecol* 1982; **59**: 133–4.
8. Scott DB, Julian DG. Observations on cardiac arrhythmias during laparoscopy. *Br Med J* 1972; **i**: 411–13.
9. Holzman M, Sharp K, Richards W. Hypercarbia during carbon dioxide gas insufflation for therapeutic laparoscopy: a note of caution. *Surg Laparosc Endosc* 1992; **2**: 11–14.
10. Morley TR. Cardiac arrhythmias during laparoscopy (letter). *Br Med J* 1972; **ii**: 295–6.
11. Motew M, Ivankovitch AD, Bieniarz J, Albrecht RF, Zahed B, Scommegna A. Cardiovascular effects and acid-base and blood gas changes during laparoscopy. *Am J Obstet Gynecol* 1973; **115**: 1002–12.
12. Kitano S, Tomikawa M, Iso Y *et al.* A safe and simple method to maintain a clear field of vision during laparoscopic cholecystectomy. *Surg Endosc* 1992; **6**: 197–8.
13. Jorgensen JO, Hanel K, Lalak NJ, Hunt DR, North L, Morris DL. Thromboembolic complications of laparoscopic cholecystectomy (letter). *Br Med J* 1993; **306**: 518–19.
14. Akhtar MS, Deere DM, Wright JT, MacRae KD. Is bladder catheterization really necessary before laparoscopy? *Br J Obstet Gynaecol* 1985; **92**: 1176–8.
15. Udwadia TE. Peritoneoscopy for surgeons. *Ann R Coll Surg Engl* 1986; **68**: 125–9.

16. Hall TJ, Donaldson DR, Brennan TG. The value of laparoscopy under local anaesthesia in 250 medical and surgical patients. *Br J Surg* 1980; **67**: 751–3.
17. Sherwood R, Berci G, Austin E, Morgenstern L. Minilaparoscopy for blunt abdominal trauma. *Arch Surg* 1980; **115**: 672–3.
18. Hasson HM. Open laparoscopy: a report of 150 cases. *J Reprod Med* 1974; **12**: 234–8.
19. Ballem RV, Rudomanski J. Techniques of pneumoperitoneum. *Surg Laparosc Endosc* 1993; **3**: 42–3.
20. East MC, Steele PRM. Laparoscopic incisions at the lower umbilical verge. *Br Med J* 1988; **296**: 753–4.
21. Gupta SP. Positioning the Veress needle. *Br J Surg* 1989; **76**: 381.
22. Dunn DC, Watson CJE. Disposable guarded trocar and cannula in laparoscopic surgery: a caveat. *Br J Surg* 1982; **79**: 927.
23. Sigel B, Golub RM, Loiacono LA *et al.* Technique of ultrasonic detection and mapping of abdominal wall adhesions. *Surg Endosc* 1991; **5**: 161–5.
24. Karatassas A, Walsh D, Hamilton DW. A safe, new approach to establishing a pneumoperitoneum at laparoscopy. *Aust NZ J Surg* 1992; **62**: 489–91.
25. Alexander JI, Hull MGR. Abdominal pain after laparoscopy: the value of a gas drain. *Br J Obstet Gynaecol* 1987; **94**: 267–9.

5.1

Expectations of Cholecystectomy

S. BANTING and D. C. CARTER

INTRODUCTION

Gallstones are a major cause of symptoms and morbidity in many countries, notably in the developed world. Prevalence studies based on cholecystography in Wales found stones in 6.2% of men and 12% of women in the age group 45–69 years,[1] while an autopsy-based study in south east England found stones in 12.4% of men and 23.7% of women of all ages.[2] A more recent study using ultrasonography in Bristol found that the prevalence of gallstones (or previous cholecystectomy) in men aged 40–69 was 6.9%, whereas in women aged 25–69 it was 8%.[3] In the age groups 60–69 years the prevalence of stones or cholecystectomy in the Bristol patients was 8.8% and 11.8% in men and women respectively. Comparable prevalence figures have been reported from a number of other European countries and from North America and the gallstones have been held responsible for the development of symptoms in 10–30% of cases in different studies.

Since 1987, the medical world has seen a dramatic transformation of the treatment of gallstones with the introduction and widespread adoption of the technique of laparoscopic cholecystectomy. In the earlier years of the last decade it looked as though surgeons were about to lose a substantial piece of their gastrointestinal territory with the inroads being made by alternative treatments for gallstones, notably dissolution therapy and extracorporeal shock wave lithotripsy. However, the promise of both techniques and their undoubted achievements was blighted by the realization that at best, they dealt only with the gallstones and did not address the underlying problem of the diseased gall bladder. The advent of laparoscopic cholecystectomy swung the pendulum back in favour of surgical cholecystectomy and there is already general recognition that the approach has an acceptably low mortality, a shorter hospital stay, a more rapid return to work and normal activity and a better cosmetic result.

Questions still surround the relative benefits and disadvantages of open and laparoscopic cholecystectomy; on the one hand the absence of a major abdominal wound has the advantage of diminishing the risk of wound complications, while on the other hand, the need to acquire the new techniques has raised questions about "surgical learning curves" and the risk of bile duct injury. In the relative absence of controlled prospective comparisons of the two techniques, these issues can now only be addressed by meticulous data collection regarding laparoscopic cholecystectomy and by audit, conducted not only by centres of excellence but by national or regional programmes, so that the true strengths and weaknesses of the new technique can be defined.

This chapter examines some of the lessons that can be learned from the experience of conventional cholecystectomy so that realistic expectations of cholecystectomy in the era of minimally invasive surgery can be defined. Three key issues will be addressed. Firstly, how safe was conventional cholecystectomy in terms of operative mortality; secondly how significant was the associated morbidity and in particular the risk of bile duct injury; and thirdly, what should one expect of cholecystectomy in the long term, particularly in respect of resolution of symptoms?

MORTALITY OF OPEN CHOLECYSTECTOMY

The operative mortality of open cholecystectomy for cholelithiasis has fallen in recent years and since 1980 many series have recorded operative mortality rates of less than 1% and in some cases, no mortality at all (Table 5.1.1). Common duct exploration is generally regarded as increasing the risk of cholecystectomy by some four to eight times,[4,5] while operations conducted on a non-elective basis were associated with a significant increase in morbidity and mortality, particularly in elderly patients (see below).

Table 5.1.1 Outcome of open cholecystectomy in some recent series

Series	n	% common duct exploration	% mortality
Lygidakis *et al.* (1983)[40]	475	34	4.2
Huber *et al.* (1983)[7]	50	20	2
Ganey *et al.* (1986)[15]	1035	29	0.5
Pickleman *et al.* (1986)[18]	269	8.6	0.4
Margiotta *et al.* (1988)[9]	119	NS	3
Heberer *et al.* (1988)[41]	544	NS	0.4
Gilliland *et al.* (1990)[17]	671	3.1	0
Herzog *et al.* (1992)[42]	1631	15.2	0.2
Clavien *et al.* (1992)[6]:			
Toronto	650	8.6	0
Geneva	602	17.9	0
Bredesen *et al.* (1992)[5]	13854	23.6*	1.2

NS = not stated
* Excludes patients undergoing additional biliary drainage procedures at the time of cholecystectomy

Clavien *et al.*[6] have recently assessed the results of elective open cholecystectomy in the years leading up to the widespread adoption of laparoscopic cholecystectomy. Data were collected retrospectively in one North American (Mount Sinai Hospital, Toronto) and one European (Geneva University Hospital) hospital and 1252 patients underwent operation in either centre in the years immediately prior to 1989. Surgery was performed in Toronto by one specialist surgeon and in Geneva by 33 different surgeons, although a surgeon with at least five years experience was present on every occasion. In both centres, the indication for surgery was symptomatic cholelithiasis and patients presenting with acute cholecystitis or cholangitis were not included. A six-week follow-up was available in all cases. There were no deaths in either centre, although 12% and 14% of patients developed complications in Toronto and Geneva respectively (see below). The bile duct was explored in 8.6% of the patients in Toronto as opposed to 17.9% in Geneva, the incidence of positive exploration being 61% and 73% respectively.

The impressive results reported from Toronto and Geneva must, however, be kept in perspective, given that they represent the modern 'gold standard' that can be achieved in a university teaching hospital or in specialist hands in patients undergoing elective cholecystectomy. Our own experience in the Lothian region of Scotland may be more representative, dealing as it does with prospectively collected audit data from the entire region (comprising a mixture of specialist and non-specialist surgical units, teaching hospitals and district general hospitals) and including all patients coming to cholecystectomy. The data show that the annual mortality rate for cholecystectomy alone has been less than 1% since 1980 (Fig. 5.1.1), despite the fact that a significant proportion of these operations (7.9% in 1989) were being undertaken on an emergency basis. The need to explore the bile duct undoubtedly increases risk, with operative mortality at the start of the decade being as high as 3.8% if choledocholithotomy was undertaken. However, in 1989 there was only one death in 79 such patients and in some intervening years there have been no deaths. This undoubtedly reflects the ready availability of ERCP and endoscopic papillotomy with stone retrieval and it is noteworthy that the number of patients undergoing cholecystectomy with CBD exploration has fallen steadily throughout the decade. The ability to use endoscopic papillotomy to overcome calculous obstruction and avoid major emergency surgery in elderly sick patients has undoubtedly made a major impact on the overall risks of biliary tract surgery.

A study of postoperative mortality following cholecystectomy in the entire female population of Denmark in the years 1977–1981 revealed a crude overall mortality rate of 1.2%, i.e. 166 deaths in 13 854 patients.[5] The 30-day mortality of simple elective cholecystectomy was similar to that of elective hysterectomy, but cholecystectomy had a higher mortality when age standardization was performed. Factors increasing risk were advancing age, acute admission, admission to hospital within three months of the index admission, number of discharge diagnoses and geographical region. The causes of death among cholecystectomy patients are shown in Table 5.1.2 and Table 5.1.3 gives a

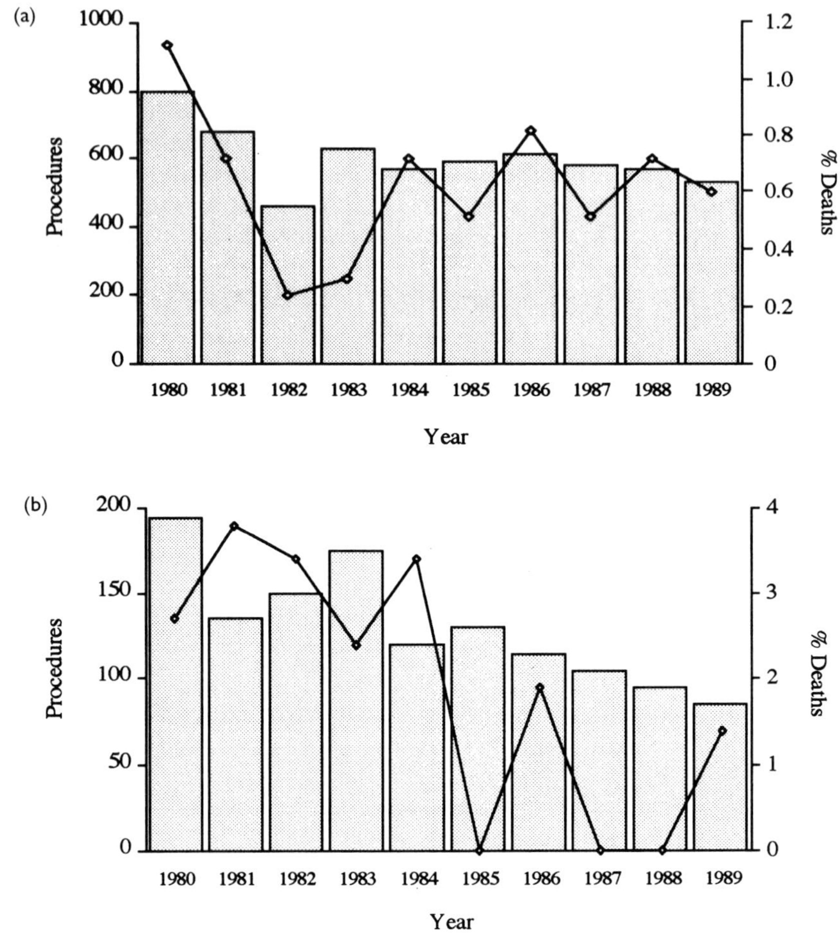

Figure 5.1.1 Rates of operation and operative mortality in Lothian, Scotland, in the years 1980–1989 for patients undergoing (a) cholecystectomy without exploration of the common bile duct, and (b) cholecystectomy with exploration of the common bile duct.

breakdown of mortality rates according to age and whether the patient underwent simple elective cholecystectomy or required exploration of the bile duct with or without biliary drainage. It is clear that mortality rises markedly once patients undergoing cholecystectomy are older than 60 years and that surgery for acute as opposed to elective conditions at least doubles mortality rates. The crude operative mortality for elective cholecystectomy with choledocholithotomy (1.6%) was four times greater than that of elective cholecystectomy alone (0.45%).

To conclude this section, it is clear that open cholecystectomy had become a safe operation in the years immediately preceding the swing towards laparoscopic removal of the gall bladder. This undoubtedly reflects refinement of

Table 5.1.2 Causes of death within 30 days of surgery in a series of 13 854 women undergoing cholecystectomy in Denmark between 1977 and 1981 (data from reference 5)

Causes of death	No. patients	(%)
Related to disease/operation	29	17.5
Thromboembolic complications	15	9
Cardiovascular disease	64	38.5
Respiratory disease	15	9
Other causes	11	6.6
Insufficient information	19	11.4
Total	166	

Table 5.1.3 Early postoperative mortality in 166 patients dying after cholecystectomy in a series of 13 854 female Danish patients (data from reference 5)

	Cholecystectomy alone		+ choledocholithotomy		+ bilary drainage	
Age (yrs)	Elective	Acute	Elective	Acute	Elective	Acute
<29	0	0.39	0	0	0	0
30–39	0	0	0	0	0	0
40–49	0.07	0.60	0.68	0	0	0
50–59	0.17	0.35	0.39	0.69	0	0
60–69	0.80	1.02	1.82	4.02	0	1.92
70–79	1.59	2.92	3.02	3.67	3.00	6.38
>80	5.56	6.75	4.71	7.14	5.00	9.68
Crude rate	0.15	1.60	1.60	3.21	1.67	5.12

perioperative care, better patient selection, improved standards of training, development of subspecialization and availability of alternative methods of treatment to deal with high risk patient groups. It can be argued that an operative mortality rate of zero was a widely attainable goal for elective open cholecystectomy, but that mortality rates of 1–2% might still be expected in elderly high risk patients undergoing surgery on a non-elective basis or when cholecystectomy had to be supplemented by bile duct exploration or bilioenteric anastomoses.

MORBIDITY OF OPEN CHOLECYSTECTOMY

The most detailed recent analysis of the spectrum of postoperative complications following open cholecystectomy comes from the Toronto–Geneva study of 1252 patients.[6] The overall complication rate in patients undergoing cholecystectomy alone was approximately 11% and this figure rose to 12–14% when patients undergoing common duct exploration were included. Overall, 72 patients (5.7%) developed grade I complications (i.e. departure from an ideal postoperative course with complications that were not life-threatening or liable to cause lasting disability) such as postoperative fever and urinary tract infection, whereas 88 (7%) developed grade II complications (potentially life-threatening but without residual disability), including four patients with bile leaks requiring reintervention. There were only two grade III complications (myocardial infarction, stroke) and no grade IV complications. The data suggest that it is better to perform surgery early in the course of symptomatic gallstone disease, not only because of the accepted increase in the risk of operation with advancing age but also because of the increased risk of postoperative complications.

Other studies have found that the elderly are at greater risk of developing complications during the treatment of acute cholecystitis,[7–9] although there is less evidence of risk increase when only those undergoing elective cholecystectomy are considered. Of interest, the two centres studied by Clavien *et al.*[6] had different patterns of individual risk factors for predicting complications, highlighting the sensitive and variable nature of risk assessment systems based on univariate and multivariate analysis. In the Geneva experience, CBD exploration was the most significant risk factor for complications, whereas in Toronto exploration incurred no greater risk, perhaps reflecting the fact that there was one operator in Toronto as opposed to a large number of surgeons in Geneva.

It should be stressed once more that these results were obtained in teaching hospitals and in the case of Toronto, by a specialist unit where all patients were referred to the care of one hepatobiliary surgeon who was involved in all operations. Furthermore, they refer to elective cholecystectomy and it is well recognized that morbidity as well as mortality is higher in patients undergoing gall bladder surgery in the face of complications such as acute cholecystitis, empyema of the gall bladder, gangrene and perforation. Although lithotripsy was not available in either centre, it seems likely that a number of patients who might have had to undergo emergency surgery because of cholangitis and obstructive jaundice were spared this intervention by ERCP and endoscopic papillotomy.

Bile Duct Injury

There is still uncertainty regarding the true incidence of bile duct injury at open cholecystectomy, let alone laparoscopic cholecystectomy. The surveys available cite figures ranging from one injury per 300–500 open cholecystectomies[10–14] to a figure of one in 1000 operations.[15–18] It may be that the incidence of bile duct injury had fallen as surgical standards and training had improved, but almost certainly there has been (and continues to be) under-reporting of the true incidence of injury, either because the surgeons concerned now feel competent to repair the problem there and then or because the injury becomes manifest late and in some cases, long after hospital discharge. In the series of 78 patients with bile duct injury reported by Blumgart *et al.*,[19] ductal damage was recognized at the time of injury in only 19% of cases and in 41% the injury declared itself by steadily progressive obstructive jaundice.

When injury does occur, there is no doubting its serious implications. Until recently, repair of bile duct strictures carried an operative mortality of around 8.3%[20] and in patients with complicated strictures, the presence of portal hypertension and liver disease may raise mortality to levels approaching 30%.[19] Assuming that the patient survives the repair, long term morbidity may result from impaired biliary drainage and periodic attacks of cholangitis, while failure to create a substantial anastomosis may cause restricture and the need for reoperation. In the experience of Blumgart *et al.*,[19] no less than 57% (46) of their patients had undergone two or more operations before referral. In our own series of patients undergoing repair of bile duct strictures, 21 of 33 patients had had a previous attempt at repair; of these, three had undergone two previous operations and two patients had undergone three procedures.

Although improved preoperative, intraoperative and postoperative care have made for safer and more effective treatment of bile duct strictures, the problem is still a major souce of short term and long term morbidity after cholecystectomy and one which threatens to be at least as significant after laparoscopic cholecystectomy. There can be no doubt that emphasis must remain on prevention, regardless of whether cholecystectomy is performed by open surgery or laparoscopic means. The persisting lesson has been that injury results from imprecise dissection and inadequate demonstration of the anatomical structures.[21] Admittedly, some patients do have anatomical anomalies or pathological changes which increase the risk of duct damage, but it is salutary to note that in the extensive Swedish review[14] the patients most at risk appeared to be young slim females who had not undergone previous surgery. One has little doubt that in many cases, a small calibre mobile common bile duct was divided in the mistaken belief that it was the cystic duct. The most significant factor appeared to be the experience of the operating surgeon in that only three of the 65 injuries were perpetrated by surgeons performing their first 25 cholecystectomies, whereas 52 injuries were the result of operation carried out by a surgeon who had undertaken between 25 and 100 cholecystectomies. Undoubtedly there is a similar danger zone on the learning curve for laparoscopic cholecystectomy and it is noteworthy that in the analysis of 1518 laparoscopic cholecystectomies reported by the Southern Surgical Club,[22] the incidence of bile duct injury in the first 13 patients operated on by each group was 2.2%, compared with 0.1% for subsequent patients.

Debate continues to surround the need for operative cholangiography during cholecystectomy, but one argument advanced by those advocating its routine use is that the risk of bile duct injury is reduced if the anatomy of the extrahepatic tree has been defined. In the Swedish experience, only three of the 65 patients did not undergo operative cholangiography at the time of cholecystectomy. However in 44% of cases, injury had occurred before a cholangiogram was obtained and in a further 52% of cases the injury was perpetrated before the films became available.

In our own series of 33 bile duct injuries, 28 occurred in patients undergoing cholecystectomy alone, the operation being performed laparoscopically in six cases. An operative cholangiogram had been performed in ten of the 28 patients, of which three were correctly interpreted, allowing primary repair of the bile duct injury. The cholangiograms were misinterpreted in six cases in that the intrahepatic biliary tree was not filled. It is clear that performing an operative cholangiogram does not confer immunity to bile duct injury, but at the time laparoscopic cholecystectomy was introduced, it was our practice to recommend routine operative cholangiography (to demonstrate anatomy as well as detect duct stones) and we see no reason to modify this practice now that minimally invasive surgery seems to be here to stay. However, there seems little point in carrying out cholangiography unless one is willing to wait to review the films before proceeding to divide ductal structures. There is no doubt that interpretation of operative cholangiography is greatly facilitated by an image intensifier (and perhaps by the availability of an immediate and objective radiological opinion) and that correct interpretation of the cholangiogram may avert catastrophe and limit the injury to the biliary tree to a degree which is immediately rectifiable.

SYMPTOM RELIEF FOLLOWING OPEN CHOLECYSTECTOMY

Relationship Between Symptoms and Gallstones

Before assessing the impact of cholecystectomy on symptoms, it is important to review the strength of the association between such symptoms and the presence of stones in a diseased gall bladder. In reality, the very basis of some of the symptoms associated with gallstone disease remains conjectural. It is clear that many patients with gallstones remain asymptomatic and conversely, that some patients without stones have symptoms which mimic those of calculous disease. It is relatively easy to understand the basis of the pain which may result from obstruction of the gall bladder in biliary colic and from acute inflammation of the gall bladder and the surrounding structures in acute cholecystitis. What is more difficult to define is the basis for the flatulent dyspepsia which traditionally has been attributed to gallstones, but its frequent aggravation by fatty foods lends support to the concept that at least in part, pain arises from a gall bladder which is being stimulated to contract in the presence of contained stones. As defined by Johnson,[23] the symptoms of flatulent dyspepsia are repeated belching, a feeling of fullness after eating a normal sized meal, inability to finish a normal sized meal, a need to loosen clothing due to abdominal distension, burning in the upper abdomen, burning discomfort in the chest (heartburn), regurgitation of bitter fluid into the mouth, nausea or vomiting.

A number of studies have examined the relationship between dyspeptic symptoms and gallstones[1,24–26] but in general, there is little difference in the prevalence of flatulent dyspeptic symptoms when patients with gallstones are compared with those without. In an ultrasonographic study of gallstone prevalence in Italy, stones were revealed in 8.2% of the male and 9.4% of the female civil servants studied.[27,28] More than two thirds of these stones had caused no symptoms. When symptoms occurred, upper abdominal pain was strongly associated with gallstones, whereas non-specific symptoms such as epigastric burning, bloating, belching, heaviness, nausea, vomiting and intolerance of fatty food were not. As Finlayson[29] has implied, studies such as this can be interpreted as showing that cholecystectomy cannot be expected to be as effective at relieving dyspeptic symptoms as it is at relieving pain.

In the Bristol ultrasonographic prevalence study conducted by Heaton *et al.*[3] very few individuals had convincing biliary symptoms; 10.4% of women had symptoms according to a questionnaire definition of biliary pain while 6.3% had symptoms on conventional history taking. No men admitted to biliary pain, although in the group who had undergone cholecystectomy, operation in men was nearly always preceded by convincing biliary symptoms. The cholecystectomy rate was significantly higher in women (43.5% versus 24%). The authors concluded that either gallstones are especially prone to cause symptoms in younger people or that there are two types of gallstone, the one being symptomatic and the other silent.

In a further prevalence study involving an unselected population in Denmark, Jorgensen[26] found that there was no significant difference in pain characteristics between individuals with a normal gall bladder and those with gall bladders that contained stones (as long as the individual concerned was unaware of their presence).

If our perceptions of gallstones as a cause of symptoms are so misguided, then it is hardly surprising that so many patients fail to find symptom relief after cholecystectomy and that there is disagreement within the medical profession about some of the indications for the operation. In a consensus development approach, Scott and Black[30] asked a panel of surgeons and a mixed panel of relevant specialists to rate a series of possible indications for cholecystectomy. Although a consensus was achieved for about two thirds of the indications, the surgical panel considered more indications to be appropriate (29% versus 13%) and fewer indications to be inappropriate (27% versus 50%) than the mixed panel.

Symptom Relief After Cholecystectomy

Various uncontrolled studies have addressed the issue of symptom relief after cholecystectomy; for example, Rhind and Watson[31] found that the operation cured or improved dyspeptic symptoms in over 80% of their gallstone patients, while Gunn and Keddie[32] found that only 19% of their patients had dyspeptic symptoms after operation and that pain was relieved or improved by operation in 93% of cases. On the other hand, Johnson[23] found that after open cholecystectomy, only 46% of patients were free from flatulent dyspepsia whereas 30% were no better. Similarly, Ros and Zambon[33] found that approximately half of their patients had complained of dyspepsia before cholecystectomy and that these symptoms persisted in half of the patients after operation. Only 53% of the patients in this study were symptom-free two years after cholecystectomy.

If the basis for symptoms before cholecystectomy remains so uncertain, it is hardly surprising that a substantial number of patients continue to experience problems after operation. Bates and his group[34] conducted a detailed analysis of 292 consecutive patients undergoing cholecystectomy for presumed biliary pain in a district general hospital in the period 1980–1985. None of the patients had asymptomatic gallstones, all had abdominal pain considered to be biliary in origin and none had flatulent dyspepsia alone. Over the following two years, 18 patients died but no others were lost to follow-up. The remaining 274 patients completed a questionnaire at one and two years after operation and their demographic characteristics and abdominal symptoms were compared with those of age and sex matched control patients admitted for elective surgery, but without a history of biliary disease or a diagnosis likely to produce abdominal symptoms.

Before operation, symptoms of flatulent dyspepsia were far more frequent in the gallstone patients, but operation markedly reduced these symptoms to an incidence almost identical to that of the control group (Table 5.1.4). However, within one year of cholecystectomy, no less than 34% of patients still suffered some abdominal pain and of 35 patients referred back to hospital for investigation, none had evidence of a retained ductal stone at a minimum follow-up of five years. Multivariate analysis showed that preoperative flatulence and long durations of attacks of pain were risk factors for postoperative dissatisfaction (as judged on a linear analogue scale). As both of these factors were common, neither was a useful predictor of outcome. One is forced to agree with the authors that it is difficult to predict outcome as far as relief of symptoms is concerned and that all patients coming to cholecystectomy, regardless of the technique employed, should be warned of the possibility of continuing symptoms.

Wilson and MacIntyre[35] have recently reported the results of a questionnaire study of patients who had undergone open or laparoscopic cholecystectomy in Lothian, the operation being performed in just over one third of cases for acute cholecystitis. After a minimum follow-up of one year, no less than 94% of patients in either group considered that the operation had cured or improved

Table 5.1.4 Pattern of symptoms recorded by patients with gallstones before and after cholecystectomy, and by age and sex matched control surgical patients without gallstone disease (data from reference 34)

	Controls n = 278	Gallstone patients Preoperative n = 278	1 year postop n = 278	2 year postop n = 274
Flatulence	30	66	44	42
Distension	33	57	37	40
Indigestion	38	71	43	42
Nausea	15	62	23	19
Vomiting	10	54	9	10
Fever	4	34	5	4
Rigor	4	30	5	2
Abdominal pain	Nil	100	34	27
Consulted GP for pain	Nil	100	23	18

Values are percentages

their preoperative symptoms and that it had been a success. The pattern of prevalence of postoperative dyspeptic symptoms and pain was similar in the two groups but less than one in five of the patients experienced such symptoms every day or on most days after operation. The proportion of patients consulting their general practitioner following laparoscopic cholecystectomy was 23% whereas it was 19% after open cholecystectomy. Whereas some earlier studies have suggested that chronic pain in the wound was the major source of abdominal pain after open cholecystectomy in about one quarter of patients, Wilson and MacIntyre found no difference between their patient groups in this regard (pain reported in 6–7% of cases), suggesting that wound-related problems are not in fact a particularly significant source of pain after cholecystectomy. The discrepancy between the results of cholecystectomy in this Scottish series and those of Bates and colleagues[34] in south east England is difficult to explain, but could represent the more stoical and accepting nature of the calvinist Scots!

Postcholecystectomy Syndromes

The term "postcholecystectomy syndrome" has been used to describe residual, recurrent or new symptoms developing after removal of the gall bladder. In truth, the term is often used as a cloak for ignorance and a convincing explanation for the problem is found in only a minority of cases. Accepted causes of the postcholecystectomy syndrome include retained common duct stones, bile duct stricture and retained gall bladder, but much more doubt surrounds the significance of a long cystic duct remnant, papillary stenosis, adhesions and painful wound neuromas. In some cases, it seems more likely that the initial symptoms were not actually arising from the gall bladder and the long list of conditions that can mimic flatulent dyspepsia and biliary pain include peptic ulceration, irritable bowel syndrome, chronic pancreatitis, liver disease, reflux oesophagitis and coronary artery disease.

Acalculous Biliary Pain

The outlook for patients with acalculous biliary pain following cholecystectomy is even less certain, given that our understanding of the mechanisms of pain production in these patients is so imperfect. There is an increasing body of evidence that some of these patients have abnormal motility not just of the gall bladder but, perhaps more importantly, of the sphincter of Oddi. It is also conceivable that in some patients with *calculous* biliary pain, the pain arises not from the stone-bearing gall bladder but from abnormal sphincter motility. Some authors have reported improvement in symptoms in as many as 85–95% of patients with acalculous biliary pain after cholecystectomy,[36,37] but controlled studies which can exclude a placebo effect of operation are still required. Controversy continues to surround the use of cholecystokinin (CCK) provocation tests as a means of reproducing symptoms and predicting which patients will benefit from having their gall bladder removed. In the experience of Lennard *et al.*[38] all 26 patients with positive CCK tests showed improvement after cholecystectomy, whereas no fewer than ten of the 16 patients with negative tests were found to have alternative explanations for their pain. However, many other authors have failed to show differences in outcome when patients with positive CCK tests were compared with those with negative tests.[39]

It is still difficult to define objective criteria on which to base the decision to recommend cholecystectomy in patients with pain thought to be consistent with a biliary tract origin but who do not have stones. One thing is certain – the advent of laparoscopic cholecystectomy should not lead to any relaxation in the indications for cholecystectomy and patients with acalculous biliary pain are no exception to this rule.

CONCLUSIONS

The morbidity and mortality of open cholecystectomy had in general reached acceptable levels by the time laparoscopic cholecystectomy was introduced and then widely adopted. The available evidence suggests that the morbidity and mortality of laparoscopic cholecystectomy will be no greater than that of open surgery and may even be lower. However, certain aspects of laparoscopic cholecystectomy will require continuing review, notably the incidence of bile duct injury. There is still considerable uncertainty about the relationship between gallstones and the symptoms traditionally attributed to them and the uncertainty is greatest in respect of the "flatulent dyspepsia" symptom complex. There is nothing to suggest that the long term outcome following laparoscopic cholecystectomy will be significantly different from that of open cholecystectomy and further study of the indications for and expectations of cholecystectomy are still required.

REFERENCES

1. Bainton D, Davies GT, Evans KT, Gravelle IH. Gallbladder disease: prevalence in a South Wales industrial town. *N Engl J Med* 1976; **294**: 1147–9.
2. Godrey PJ, Bates T, Harrison M, King MB, Padley NR. Gall stones and mortality: a study of all gall stone related deaths in a single health district. *Gut* 1984; **25**: 1029–33.
3. Heaton KW, Braddon FEM, Mountford RA, Hughes AO, Emmett PM. Symptomatic and silent gall stones in the community. *Gut* 1991; **32**: 316–20.
4. Martin JK Jr, van Heerden JA. Surgery of the liver, biliary tract and pancreas. *Mayo Clin Proc* 1980; **55**: 333–7.
5. Bredesen J, Jorgensen T, Andersen TF *et al.* Early postoperative mortality following cholecystectomy in the entire female population of Denmark, 1977–1981. *World J Surg* 1992; **16**: 530–5.
6. Clavien PA, Sanabria JR, Mentha G *et al.* Recent results of elective open cholecystectomy in a North American and a European center – comparison of complications and risk factors. *Ann Surg* 1992; **216**: 618–26.
7. Huber DF, Martin EW, Cooperman M. Cholecystectomy in elderly patients. *Am J Surg* 1983; **146**: 719–22.
8. Houghton PW, Jenkinson LR, Donaldson LA. Cholecystectomy in the elderly: a prospective study. *Br J Surg* 1985; **72**: 220–2.
9. Margiotta SJ Jr, Horwitz JR, Willis IH, Wallack MK. Cholecystectomy in the elderly. *Am J Surg* 1988; **156**: 509–12.
10. Bismuth H. Post-operative strictures of the bile duct. In: *The Biliary Tract*, Clinical Surgery International Vol. 5 (ed. Blumgart LH). Edinburgh, Churchill Livingstone, 1982.
11. Kune GA. Bile duct injury during cholecystectomy. Causes, prevention and surgical repair in 1979. *Aust NZ J Surg* 1979; **49**: 35–40.
12. Madsen CM, Sorensen HR, Truelsen F. The frequency of bile duct injuries, illustrated by a Danish county survey. *Acta Chir Scand* 1960; **119**: 110–11.
13. Rosenqvist H, Myrin SO. Operative injuries to the bile ducts. *Acta Chir Scand* 1960; **119**: 92–107.
14. Andren-Sandberg A, Alinder A, Bengmark S. Accidental lesions of the common bile duct at cholecystectomy: pre- and per-operative factors of importance. *Ann Surg* 1985; **201**(3): 328–33.
15. Ganey JB, Johnson PA, Prillaman PE, McSwain GR. Cholecystectomy: clinical experience with a large series. *Am J Surg* 1986; **151**: 352–7.
16. McSherry CK. Cholecystectomy: the gold standard. *Am J Surg* 1989; **158**: 174–8.

17. Gilliland TM, Traverso LW. Modern standards for comparison of cholecystectomy with alternative treatments for symptomatic cholelithiasis with emphasis on long term relief of symptoms. *Surg Gynecol Obstet* 1990; **170**: 39–44.
18. Pickleman J. Controversies in biliary tract surgery. *Can J Surg* 1986; **29**: 429–423.
19. Blumgart LH, Kelley CJ, Benjamin IS. Benign bile duct stricture following cholecystectomy: critical factors in management. *Br J Surg* 1984; **71**: 836–43.
20. Warren KW, Christophi C, Armendariz R. The evolution and current perspectives of the treatment of benign bile duct strictures: a review. *Surg Gastroenterol* 1982; **1**: 141–54.
21. Garden OJ. Iatrogenic injury to the bile duct. *Br J Surg* 1991; **78**: 1412–13.
22. The Southern Surgeons Club. A prospective analysis of 1518 laparoscopic cholecystectomies. *N Engl J Med* 1991; **324**: 1074–8.
23. Johnson AG. Gallstones and flatulent dyspepsia: cause or coincidence? *Postgrad Med J* 1971; **47**: 767–72.
24. Price WH. Gallbladder dyspepsia. *Br Med J* 1963; **iii**: 138–41.
25. Pixley F, Mann J. Dietary factors in the aetiology of gallstones: a case control study. *Gut* 1988; **29**: 1511–15.
26. Jorgensen T. Abdominal symptoms and gallstone disease: an epidemiological investigation. *Hepatology* 1989; **9**: 856–60.
27. Rome Group for the Epidemiology and Prevention of Cholelithiasis (GREPCO). Prevalence of gallstone disease in an Italian adult female population. *Am J Epidemiol* 1984; **119**: 796–805.
28. Rome Group for the Epidemiology and Prevention of Cholelithiasis (GREPCO). The epidemiology of gallstone disease in Rome, Italy. Prevalence data in men. *Hepatology* 1988; **8**: 904–6.
29. Finlayson N. Cholecystectomy for gall stones. *Br Med J* 1989; **298**: 133–4.
30. Scott EA, Black N. Appropriateness of cholecystectomy in the United Kingdom – a consensus panel approach. *Gut* 1991; **32**: 1066–70.
31. Rhind JA, Watson L. Gall stone dyspepsia. *Br Med J* 1968; **1**: 32.
32. Gunn A, Keddie N. Some clinical observations on patients with gallstones. *Lancet* 1972; **ii**: 239–41.
33. Ros E, Zambon D. Postcholecystectomy symptoms. A prospective study of gallstone patients before and two years after surgery. *Gut* 1987; **28**: 1500–4.
34. Bates T, Ebbs SR, Harrison M, A'Hern RP. Influence of cholecystectomy on symptoms. *Br J Surg* 1991; **78**: 964–7.
35. Wilson RG, MacIntyre IMC. Symptomatic outcome after laparoscopic cholecystectomy. *Br J Surg* 1993; **80**: 439–41.
36. Dunn FH, Christensen EC, Reynolds J. Cholecystokinin cholecystography. *JAMA* 1974; **228**: 997–1003.
37. Nathan MH, Newman A, Murray DJ, Camponovo R. Cholecystokinin cholecystography. Four years evaluation. *Am J Roentgenol* 1970; **110**: 240–51.
38. Lennard TWJ, Farndon JR, Taylor RMR. Acalculous biliary pain: diagnosis and selection for cholecystectomy using the cholecystokinin test for pain reproduction. *Br J Surg* 1984; **71**: 368–70.
39. Sunderland GT, Carter DC. Clinical application of the cholecystokinin provocation test. *Br J Surg* 1988; **75**: 444–9.
40. Lygidakis NJ. Operative risk factors of cholecystectomy–choledochotomy in the elderly. *Surg Gynecol Obstet* 1983; **157**: 15–19.
41. Heberer G, Paumgartner G, Sauerbruch T *et al.* A retrospective analysis of 3 years' experience of an interdisciplinary approach to gallstone disease including shockwaves. *Ann Surg* 1988; **208**: 274–8.
42. Herzog U, Messmer P, Sutter M, Tondelli P. Surgical treatment for cholelithiasis. *Surg Gynecol Obstet* 1992; **175**: 238–42.

5.2

Laparoscopic Cholecystectomy

S. PATERSON-BROWN, A. DE BEAUX, J. D. GREIG and O. J. GARDEN

INTRODUCTION

The recent introduction of laparoscopic cholecystectomy[1–4] has become almost universally accepted by the surgical fraternity.[5,6] However sporadic reports of operative complications and a potential increase in the incidence of common bile duct injuries[7] have led to some words of caution.[8,9] Many reports of bile duct injury remain anecdotal[9,10] and anxieties have not been substantiated by recent multicentre studies from Europe[11] and the United States[12] which report an incidence of injury to the common bile duct of between one in 200–300. This figure is slightly higher than the accepted incidence of one in 300–500 following open cholecystectomy[13–15] although the true morbidity and mortality of laparoscopic cholecystectomy will only be known when truly multicentre prospective audit data become available.

Debate regarding training in laparoscopic cholecystectomy continues[16] and it remains difficult for each surgical unit to gauge their success against others and, more importantly, to recognize the length and incline of the learning curve which all surgeons must climb. Furthermore, specialties other than surgery could well become involved in the management of these patients, if the previous reliance on operative cholangiography is to be replaced by preoperative intravenous cholangiography or endoscopic retrograde cholangiography.[17]

This chapter not only describes the operative details for laparoscopic cholecystectomy but attempts to answer some of these additional questions.

TECHNIQUE OF LAPAROSCOPIC CHOLECYSTECTOMY

We consider that all patients with symptomatic gallstones should be considered for laparoscopic cholecystectomy providing their cardiorespiratory status does not preclude laparoscopy. Previous upper abdominal incisions do not constitute

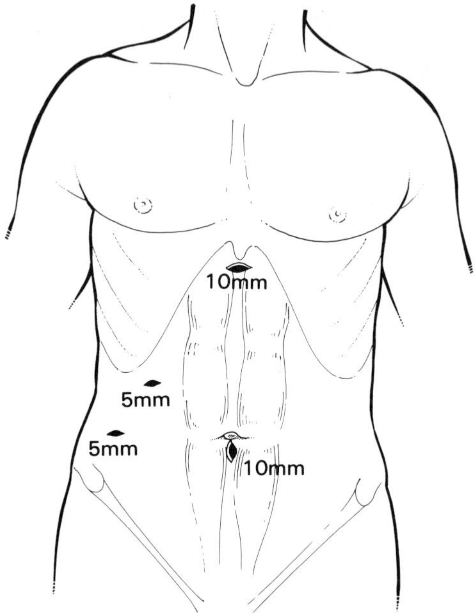

Figure 5.2.1 Position of the ports for laparoscopic cholecystectomy.

a contraindication, particularly if an open technique of laparoscopy is used (Chapter 4). Similarly patients with acute cholecystitis should be offered laparoscopic cholecystectomy provided their overall condition is stable. Preoperative investigations include ultrasonography and liver function tests to confirm the diagnosis of gallstones and evaluate the relative risks of choledocholithiasis. It is our practice to refer patients for endoscopic retrograde cholangiography (ERC) preoperatively only if there is strong evidence of common bile duct stones (elevated serum bilirubin *and* alkaline phosphatase levels; a dilated common bile duct with stones seen on ultrasonography).

Patients are prepared for theatre and, under full general anaesthesia with endotracheal intubation, placed supine on the operating table. Pneumoperitoneum and insertion of instruments are performed as previously described (Chapter 4) and the position of the ports is shown in Figure 5.2.1. Some surgeons now routinely attempt the operation with three ports (leaving out the most lateral of the rightsided ports normally used to grasp and elevate the fundus of the gall bladder) but the authors usually use four. Once the instruments have been inserted the patient is placed in the reverse Trendelenburg position with the right side up. A nasogastric tube may be passed at this point if the stomach and duodenum are excessively distended.

Before dissection commences the fundus of the gall bladder is grasped by grasping forceps passed down the most lateral rightsided port. They are then pushed upwards over the liver edge, thereby exposing the length of the gall

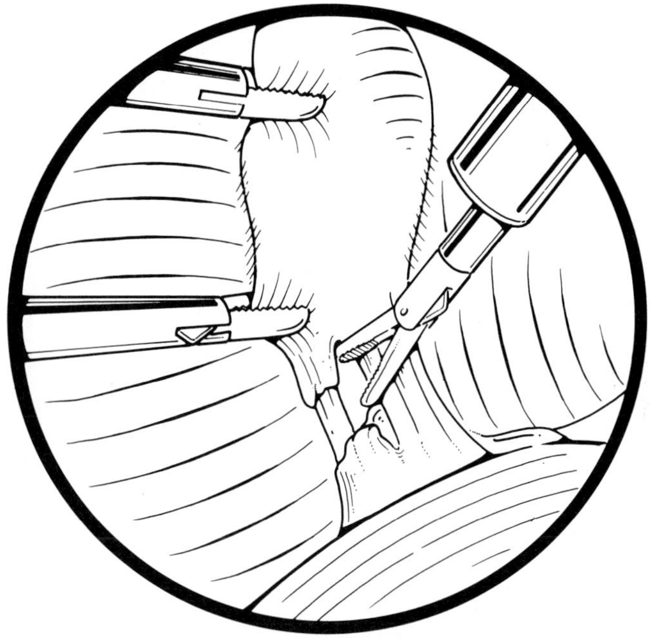

Figure 5.2.2 The peritoneum over the anterior surface of Calot's triangle is opened, starting over Hartmann's pouch and staying close to the gall bladder.

bladder down to the area of Hartmann's pouch and the cystic duct. The second pair of grasping forceps passed down the medial right upper quadrant port grasps Hartmann's pouch; if the gall bladder is very long it may be necessary to 'walk down' the proximal part with these grasping forceps and another pair inserted down the epigastric port, in order to reach a suitable point.

Once Hartmann's pouch has been grasped and pulled away from the free edge of the lesser omentum – and the common bile duct – the peritoneum over the anterior and then posterior surfaces of Calot's triangle are gently divided (Fig. 5.2.2). Care should be taken to start close to the gall bladder, first with blunt dissection and then using the hook with electrocautery. Once the cystic duct has been identified and dissected free a titanium clip is placed across the distal portion and an operative cholangiogram performed. There are now a multitude of instruments and techniques available to assist this procedure; however, we prefer to use a venous canula (size 14G) through which is inserted a 3.5 Ch umbilical catheter (Argyle, Petit-Rochain, Belgium). After an incision has been made in the cystic duct just proximal to the clip, the catheter is inserted and secured in position by a half-closed titanium clip (Fig. 5.2.3). Once the cholangiogram is completed, this clip is removed, the catheter withdrawn and the proximal cystic duct clipped with an additional two clips. At this time, if the cystic artery is visible and has been dissected free, it is also clipped and then both are divided.

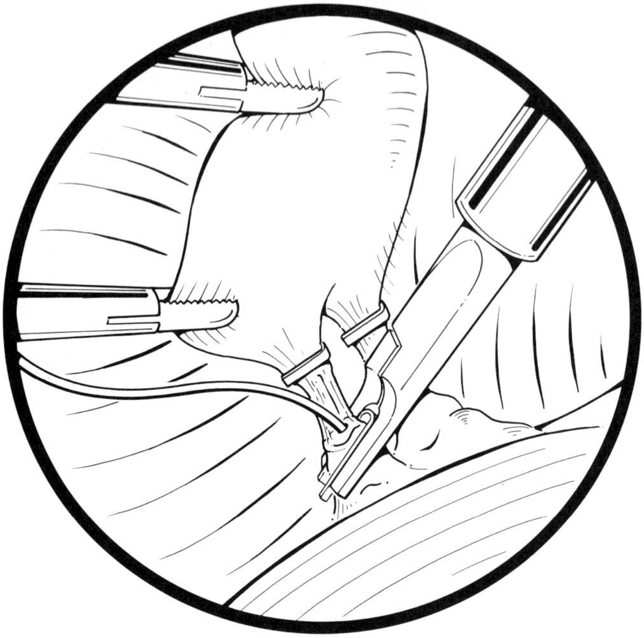

Figure 5.2.3 The cholangiogram catheter secured in place by a partially closed titanium clip.

The gall bladder is then dissected from the undersurface of the liver using the hook and electrocautery (Fig. 5.2.4). Before completing the dissection it is useful to irrigate and suction out the fluid in the gall bladder fossa while the liver is still elevated. The dissection is then completed, the gall bladder removed through the epigastric port and a final inspection and irrigation of the undersurface of the liver carried out. The gall bladder is removed through the epigastric port in preference to the umbilical one as there is less risk of herniation if the incision needs to be extended and subsequent closure – particularly in obese patients – is difficult. The authors routinely insert a soft silastic drain into the gall bladder bed through one of the right upper quadrant ports at the end of the procedure. The ports are then removed, the umbilical and epigastric incisions closed with deep sutures and all skin incisions closed with subcuticular dissolvable sutures. Local anaesthetic is infiltrated into the wounds.

Oral fluids are introduced once the patient has regained full consciousness, the drain is removed after six hours (or the following morning) if there is no bile and the patient is discharged home.

During the operation in the first 130 patients the total operating time (drapes on to drapes off), dissection time (start of gall bladder dissection to removal of gall bladder from gall bladder bed) and gall bladder removal time were determined. The time taken from drapes on to start of dissection represents the time taken for insufflation, insertion of ports and exposure of the gall bladder.

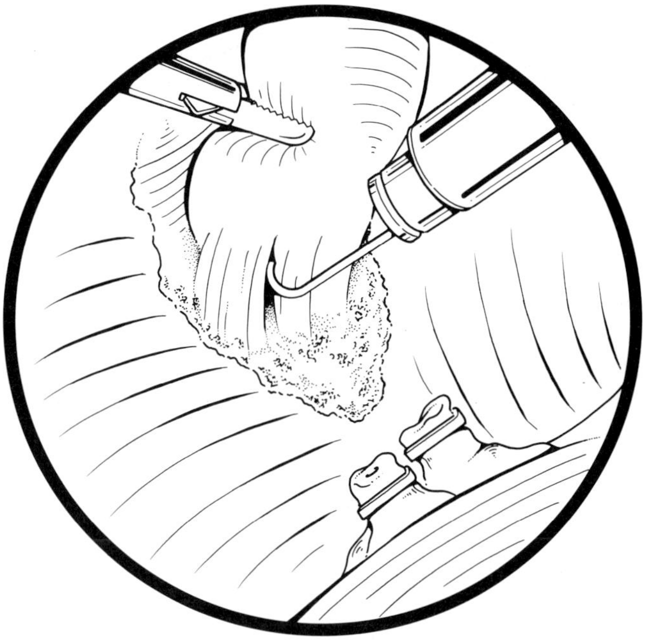

Figure 5.2.4 Dissection of the gall bladder from the liver bed using hook diathermy.

ADDITIONAL TECHNIQUES FOR DIFFICULT CIRCUMSTANCES

Improvements in the visualization of Calot's triangle and dissection of the structures within it involve accurate positioning of ports and if necessary, the use of endoretractors. Obstruction to the view from a prominent left lobe of the liver or distended duodenum may require the insertion of a port in the left upper quadrant. Instruments for dissection can then be inserted through this port with the epigastric port being used to insert instruments for retraction of the liver, either an endoretractor or a suction tube. We now routinely use a 30° oblique-viewing laparoscope which improves the view of Calot's triangle and the common bile duct.

Adequate closure of a large diameter cystic duct may require ligatures and these may be tied before dividing the cystic duct using either intracorporeal or extracorporeal knots. Alternatively the cystic duct can be divided (it is best to attempt partial closure with metal clips first) and then a pretied Roeder knot (Endoloop, Ethicon Ltd, UK) applied. The Endoloop is passed down the epigastric port and the cystic duct stump grasped by forceps passed down the medial right upper quadrant port. As in open surgery, a short cystic duct may occasionally need to be closed with sutures, using intracorporeal knotting.

If the gall bladder is very distended it should be decompressed, either by percutaneous insertion of a needle or by inserting the suction tube into a hole in the fundus. In cases of acute cholecystitis, decompression is invariably required before grasping forceps can be applied to the gall bladder. The hole can be closed by suture, a pretied loop ligature with a Roeder knot or simply by careful positioning of the retracting forceps.

Dissection using the electrocoagulation hook, scissors or spatula is the most common method of removing the gall bladder from the liver. Laser dissection provides little advantage over electrocoagulation in straightforward cases, but greatly facilitates the operation in cases of severe chronic inflammation and particularly when the gall bladder is partly intrahepatic.

Problems resulting from a stoneladen gall bladder include stone spillage and subsequent retrieval. Various forms of pouches have been developed into which either retrieved stones or the gall bladder can be placed. However, removal through the abdominal incision usually remains difficult and the use of an electromechanical stone crusher (Laprolith, Baxter Health Care, USA) greatly facilitates removal of the stoneladen gall bladder.

RESULTS

We have now attempted laparoscopic cholecystectomy in 290 patients and have been successful on 269 (93%) occasions. The reasons for conversion to open operation are given in Table 5.2.1 and the underlying diagnoses in Table 5.2.2.

Table 5.2.1 Reasons for conversion to open cholecystectomy (n = 21)

Severe chronic inflammation, gall bladder adhesions or intra-abdominal adhesions	12
Acute cholecystitis	7
Bile duct injury	1
Choledocholithiasis	1

Table 5.2.2 Diagnoses (n = 290)

Chronic cholecystitis (one of which had previously undergone percutaneous drainage of a liver abscess)	232
Acute cholecystitis	30
Gallstone pancreatitis	23
Acalculous gall bladder disease	5

Table 5.2.3 Complications

Requiring operation:	
Bile duct injury	1
Major bile leak (from duct of Luschka)	1
Obstructed umbilical hernia	1
Operation not required:	
Minor bile leak (settled over 48 hours)	2
Chest infection	1
Wound infection/haematoma	1
Urinary tract infection (these occurred in the first 100 patients following which routine urinary catheterization was abandoned)	6
Deep vein thrombosis	1
Pulmonary thromboembolism	1

After the first five patients, attempts were made to perform intraoperative cholangiography in most patients and this was successful in 196 of 217 (90%) patients in whom it was attempted.

Overall there were 15 complications (Table 5.2.3) and no deaths in the patients submitted to laparoscopic cholecystectomy. There were two major biliary complications: one bile leak from the gall bladder bed (duct of Luschka) and a bile duct injury recognized immediately and repaired at laparotomy. In the former, the patient re-presented with abdominal pain seven days after surgery. No drain had been used in this patient and he required a laparotomy for biliary peritonitis, from which he made a full recovery. The second patient had experienced several episodes of acute cholecystitis in the preceding few years and severe chronic inflammation of the gall bladder complicated the laparoscopic dissection. There were bile leaks detected in the drain fluid of another two patients – both resolved spontaneously, one after 24 hours and the other after 48 hours and a normal ERC. Significant additional complications were observed in a further three patients: one patient developed an obstructed umbilical hernia three days postoperatively in a wound which had been extended and where obesity had made closure difficult; a second patient developed a deep vein thrombosis requiring anticoagulation. The remaining patient was readmitted to another hospital four days after laparoscopic cholecystectomy with a pulmonary thromboembolism, but made a full recovery following treatment.

The mean total operating and dissection times for the first 130 patients are shown in Figure 5.2.5. The dissection time reflects the acquisition of experience during the learning curve and represents the experience of the team as a whole rather than individual operators. The learning curve for one operator (OJG) starting from case number one is perhaps a better indication of the learning curve (Fig. 5.2.6) as all subsequent operators had "experienced" assistants. It can be seen that the mean dissection time for the first ten patients (120 minutes, range 60–320 minutes) is much slower than subsequent groups of ten. Operative

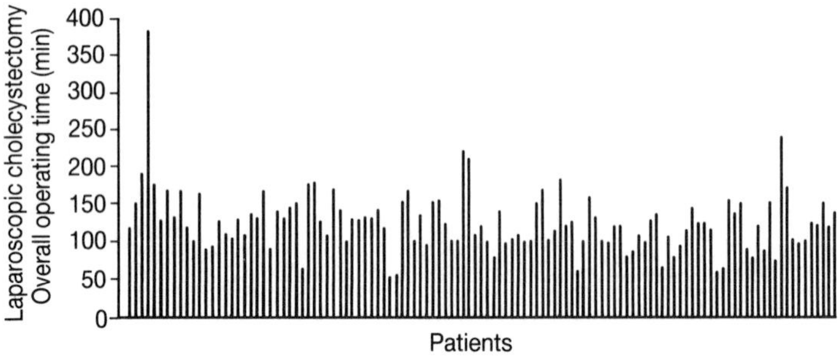

Figure 5.2.5 Overall operating time for laparoscopic cholecystectomy.

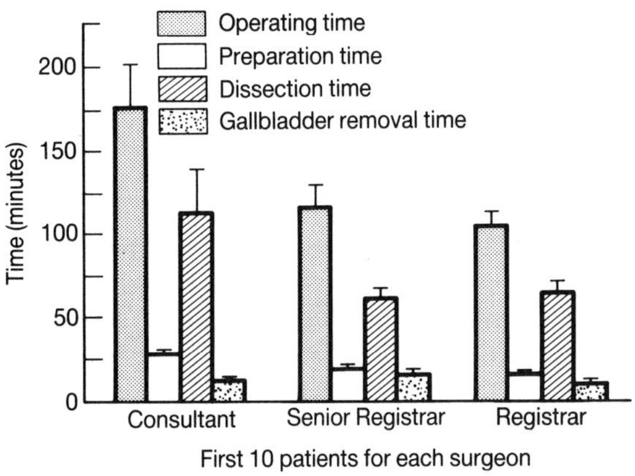

Figure 5.2.6 Operating times for the first ten patients for each surgeon.

cholangiography added only an average of ten minutes to the dissection time compared with those patients in whom it was not attempted.

Abnormal cholangiograms suggestive of possible common bile duct stones were obtained in 21 patients (16 with preoperative risk factors for choledocholithiasis and five with no risk factors). Sixteen patients underwent postoperative ERC which confirmed stones in 12 (all of which were successfully removed endoscopically) and refuted stones in four. Two patients underwent transcystic exploration and removal of the common bile duct stone, one patient underwent laparoscopic common bile duct exploration and removal of two stones measuring 2 cm in diameter. One patient was converted to open surgery for exploration of the common bile duct and one patient was managed expectantly as the filling defect was thought to be an air bubble. Serial liver function tests were performed during early follow-up of this patient and have remained normal.

In this series of laparoscopic cholecystectomies the Laprolith (Baxter Health Care, USA) successfully destroyed all stones within the gall bladder in 20 of 23 patients in whom it was used, with a mean "grinding" time of only 38 seconds.[18]

DISCUSSION

This chapter reports our technique and results of laparoscopic cholecystectomy which are very similar to those reported by a recent multicentre study from seven European centres:[11] laparoscopic cholecystectomy was successfully performed in all but 45 of 1236 patients (96%), with only four bile duct injuries in the 1203 successful laparoscopic procedures. They reported no deaths and a median hospital stay of three days with a median return to normal activities of only 11 days. Although our learning curve appeared to flatten out after the first ten patients it must be remembered that in all operations at least one of the two original surgeons (SPB and OJG) was present. Whether attending courses and training on pelvic simulators alters this curve is open to debate, but observations from our own training courses suggest that those surgeons who have acquired some basic laparoscopic skills on a simulator perform more competently from the outset than those who have not.

The debate regarding the use of operative cholangiography remains unresolved.[17] Although there are good data supporting a selective approach to intraoperative cholangiography at open cholecystectomy[19,20] the same is not yet true for the laparoscopic procedure. Although studies examining the risk factors for choledocholithiasis have demonstrated various risk factors suggesting underlying choledocholithiasis, on multivariate analysis it would appear that only an increased diameter of common bile duct and the presence of multiple (more than ten) gallstones were significant independent indicators.[21] The main problem in converting these data to laparoscopic cholecystectomy is the inability of the surgeon to measure the size of the common bile duct or to palpate the extrahepatic biliary tree which some surgeons consider a useful adjunct to detecting common bile duct stones.[22] Although percutaneous ultrasonography may be helpful in the assessment of common bile duct diameter, the emergence of ultrasound probes which can be passed down the laparoscopic ports may further improve upon the accurate measurement of common bile duct diameter as well as the stone load within the gall bladder.

Our own experience with both mechanical sectoral and linear array laparoscopic ultrasound probes has shown that these are as useful as cholangiography in the detection of common bile duct stones.[23] It remains to be seen, however, whether the biliary anatomy can be as well demonstrated as with cholangiography. It is possible, nonetheless, that laparoscopic ultrasonography may facilitate a policy of selective cholangiography.

The addition of cholangiography to our dissection time was only ten minutes on average. Furthermore, our success rate of 90% includes the learning curve and represents our policy of "almost routine" cholangiography. On the premise that the best time to learn operative cholangiography is not during the mandatory situation, such as following failed preoperative ERCP in cases of suspected choledocholithiasis or when the biliary anatomy is difficult, we recommend that it should be performed as a routine. Not only will the surgeon become competent in the technique but the biliary anatomy will be displayed in all patients, knowledge of the path of the right hepatic duct being particularly useful in patients with biliary anomalies. The narrow calibre common bile duct in the slim female patient appears to be at most risk of damage at open cholecystectomy,[14] and there is no reason to suppose that this will not remain the case for laparoscopic cholecystectomy.

There has been some doubt as to the role of laparoscopic cholecystectomy in the management of acute cholecystitis. Our own experience has confirmed that recognition of the anatomical structures and dissection can be challenging in the presence of acute inflammation. Fears that there would be an unacceptable risk of disseminating infection or of perpetrating an injury to the bile duct appear unfounded[24] and recent reports have demonstrated a significant benefit in terms of recovery and cost benefit when the laparoscopic approach is employed in preference to the open operation.[25] This approach to acute cholecystitis merely serves to underline the fact that the advent of laparoscopic surgery should not be allowed to modify well-established and proven methods of surgical treatment of gallstone disease.

REFERENCES

1. Reddick EJ, Olsen DO. Laparoscopic laser cholecystectomy. *Surg Endosc* 1989; **3**: 131–3.
2. Dubois F, Icard P, Berthelot G, Levard H. Coelioscopic cholecystectomy. *Ann Surg* 1990; **211**: 60–2.
3. Perissat J, Collet D, Belliard R. Gallstones: laparoscopic treatment – cholecystectomy, cholecystostomy and lithotripsy. *Surg Endosc* 1990; **4**: 1–5.
4. Nathanson LK, Shimi S, Cuschieri A. Laparoscopic cholecystectomy: the Dundee technique. *Br J Surg* 1991; **78**: 155–9.
5. Wastell C. Laparoscopic cholecystectomy. *Br Med J* 1991; **302**: 303–4.
6. Thompson JN. Laparoscopic cholecystectomy. *Br Med J* 1991; **302**: 533.
7. Garden OJ. Iatrogenic injury to the bile duct. *Br J Surg* 1991; **78**: 1412–13.
8. Smith R. Laparoscopic cholecystectomy (letter). *Br Med J* 1991; **302**: 593.
9. Smith R. Injuries to common bile duct during laparoscopic cholecystectomy (letter). *Br Med J* 1991; **303**: 1475.
10. Cameron JL, Gadacz TR. Laparoscopic surgery. *Ann Surg* 1991; **213**: 1–2.

11. Cuschieri A, Dubois F, Mouiel J *et al.* The European experience with laparoscopic cholecystectomy. *Am J Surg* 1991; **161**: 385–7.
12. The Southern Surgeons Club. A prospective analysis of 1518 laparoscopic cholecystectomies. *New Engl J Med* 1991; **324**: 1073–8.
13. Kune GA. Bile duct injury during cholecystectomy. Causes, prevention and surgical repair in 1979. *Aust NZ J Surg* 1979; **49**: 35–40.
14. Andren-Sandberg A, Johansson S, Bengmark S. Accidental lesions of the common bile duct at cholecystectomy. *Ann Surg* 1985; **201**: 452–5.
15. Bismuth H. Post-operative strictures of the bile duct. In: *The Biliary Tract*, Clinical Surgery International. (ed. Blumgart LH), pp. 209–18. Edinburgh, Churchill Livingstone, 1982.
16. Paterson-Brown S, Garden OJ, Carter DC. Laparoscopic cholecystectomy. *Br J Surg* 1991; **78**: 131–2.
17. Scott-Coombes D, Thompson JN. Bile duct stones and laparoscopic cholecystectomy. *Br Med J* 1991; **303**: 1281–2.
18. Cuschieri A, Garden OJ, Sackier J, Buess GF. Clinical evaluation of the Laprolith intra-operative lithotripter. *Br J Surg* 1992; **79**: 1350–1.
19. Wilson TG, Hall JC, Watts JM. Is operative cholangiography always necessary? *Br J Surg* 1986; **73**: 637–40.
20. Levine S, Lerner HJ, Leifer ED, Lindheim SR. Intraoperative cholangiography: a review of indications and analysis of age–sex groups. *Ann Surg* 1983; **198**: 692–7.
21. Taylor TV, Torrance B, Rimmer S, Hillier V, Lucas SB. Operative cholangiography: is there a statistical alternative? *Am J Surg* 1983; **145**: 640–3.
22. Cassie GF, Kapadia CR. Operative cholangiography or extra-ductal palpation: an analysis of 418 cholecystectomies. *Br J Surg* 1981; **68**: 516–17.
23. Windsor JA, Garden OJ. Laparoscopic ultrasonography. *Aust NZ J Surg* 1993; **63**: 1–2.
24. Wilson P, Leese T, Morgan WP, Kelly JF, Brigg J. Elective laparoscopic cholecystectomy for "all-comers". *Lancet* 1991; **338**: 795–7.
25. Unger SW, Rosenbaum G, Unger HM, Edelman DS. A comparison of laparoscopic and open treatment of acute cholecystitis. *Surg Endosc* 1993; **7**: 408–11.

Overview

Cholecystectomy

Cholecystectomy was one of the first procedures to benefit from the introduction of laparoscopic surgery and there is no doubt that the success of laparoscopic cholecystectomy has been the main driving force behind the development of laparoscopic surgery. The expectations following open cholecystectomy are eloquently described by Banting and Carter, particularly with regard to symptom relief, complication rates and mortality, and these should be no different following the laparoscopic procedure. The large amount of data which are now available from laparoscopic cholecystectomy would suggest that the laparoscopic approach is now regarded by most surgeons as the correct first treatment option for symptomatic gall bladder stones. It therefore seems unlikely that this procedure will be subjected to satisfactory evaluation by means of a prospective controlled clinical trial, and therefore direct comparisons with retrospective data must be made. Early reports of an increase in common bile duct injuries associated with the learning process have not been confirmed but this may be due to under-reporting, and continuing audit of complications will be required in the future. As surgeons have become experienced in the technique, the indications for laparoscopic cholecystectomy have expanded to include acutely inflamed gall bladders, although the incidence of conversion to open operation remains higher for these more complex cases.

The arguments for and against operative cholangiography have not diminished with the introduction of the laparoscopic procedure and, if anything, have become more heated. There remains a substantial body of opinion which supports selective cholangiography in patients with increased risk of choledocholithiasis. This seems to be more reasonable than either selective pre-operative endoscopic retrograde or intravenous cholangiography. Both have an inherent morbidity and are associated with a high incidence of normal examinations unless the criteria are exceedingly strict. Most surgeons would agree that intra-operative cholangiography is occasionally essential (difficult anatomy and failed pre-operative ERC for suspected choledocholithiasis), and on the premise that the time to learn is not in these difficult cases, all surgeons should become proficient in the technique before deciding whether to abandon it, adopt a selective policy or perform it as a routine. It is an essential technique if the surgeon wishes to progress to the laparoscopic removal of common bile duct stones.

6.1

Choledocholithiasis – Detection and Open Management

D. MENZIES and R. W. MOTSON

INTRODUCTION

Cholecystectomy is one of the commonest operations performed. In the USA approximately 502 000 operations are performed each year[1] and in the UK more than 40 000 procedures are performed annually.[2] The incidence of common bile duct stones in these patients varies from 6–19%,[3–8] though the mean incidence is 11.7%. The detection of common bile duct stones relies upon clinical suspicion, abnormal laboratory and radiological investigations, endoscopic retrograde cholangiopancreatography (ERCP) and detection at the time of surgery either by inspection or the use of peroperative cholangiography. The failure of identification and treatment of common bile duct stones will result in increased morbidity and mortality among these patients.[9]

DETECTION OF COMMON BILE DUCT STONES

It is generally accepted that peroperative cholangiography is the most reliable method of identifying choledocholithiasis. Though this method of stone detection is not infallible there is no other method of common duct imaging, other than direct duct exploration, that is comparable. Additional information that may be of benefit to the surgeon in interpreting operative cholangiograms or in selecting patients for peroperative cholangiography can be gained from preoperative patient assessment.

Preoperative Detection of Common Bile Duct Stones

The preoperative indications of choledocholithiasis are shown in Table 6.1.1.

Table 6.1.1 The indicators which are suggestive of a possible stone in the common bile duct

Clinical	History	Jaundice Pancreatitis Cholangitis
	Examination	Jaundice
Laboratory	Abnormal LFT	Elevated AST, ALT, ALP, bilirubin
Radiological	Ultrasound	Dilated CBD Stone in CBD
	IV cholangiogram	Stone in CBD
	CT scan	Stone in CBD
	ERCP	Stone in CBD

Clinical

A previous history or the presence of jaundice, pancreatitis or cholangitis suggest that common bile duct stones may be present. The reliability of these clinical indicators is poor. Exploration of the common bile duct in these patients will identify stones in only 9%.[10] While it has been reported that choledocholithiasis will be present in only 3–8% of those patients who have never been jaundiced or had pancreatitis,[5,11] only 45% of patients with common bile duct stones have positive clinical indications of their stones.[8]

Laboratory Investigations

The laboratory investigations listed in Table 6.1 are probably the most sensitive indicators of common bile duct stones. In a series of common bile duct explorations 62% of positive explorations were accompanied by abnormal liver function tests.[8] Around 25% of patients with raised liver function tests have common duct stones.[5]

Radiological Investigations

The commonest modalities of biliary tract radiology are ultrasound, IV cholangiography, ERCP and, less frequently, CT scanning.

Ultrasonography. The mainstay of radiological investigation of the biliary tract is ultrasound. There is no doubt that this form of imaging is admirable at detecting cholelithiasis and is now the commonest diagnostic procedure performed for gall bladder stones. Ultrasound is less accurate at identifying stones in the common bile duct and studies from the early 1980s demonstrated that this investigation only identified common bile duct stones correctly in approximately 20%.[12,13] It has since been suggested that with more modern real-time ultrasonography a greater sensitivity may be achieved[14] though with the use of real-time scanning only 23% of common duct stones which were causing obstruction were identified.[15] While ultrasound has many advantages – it is widely available, simple and quick to perform, has no radiation risk and is inexpensive – it has limitations in that it is dependent upon the build of the patient, the absence of bowel gas and the expertise of the operator.

CT scanning. Although CT scanning is less commonly used to identify common bile duct stones it has been reported as an accurate non-invasive method of common duct stone detection. Sensitivities of between 75–90% have been reported.[16–19] Over the last five years the resolution capacity of CT scanners has improved and one might expect an even higher sensitivity, although in a study in 1992, CT scanning correctly identified stones as the cause of obstructive jaundice in only 23%.[15] Stones within the common bile duct may be difficult to image with CT since most stones within the common duct are predominantly cholesterol (80%)[20] and are nearly isodense with bile. CT is expensive and time-consuming to perform and is not practical to use as a routine test for the detection of choledocholithiasis.

Endoscopic retrograde cholangiopancreatography. ERCP is considered to be the most sensitive method of detecting common bile duct stones. The accuracy of stone detection in jaundiced patients has been reported to be between 79–90%.[15,21,22] The false-negative results are usually due to either a technically unsatisfactory study or misinterpretation of the X-rays. The disadvantages of ERCP are that it is expensive, time-consuming, invasive, requires technical expertise of more than one hospital department and has a significant complication rate. Apart from the accuracy of ERCP the advantages are that at the time of the study, if stones are seen within the common bile duct, a sphincterotomy can be performed and the stones extracted or left to pass spontaneously.

The advent of laparoscopic cholecystectomy has highlighted the need to detect common bile duct stones prior to surgery. Although laparoscopic exploration of the common bile duct is possible it requires some degree of expertise and the appropriate instruments which may not be available to the general surgeon performing laparoscopic cholecystectomies. The clearance of the common bile duct with ERCP and sphincterotomy will avoid the need to explore the common duct at operation.

Studies which compare the mortality and morbidity of endoscopic sphincterotomy versus open common bile duct exploration are generally agreed that endoscopic treatment has a lower morbidity and mortality rate than open surgery in patients over 60 years of age. Under the age of 60 there is no difference.[23,24] The retained stone rate after endoscopic sphincterotomy is higher than that after open surgery and several repeated endoscopic procedures may be needed before the bile ducts are cleared.[24–26] The dilemma is compounded when stones are found within a normal sized duct when endoscopic sphincterotomy has an even higher complication rate.[27,28]

Intravenous cholangiography. Over the last ten years the use of IV cholangiography has fallen from favour. In the early 1980s reports appeared which suggested that IV cholangiography should be discouraged or abandoned due to its

Table 6.1.2 Features at operation which indicate possible common bile duct stones

Gall bladder	Multiple small stones Single faceted stone Dilated cystic duct
Common bile duct	Dilated common bile duct Palpable stones

associated toxicity and high diagnostic error rate.[29–31] Minor reactions occurred in 4–24% of cases[32] and deaths were reported to happen in 1/3000 to 1/5000 cases.[33,34] There has recently been a revival of the use of IV cholangiography[35] with the introduction of a safer contrast medium – meglumine iotroxate. This is used with tomography of the right upper quadrant after infusion over 30 minutes. Two recent reports have suggested that IV cholangiography is an acceptable substitute for peroperative cholangiography and that this can be avoided at laparoscopic cholecystectomy; however, both series were small and reported a missed stone rate of 12.5%.[36,37]

Operative Detection of Common Bile Duct Stones

The indication of the need to explore the common bile duct at the time of surgery relies upon the findings of an operative cholangiogram. The suspicion of the presence of duct stones may be supported by manual inspection of the gall bladder and the common bile duct.

Manual Detection

Features which raise the possibility of common bile duct stones are listed in Table 6.1.2. Abnormalities within the gall bladder are poor indicators of the presence of choledocholithiasis. Between 5–15% of patients with either multiple small stones or a dilated cystic duct have stones within the common bile duct.[10] Abnormalities of the common bile duct are far more sensitive as indicators of the presence of stones; 34–84% of patients with a dilated common bile duct have stones and not surprisingly, 100% of patients thought to have palpable common duct stones had these confirmed at exploration.[5,6]

Operative Cholangiography

There are many methods of performing operative cholangiography. The most popular is by cannulation of the cystic duct. Abnormal features of operative cholangiography are listed in Table 6.1.3.

Table 6.1.3 Abnormal features suggesting common bile duct stones at operative cholangiography

Abnormal findings at operative cholangiography	Filling defect Dilated common bile duct No flow into duodenum No flow into right and left hepatic ducts Interstitial portion of the common bile duct not demonstrated

The success of common bile duct clearance relies on the accuracy of the method by which the stones are detected. It is therefore important to produce high quality operative cholangiograms. The method favoured by the authors has been described elsewhere.[38] Briefly this involves cannulation of the cystic duct and the production of three cholangiograms after the injection of 1, 3 and 5 ml of contrast medium. The exposure for radiography is calculated according to the patient's anteroposterior diameter measured immediately before surgery. The initial injection of 1 ml of contrast medium will not overfill a small duct and after the injection of the third volume, even a large duct system is filled. With this method of cholangiography, only 1.4% false-positive examinations resulted.[8]

Routine Versus Selective Cholangiography

Over the last few years there has been a move away from performing routine preoperative cholangiography to performing selective peroperative cholangiography.[5,7,10,39–42] Selective cholangiography involves the performance of peroperative cholangiography only in those patients who are likely to have choledocholithiasis. The indicators of those at risk of common bile duct stones are listed in Tables 6.1.1 and 6.1.2 and are discussed above. The arguments for this type of policy are that it avoids wasted time at surgery, reduces the number of false-positive bile duct explorations and detects nearly all clinically significant common duct stones.

The case for selective cholangiography is still not clearcut and there is considerable disagreement in the literature. It is reported that 40–50% of unnecessary common bile duct explorations may be avoided if selective cholangiography is used.[5,41] In the authors' own series only one out of nine unnecessary common bile duct explorations would have been avoided with the use of selective cholangiography in a series of 99 patients.[8] While there are reports of selective operative cholangiography having a 0% retained stone rate,[5,40] these studies were relatively small and gave no indication of the method or length of follow-up. Other studies have found clinically unsuspected stones in 1–5% of cholecystectomies that would have been missed with the use of selective cholangiography.[6,7,8,41] In one study 40% of common bile duct stones would have been missed if selective operative cholangiography had been employed.[41]

Whether these missed common bile duct stones would be of clinical significance is unknown. It is estimated that as few as 0.3% of patients will return with symptomatic choledocholithiasis after cholecystectomy and selective cholangiography,[43] although in a recent series 1.5% of patients returned with symptomatic common bile duct stones after only one month follow-up.[42] It seems unlikely that all missed common bile duct stones will become symptomatic and it has been estimated that only one in 20 will cause problems.[44] However, the only study to prospectively follow 152 patients with untreated, known retained common bile duct stones after cholecystectomy and exploration of the common bile duct found that 96% required surgery for their stones within five years.[45]

A further argument for performing routine operative cholangiography is that this will provide a road map of the biliary tree and help prevent inadvertent major bile duct injuries. Series of patients with operative bile duct injuries have a low incidence of operative cholangiography being performed.[46,47] It is not recommended that operative cholangiography should be performed for this reason alone. Bile duct injury can only be prevented by careful dissection of the operative field; an operative cholangiogram should not be relied upon to prove that the dissection has been safe as a number of injuries will occur *before* the cholangiogram is performed.

Cholecystectomy without a policy of operative cholangiography is unwise. The individual surgeon must decide whether they will use routine or selective cholangiography and whether or not the cost and time benefit of performing selective imaging and reducing negative common bile duct exploration with its high morbidity outweighs the risks of leaving stones within the common bile duct. Prior to the establishment of laparoscopic cholecystectomy 84% of surgeons in the UK performed routine operative cholangiography.[48] The authors feel that while selective cholangiography seems attractive its benefit has not been clearly demonstrated. In an efficiently run operating department the time taken to perform cholangiography is minimal, high quality X-rays can be easily achieved with a little care and the incidence of false-positive results can be low enough to be insignificant. The benefits from detecting all common bile duct stones outweighs the risks of leaving them behind.

THE OPEN MANAGEMENT OF COMMON BILE DUCT STONES

Exploration of the Common Bile Duct

Once common bile duct stones have been identified at open surgery their treatment relies on exploration of the common bile duct. This can be performed either via the cystic duct, a supraduodenal choledochotomy or a transduodenal approach. Cystic duct exploration is only possible if the duct is large enough to admit an exploring instrument or the choledochoscope. It may not be possible to remove large common bile duct stones via the cystic duct even though instrumental access is achieved. In such cases and in the majority of other cases, the route of choice is via a supraduodenal choledochotomy.

Supraduodenal Choledochotomy – Operative Technique

A detailed account of the method of duct exploration is given elsewhere.[49] At the time of duct exploration the gall bladder has usually been removed. The anterior surface of the common bile duct is exposed. It is this portion of the duct which is relatively free from blood vessels as the blood supply to the duct is on its lateral aspect.[50] Stay sutures are inserted and a vertical choledochotomy is made in the lowest portion of the duct immediately above the duodenum. This is the easiest site for access with the choledochoscope and should a choledochoduodenostomy be necessary then the bile duct incision is in an appropriate place.

On making the choledochotomy, stones may be expressed immediately. Further stones may be retrieved by a combination of flushing, the use of Desjardins forceps or a balloon catheter. The proximal bile ducts should be explored first. While exploration of the distal duct is undertaken it is wise to occlude the proximal ducts by inserting a dental role tied to a suture. This will prevent stones being flushed from the distal common bile duct into the proximal ducts.

Postexploration examination. Once it is considered that all the stones have been removed then a postexploratory check of the common bile duct should be made. Omission of a postexploratory examination will lead to a higher incidence of retained common bile duct stones.[51] The examination can be made either by a further cholangiogram or, more preferably, by a completion choledochoscopy.

Completion cholangiography can be performed before the common bile duct is closed or after a T-tube has been inserted. Examination prior to closure of the duct requires the insertion of two small Foley catheters into the common bile duct, one passed distally and one proximally. The balloons are inflated with a few ml of saline to occlude the duct and prevent leakage from the choledochotomy. Contrast medium can be injected beyond the balloons through the catheter lumen.[52]

Examination after the insertion of a T-tube can be performed through the T-tube but it is essential that all air bubbles be excluded from the T-tube prior to the administration of the contrast medium or they may be mistaken for retained stones. This can be achieved by aspirating bile back into the T-tube and then clamping the tube below the head of bile; a 23 gauge needle can be inserted into the T-tube above the T-tube clamp and saline flushed through to remove the air from the tube without flushing it into the common bile duct.[53]

Postexploratory cholangiography frequently demonstrates failure of passage of contrast into the duodenum. This is due to sphincter of Oddi spasm induced by the common bile duct exploration and should not be interpreted as being due to a retained stone unless an obvious filling defect is seen.[49]

The use of T-tube drainage. The standard closure of the common bile duct is over a T-tube. This is to prevent bile leakage from the choledochotomy secondary to the presence of oedema or spasm of the sphincter of Oddi. The intraduct portion of the tube should be kept to minimum length. The proximal limb should not be so long as to occlude the right or left hepatic ducts and the distal limb should not encroach upon or pass through the ampulla. The T-junction of the T-tube can be sculpted to permit easier removal.[54] A large T-tube should be used, preferably 16 Ch or larger. The size of the T-tube is important as, in the event of any retained stones being detected at a postoperative T-tube cholangiogram, then the T-tube tract can act as access to the common bile duct for removal of the stones either by percutaneous choledochoscopy[55,56] or fluoroscopic steerable catheter extraction.[57]

The choledochotomy can be closed with either interrupted or continuous sutures. A T-tube cholangiogram is taken around day 8–10 and if the ducts are clear then the T-tube can be removed. The presence of a T-tube can increase the incidence of wound infection, lengthen hospital stay and cause complications such as biliary peritonitis on removal.[58–60] It is therefore argued that the common bile duct can be closed primarily and any bile leakage can be controlled with a nearby drain. This does exclude the possibility of postoperative cholangiography and the early detection of retained stones and denies access to treat them. Overall, the complications of T-tube drainage are small[8] and the benefits outweigh the disadvantages except in the hands of an experienced choledochoscopist who can be confident that the bile ducts have been completely cleared of stones prior to primary closure.

Transduodenal Exploration of the Common Bile Duct

This method of common duct exploration is best for stones impacted at the lower end of the common bile duct that are not so easily accessible via a supraduodenal route, though with the modern flexible choledochoscope the retrieval of impacted stones is relatively simple to achieve using a Dormia basket via the working channel of the choledochoscope. A transduodenal approach will complement a supraduodenal approach in a difficult common bile duct exploration and may be used to treat an ampullary stenosis or achieve drainage of the common duct by allowing the creation of a sphincteroplasty.

Operative technique. The duodenum should be formally mobilized by Kocher's manoeuvre and the head of the pancreas mobilized. This will allow easier access to the ampulla. It is useful to identify the ampulla prior to opening the duodenum as this will limit the size of the duodenostomy that will be required. Identification of the ampulla may be achieved by passing a fine catheter down the cystic duct and palpating it within the duodenum. A longitudinal duodenotomy can then be made along the lateral border of the second part of the duodenum and the ampulla identified. If the duodenum has been opened blindly then flushing normal saline down the cystic duct may help locate the papilla.

Once the papilla has been identified a grooved director is passed through the ampulla into the common bile duct and the ampulla opened along its superior border. Once the lower end of the common bile duct has been opened the duct can be explored from below with Desjardins forceps, a balloon catheter or flushing catheter as in the supraduodenal approach. The flexible choledochoscope may be used as the exploring instrument and stones removed with a Dormia basket. The open ampulla can be left unsutured as a sphincterotomy or sutures inserted to appose the mucosal surfaces of the duodema and common bile duct as a sphincteroplasty. In performing a sphincteroplasty particular attention is given to placement of the apical suture. A synthetic soluble 000 suture is most appropriate.

The benefits of sphincteroplasty over sphincterotomy are that by inserting mucosal sutures the likelihood of a subsequent stenosis is reduced and that extravasation of bile into the retroperitoneal tissues is prevented.[61,62] However, in omitting the mucosal sutures the chances of causing pancreatic duct damage are less.[63] Overall, there is probably little to choose between the two techniques.[49]

T-tube drainage after a transduodenal exploration and sphincterotomy/sphincteroplasty is probably unnecessary as this may lead to additional complications and any retained stones should be able to pass unhindered into the duodenum via the sphincterotomy.[61]

Common Bile Duct Drainage

At the time of common bile duct exploration it should be considered whether the patient requires permanent common bile duct drainage or not. In cases where there are multiple common bile duct stones, in the presence of biliary sludge and in explorations after previous cholecystectomy for recurrent or retained common duct stones, a duct drainage procedure may be appropriate. This can either be achieved with a transduodenal exploration with a sphincterotomy or sphincteroplasty, as above, or a choledochoduodenostomy.

The operative technique for choledochoduodenostomy is well described elsewhere.[49] The important aspects of the procedure are a full mobilization of the duodenum so that the anastomosis can be made with no tension and an adequate sized stoma (2–2.5 cm) created. The main criticism of the operation is the occurrence of "sump syndrome". In these cases food debris rests within the distal common bile duct giving rise to pain and repeated episodes of cholangitis. The incidence of this complication is very low and its occurrence can be further reduced by ensuring that the stoma is of an adequate size. Problems are only likely to arise when there is a stenosis at the anastomosis. Reflux of duodenal contents occurs with sphincterotomies/sphincteroplasties but again this complication is unlikely to arise unless there is a stenosis at the papilla.

Tables 6.1.4–6 list the major series of the three procedures along with their mortality and incidence of postoperative cholangitis. There is little difference

Table 6.1.4 Transduodenal sphincterotomy (reproduced with permission from Motson R. W. (ed) *Retained Common Duct Stones. Prevention and Treatment*, Grune and Stratton, London, 1985)

			Mortality		Cholangitis	
Authors	**Year**	**N**	**No.**	**%**	**No.**	**%**
Thomas *et al.*[64]	1971	53	4	7.6	—	—
Stuart & Hoerr[65]	1972	18	1	5.6	—	—
Peel *et al.*[63]	1974	82	2	2.4	0	0.0
Partington[66]	1977	47	2	4.3	—	—
Vellacott & Powell[67]	1979	32	3	9.4	1	3.1
Panahy & Ritchie[68]	1982	109	2	1.8	1	0.9
Peel[69]	1984	83	0	0.0	3	3.6
Total		424	14	3.3	5	1.6

Table 6.1.5 Transduodenal sphincteroplasty (reproduced with permission from Motson R. W. (ed) *Retained Common Duct Stones. Prevention and Treatment*, Grune and Stratton, London, 1985)

			Mortality		Cholangitis	
Authors	**Year**	**N**	**No.**	**%**	**No.**	**%**
Stefanini *et al.*[70]	1974	712	7	1.1	—	—
Rutledge[71]	1976	60	0	0.0	—	—
Partington[66]	1977	87	2	2.3	—	—
Jones[61]	1978	312	3	1.0	—	—
Vogt & Hermann[72]	1981	37	0	0.0	—	—
Choi *et al.*[73]	1982	42	1	2.4	3	7.1
Strom & Stone[74]	1982	123	3	2.4	—	—
Leckie *et al.*[75]	1982	21	1	4.8	—	—
Nardi *et al.*[76]	1983	95	4	4.2	—	—
Carter[77]	1983	212	12	5.7	0	0.0
Antrum & Hall[78]	1984	118	3	2.5	—	—
Total		1819	36	2.0	3	1.2

between each technique. A randomized prospective trial comparing patients who underwent a choledochotomy and T-tube drainage with a transduodenal sphincteroplasty and patients who had a choledochoduodenostomy found that early morbidity and mortality and late complications were lower in the choledochoduodenostomy group.[156]

The various methods of common bile duct exploration should not be considered as being in competition with each other as each approach has its own particular indication for application. The supraduodenal choledochotomy with

Table 6.1.6 Choledochoduodenostomy (reproduced with permission from Motson R. W. (ed) *Retained Common Duct Stones. Prevention and Treatment*, Grune and Stratton, London, 1985)

			Mortality		Cholangitis	
Authors	**Year**	**N**	**No.**	**%**	**No.**	**%**
Madden *et al.*[79]	1970	100	4	4.0	0	0.0
Thomas *et al.*[64]	1971	57	2	3.5	—	—
Stuart & Hoerr[65]	1972	13	0	0.0	—	—
Degenshein[80]	1974	175	7	4.0	2	1.1
Rutledge[71]	1976	13	0	0.0	1	7.7
Keighley *et al.*[81]	1976	28	0	0.0	—	—
Schein & Gliedman[82]	1978	100	3	3.0	0	0.0
Kaminski *et al.*[83]	1979	25	1	4.0	—	—
Lygidakis[84]	1981	342	0	0.0	0	—
Vogt & Hermann[72]	1981	88	4	4.6	4	4.6
Lygidakis[85]	1982	92	0	0.0	—	—
de Almeida[86]	1984	70	1	1.4	—	—
Total		1103	22	2.0	7	0.9

completion choledochoscopy is adequate for most cases of choledocholithiasis. Stones impacted at the lower end of the common bile duct are best approached transduodenally if they cannot be removed with the flexible choledochoscope. In the event of a duct drainage procedure being necessary then there is little to choose between a choledochoduodenostomy, transduodenal sphincterotomy or sphincteroplasty.

Operative Choledochoscopy

When the common bile duct is explored, one of three methods of exploration can be used. This may be a blind exploration with the passage of a flushing catheter, Desjardins forceps or a balloon catheter and a completion cholangiogram. Alternatively, after instrumentation a direct visual examination can be performed with a rigid or a flexible choledochoscope.

The Choledochoscope

Development. The first direct visual inspection of the common bile duct was performed in the 1880s with the use of a glass speculum.[87] In 1923, a speculum with a proximal mirror was used which reflected light from a surgeon's headlamp.[88] By 1941 a rigid optical choledochoscope was developed by modifying a cystoscope.[89] Wildegans continued to improve on a rigid choledochoscope that he developed in 1953 until it was commercially available in 1958.[90] In the 1970s the Hopkins rod lens system was developed and incorporated in the Karl Stortz rigid choledochoscope. This gave good quality views of the common bile duct with minimal distortion of the image. There has been little improvement in rigid systems since.

The flexible choledochoscope was introduced in 1965.[91] The advantage of the flexible system over the rigid choledochoscope was its greater manoeuvrability; however, the optical image was poorer. From then until the present day, the flexible choledochoscope has been continually improved. The current range of flexible choledochoscopes produce excellent images on a par with the rigid choledochoscope and have, in addition to their irrigation channel, an instrumentation channel for the insertion of a variety of instruments that can be used within the common bile duct. Fine calibre choledochoscopes have been manufactured which measure between 0.8–2 mm. These are too narrow to incorporate an instrument channel but allow inspection of the interior of the common bile duct and can be introduced percutaneously,[92,93] via the cystic duct[94,95] or through the working channel of the duodenoscope.[96]

The rigid choledochoscope. This instrument contains a Hopkins rod lens system housed in a metal shaft with a distal viewing limb. This limb is angulated in relation to the shaft. The usual angle is 90° though a 120° angle is available. There is a proximal lens housed in the eyepiece. Instrumentation with the choledochoscope is possible by passage of instruments either down the irrigation channel or down an attachment that fits onto the shaft of the choledochoscope. The rigid choledochoscope produces excellent optical images and, due to its rigidity, it is easier to manipulate in the ducts. The fixed length viewing limb limits the degree of access that can be achieved within the bile ducts, especially in viewing the proximal bile ducts. Instrumentation with the rigid choledochoscope is cumbersome, particularly with the external attachment which increases the diameter of the instrument. Despite these drawbacks the rigid scope is cheaper than the flexible choledochoscope and is easier to use in inexperienced hands.

The flexible choledochoscope. The instrument consists of an upper control unit which houses the eye piece and lever to control angulation at the tip via control wires. The working shaft is 40 cm long and contains the viewing and illumination fibreoptic bundles, an irrigation channel, which doubles as an instrument channel, and the control wires. The angulation at the tip ranges through 290° in one plane, but a full range of movement can be achieved by rotating the instrument. Improvements in the optical system now allow the production of an image of similar quality to that of the rigid choledochoscope. The manoeuvrability of the flexible choledochoscope is superior to that of the rigid version and enables better access to the proximal biliary tree. It is possible to reach the second or third generation ducts within the liver. The distal common bile duct can be inspected without mobilizing the duodenum, which is usually necessary with the rigid scope.[97]

The instruments available for use with the choledochoscope pass down the irrigation channel and therefore reduce the flow of irrigant, which can be a disadvantage. These instruments consist of a Dormia basket, a quadrangular basket, a double-jointed curette, a balloon catheter and grasping or biopsy forceps.

Although the flexible choledochoscope is more expensive and the repair and service costs are higher than the rigid scopes, its versatility and suitability for percutaneous use via a T-tube track and laparoscopic use via a cannula makes the flexible choledochoscope the instrument of choice.

Operative Technique

The initial choledochotomy and exploration are made as described above. An experienced operator may use the choledochoscope as the initial instrument of exploration and stones can be retrieved under direct vision, thereby avoiding the possibility of trauma to the ducts which can be created by blind instrumentation.

The choledochoscope is introduced through the choledochotomy and the stay sutures are crossed over the choledochoscope to maintain some pressure within the ducts and help their distention. A systematic examination is essential to ensure that all the accessible ducts have been inspected. Initially a proximal duct examination should be performed. This will reduce the chance of stones being washed from the distal duct up into the proximal system where they may be lost. The second or third generation ducts can be inspected, especially in a dilated system. After this examination the choledochoscope is withdrawn and reinserted into the distal common bile duct. A complete examination includes the identification and inspection of the sphincter of Oddi with its typical rosette appearance. If there is any doubt about the identification of the sphincter then a balloon catheter can be passed into the duodenum and the balloon inflated. The catheter is then withdrawn until the 1 cm mark comes into view; when this is seen, the sphincter is in view.

If stones are found they can be removed with the Dormia basket or balloon catheter. If the stone is impacted and cannot be dislodged it can be crushed with a specially reinforced basket or it can be fragmented with ultrasound lithotripsy[98] or by laser.[99]

Complications. It is difficult to attribute a higher incidence of standard complications, such as bile leak from the choledochotomy, pancreatitis or wound infection, to the use of the choledochoscope. These complications occur without choledochoscopy and there is no increased incidence after its use.[49,100–102] An episode of septicaemia has been reported after choledochoscopy with a high irrigation pressure.[103] Injury to the common bile duct is very rare. There is only one report of a duct injury after rigid choledochoscopy with a 120° choledochoscope.[101] There are no reports of duct injuries due to the 90° or flexible choledochoscope. Aspiration of infused saline has been reported on two occasions.[105,106] These occurred after prolonged choledochoscopy in which large volumes of fluid were used, which refluxed into the stomach. It seems reasonable in such cases to insert a nasogastric tube at the time of choledochoscopy to prevent this problem. Overall, the technique must be regarded as safe and it does not increase morbidity once the common bile duct has been opened.

A Comparison of Blind Exploration of the Common Bile Duct with Rigid and Flexible Choledochoscopy

The results of a number of series of common bile duct explorations are shown in Tables 6.1.7–9. In these tables the percentage of retained stones is given. This is calculated from the number of retained stones as a proportion of the number of stone-positive explorations performed, *not* as a proportion of the total number of common bile duct explorations that were carried out in each series. If the latter figure were used then the retained stone rates would be misleading especially in the event of a large number of stone-negative explorations. The data given here therefore may not be identical to the original article.

Blind exploration (Table 6.1.7). The mean retained stone rate for this type of exploration is 10.6%. Over the period covered by the publications there has not been any improvement on the incidence of retained stones.

Rigid choledochoscopy (Table 6.1.8). In these series the incidence of retained stones is much lower than with blind exploration. The mean retained stone rate is 3.6%. Two of these publications report a retained stone rate of 13%.[102,103] These appear to be unusually high and the results cannot be explained. A graph of the retained stone rate plotted against the year of publication is given in Figure 6.1.1. The two reports with high retained stone rates fall outside the 99% confidence limits for the whole group; if these two studies are excluded then the retained stone rate is 3.3%. It is also seen, in Figure 6.1.1. that there appears to have been a steady increase in the retained stone rate in the later years. The fixed length of the viewing limb of the rigid choledochoscope may have resulted

Table 6.1.7 The results of blind exploration of the common bile duct

Reference	Year	Stone-positive exploration	No. retained stones	% of retained stones
Isaacs & Davies[107]	1960	—	—	5.0
Way *et al.*[51]	1972	—	—	10.0
Faris *et al.*[108]	1975	78	1	1.3
Stubbs & Blumgart[109]	1984	23	3	13.0
Gartell & McGinn[110]	1984	32	6	18.7
Rogers *et al.*[111]	1985	55	7	12.7
Jakimowicz *et al.*[112]	1986	40	3	7.5
Neoptolemos *et al.*[23]	1987	59	5	8.5
Sheridan *et al.*[113]	1987	191	37	19.4
Mean retained stone rate (%)				10.6

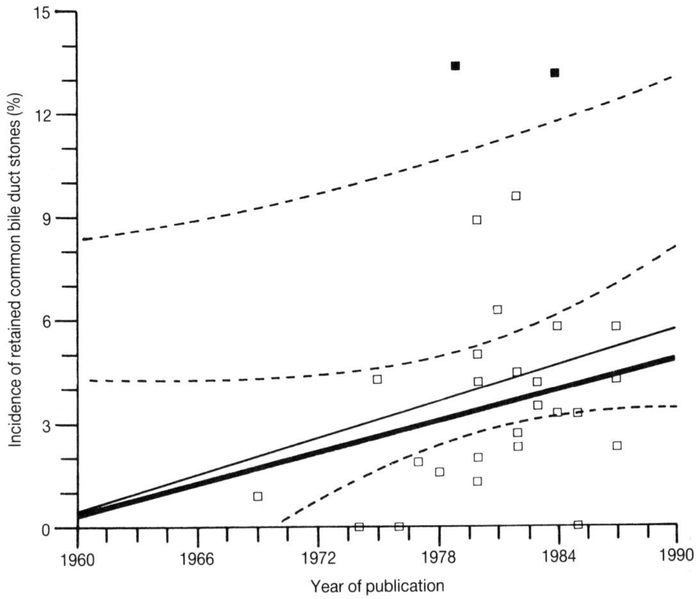

Figure 6.1.1. 30 series of rigid choledochoscopies. ——, Regression line for whole series; ——, regression line for studies within 99% confidence intervals; - - - (outer), 95% confidence interval for series; - - - (inner), 99% confidence interval; ■, studies outside 99% confidence interval.

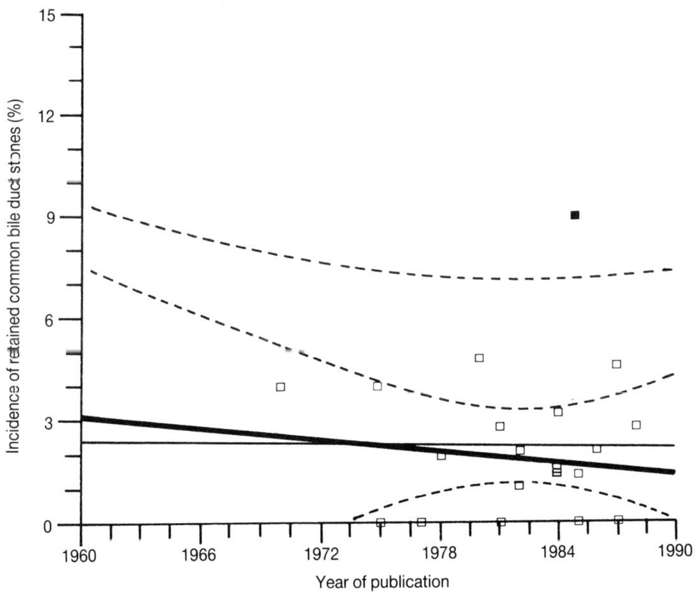

Figure 6.1.2. 22 series of flexible choledochoscopies. ——, Regression line for whole series; ——, regression line for studies within 99% confidence intervals; - - - (outer), 95% confidence interval for series; - - - (inner), 99% confidence interval; ■, studies outside 99% confidence interval.

Table 6.1.8 The results of rigid choledochoscopy

Reference	Year	Stone-positive exploration	No. retained stones	% of retained stones
Wildegans[90]	1958	94	1	1.1
Brocks[114]	1959	14	0	0.0
Schein[115]	1969	117	1	0.9
Leslie[116]	1974	71	0	0.0
Shore *et al.*[117]	1975	70	3	4.3
Griffin[118]	1976	25	0	0.0
Nora *et al.*[119]	1977	208	4	1.9
Fourtanier[120]	1978	60	1	1.6
Kappas *et al.*[103]	1979	67	9	13.4
Botticher & Knoch[121]	1980	76	1	1.3
Boulenger *et al.*[122]	1979	78	1	1.3
Motson *et al.*[104]	1980	40	2	5.0
Lennert[123]	1976	148	3	2.0
Feliciano[124]	1980	79	7	8.9
Rattner & Warshaw[125]	1981	144	6	4.2
Broadie *et al.*[101]	1981	32	2	6.3
Ernst & Windsor[126]	1982	38	1	2.7
Kappes *et al.*[127]	1982	87	2	2.3
Pott[128]	1982	200	9	4.5
Heuman[129]	1982	73	7	9.6
Broe *et al.*[130]	1983	88	4	3.5
King & String[131]	1983	24	1	4.2
Dayton *et al.*[102]	1984	53	7	13.2
Escat *et al.*[132]	1985	303	10	3.3
Stubbs & Blumgart[109]	1984	17	1	5.8
Leahy & Peel[133]	1985	33	0	0.0
Elftheriadis[134]	1985	30	1	3.3
Lau *et al.*[135]	1987	23	1	4.3
Johnson & Hosking[136]	1987	68	4	5.8
Lennert[137]	1987	352	8	2.3
Total		2712	97	3.6

in stones being missed at the end of a long common bile duct or in the proximal branches of the biliary tree.

Flexible choledochoscopy (Table 6.1.9). The results of these series show that after flexible choledochoscopy the retained stone rate is even lower than that after rigid choledochoscopy. The mean retained stone rate is 1.9%. Within this group there are seven studies with no retained stones. One study[150] reported a retained stone rate of 9% which is twice as much as the next highest rate. From Figure 6.1.2, it can be seen that this study lies outside the 99% confidence interval for the group. This result cannot be accounted for. In the later years of the series there is a convincing reduction in the retained stone rates. This may be due to increasing experience with the flexible choledochoscope.

Table 6.1.9 The results of flexible choledochoscopy

Reference	Year	Stone-positive exploration	No. retained stones	% of retained stones
Shore & Shore[138]	1970	100	4	4.0
Longland[139]	1975	49	2	4.1
Stotter *et al.*[140]	1975	20	0	0.0
Finnis & Rowntree[141]	1977	70	0	0.0
Legrand *et al.*[142]	1978	200	4	2.0
Yap *et al.*[143]	1980	84	4	4.8
Bauer *et al.*[144]	1981	36	1	2.8
Grange & Maillard[145]	1981	47	0	0.0
Wang[146]	1982	47	1	2.1
Chen *et al.*[147]	1983	184	2	1.1
Gartell & McGinn[110]	1984	31	1	3.2
Leggeri *et al.*[148]	1984	128	2	1.6
Ashby[149]	1984	65	1	1.5
May & Corfield[150]	1985	33	3	9.0
Elftheriadis[134]	1985	88	0	0.0
Ashby[151]	1985	70	1	1.4
Jakimowicz *et al.*[152]	1985	26	0	0.0
Jakimowicz *et al.*[112]	1986	238	5	2.1
Choi *et al.*[153]	1987	65	3	4.6
Markowitz[154]	1987	102	0	0.0
Molina *et al.*[155]	1988	36	1	2.8
Menzies & Motson[8]	1992	97	0	0.0
Total		1816	35	1.9

CONCLUSIONS

Since cholecystectomy was first performed, surgical success has been marred by the problems of retained stones. With the introduction of choledochoscopy the incidence of retained stones has fallen. Improvements in the design of the modern flexible choledochoscope, increasing availability and expertise in its use have reduced the incidence of retained stones, after open surgery, to negligible levels. With the advent of laparoscopic surgery it remains to be seen if laparoscopic cholecystectomy and ERCP or laparoscopic exploration of the common bile duct will be able to match the results of open exploration of the common bile duct painstakingly improved over the last decade.

REFERENCES

1. *Socio-economic Fact Book for Surgery 1988*. Socio-economic Affairs Department, American College of Surgeons.

2. *Hospital In-patient Inquiry 1980; Main Tables.* Department of Health and Social Security/Office of Population Census and Surveys, London, HMSO.
3. Lieber MM. Incidence of gall stones and their correlation with other diseases. *Ann. Surg* 1952; **135**: 394–405.
4. Motson RW. Operative cholangiography. In: *Retained Common Duct Stones. Prevention and Treatment* (ed. Motson RW), pp. 8–9. London, Grune and Stratton, 1985.
5. Yip A, Lam KH, An evaluation of routine operative cholangiography. *Aust NZ J Surg* 1988; **58**: 391–5.
6. Shivley EH, Wieman TJ, Adams AL, Romines RB. Operative cholangiography. *Am J Surg* 1990; **159**: 380–4.
7. Pace BW, Cosgrove J, Breuer B, Margolis IB. Intraoperative cholangiography revisited. *Arch Surg* 1992; **127**: 448–50.
8. Menzies D, Motson RW. Operative common bile duct imaging by operative cholangiography and flexible choledochoscopy. *Br J Surg* 1992; **79**: 815–17.
9. McSherry CK, Glenn F. The incidence and cause of death following surgery for non-malignant biliary tract disease. *Ann Surg* 1980; **191**: 271–5.
10. Frazee RC, van Heerden JA. Cholecystectomy with concomitant exploration of the common bile duct. *Surg Gynecol Obstet* 1989; **168**: 513–16.
11. Ijzermans JNM, de Waard P, Merkelbach JW. Cholangiography during cholecystectomy: a plea for selective use. *Neth J Surg* 1989; **41**: 79–81.
12. Cronan JJ, Mueller PR, Simeone JF, O'Connell RS, van Sonnenberg E, Whittenberg J. Prospective diagnosis of choledocholithiasis. *Radiology* 1983; **146**: 467–9.
13. Einstein DM, Lapin SA, Ralls PW, Halls JM. The insensitivity of sonography in the detection of choledocholithiasis. *Am J Radiol* 1984; **142**: 725–8.
14. Lindsell DRM. Ultrasound imaging of the pancreas and biliary tract. *Lancet* 1990; **335**: 390–3.
15. Pasanen P, Partanen K, Pikkarainen P, Achava E, Pirinen A, Janatuinen E. Ultrasonography, CT and ERCP in the diagnosis of choledochal stones. *Acta Radiol* 1992; **33**: 53–6.
16. Baron RL, Stanley RJ, Lee JKT *et al.* Prospective comparison of the evaluation of biliary obstruction using computed tomography and ultrasonography. *Radiology* 1982; **145**: 91–8.
17. Jeffrey RB, Federle MP, Laing FC, Wall IS, Rego J, Moss AA. Computed tomography in choledocholithiasis. *Am J Radiol* 1983; **140**: 1179–83.
18. Mitchell SE, Clark RA. A comparison of computed tomography and sonography in choledocholithiasis. *Am J Radiol* 1984; **142**: 729–33.
19. Baron RL. Common bile duct stones. Reassessment of criteria for CT diagnosis. *Radiology* 1987; **162**: 419–24.
20. Whiting MJ, Watts JM. Chemical composition of common bile duct stones. *Br J Surg* 1986; **73**: 229–32.
21. Kullman E, Borch K, Tarpila E, Liedberg G. Endoscopic retrograde cholangiopancreatography (ERCP) in patients with jaundice and suspected biliary obstruction. *Acta Chir Scand* 1984; **150**: 657–63.
22. Matzen P, Malchow-Muller A, Lejertofte J, Stage P. Endoscopic retrograde cholangiopancreatography and transhepatic cholangiography in patients with suspected obstructive jaundice. *Scand J Gastroenterol* 1982; **17**: 731–5.
23. Neoptolemos JP, Carr-Locke DL, Fossard DP. Prospective randomised study of preoperative endoscopic sphincterotomy versus surgery alone for common bile duct stones. *Br Med J* 1987; **294**: 470–4.
24. Schwab G, Pointer R, Wetscher G, Glaser K, Foltin E, Bodner E. Treatment of calculi of the common bile duct. *Surg Gynecol Obstet* 1992; **175**: 115–20.
25. Stain SC, Cohen H, Tsuishoysha M, Donovan AJ. Choledocholithiasis. Endoscopic sphincterotomy or common bile duct exploration. *Ann Surg* 1991; **213**: 627–33.

26. Stiegman GV, Goff JS, Mansour A, Pearlman N, Reveille RM, Norton L. Precholecystectomy endoscopic cholangiography and stone removal is not superior to cholecystectomy cholangiography and common duct exploration. *Am J Surg* 1992; **163**: 227–30.
27. Bell RCW, Steigman GV, Goff JS, Reveille M, Norton LW, Pearlman N. Decision for surgical management of perforation following endoscopic sphincterotomy. *Am Surg* 1991; **57**: 237–40.
28. Cotton PB, Baillie J, Pappas TN, Meyers WS. Laparoscopic cholecystectomy and the biliary endoscopist. *Gastrointest Endosc* 1991; **37**: 94–6.
29. Rholl KS, Smathers R, McClennean BL, Lee JK. Intravenous cholangiography in the CT era. *Gastrointest Radiol* 1985; **10**: 69–74.
30. Eubanks B, Martinez C, Mehigan D, Cameron J. Current role of intravenous cholangiography. *Am J Surg* 1982; **143**: 731–3.
31. Goodman MW, Ansel HJ, Vennes J, Lasser, Silvis S. Is intravenous cholangiography still useful? *Gastroenterology* 1980; **709**: 642–5.
32. Ott G, Gelfand D. Complications of gastrointestinal radiologic procedures. II. Complications related to biliary tract studies. *Gastrointest Radiol* 1981; **6**: 47–56.
33. Shehadi W, Toniollo G. Adverse reactions to contrast media. *Radiology* 1980; **137**: 299–302.
34. Ansell G. Adverse reactions to contrast agents. Scope of problem. *Invest Radiol* 1970; **5**: 374–84.
35. Scott IR, Gibney RG, Becker CD, Fache JS, Burhenne HJ. The use of intravenous cholangiography in teaching hospitals: A survey. *Gastrointest Radiol* 1989; **14**: 148–50.
36. Huddy SPJ, Southam JA. Is intravenous cholangiography an alternative to the routine per-operative cholangiogram? *Postgrad Med J* 1986; **65**: 896–9.
37. Joyce WP, Keana R, Burke GJ *et al.* Identification of common bile duct stones in patients undergoing laparoscopic cholecystectomy. *Br J Surg* 1991; **78**: 1174–6.
38. Hallan RI, Loosemore TM, Motson RW. Preoperative prediction of exposure for operative cholangiography. *Br J Surg* 1986; **73**: 782.
39. Gregg RO. The case for selective cholangiography. *Am J Surg* 1988; **155**: 540–4.
40. Pernthaler H, Sandbichler P, Schmid TH, Margreiter R. Operative cholangiography in elective cholecystectomy. *Br J Surg* 1990; **77**: 399–400.
41. Pasquale MD, Nauta RJ. Selective vs routine use of intraoperative cholangiography. *Arch Surg* 1989; **124**: 1041–2.
42. Lillemore KD, Yeo CJ, Talamini MA, Wang BH, Pitt HA, Gadacz TR. Selective cholangiography. Current role in laparoscopic cholecystectomy. *Ann Surg* 1992; **215**: 669–74.
43. Bogokowsky H, Slutzki S, Zaidenstein L, Halpern Z, Negri M, Abramsohn R. Selective operative cholangiography. *Surg Gynecol Obstet* 1987; **164**: 124–6.
44. Mansberger JA, Davis JB, Scarborough C, Bowden TA. Selective intra-operative cholangiography: a case for its use on an anatomic basis. *Am Surg* 1988; **54**: 31–3.
45. Hicken NF, McAllister AJ. Operative cholangiography as an aid in reducing the incidence of "overlooked" common bile duct stones: a study of 1293 choledochotomies. *Surgery* 1964; **55**: 753–8.
46. Kelly CJ, Blumgart LH. Peroperative cholangiography and postcholecystectomy biliary strictures. *Ann R Coll Surg Engl* 1985; **67**: 93–5.
47. Moosa AR, Mayer AD, Stabile B. Iatrogenic injury to the bile ducts. *Arch Surg* 1990; **125**: 1028–30.
48. Cahill CJ, Pain JA. Current practice in biliary surgery. *Br J Surg* 1988; **75**: 1169–72.
49. Motson RW. Exploration of the common bile duct. In: *Retained Common Duct Stones. Prevention and Treatment* (ed. Motson RW) pp. 23–35. London, Grune and Stratton, 1985.

50. Northover JMA, Terblanche J. A new look at the arterial blood supply in man and its surgical implications. *Br J Surg* 1979; **66**: 379–84.
51. Way LW, Admirand WH, Dunphy JE. Management of choledocholithiasis. *Ann Surg* 1972; **176**: 347–59.
52. Gervin AS, Fischer RP. Simple technique for operative assessment of retained stones in the common bile duct. *Surg Gynecol Obstet* 1983; **155**: 251–2.
53. Van Heerden JA. A technique for T-tube cholangiography. *Arch Surg* 1976; **111**: 85.
54. Crnojevic L, Thompson JN, Dudley HAF. T-tubes: virgin, slit, guttered or sculpted. *Br J Surg* 1988; **75**: 615–16.
55. Menzies D, Motson RW. Percutaneous flexible choledochoscopy – a simple method of retained common bile duct stone removal. *Br J Surg* 1991; **78**: 959–60.
56. Berci G, Morgenstern L. Paz-Partlow M. Intraoperative and postoperative biliary endoscopy (choledochoscopy). The role of the surgeon. *Am Surg* 1989; **55**: 267–72.
57. Burhenne HJ. Percutaneous extraction of retained common bile duct stones: 661 patients. *Am J Roentgenol* 1980; **134**: 888–98.
58. Lygidakis NJ. Choledochotomy for biliary lithiasis: T-tube drainage or primary closure. Effects on postoperative bacteraemia and T-tube bile infection. *Am J Surg* 1983; **146**: 254–6.
59. Gilliat DA, May RE, Kennedy R, Longstaff AJ. Complications of T-tube drainage of the common bile duct. *Ann R Coll Surg Engl* 1985; **67**: 370–1.
60. Payne RA, Woods WGA. Primary suture or T-tube drainage after choledochotomy? *Ann R Coll Surg Engl* 1986; **68**: 196–8.
61. Jones SA. The prevention and treatment of recurrent bile duct stones by transduodenal sphincteroplasty. *World J Surg* 1978; **2**: 473–85.
62. Jones SA, Steedman RA, Keller TB, Smith LL. Transduodenal sphincteroplasty (not sphincterotomy) for biliary and pancreatic disease. *Am J Surg* 1969; **118**: 292–306.
63. Peel AG, Bourke JB, Hermann-Taylor J, Maclean ADW, Mann CV, Ritchie HD. How should the common bile duct be explored? *Ann R Coll Surg Engl* 1975; **56**: 125–34.
64. Thomas CG Jr, Nicholson CP, Owen J. Effectiveness of choledochoduodenostomy and transduodenal sphincterotomy in the treatment of benign obstruction of the common bile duct. *Ann Surg* 1971; **173**: 845–56.
65. Stuart M, Hoerr SO. Late results of side-to-side choledochoduodenostomy and transduodenal sphincterotomy for benign disorders. A twenty year comparative study. *Am J Surg* 1972; **123**: 67–72.
66. Partington PF. Twenty-three years of experience with sphincterotomy and sphincteroplasty for stenosis of the sphincter of Oddi. *Surg Gynecol Obstet* 1977; **145**: 161–8.
67. Vellacott KD, Powell PH. Exploration of the common bile duct: a comparative study. *Br J Surg* 1979; **66**: 389–91.
68. Panahy C, Ritchie HD. Personal communication, 1983.
69. Peel ALG. Personal communication, 1984.
70. Stefanini P, Carboni M, Patrassi N, de Bernardinnis G, Negro P, Loriga P. Transduodenal sphincteroplasty: its use in the treatment of lithiasis and benign obstruction of the common bile duct. *Am J Surg* 1974; **128**: 672–7.
71. Rutledge RH. Sphincteroplasty and choledochoduodenostomy for benign biliary obstructions. *Ann Surg* 1976; **183**: 476–87.
72. Vogt DP, Hermann RE. Choledochoduodenostomy, choledochojejunostomy or sphincteroplasty for biliary and pancreatic disease. *Ann Surg* 1981; **193**: 161–8.
73. Choi TK, Lee NW, Wong J, Ong GB. Extraperitoneal sphincteroplasty for residual stones – an update. *Ann Surg* 1982; **196**: 26–9.
74. Strom PR, Stone HH. A technique for transduodenal sphincteroplasty. *Surgery* 1982; **92**: 546–9.

75. Leckie PA, Schmidt N, Taylor R. Impacted common bile duct stones. *Am J Surg* 1982; **143**: 540–1.
76. Nardi JL, Michelassi F, Zannini P. Transduodenal sphincteroplasty. 5–25 year follow-up of 89 patients. *Ann Surg* 1983; **198**: 453–61.
77. Carter AE. The transduodenal per-ampullary approach to common bile duct calculi. *Ann R Coll Surg Engl* 1983; **65**: 183–4.
78. Antrum RM, Hall R. Transduodenal sphincteroplasty: an analysis of 118 consecutive cases. *Br J Surg* 1984; **71**: 446–8.
79. Madden JL, Chan JY, Kandalaft S, Parekh M. Choledochoduodenostomy. An unjustly maligned surgical procedure? *Am J Surg* 1970; **119**: 45–54.
80. Degenshein GA. Choledochoduodenostomy: an 18 year study of 175 consecutive cases. *Surgery* 1974; **76**: 319–24.
81. Keighley MRB, Burdon DW, Baddeley RM *et al.* Complications of supraduodenal choledochotomy: a comparison of three methods of management. *Br J Surg* 1976; **63**: 754–8.
82. Schein CJ, Gliedman ML. Choledochoduodenostomy as an adjunct to choledocholithotomy. *Surg Gynecol Obstet* 1978; **146**: 25–32.
83. Kaminski DL, Burner HB, Codd JE, Wolfe BM. Evaluation of the results of external choledochoduodenostomy for retained, recurrent or primary common duct stones. *Am J Surg* 1979; **137**: 162–6.
84. Lygidakis NJ. Choledochoduodenostomy in calculous biliary tract disease. *Br J Surg* 1981; **68**: 762–5.
85. Lygidakis NJ. Surgical approaches to postcholecystectomy choledocholithiasis. *Arch Surg* 1982; **117**: 481–4.
86. De Almeida AM, Cruz AG, Aldeia FJ. Side-to-side choledochoduodenostomy in the management of choledocholithiasis and associated diseases. *Am J Surg* 1984; **147**: 253–9.
87. Ashby BS. Choledochoscopy. *Clin Gastroenterol* 1978; **7**: 685–700.
88. Bakes J. Die choledochpapilloskopie hebst bemerkungen uder hepaticus-drainage und dilatation der papille. *Arch Klin Chir* 1923; **126**: 473–83.
89. MacIver MA. An instrument for visualising the interior of the common bile duct at operation. Preliminary note. *Surgery* 1941; **9**: 112–14.
90. Wildegans H. Endoscopy of the biliary tract. *German Med Monthly* 1958; **3**: 377–80.
91. Shore JM, Lippman HN. A flexible choledochoscope. *Lancet* 1965; **i**: 1200–1.
92. Chen MF, Jan YY. Percutaneous transhepatic removal of common bile duct stones with a fibreoptic choledochoscope. *Gastrointest Endosc* 1986; **32**: 347–9.
93. Shimada H, Nishmoto S, Matsuba A, Nakagawara G, Kobayashi M. Experience with percutaneous transhepatic fibreoptic choledochoscopy for retained stones in the biliary tract. *Surg Endosc* 1987; **1**: 189–94.
94. Morris DL, Harrison J, Balfour T, Wherry DC. Operative choledochoscopy via the cystic duct: a pilot study with an ultra-thin fibreoptic endoscope. *Br J Surg* 1987; **74**: 613.
95. Nghiem DD. Choledochoscopy without choledochotomy. *Surg Gynecol Obstet* 1987; **164**: 377–8.
96. Miller BM, Korazek RA, Ryan JA, Ball TJ, Traverso HW. Surgical versus endoscopic management of common bile duct stones. *Ann Surg* 1988; **207**: 135–41.
97. Iseli A, Marshal VC. Choledochoscopy: a comparison of a rigid and a flexible fibre optic instrument. *Med J Aust* 1978; **1**: 131–2.
98. Matsumoto S, Tanaka M, Yoshimoto M, Miyazaki K, Ikeda S, Nakayama F. Electrohydraulic lithotripsy of intrahepatic stones during choledochoscopy. *Surgery* 1987; **102**: 852–6.
99. Ell CH, Lux G, Hochberger J, Muller D, Demling L. Laser lithotripsy of common bile duct stones. *Gut* 1988; **29**: 746–51.
100. Griffin WT. Choledochoscopy. *Am J Surg* 1976; **132**: 697–8.

101. Broadie TA, Lowe DK, Glover JL, Yaw PB, Jesseph JE. Intraoperative choledochoscopy: an efficacious adjunct to common duct exploration in calculous biliary tract disease. *Am Surg* 1981; **47**: 121–4.
102. Dayton MT, Conter R, Tompkins RK. Incidence of complications with operative choledochoscopy. *Am J Surg* 1984; **147**, 139–45.
103. Kappas A, Alexander-Williams J, Keighly MRB, Watts GT. Operative choledochoscopy. *Br J Surg* 1979; **66**: 177–9.
104. Motson RW, Woods AJ, de Jode LR. Operative choledochoscopy. Experience with a rigid choledochoscope. *Br J Surg* 1980; **67**: 406–9.
105. Weller RM. The choledochoscope – two hazards. *Anaesthesia* 1982; **37**: 606.
106. Schebesta AG, Sporr D, O'Leary J, Moulton J. Gastric aspiration associated with choledochoscopy. *Anaesth Int Care* 1983; **11**: 257–8.
107. Issacs JP, Davies ML. Technique and evaluation of operative cholangiography. *Surg Gynecol Obstet* 1960; **111**: 103–12.
108. Faris I, Thomson JPS, Grundy DJ, le Quesne LP. Operative cholangiography: a reappraisal based on a review of 400 cholangiograms. *Br J Surg* 1975; **62**: 960–72.
109. Stubbs RS, Blumgart LH. Exploration of the common bile duct: effect of a change of policy in one surgical unit. *J R Coll Surg Edinb* 1984; **29**: 76–80.
110. Gartell PC, McGinn FP. Choledochoscopy: are stones missed? A prospective controlled study. *Br J Surg* 1984; **71**: 767–9.
111. Rogers AL, Farha GJ, Beamer RL, Chang FC. Incidence and associated mortality of retained common bile duct stones. *Am J Surg* 1985; **150**: 690–3.
112. Jakimowicz JJ, Carol EJ, Mak B, Roukema A. An operative choledochoscopy using the flexible choledochoscope. *Surg Gynecol Obstet* 1986; **162**: 215–21.
113. Sheridan WG, Williams HO, Lewis MH. Morbidity and mortality of common bile duct explorations. *Br J Surg* 1984; **74**: 1095–9.
114. Brocks H. Choledochoscopy versus cholangiography. Experience of a twelve month trial. *Acta Chir Scand* 1959; **118**: 434–8.
115. Schein CJ. Biliary endoscopy: an appraisal of its value in biliary lithiasis. *Surgery* 1969; **65**: 1004–6.
116. Leslie D. Endoscopy of the bile duct: an evaluation. *Aust NZ J Surg* 1974; **44**: 340–2.
117. Shore JM, Berci G, Morgenstern L. The value of biliary endoscopy. *Surg Gynecol Obstet* 1975; **140**: 601–4.
118. Griffin WT. Choledochoscopy. *Am J Surg* 1976; **132**: 697–8.
119. Nora PF, Berci G, Dorazio RA *et al.* Operative choledochoscopy. Results of a prospective study in several institutions. *Am J Surg* 1977; **133**: 105–10.
120. Foutanier G, Lacroix A, Escat J. L'interet de la choledochoscopie au cours de l'exploration de la voie biliare principal pour lithiase. *Ann Chir* 1978; **32**: 122–5.
121. Botticher R, Knoch M. Diagnostoscher und therapeutischer stellenwert der intraoperative choledochoscopie. *Langenbecks Arch Chir* 1980; **351**: 17–22.
122. Boulenger M, Solente JJ, Moline J *et al.* La choledochoscopie per-operatoire. A propos de 120 cas. *Lyon Chir* 1979; **75**: 166–7.
123. Lennert KA. Die interoperative choledochoskopie. Erfahrungen mit einem neuen Choledochoskop. *Chirug* 1976; **47**: 248–9.
124. Feliciano DV, Mattox KL, Jordan GL Jr. The value of choledochoscopy in exploration of the common bile duct. *Ann Surg* 1980; **191**: 649–54.
125. Rattner DW, Warshaw AL. Impact of choledochoscopy on the management of choledocholithiasis. Experience with 499 common duct exploration at the Massachusetts General Hospital. *Ann Surg* 1981; **194**: 76–9.
126. Ernst D, Windsor CWO. The use of the rigid choledochoscope in exploration of the common bile duct. *Br J Surg* 1982; **69**: 463–4.
127. Kappes SK, Adams MB, Wilson SD. Intraoperative biliary endoscopy. Mandatory for common bile duct explorations? *Arch Surg* 1982; **117**: 603–7.

128. Pott JH. *Peroperative Investigation with a Rigid Choledochoscope*. Association of Surgeons, Manchester, 1982.
129. Heuman R, Smeds S, Hellgren E, Sjodahl R, Wettersfors J. Evaluation of factors affecting the incidence of retained calculi in the bile ducts. *Acta Chir Scand* 1982; **145**: 185–7.
130. Broe PG, Magee DJ, Kirwan WO. Value of choledochoscopy in exploration of the common bile duct. *Gut* 1983; **24**: 503.
131. King ML, String ST. Extent of choledochoscopic utilization in common bile duct exploration. *Am J Surg* 1983; **146**: 322–4.
132. Escat J, Fourtanier G, Maigne C, Vaislic L, Fournier D, Prevost F. Choledochoscopy in common bile duct surgery for choledocholithiasis: a must. Eight years experience in 441 consecutive patients. *Am Surg* 1985; **51**: 166–7.
133. Leahy AL, Peel ALG. Choledochoscopy, post-exploratory fluorocholangiography, or both? *Ann R Coll Surg Engl* 1985; **67**: 99–100.
134. Elftheriadis E, Zissiadis A, Kotzampassi K, Aletras H. Rigid or flexible choledochoscopy? *Endoscopy* 1985; **17**: 212–13.
135. Lau WY, Chong KK, Tan ST *et al.* A scientific evaluation of operative choledochoscopy in acute cholangitis. *Ann Surg* 1987; **206**: 142–7.
136. Johnson AG, Hosking SW. Appraisal of the management of bile duct stones. *Br J Surg* 1987; **74**: 555–60.
137. Lennert KA. Technique and result of intraoperative choledochoscopy. *Surg Endosc* 1987; **1**: 51–4.
138. Shore JM, Shore E. Operative biliary endoscopy: experience with the flexible choledochoscope in 100 consecutive choledocholithotomies. *Ann Surg* 1970; **71**: 269–78.
139. Longland CJ, cited by Ashby BS. Choledochoscopy. *Clin Gastroenterol* 1978; **7**: 685–700.
140. Stotter I, Wiendl HJ, Ultsch B. An improved flexible cholangioscope. *Endoscopy* 1975; **7**: 150–3.
141. Finnis D. Rowntree D. Choledochoscopy in exploration of the common bile duct. *Br J Surg* 1977; **64**: 661–4.
142. Legrand G, Izard G, Cave C *et al.* La choledochoscopie per-operatoire dans la chirurgie de la lithiasise de la voie principal. A propos de 200 cas. *Lyon Chir* 1978; **74**: 321–4.
143. Yap PC, Atacador M, Yap AG, Yap RG. Choledochoscopy as a complementary procedure to operative cholangiography in biliary surgery. *Am J Surg* 1980; **140**: 648–52.
144. Bauer JJ, Salky BA, Gelernt IM, Kreel I. Experience with the flexible fibreoptic choledochoscope. *Ann Surg* 1982; **196**: 161–8.
145. Grange D, Maillard JN. La choledochoscopie peroperatoire. *Gastroenterol Clin Biol* 1981; **5**: 857–65.
146. Wang YH. The use of operative choledochoscope. *J Formosan Med Ass* 1982; **81**: 1140–3.
147. Chen MF, Chan YY, Chou FF, Wang CS, Jeng LB, Chen CW. Use of fibreoptic choledochoscope in common bile duct and intrahepatic duct exploration. *Gastrointest Endosc* 1983; **29**: 276–8.
148. Leggeri A, Liguori G, Umeri F. *Intraoperative Choledochoscopy*. Puccin & Butterworth; Padua 1984; pp. 83–8.
149. Ashby BS. Cited by Motson RW, Operative choledochoscopy. In: *Retained Common Duct Stones. Prevention and Treatment* (ed. Motson RW), p. 49. London, Grune and Stratton, 1985.
150. May RE, Corfield A. An assessment of operative choledochoscopy – a worthwhile procedure or not? *Ann R Coll Surg Engl* 1985; **67**: 96–8.

151. Ashby BS. Operative choledochoscopy in common bile duct surgery. *Ann R Coll Surg Engl* 1985; **67**: 279–83.
152. Jakimowicz JJ, Carol EJ, Haeck L. Adkin SK. A new improved flexible choledochoscope: preliminary experience. *Dig Surg* 1985; **2**: 49–52.
153. Choi S, Choi TK, Wong J. Intraoperative flexible choledochoscopy for intrahepatic and extrahepatic biliary calculi. *Surgery* 1987; **101**: 571–6.
154. Markowitz I, Overby JL, Kappelman MD, Webb WR. Choledochoscopy in prevention of retained common bile duct stones. *Am Surg* 1987; **53**: 558–61.
155. Molina LM, de Diego JA, de Frutos L *et al.* Operative choledochoscopy in biliary surgery. *Hepatogastroenterology* 1988; **35**: 162–6.
156. Lygidakis NJ. Prospective randomised study of recurrent choledocholithiasis. *Surg Gynecol Obstet* 1982; **155**: 679–84.

6.2

Closed Treatment of Choledocholithiasis

D. LICHTENSTEIN and D. CARR-LOCKE

INTRODUCTION

Endoscopic retrograde cholangiopancreatography (ERCP) was first introduced as a diagnostic procedure in 1968 and has since evolved into a widely accepted safe and effective technique for the evaluation and treatment of pancreatic and biliary tract disorders. Endoscopic treatment of choledocholithiasis has gained widespread acceptance since the first independent reports of endoscopic sphincterotomy (ES) by Kawai[1] and Classen in 1974.[2] Endoscopic sphincterotomy was initially considered justifiable only in elderly postcholecystectomy patients with recurrent or retained common bile duct (CBD) stones who were at high risk of serious complications from conventional surgical CBD exploration.

With improved efficacy, demand and training in therapeutic biliary endoscopic techniques, however, there has been an expanding role for the endoscopic management of choledocholithiasis. There is now general agreement among surgeons and gastroenterologists that endoscopic removal of CBD stones is preferable to surgery in (a) patients who have undergone previous cholecystectomy, (b) in the high-risk surgical patient when the gall bladder is still present, (c) in patients with severe acute cholangitis, (d) in selected patients with acute biliary pancreatitis, and (e) in special circumstances for the average risk surgical patient with suspected choledocholithiasis prior to laparoscopic cholecystectomy. Up to 15% of patients undergoing cholecystectomy have common duct stones. Unlike gall bladder stones, the majority of individuals with asymptomatic common duct stones will ultimately become symptomatic with the development of one or a combination of presentations including biliary pain, jaundice, cholangitis or pancreatitis. This natural history has militated in favour of an active treatment approach rather than expectant management for all patients with detected CBD stones.

ENDOSCOPIC TECHNIQUES

Centres providing endoscopic services for the treatment of bile duct stones must be fully equipped with appropriate endoscopic and fluoroscopic equipment and a team comprising endoscopist, radiologist and GI nursing staff trained in all aspects of the procedures including proper handling and disinfection of the endoscopic equipment, as well as management of potential procedural complications. A basic tenet that underlies the recommendations for endoscopic therapy is the understanding that the techniques discussed are performed by skilled endoscopists who have appropriate training and experience, as the overall results and attendant procedure related complications are to a significant degree dependent upon these factors.

A detailed description of the procedure including the advantages, hazards and alternatives is discussed with the patient and a complete blood count, liver function tests and coagulation studies are obtained. Coagulopathy should be corrected when possible prior to ERCP. Antibiotic prophylaxis is routinely administered one hour prior to therapeutic biliary procedures, although this is not necessarily required if adequate biliary decompression is achieved.[3] Under conscious sedation, a side-viewing duodenoscope is passed to the level of the major papilla. The ampullary orifice is cannulated with a 5 or 6 French diameter catheter and radio-opaque contrast is injected into the biliary and pancreatic ducts (Fig. 6.2.1). In expert hands, the sensitivity of diagnostic ERCP for detecting choledocholithiasis approaches 100%.

Endoscopic Sphincterotomy and Precut Papillotomy

Once choledocholithiasis has been documented, sphincterotomy is usually required to facilitate stone removal. For small stones, however, it may be possible to perform extraction with a basket catheter through the intact papilla without the need for initial ES. Undue resistance at the choledochal sphincter may be alleviated by the lingual application of a nitrate spray together with intravenous glucagon, routinely employed for inhibition of duodenal motility during ERCP.

Sphincterotomy utilizes a specialized catheter equipped with a diathermy wire close to its tip through which a radiofrequency current is passed to achieve cutting and electrocautery (Fig. 6.2.2). Bowing of the wire and elevation and/or traction on the sphincterotome allow the endoscopist to produce an incision through the biliary sphincter in a cephalad direction along the intramural course of the CBD. Sphincterotomy is performed in a controlled stepwise fashion through the application of a blended (cutting and coagulation) electrocautery current. The length of the sphincterotomy is dependent upon the degree of CBD dilatation and the size of the stone to be removed. Selective cannulation of the CBD, which is confirmed fluoroscopically, is a fundamental requirement for safe

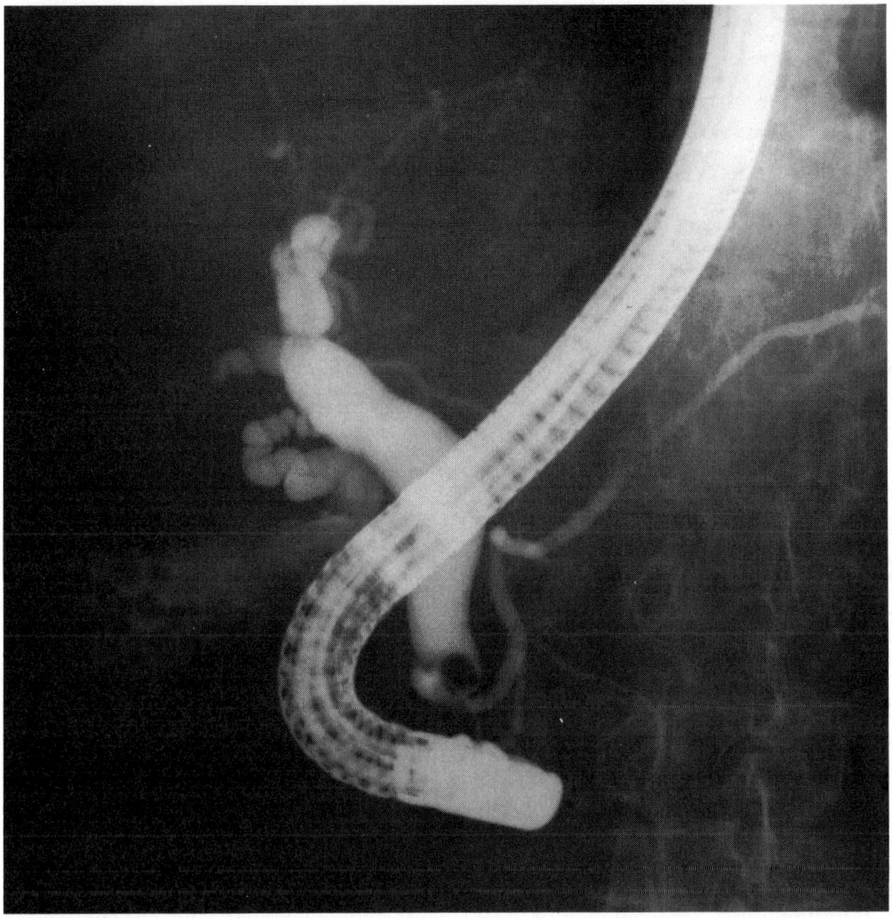

Figure 6.2.1 Diagnostic ERCP demonstrating choledocholithiasis and cholelithiasis.

ES. In experienced hands, this can be achieved in at least 95% of patients with the aid of a variety of accessory cannulas, papillotomes and guidewires.[4,5]

In the 5% where selective cannulation fails, access to the CBD can often be obtained with the use of a precut papillotomy[6] or a combined percutaneous endoscopic technique.[7] The technique of precut papillotomy involves cutting the roof of the papilla with a needle-knife or a specifically designed precut papillotome, thereby revealing the opening to the common bile duct. The needle-knife, which is the more popular of the two instruments, consists of an exposed diathermy wire which can be extended several millimetres beyond the surrounding plastic catheter whereas the precut papillotome is a modified standard papillotome with the cutting wire inserting into the distal tip of the catheter. The technique of precut papillotomy should only be performed in situations of known biliary tract pathology requiring endoscopic therapy and only in the

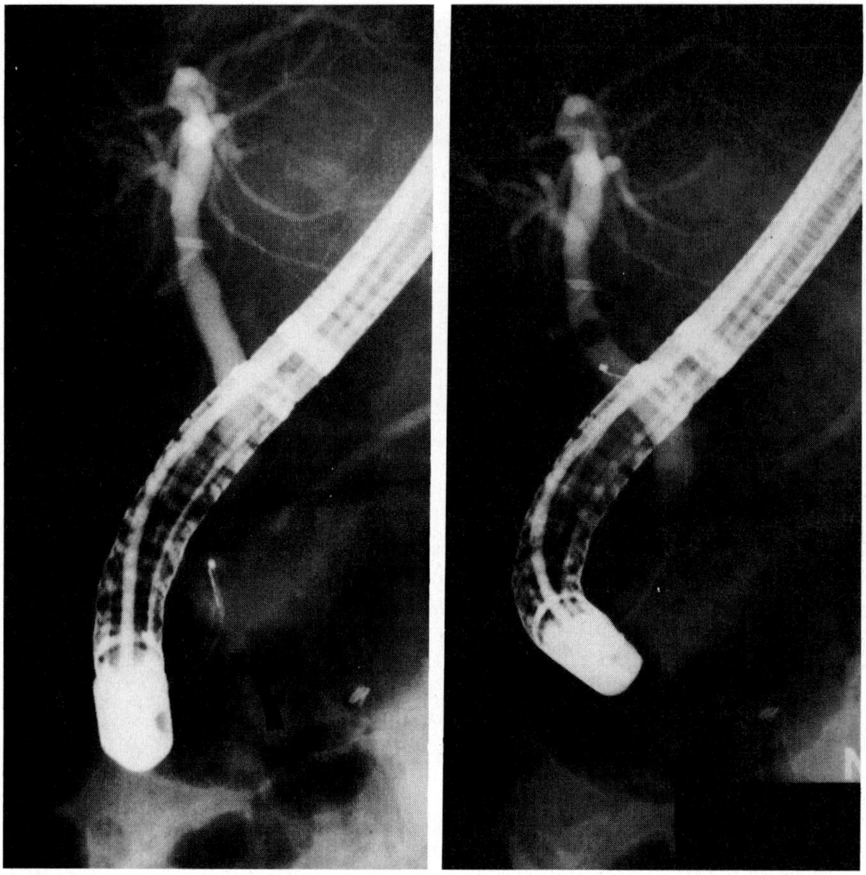

Figure 6.2.2 Position of standard papillotome (arrow) during sphincterotomy (left) and during initial deep cannulation (right) with single bile duct stone and cholecystectomy clips.

hands of a skilled endoscopist, as the complication rates are higher when this technique is compared with standard sphincterotomy.[6–9] It is most useful when cannulation is prevented by a stone impacted in the ampulla, as the intramural CBD is usually dilated and easily incised to form a choledochoduodenal fistulotomy.[10]

A major bleeding diathesis is a contraindication to ES. Such individuals with common duct stones identified on endoscopic cholangiography can be temporarily managed by achieving biliary decompression with a nasobiliary tube (Fig. 6.2.3) or endoprosthesis (Fig. 6.2.4) placement to prevent stone impaction at the ampulla. Once the coagulopathy has been corrected and sepsis has been controlled by administration of antibiotics, safe ES can be performed and common duct stones removed.

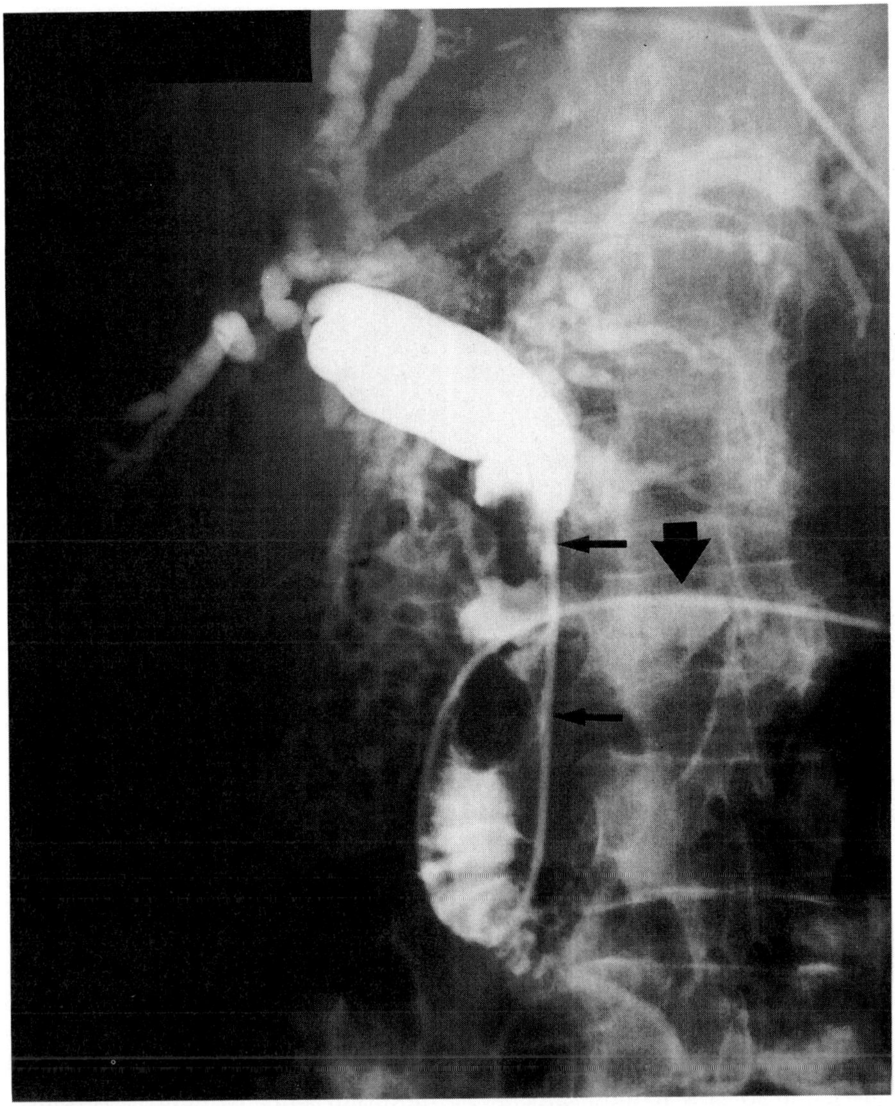

Figure 6.2.3 Nasobiliary tube (broad arrow) in place for two bile duct stones (narrow arrows) and cholangitis with concomitant cholelithiasis.

Stone Extraction

Many stones, particularly those under 1 cm diameter, will pass spontaneously after standard ES. Nevertheless, most experts will attempt stone extraction from the CBD immediately following ES as this will reduce the incidence of retained stones and complications. The incision must be of sufficient size to provide an

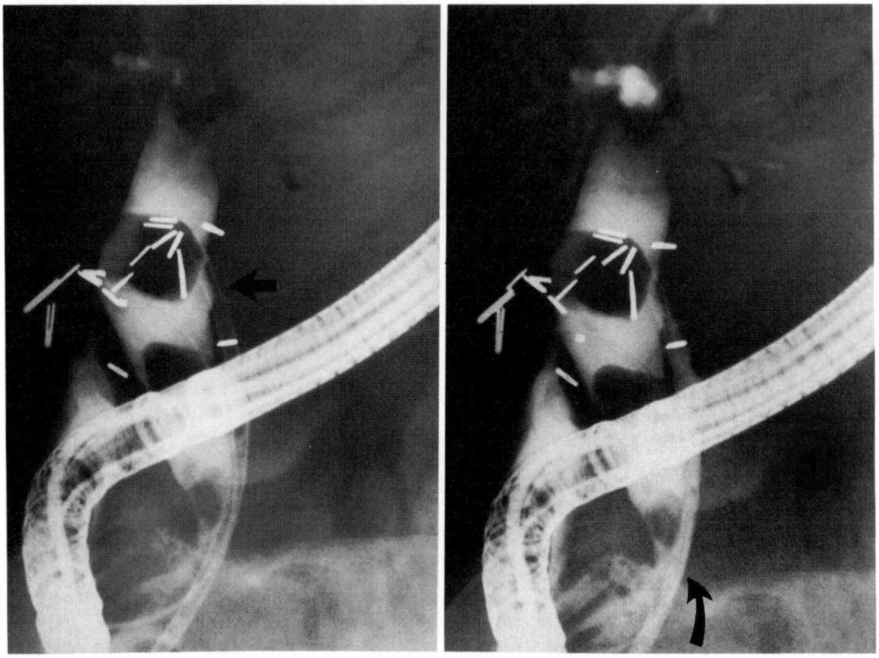

Figure 6.2.4 Biliary endoprosthesis (arrow) for difficult bile duct stones in a postcholecystectomy patient.

opening large enough to allow stone extraction and thereby avoid stone impaction. Stones which are larger than the endoscope on radiographic imaging are likely to be more difficult to extract and therefore require adjuvant techniques.

A Dormia basket is a popular device for entrapping and removing stones (Fig. 6.2.5). Care and good judgement must be utilized to avoid impaling the basket wires into the stone surface as this can result in basket impaction. Stone extraction can alternatively be accomplished with a Fogarty-type balloon catheter which avoids the possibility of instrument impaction (Fig. 6.2.6). The balloon is particularly useful in individuals with small diameter common bile ducts or when multiple stones are present. Overall duct clearance can be expected in 90–95% of those undergoing successful sphincterotomy, resulting in an overall therapeutic success rate of endoscopic stone clearance approximating 80–95%, with the highest success rates noted as experience increases.[11–16] Patients are usually hospitalized overnight for routine observation and discharged the following day if complications are not encountered.

Complications

Early complications encountered with endoscopic sphincterotomy are well described and can be divided into those inherent to all endoscopic procedures such

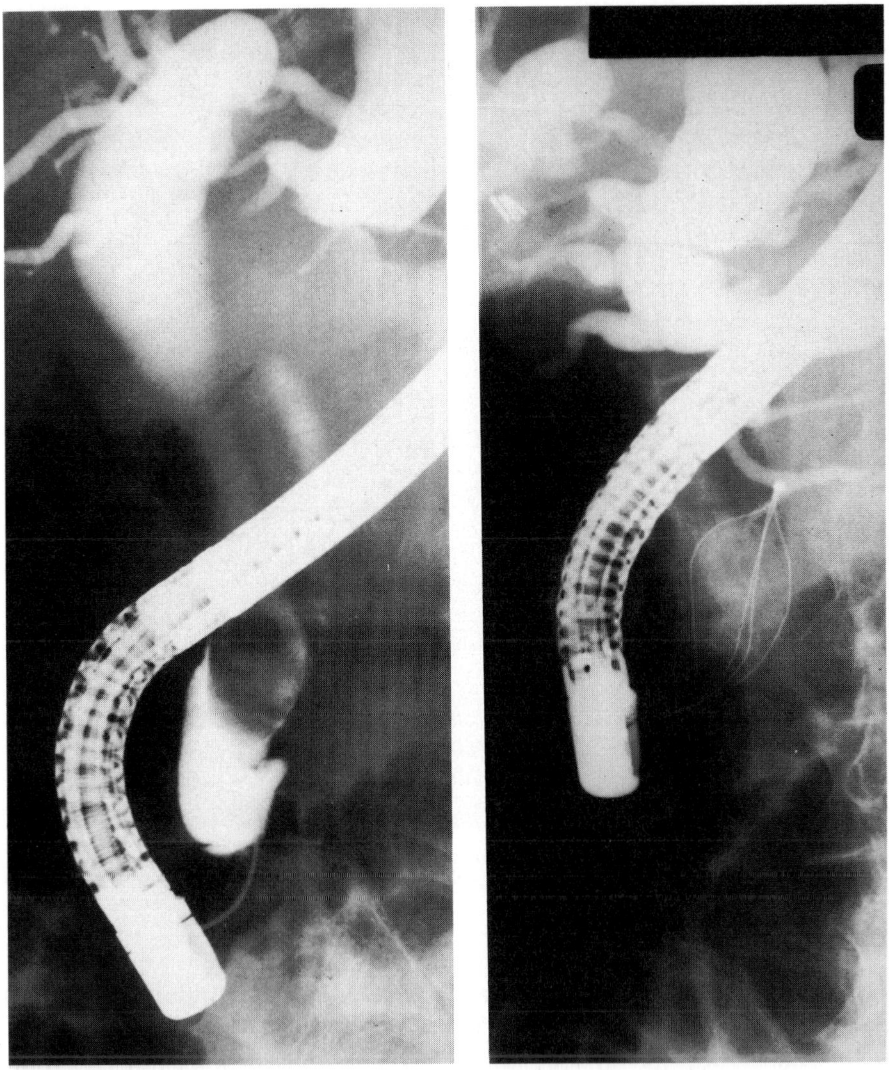

Figure 6.2.5 Basket extraction (right) of single large bile duct stone.

as drug reactions or cardiorespiratory compromise and those complications arising specifically from the sphincterotomy. The ES complication rate of 8–10% is remarkably similar among various centres despite great differences in procedure indications and patient selection. The major complications include haemorrhage in 2–3%, acute pancreatitis in 1–4%, cholangitis in 1–3% and retroduodenal perforation in 1%.[11,14,16–18] The overall mortality from the procedure approximates 0.5–1.0%[11,14,16–18] with a 30-day mortality of 3–16%[15,18,20] which is a reflection of the severity of underlying illness at the time of the procedure. Emergency surgery is required in less than 20% of these

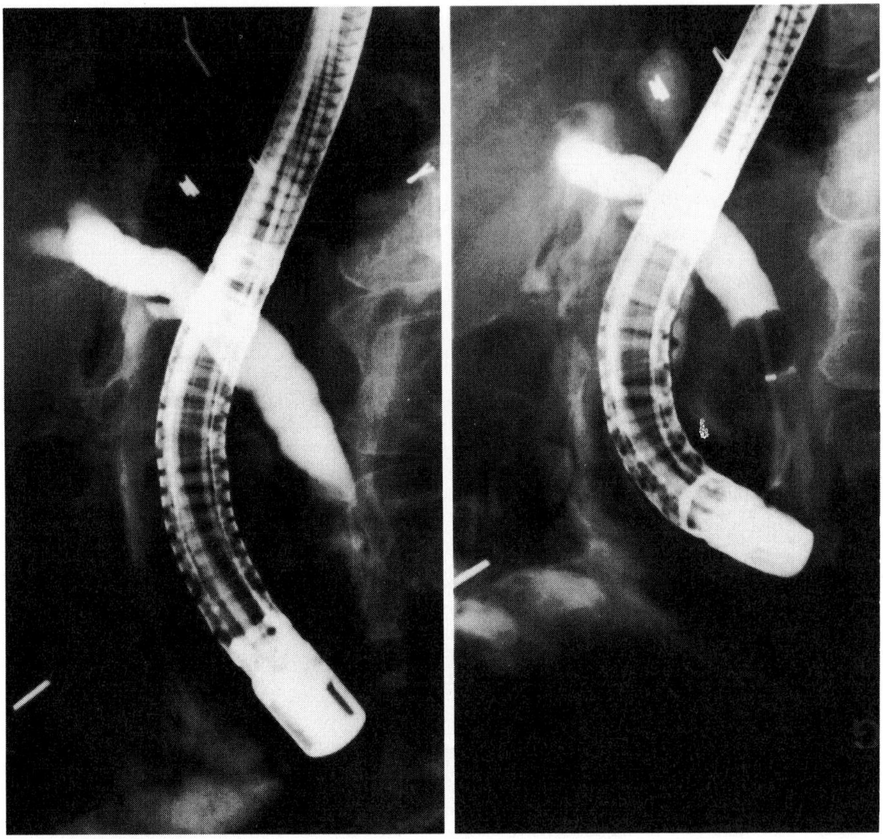

Figure 6.2.6 Balloon extraction (right) of an impacted bile duct stone.

complications with bleeding, cholangitis, perforation and pancreatitis being the reasons for intervention in decreasing order of frequency. Additional problems rarely encountered include impaction of a retrieval basket, gallstone ileus,[19] acute cholecystitis, splenic trauma[20] and subcutaneous emphysema.[21]

Complication rates are largely dependent upon the definition of "complication" which varies among studies, as do the degrees of severity of each complication which can vary from trivial to life-threatening. Higher complication rates can be anticipated early in an endoscopist's experience although this factor has not been well studied.[22] Perforation and pancreatitis appear to occur more often in patients with small bile duct diameters[23] and when precutting techniques are utilized.[8,9] The incidence of complications is not influenced by the clinical indication for the procedure (e.g. pancreatitis, biliary pain, cholangitis), although the development or progression of cholangitis is more likely if cholangitis exists prior to the procedure. The incidence of complications is also unaffected by patient age, presence of a gall bladder or T-tube drain, prior biliary surgery or the presence of a periampullary diverticulum,[22,24,25] although these factors may render the procedure technically more difficult. Transmission of hepatitis B or HIV infection has not occurred as these viruses are readily destroyed by current disinfection procedures.[26]

Most *bleeding* occurs immediately or within several hours of sphincterotomy, although delayed haemorrhage may occur up to two weeks following the procedure.[22] Sphincterotomy technique with a controlled cut to ensure adequate coagulation and with avoidance of an uncontrolled incision "zipper cut" will reduce the risk of haemorrhage. Although it is advisable to stop all non-steroidal anti-inflammatory medications several days prior to planned sphincterotomy, there are no controlled data to indicate an appreciable increased risk with continued usage.[22] Portal hypertension and renal failure with their associated bleeding diathesis may add to the risk of sphincterotomy.[27] Most episodes of haemorrhage are managed non-operatively. Endoscopic methods utilized to control bleeding include completion of the sphincterotomy in order to apply additional coagulating current at the upper margin of the sphincterotomy and allow full retraction of a partly severed vessel, temporary tamponade of the freshly cut papilla with a balloon catheter, submucosal injection of adrenaline at the site of bleeding and direct application of multipolar electrocoagulation.[22,28]

The endoscopic view may be completely obscured by blood in circumstances of severe arterial bleeding making endoscopic therapy impossible. Angiographic transcatheter embolization may be attempted when endoscopic methods fail to control bleeding.[19] Surgery should be performed for medical treatment failures and those in whom the endoscopic biliary procedure has failed to provide CBD clearance. The surgical procedure consists of conversion of the sphincterotomy into a formal surgical sphincteroplasty which oversews the bleeding artery typically located at the apex of the incision.

Post-ERCP *pancreatitis* is defined as a clinical syndrome of hyperamylasaemia and abdominal pain requiring hospital admission. Hyperamylasaemia in the absence of abdominal pain is not sufficient to diagnose pancreatitis, as amylase elevations can be expected following routine ERCP in 30–75% of patients.[22] Fortunately, the majority of patients develop mild self-limiting pancreatitis but severe pancreatitis and death can occur. The management is similar to other forms of pancreatitis. The incidence is no higher after ES compared with diagnostic ERCP alone.

The pathogenesis of ERCP induced pancreatitis is not well understood. A number of aetiological factors have been proposed including mechanical, chemical, hydrostatic, enzymatic, microbiological, thermal and allergic ductal trauma. Hydrostatic and mechanical trauma from sphincter of Oddi manometry, overfilling of the duct with contrast manifested by acinarization and repeated pancreatic duct cannulation have been the only identified risk factors for pancreatitis during ERCP.[29] A number of agents shown to be of benefit in experimental pancreatitis models have been clinically studied to determine if prophylactic administration will reduce the incidence or severity of ERCP induced pancreatitis. Performance of ERCP with low osmolality contrast agents[30,31] and prophylactic use of antibiotics, glucagon, calcitonin and somatostatin or its analogue octreotide may reduce the elevation in serum amylase following the procedure, but these agents have not resulted in a reduced incidence of pancreatitis and therefore cannot be recommended.[32–34]

Pre-existing *cholangitis* increases the risk of ERCP induced sepsis. Care must be taken not to overfill an already infected biliary system as this can lead to cholangiovenous reflux of infected bile and thereby exacerbate or precipitate systemic sepsis.[35] In the patient with cholangitis, the biliary system is decompressed first by aspirating bile prior to contrast injection and the least amount of contrast necessary to define the site and level of obstruction is injected. Cholangitis results from biliary stasis, therefore measures should be directed at providing good bile drainage before terminating the endoscopic procedure. If a stricture is present or the CBD is not cleared of calculous material, a stent or nasobiliary catheter may be necessary to provide drainage. Antibiotics should be continued until infection is resolved and there is certainty regarding bile flow. Percutaneous drainage or immediate surgery are additional options for circumstances when adequate drainage is not achieved endoscopically.

Retroperitoneal perforation results from a sphincterotomy that extends beyond the intramural segment of bile duct. This intramural segment may be shorter in patients with normal calibre bile ducts, placing these individuals at greater risk for perforation.[23] A diagnosis of perforation can be made if retroperitoneal structures are seen during the procedure or if retroperitoneal gas or extravasation of contrast is observed at the time of ERCP. Postprocedure diagnosis relies on radiological demonstration of retroperitoneal air on an abdominal flat plate, extravasation of contrast outside the duodenal lumen on upper GI series or, most accurately, the presence of air in the retroperitoneal space on abdominal CT scanning (Fig. 6.2.7). The initial approach is non-surgical with antibiotics, intravenous fluids and close monitoring with surgical colleagues. If deterioration ensues or an abscess forms, percutaneous or operative drainage is required.

Long term complications from follow-up studies for up to 11 years after sphincterotomy have documented a 10–15% incidence of subsequent biliary complications,[36,37] a figure which compares favourably with those seen following surgical common bile duct exploration and drainage procedures.[38,39] The significant complications include recurrent stones, sphincter stenosis and cholangitis. The majority of these can be managed through additional endoscopic therapy. Longer follow-up will be necessary before we can become confident with performing this procedure in the younger population.

DIFFICULT BILE DUCT STONES

Most experts would agree that the most difficult circumstances encountered during endoscopic stone removal are the result of technical difficulties with

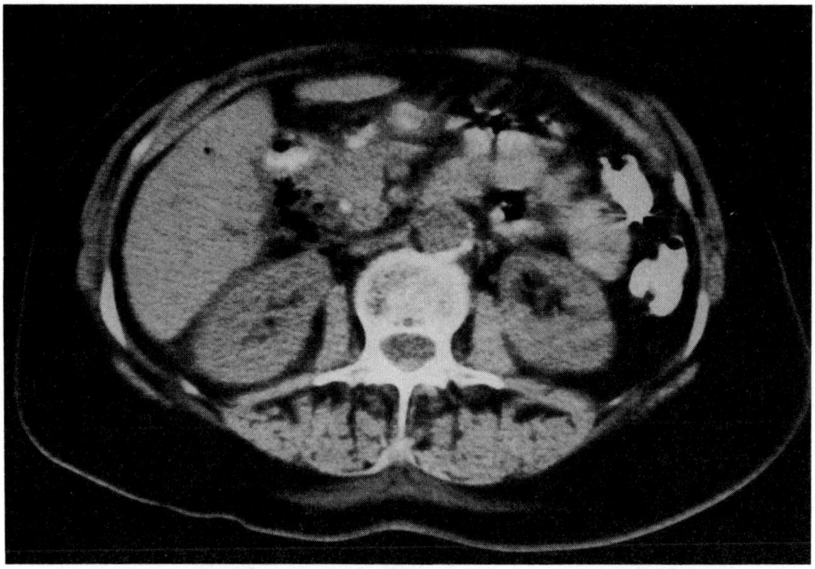

Figure 6.2.7 CT scan after retroperitoneal perforation showing air anterior to the right kidney.

achieving deep biliary cannulation or performing ES, sometimes due to inaccessibility of the papilla and related to aberrant anatomy or unfavourable duodenal or papillary structures such as a periampullary diverticulum, or prior surgery such as a Billroth II or Roux-en-Y reconstruction. As previously discussed, adjuvant techniques with precutting and combined percutaneous–endoscopic procedures will increase the success rates in these difficult circumstances.[6,7] The patient with a Billroth II partial gastrectomy poses a unique challenge with regard to selective bile duct cannulation and the performance of ES, as the visualized anatomy is reversed (Fig. 6.2.8). When difficulty is encountered with the Billroth II patient, alternative techniques can be employed including needle-knife sphincterotomy with either a stent or nasobiliary drain used as a guide for cutting[40] or use of specially designed reverse direction accessories.

Once ES is performed successfully a variety of factors may hinder stone extraction including a disproportionately narrow lower bile duct segment, a large stone of greater than 15 mm, intrahepatic stones, a stone located proximal to a stricture or a large number of stones (Table 6.2.1). Stones which appear larger than the endoscope on radiographic imaging are likely to be more difficult to extract and therefore may require adjuvant techniques to remove them. Stone consistency (e.g. hard) and shape (e.g. "piston stone") may also adversely influence extraction success. Adjuvant techniques that have been developed to reduce stone size prior to endoscopic removal include mechanical lithotripsy, extracorporeal shock wave lithotripsy (ESWL), intracorporeal lithotripsy with laser or electrohydraulic probes and chemical dissolution. Treatment options

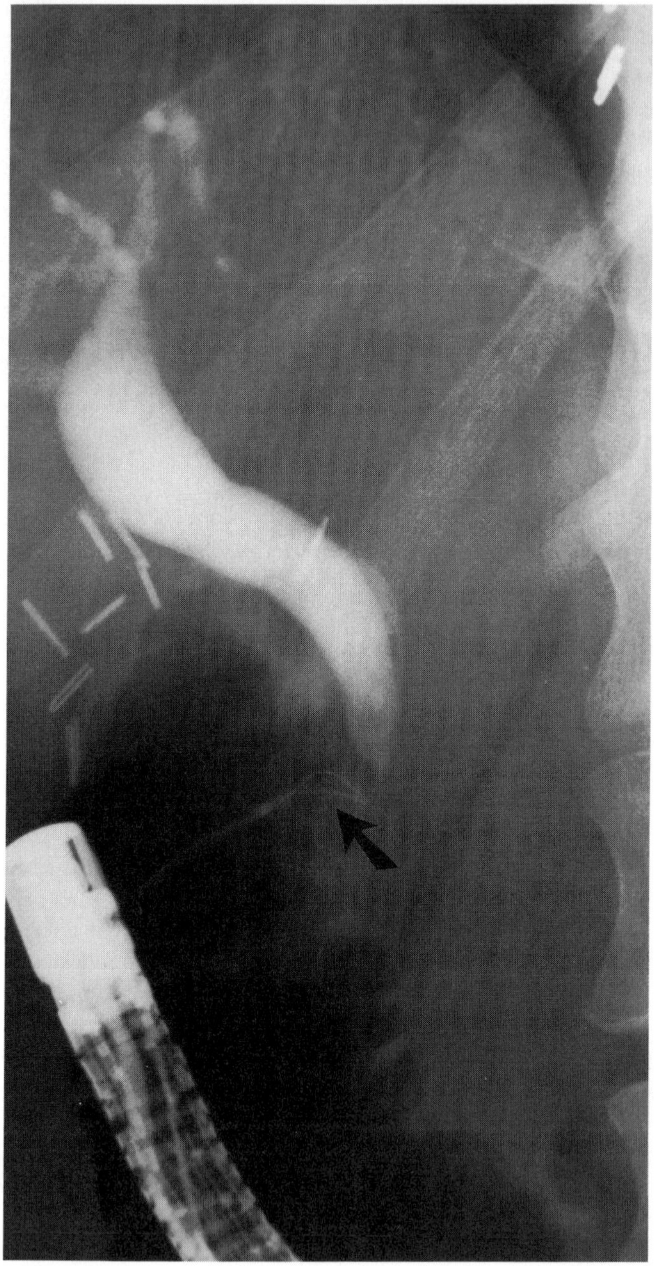

Figure 6.2.8 Sphincterotomy in Billroth II anatomy using a 'reverse' papillotome (arrow) with the cautery wire cephalad.

Table 6.2.1 Difficult bile duct stones

Stones greater than 15 mm
Intrahepatic stones
Multiple stones
Impacted stones
Stone proximal to a biliary stricture
Tortuous bile duct
Disproportionate size of the bile duct stone
Duodenal diverticulum
Billroth II reconstruction
Surgical duodenotomy

must be discussed jointly by endoscopists, surgeons and interventional radiologists when difficulties are encountered with CBD stone therapy (Fig. 6.2.9).

Mechanical Lithotripsy

Removal of large common duct stones remains a challenge for the most skilled endoscopist. Mechanical lithotripsy has evolved and remains the best initial option for stones which cannot be removed by conventional techniques, as it can be applied safely and effectively during the initial endoscopic procedure. Standard retrieval baskets contained within a Teflon sheath may fail to crush large stones, as most exceed the breaking strength of the catheter leading to buckling of the Teflon as the wires are tightened around the stone which thus remains intact and entrapped. Mechanical lithotripters which are modifications of standard Dormia baskets are of greater tensile strength and have greatly improved the success of stone fragmentation (Fig. 6.2.10). The reinforced basket is opened in the bile duct and the stone entrapped within the braided wires. This can either be performed most simply through the endoscope instrumentation channel or after the endoscope has been removed from the patient and a metal sheath is extended over the inner Teflon catheter whose outer end is attached to a winding mechanism at the end of the metal sheath. When cranked, this system retracts the basket and captured stone against the rigid distal end of the metal sheath leading to stone fracturing. The stone fragments can then be removed with the basket or a retrieval balloon. This technique allows removal of 80–94% of difficult bile duct stones which are refractory to standard extraction techniques.[41–45] Failures are typically secondary to the inability to engage the stone within the basket.

Non-Mechanical Lithotripsy

Shockwave lithotripsy with extracorporeal (ESWL) and intracorporeal techniques (laser or electrohydraulic probes) appear to be acceptable adjuncts to other

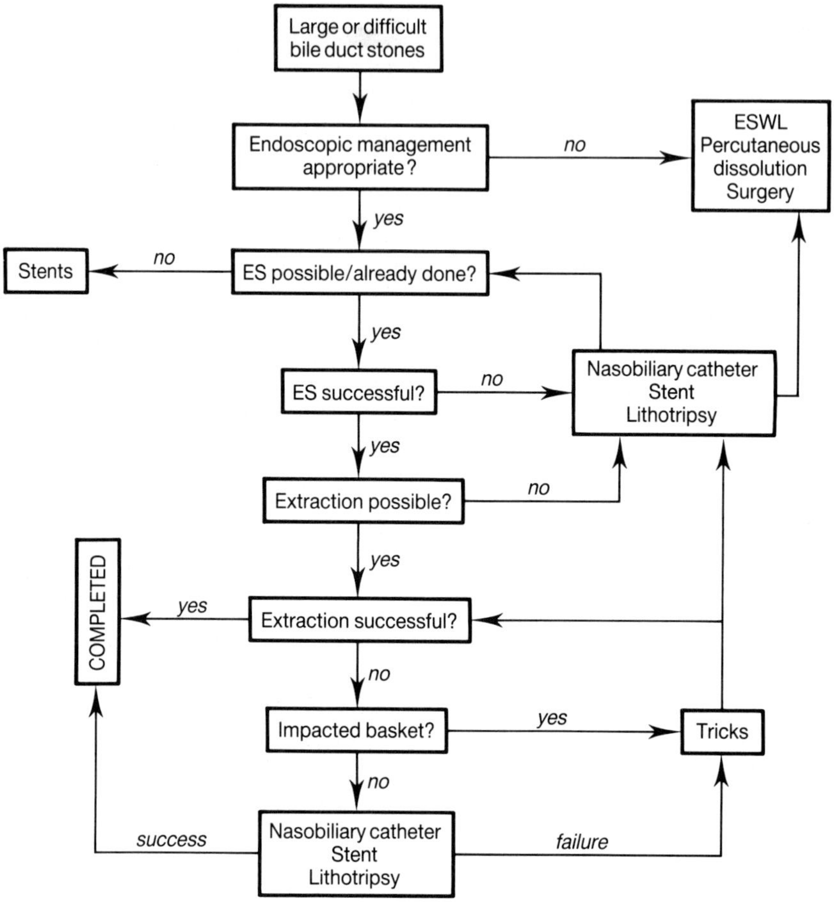

Figure 6.2.9 Algorithm of difficult stone therapy

techniques used to achieve common duct stone fragmentation and removal. The choice between these various methods or surgery largely depends on local expertise, as high success rates and low morbidity are reported in well-trained hands. Targeting of stones appears to be the major technically difficult aspect of applying these methods. Focusing of shockwaves can be accomplished under direct visualization with the "mother–daughter" endoscope design and through intra- or extraductal ultrasonographic or fluoroscopic targeting. Multiple treatment sessions may be required and additional endoscopic procedures are often necessary to remove stone fragments, adding to treatment costs and patient discomfort.

The use of *laser energy* for gallstone fragmentation has been developed in recent years at specialist centres.[46] The first generation laser systems using continuous wave energy neodymium:Yttrium aluminium garnet (Nd.Yag) devices were both ineffective in stone fragmentation and of high risk for thermal bile duct

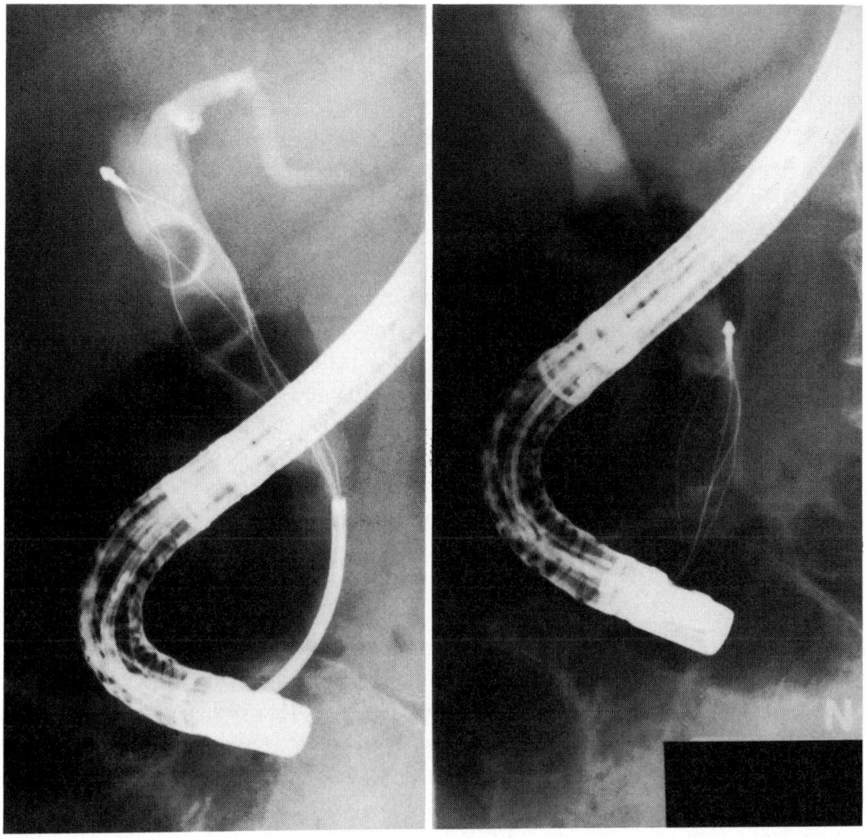

Figure 6.2.10 Mechanical lithotripsy of three bile duct stones showing capture (left) and fragmentation against the metallic sheath (right).

injury.[47] Second generation devices which have gained acceptance are based on high energy flashlamp pulsed dye laser technology. These devices deliver low pulse energies and generate little thermal energy, minimizing the risk of bile duct injury. The application of the laser pulse leads to rapid expansion and collapse of plasma on the stone surface, resulting in a mechanical shock wave. Initially, under direct visualization, laser–stone contact was ensured during ERCP through the use of the dual "mother and baby" endoscope system but, more recently, several groups have performed laser lithotripsy under fluoroscopic guidance with the use of devices that facilitate laser–stone contact and maintain the laser tip centrally located in the bile duct lumen.[48,49] These devices consist of a laser basket, a balloon catheter system, or a three-layer sleeve system through which the laser fibre is passed. Several series describe an overall success rate for laser lithotripsy ranging from 80–90% for clearing bile duct stones refractory to standard extraction techniques.[47–49] No major complication directly attributable to the laser lithotripsy was reported. The entire technique of sphincterotomy, laser lithotripsy procedure and extraction of stone fragments is often achieved in a single endoscopic session.

Since its development during the 1950s in the Soviet Union as a method to fragment rocks during mining, electrohydraulic lithotripsy (EHL) has been adopted for medical use for the treatment of nephrolithiasis and more recently biliary tract calculi.[50] The electrohydraulic probe consists of two coaxially isolated electrodes at the tip of a flexible catheter which is capable of delivering electric sparks in short rapid pulses leading to sudden expansion of the surrounding liquid environment, thereby generating pressure waves which result in stone fragmentation.[50] Stone contact with the electrode is achieved through the use of the basket or balloon catheter systems[51] or under direct visual targeting through the working channel of a mother–daughter endoscope,[52,53] thus minimizing the risk of bile duct injury and perforation. Cumulative experience with EHL is limited, with published reports documenting complete stone clearance following multiple treatment sessions in up to 86%.[51–54] Its main advantage over laser technology is its low cost.

ESWL with a variety of lithotripsy devices is now accepted as an alternative to fragmenting the difficult bile duct stone. In contrast to other lithotripsy techniques, direct contact with the stone is not necessary. Most centres have localized stones with fluoroscopic focusing during contrast perfusion of the CBD through an endoscopically placed nasobiliary catheter or percutaneous drain.[55] Ponchon and colleagues[56] have recently reported ESWL success with an ultrasonographic localization system, although it was less effective when multiple stones were present. Several large series[54,56–59] indicate success rates for ESWL stone fragmentation of 53–91% and duct clearance in 58–86%. The major drawback has been the need by most patients for multiple treatment sessions and at least one subsequent ERCP for extraction of stone fragments. Minor complications are common, including haematuria, biliary pain, haemobilia, transient LFT elevations and cutaneous petechiae.

Chemical dissolution of biliary stones has been attempted by perfusing the common bile duct with solvents administered via an indwelling nasobiliary tube (NBT), percutaneous transhepatic catheter, cholecystostomy tube or through an existing T-tube. The initial results with these agents have been disappointing due to incomplete stone dissolution and the potential for complications. A semisynthetic vegetable oil, mono-octanoin, composed of 70% glycerol-1-mono-octanoate and 30% glycerol-1,2 di-octanoate has been used experimentally for the dissolution of bile duct stones since 1977. Results collected from 222 clinicians treating 343 patients with CBD stones between 1977 and 1983 were disappointing with a success rate for complete stone dissolution of only 25.6% and an additional partial success rate of 28%, defined as incomplete stone dissolution or facilitation of other extraction methods.[60] Serious adverse effects leading to discontinuation of treatment occurred in 5%, including haemorrhage from duodenal ulceration, acute pancreatitis, jaundice, pulmonary oedema, acidosis, anaphylaxis, septicaemia and leucopenia but no deaths were reported.

The use of newer organic solvents such as aliphatic ether and methyl-tert-butyl ether (MTBE) have also been disappointing with complete stone dissolution in only 30–45% and unacceptably high complication rates related to systemic absorption from spillover of solvent into the duodenum and intrahepatic bile ducts.[61–64] Total success with cholesterol solvents for large CBD stones is unlikely to be achieved, as these stones are primarily composed of bile pigments with small concentrations of cholesterol. The addition of metal chelators (EDTA) may improve the dissolution of calcium containing stones.[65,66] Therefore, due to its low efficacy and high morbidity, contact chemical dissolution therapy has not assumed an important role in patients with refractory CBD stones and should be reserved for patients who have failed other adjuvant endoscopic techniques and are poor operative candidates. Newer agents with better methods for instillation are awaited.

Nasobiliary Tube and Biliary Endoprosthesis

In the 5% or less of situations where stone extraction is incomplete or impossible because of stone size, local anatomy, bleeding diathesis or technical difficulty leading to incomplete ES, a nasobiliary tube[67] should be inserted to provide biliary decompression and prevent stone impaction in the distal CBD. This serves as a temporizing therapy allowing for improvement in the patient's clinical condition until complete stone clearance is achieved either via additional endoscopic manoeuvres or subsequent surgery. This is of paramount importance for those individuals with established cholangitis where the requirement for emergency surgery can be transformed into a semielective procedure. This is also of major importance in situations of biliary ductal obstruction where incomplete duct clearance and poor biliary drainage can lead to the development of cholangitis, a complication which can be avoided by the routine use of a NBT. Antibiotics should be administered for the duration of NBT drainage. The nasobiliary tube (Fig. 6.2.3) consists of a 300 cm long 5 or 7 French gauge catheter placed in the biliary system with the proximal end exiting through the ampulla then traversing the nose and draining into a collection bag. In those with uncertain duct clearance, a follow-up cholangiogram can be obtained via the NBT without the need for repeat ERCP. NBTs are tolerated remarkably well for periods of several days. The primary problem with NBT placement has been the accidental or intentional dislodgement of the catheter by the confused or unco-operative patient. This has led to the alternative therapy of temporary biliary endoprosthesis placement (Fig. 6.2.4) for those in whom ES and attempts to remove CBD stones are unsuccessful.[68,69]

Surgery is usually recommended when aggressive endoscopic methods fail to remove bile duct stones. In the poor surgical risk patient, an acceptable non-surgical alternative is ES and long term placement of a biliary endoprosthesis.[70–73] Stent patency is not of major clinical importance in this situation, as the sphincterotomy typically provides an adequate conduit for bile flow around the prosthesis which serves principally to prevent stone impaction at the ampulla of Vater. In three series totalling 53 elderly high risk patients,[71–73] with up to five years follow-up, only three required surgery for biliary complications and four were operated on electively for treatment of stent occlusion or migration. An additional 16 patients had already died from non-biliary causes. The addition of ursodeoxycholic acid to such patients can result in CBD stone dissolution although additional studies are necessary to determine the true efficacy of this treatment in this setting.[74]

CLINICAL INDICATIONS

Postcholecystectomy with T-tube in situ

Bile duct stones detected in the early postoperative period on T-tube cholangiography of less than 10 mm diameter may pass spontaneously or with hydrostatic pressure from flushing or perfusing the T-tube. However, the majority of these stones will require additional mechanical manipulation. Increased morbidity and mortality with secondary bile duct explorations has stimulated the development of alternative techniques including hydraulic T-tube irrigation with or without pharmacologic relaxation of the sphincter of Oddi with glucagon or nitrates,[75] T-tube infusion of cholesterol solvents,[75] T-tube tract choledochoscopy and lithotripsy[76] or percutaneous extraction of stones through a mature T-tube track. Results with this latter technique have ranged from 77–96% success but multiple sessions are often required and the technique can be complicated by sepsis, biliary trauma and biliary leakage in 4–8%.[75,77–80] Delays of four to six weeks are required prior to manipulation to allow maturation of the T-tube track. Alternatively, early ES can be safely and effectively applied after stone detection without the need for T-tube maturation allowing timely discharge from hospital.

The results from eight endoscopic series totalling 337 patients indicate an overall endoscopic success rate of 90% with a morbidity of 7% and mortality of 0.6%.[80–87] The choice between these two techniques of similar efficacy and safety depends upon local expertise, as direct comparisons have not been made in controlled trials.

Pregnancy

Symptomatic choledocholithiasis during pregnancy poses a diagnostic and therapeutic challenge. Endoscopic treatment can be performed provided certain precautions are taken to minimize fetal exposure to radiation.[88–90] During ERCP, the fetus is shielded with an abdominal lead apron, no radiographs are taken and dosimetry should be performed to estimate the amount of radiation exposure to the fetus. These patients should undergo elective cholecystectomy upon completion of pregnancy to prevent recurrence.

Postcholecystectomy without T-tube

Common bile duct stones are present in 10–15% of patients undergoing cholecystectomy for symptomatic cholelithiasis. The incidence of retained common bile duct stones remains at approximately 2–5% following conventional and laparoscopic cholecystectomy with an incidence as high as 5–15% following common duct exploration.[91] Endoscopic sphincterotomy remains the treatment of choice for the elderly patient presenting days to years after cholecystectomy[92] as these individuals are at high risk from further abdominal surgery.[93,94] ES is also recommended in the young, fit postcholecystectomy individual. Long term follow-up will be necessary in this group of individuals as the post-ES follow-up data largely reflect results of endoscopic procedures performed in elderly patients although there is no compelling reason to suspect that the results will differ.

Selected Patients with Gall Bladder In Situ

In the elderly, a deliberate decision is often made to leave the gall bladder in situ following ES and CBD stone removal. The short and long term results and complications of ES in patients with a gall bladder do not differ from those in the postcholecystectomy patient. These patients, in view of their shorter life expectancy, can be managed expectantly unless symptoms dictate otherwise. Careful follow-up for five to ten years in these patients with intact gall bladders indicates that approximately 10% will develop gall bladder symptoms or complications sufficient to warrant cholecystectomy, the majority of which occur in the first year.[95–100] This risk for developing gall bladder symptoms is similar to that of patients with asymptomatic cholelithiasis.[101] Furthermore, the majority of the patients requiring cholecystectomy have not presented on an emergency basis.

The risk for developing biliary symptoms appears to be dependent on the continuing presence of stones in the gall bladder. In two reports,[96–100] none of 155 patients with acalculous gall bladders at initial ES developed symptoms or complications that subsequently required cholecystectomy. In those with gallstones, there do not appear to be any reliable predictors to identify those patients with cholelithiasis who are likely to develop gall bladder complications following ES. Non-filling of the gall bladder with radiographic contrast at ERCP[102] or with radiotracer by nuclear scintigraphy[103] may confer a higher likelihood for developing symptoms, although results from other series do not concur.[95,98]

These results suggest that the low risk of subsequent gall bladder complications after ES and bile duct clearance, when patients are kept under supervision, outweighs the known higher mortality for cholecystectomy in the elderly and militates against routine cholecystectomy in this group. Few physicians would recommend this approach in the fit patient under age 60 where the expectation for long term survival and therefore development of symptoms necessitating cholecystectomy is great. The risk of elective cholecystectomy is probably smaller than the risk of subsequently developing gall bladder symptoms in this group and therefore elective cholecystectomy would seem most appropriate for these patients.

The place of preoperative ES in young, low surgical risk patients with suspected choledocholithiasis has been examined to determine if preoperative ERCP and ES confer an advantage in terms of morbidity, mortality and length of hospital stay compared with a conventional approach of open cholecystectomy, operative cholangiography and common bile duct exploration. Two prospective, randomized controlled trials[104,105] have addressed this question with the conclusion that no advantage is conferred by initial endoscopic bile duct clearance prior to cholecystectomy. High risk surgical patients were excluded from these studies and both were conducted in the era of open cholecystectomy. With the recent developments in laparoscopic cholecystectomy, these conclusions must be re-evaluated.

Laparoscopic Cholecystectomy

Laparoscopic cholecystectomy has now replaced open cholecystectomy as the procedure of choice for gall bladder removal in the vast majority of individuals with symptomatic cholelithiasis.[106,107] Optimal management of patients with suspected common bile duct stones has yet to be determined in those undergoing laparoscopic cholecystectomy. The approach to CBD stones in the laparoscopic cholecystectomy patient is quite varied with an expanding array of available treatment options as improvements occur in endoscopic, surgical and percutaneous procedures. Laparoscopic transcystic cholangiography[108,109] and choledochoscopy with stone extraction[110] can be performed at the time of laparoscopic cholecystectomy but the latter technique requires specialized equipment and is currently in a developmental stage only applied in a limited form at specialized surgical centres. Laparoscopic transcystic choledochoscopy is hindered by the small size and tortuosity of the cystic duct, making instrument passage and stone lithotripsy and removal potentially difficult. Thus a need for endoscopic management has evolved, with ERCP playing a central role in preoperative and postoperative CBD stone detection and removal.

We and others[111] have found it useful to stratify patients preoperatively into low, intermediate and high likelihood for CBD stones (Table 6.2.2) based on established clinical and biochemical indicators including elevated liver function studies (LFTs), a dilated CBD greater than 8 mm on ultrasound and a history of

Table 6.2.2 Cholangiography stratification for risk of choledocholithiasis

High likelihood = preoperative ERCP
Bilirubin >2 mg dl^{-1}
Alkaline phosphatase >150 ul^{-1}
Presence/recent history of jaundice/pancreatitis
Dilated CBD/stone on sonography
Intermediate likelihood = IOC
Bilirubin 1.5–2.0 mg dl^{-1}
Alkaline phosphatase 110–150 ul^{-1}
Transaminases >2 × normal
Remote jaundice/pancreatitis
Low likelihood = no ERCP/IOC
Normal LFTs
No ductal dilatation
No jaundice/pancreatitis

IOC = Intra-operative cholangiography.

jaundice or pancreatitis.[112–114] Some centres have advocated routine preoperative or intraoperative cholangiography to document aberrant ductal anatomy and detect asymptomatic CBD stones. We would not support this recommendation as aberrant ductal anatomy is infrequently identified and rarely contributes to operative ductal injury. Furthermore, in the absence of clinical or biochemical indicators ("low likelihood" category), CBD stones will be present in only 2–3% of individuals, a yield which would probably be offset by the risks of the ERCP itself.[115] Small asymptomatic stones may be of minor clinical relevance as their natural history is not known and conceivably many, if not most, of these calculi would pass spontaneously without ever coming to clinical attention.

To date, we have favoured selective cholangiography for patients only with risk factors for choledocholithiasis. We have proposed three general strategies (Fig. 6.2.11a–c) to manage these individuals with "suspected" CBD stones. Algorithm (a) offers the advantage of complete surgical management with a single procedure without the need for additional postoperative attempts at stone extraction. The major disadvantage is the high rate of conversion to an open procedure which is not in keeping with the desire to maintain minimally invasive therapy. This strategy has not gained widespread acceptance but would be a reasonable approach either in centres not capable of providing adequate endoscopic therapy or when reliable techniques are achieved for performing laparoscopic CBD exploration. Algorithm (b) focuses on endoscopic cholangiography and stone clearance prior to performance of laparoscopic cholecystectomy. This approach appears justified in the patient with a "high likelihood" of a CBD stone in order to avoid prolonging the operative procedure with intraoperative cholangiography while maintaining the minimally invasive approach and reducing the need for conversion to an open common bile duct exploration

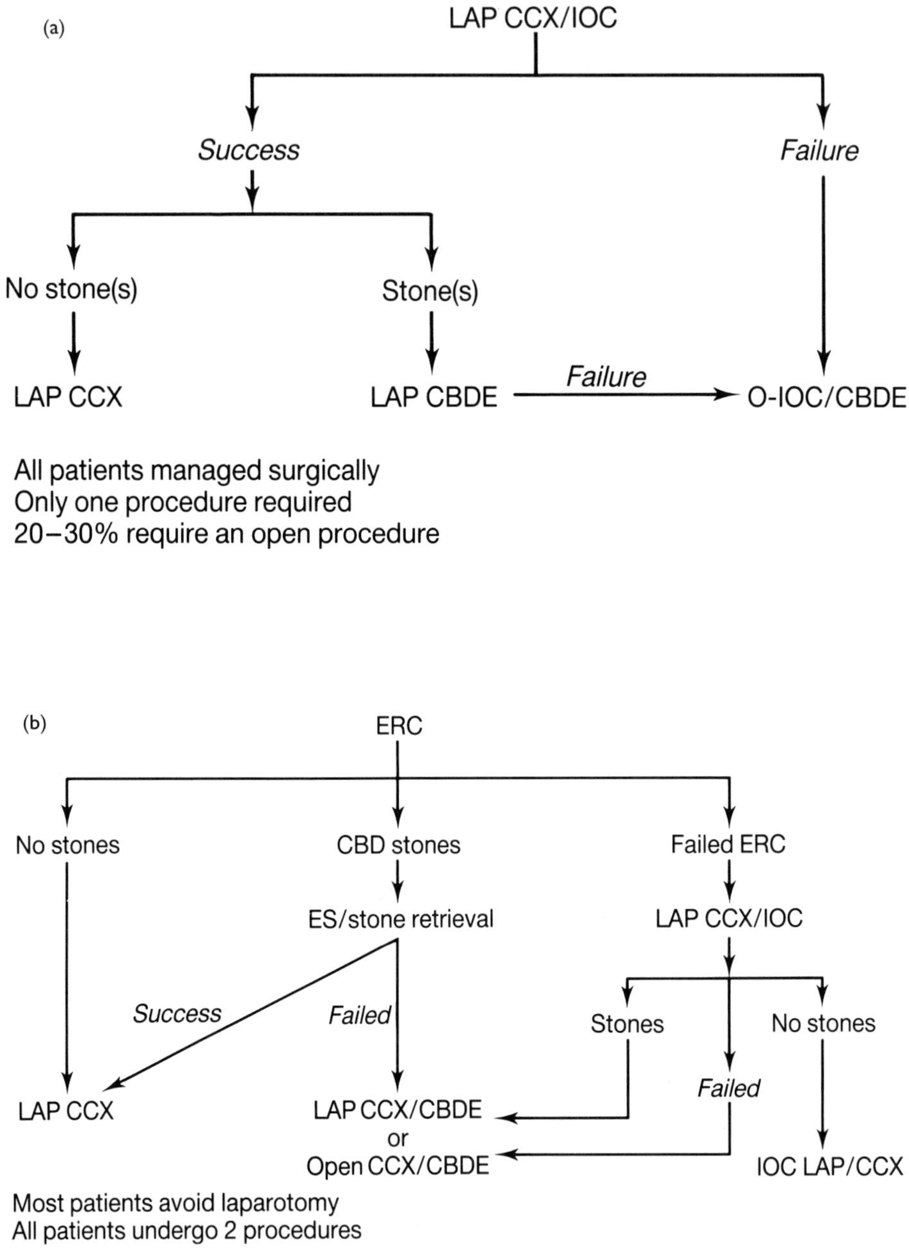

Figure 6.2.11 Algorithms for managing bile duct stones associated with laparoscopic cholecystectomy. (a) Laparoscopic cholecystectomy + IOC proceeding to laparoscopic CBD exploration and open CBD exploration for failures; (b) Preop ERC; (c) Laparoscopic cholecystectomy + IOC and post-op ERC for failures. Open explanation of CBD for ERC failures.

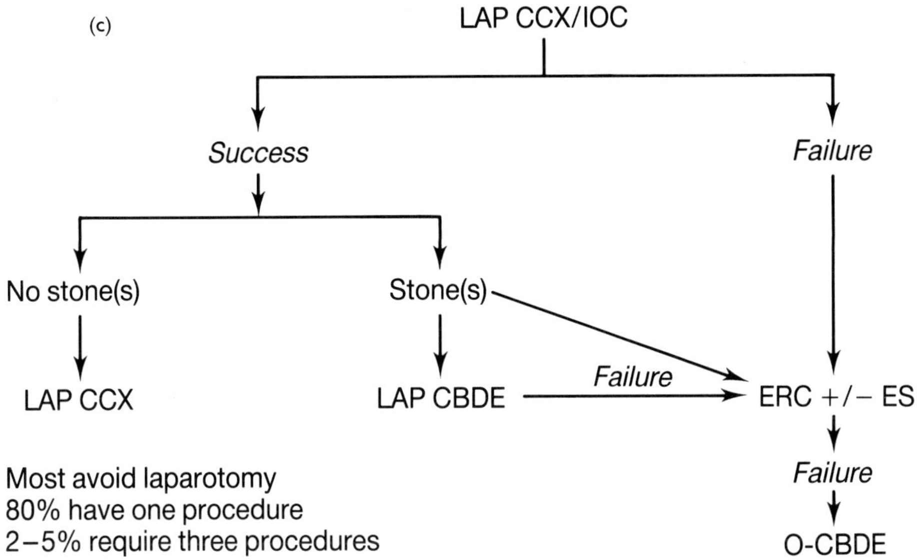

Figure 6.2.11(c)

for laparoscopic failures.[115–117] It is often possible to remove small stones (up to 3 mm diameter) during ERCP through the intact papilla with appropriate balloon catheters and baskets, thereby sparing the patient the potential short term and long term risks of ES.[118–120] Algorithm (c) utilizes laparoscopic transcystic cholangiography to detect CBD stones with postoperative ERCP to remove stones in those with positive cholangiograms. This strategy relies heavily on ERCP in a back-up role requiring endoscopic expertise, as failed stone removal will necessitate referral to a more experienced endoscopist or a second open operative procedure. The choice among these various strategies for the patient felt to be of "intermediate likelihood" should be strongly influenced by the quality of the surgical and endoscopic therapy available.

At our institution, in a prospective series of 750 consecutive laparoscopic cholecystectomies (Table 6.2.3), preoperative ERCP (algorithm b) was performed in 36 (4.8%) considered likely to have CBD stones based on indicators of a total bilirubin greater than 2 mg dl^{-1}, alkaline phosphatase greater than 150 ul^{-1}, a dilated CBD on ultrasound or a recent history of jaundice or pancreatitis. ERC was successful in 35 (97%) and nine (25%) were positive. All stones were removed following sphincterotomy with only one complication of mild pancreatitis which delayed surgery by three days. Aberrant ductal anatomy was present in two, Mirrizzi's syndrome in one and 23 were normal. Only one of nine patients with pancreatitis as the indicator for cholangiography had a CBD stone, questioning the utility of pancreatitis as a predictor of choledocholithiasis.

We suggest performance of prelaparoscopic cholecystectomy ERCP 24–48 hours prior to the planned surgery[117] whenever logistically feasible to avoid the

Table 6.2.3 ERCP in 750 laparoscopic cholecystectomies at Brigham and Women's Hospital, 1990–1992

Pre-operative ERCP	36 (4.8%)
Normal	23 (64%)
Stones	9 (25%)
Mirizzi's syndrome	1 (2.8%)
Aberrant anatomy	2 (5.6%)
Failed ERC	1 (2.8%)
Intraoperative cholangiography	45 (6.0%)
Successful	39 (87%)
Stones	2 (5.1%)
Not attempted	705 (94%)

infrequent occurrence of stone migration from the gall bladder into the CBD during the ERCP–laparoscopic cholecystectomy interval, resulting in the possibility of a retained CBD stone. This sequence of events occurred early in our series in one patient who passed a stone from the gall bladder into the CBD during a three week interval between the preoperative ERCP and laparoscopy. It has not recurred with subsequent performance of preoperative ERCP at the recommended 24–48 hour interval. Selective intraoperative cholangiography (algorithm c) was performed in 45 (6%) patients felt to be of "intermediate risk" for CBD stones based on preoperative indicators that included a total bilirubin elevation of 1.5–2.0 mg dl^{-1}, alkaline phosphatase of 110–150 ul^{-1}, transaminases greater than twice normal or a remote history of jaundice or pancreatitis. Only two (4.4%) of these studies were positive. Patients without preoperative indicators (669 patients) considered "low risk" did not undergo cholangiography and 11 (1.6%) have subsequently been found to have retained stones, all managed successfully by ERCP and ES.

Further studies are needed to clarify preoperative indicators for CBD stones and thereby better define the preoperative likelihood of CBD stones in individual patients. Many questions remain unanswered. There is limited experience with intraoperative ERCP[121] which is most appealing and convenient for the patient but requires a great deal of effort to co-ordinate. It may be awkward for the endoscopist due to patient positioning and may have deleterious consequences on the subsequent cholecystectomy due to bowel distention from air insufflation during endoscopy.

What is the risk of sphincterotomy in patients with non-dilated bile ducts? Will long-term complication rates following ES of 10–15% parallel those already reported in the elderly? What is the natural history of small asymptomatic stones incidentally detected at cholangiography and should they be left alone unless symptoms develop? Will intravenous cholangiography become an accurate diagnostic study? Careful prospective studies will be required to answer many of these questions and randomized trials need to be performed to establish the proper strategies for managing these patients. Until laparoscopic techniques are developed that permit duct exploration and stone removal, the main choices for CBD stone management will remain pre- and postlaparoscopic cholecystectomy ES and duct clearance or conversion to an open operation with standard cholecystectomy and CBD exploration.

Gallstone Pancreatitis

Acute pancreatitis due to impaction of gallstones in the ampulla of Vater was first reported by Opie in 1901.[122] From this observation derived the "obstructive theory" to explain the mechanisms responsible for gallstone pancreatitis. Stone impaction in the common channel of the pancreatic and common bile duct is postulated to result in obstruction of the two systems and resultant reflux of bile into the pancreatic duct.[123] In support of the (transient) obstructive theory, gallstones can be recovered from the faeces of 85–89% of patients[124,125] and the incidence of common bile duct stones is as high as 80% in those undergoing urgent operative or endoscopic intervention compared with a 5–30% incidence when the procedure is delayed.[125–127]

There are now well-established criteria (e.g. Ranson, Imrie, Glasgow, APACHE II) for assessing severity of pancreatitis and thereby predicting local adverse events of necrosis, haemorrhage, infection and pseudocyst formation as well as systemic complications of adult respiratory distress syndrome, disseminated intravascular coagulation, distant fat necrosis and renal failure.[128] Stratifying patients into severity of illness based on these criteria has been helpful in directing appropriate management. The majority of patients experience mild pancreatitis due to transient impaction of a stone in the ampulla followed by spontaneous migration into the duodenum. These individuals do well with conservative therapy alone and are unlikely to benefit from urgent intervention. In contrast, it has been proposed that the more severe cases of pancreatitis result from persistent stone impaction or choledocholithiasis with infected bile, offering the hope that early stone extraction by surgical or endoscopic techniques would halt progression of the acute event and prevent the development of future attacks.

The use of early surgical therapy in cases of acute gallstone pancreatitis has been challenged due to the high operative morbidity and mortality. Results and conclusions from numerous series comparing early and late surgical therapy in gallstone pancreatitis are difficult to interpret. The mortality rates range from 2–67%, the studies are retrospective with frequent comparisons with historical controls and stratification for severity of illness has not been utilized.[127,129–131] In the most recent series, Kelly and Wagner[132] prospectively randomized 165 patients with gallstone pancreatitis to early or delayed surgery. In the group with severe pancreatitis, they found a 48% mortality following urgent operative intervention, compared with an 11% mortality in patients in whom surgery was delayed for more than 48 hours. In contrast, those patients with mild pancreatitis had mortalities of 3.3% and 0%, respectively. These results would favour avoidance of early operative intervention in the acute phase of biliary pancreatitis unless local complications from necrotizing disease dictate otherwise.

An endoscopic approach to gallstone pancreatitis offers the theoretical advantage of immediate relief of ampullary obstruction and ductal clearance without the risks of general anaesthesia or the surgical procedure. There was initial reluctance to perform ERCP in patients with acute pancreatitis due to concerns that the procedure would exacerbate the illness and lead to patient demise. Safrany and Cotton[133] were the first to report ES in 11 patients with "severe" gallstone pancreatitis. The procedure was performed within 24 hours of hospitalization and common duct stones were found in all patients with stone impaction at the ampulla in six individuals. Endoscopic removal of common duct stones resulted in "prompt clinical and biochemical improvement" in ten of the 11 patients. Subsequent clinical studies supported the safety and efficacy of ERCP in the setting of acute biliary pancreatitis[134,135] but these reports were inconclusive due to study flaws including non-randomization in patient selection, variation in timing of the procedure and failure to stratify for severity of pancreatitis.

The Leicester group[136] were the first to perform a controlled study to evaluate the efficacy of ERCP in biliary pancreatitis. A group of 121 patients with suspected gallstone pancreatitis were randomized to urgent (within 72 hours of hospitalization) ERCP and ES if stones were present or conventional non-endoscopic management. Common bile duct stones were found in 63% of the predicted severe group and only 26% of those with predicted mild attacks. Those with mild pancreatitis have favourable outcomes regardless of treatment strategy, with a similar incidence of complications and no deaths. In the group of patients with "severe" pancreatitis defined by modified Glasgow criteria, urgent ES significantly reduced the morbidity (pseudocyst formation or systemic complications) from 61% to 24% and length of hospitalization from 17 days to 9.5 days compared with conservatively managed patients. Mortality was lower in the ERCP group (4% vs 18%); however the difference did not reach statistical significance.

A second study recently published by the Hong Kong group[137] prospectively randomized 195 consecutive patients with suspected gallstone pancreatitis to urgent (within 24 hours of hospital admission) ERCP with papillotomy or initial conservative treatment with selective ERCP only if their condition deteriorated. In this region of the world, where choledocholithiasis is frequently responsible for acute pancreatitis, emergency ERCP resulted in a reduction in biliary sepsis from 12% in the conservatively treated patients to 0% in those undergoing endoscopic papillotomy and stone extraction. Overall, there were no significant differences in the incidence of either local (10.3% vs. 12.2%) or systemic complications (10.3% vs. 14.3%). However, in the subset of patients with "severe" pancreatitis and common duct stones, urgent endoscopic sphincterotomy resulted in a decrease in the combined incidence of local and systemic complications of 21% and mortality rate of 5.3% compared with the conservatively managed group where the rates were 68.8% and 25%, respectively.

These studies demonstrate that ERCP and endoscopic stone extraction can be safely performed in the setting of acute biliary pancreatitis. Furthermore, urgent ERCP and ES can be performed with good rationale in those patients with severe or progressive pancreatitis due to the resultant reduction in major local peripancreatic complications and the increasingly recognized coexistence of acute cholangitis potentially translating into a reduced mortality. Subsequent elective cholecystectomy should be performed although in the high risk patient the gall bladder may be left in situ. In the patient with mild pancreatitis, no immediate intervention is advised. If later proven to have gallstones or microlithiasis,[138,139] elective laparoscopic cholecystectomy with preoperative ERCP or intraoperative cholangiography should be performed during the same hospitalization. In the postcholecystectomy patient, endoscopic therapy is definitive. The role of endoscopic sphincterotomy in lieu of cholecystectomy for the high risk patient with an intact gall bladder and gallstone pancreatitis in the absence of choledocholithiasis requires further evaluation.[140]

Cholangitis

The most common cause of suppurative cholangitis is obstruction of the biliary system by a common bile duct stone leading to raised intrabiliary pressure and cholangiovenous reflux.[141] The majority of patients with calculous cholangitis will present with mild disease and a clinical picture of pain, fever and jaundice, termed "Charcot's triad". They typically respond rapidly to conservative therapy consisting of intravenous fluids and antibiotics. For these individuals further treatment should be based on their fitness for surgery. The poor risk surgical patient should undergo ES and stone extraction leaving the gall bladder in situ. The younger, low operative risk patient should undergo definitive treatment with the option of either ES followed by laparoscopic cholecystectomy or conventional cholecystectomy and CBD exploration.

Reynolds and Dargan in 1959 described a particularly lethal form of acute suppurative cholangitis in which shock and mental confusion were additional clinical features.[142] Emergency ERCP is the treatment of choice for these individuals with severe cholangitis at presentation, as well as for those individuals not responding within 24 hours to conservative treatment. Emergency surgery should be reserved for those in whom endoscopic therapy fails, as conventional surgical treatment is associated with a morbidity and mortality of 10–50% depending upon the severity of illness and the presence of other illnesses.[143] Endoscopic decompression can be performed successfully in 85–95% of cases, with a lower morbidity and mortality compared with percutaneous transhepatic[144–146] or surgical drainage.[147–153] This can be a most gratifying experience for the medical team involved, as purulent bile draining from the biliary tree following successful ES is typically followed by rapid clinical improvement. In a critically ill patient only brief attempts should be made to remove CBD stones endoscopically. Decompression of the biliary system with a NBT or endoprosthesis can temporize matters in such a patient with cholangitis and failed endoscopic duct clearance, such that subsequent attempts at endoscopic stone removal can be performed safely on a semielective rather than emergency basis.[15,68] Moreover, a nasobiliary tube can be placed without ES, thus avoiding the risk of haemorrhage due to coagulopathy which frequently accompanies severe cholangitis.

Leese *et al.*[148] performed the first retrospective, uncontrolled comparison of endoscopic and surgical biliary decompression in 71 patients with acute calculous cholangitis. ES was performed in 43 and surgery in 28 with 30 day mortalities of 4.7% and 21.4%, respectively. These results were impressive considering that the ES group was older (mean age 75 vs. 66.5 years) and had a significantly greater number of associated medical illnesses. Similarly, Leung *et al.*[149] reported their results of urgent endoscopic biliary drainage in 105 patients with acute calculous cholangitis who did not rapidly respond to conservative management. Endoscopic treatment was successful in 102 (97%) of the patients and the overall mortality was only 4.7%, a figure which compares very favourably with historical surgical controls.[149] Three patients died of uncontrolled sepsis despite successful endoscopic drainage, one patient died of a stroke and one death occurred among the three patients who underwent emergency surgery following unsuccessful endoscopic therapy.

In the only prospective, randomized, controlled trial published to date,[153] 82 consecutive patients with severe acute cholangitis due to choledocholithiasis were randomly assigned to undergo emergency endoscopic biliary drainage or surgical decompression. The hospital mortality rate was significantly lower in the endoscopically treated group (10%) compared with those treated surgically (32%). Furthermore, patients in the surgery group had more complications (66% vs. 34%), greater need for mechanical ventilatory support (63% vs. 29%) and a higher rate of retained common duct stones (29% vs. 7%). Therefore, endoscopic drainage is safer and more effective than surgery for severe acute cholangitis related to choledocholithiasis. In the presence of mild disease, urgent biliary decompression can also be considered to prevent progression to more severe disease, although controlled trials in this group have not been reported.

CONCLUSIONS

Endoscopic sphincterotomy has been enthusiastically accepted since its birth 20 years ago, largely owing to physician and patient acceptance as a safe and effective means of managing common bile duct stones. Endoscopic techniques are well established and with continued development and improvements in supporting equipment, we suspect that the endoscopist's ability to remove stones will continue to improve. Optimal management of individuals with calculous biliary tract disease continues to require an integrated approach between endoscopists, surgeons and interventional radiologists. Based on current evidence, there seems to be little doubt that endoscopic therapy is the treatment of choice for elderly patients with bile duct stones regardless of their clinical presentation or gall bladder status, and for patients of all ages when presenting with cholangitis or severe gallstone pancreatitis. Furthermore, early postoperative patients with retained stones can safely be treated by ES without the need to await maturation of a T-tube track.

The place of ERCP remains to be defined in the new era of minimally invasive surgery where a number of acceptable algorithms have been proposed to manage the laparoscopic cholecystectomy patient suspected of harbouring common bile duct stones.

REFERENCES

1. Kawai K, Akasaka Y, Murakami K, Tada M, Kohle Y, Nakajima M. Endoscopic sphincterotomy of the ampulla of Vater. *Gastrointest Endosc* 1974; **20**: 148–51.
2. Classen M, Demling L. Endokopische sphinkterotomie der papilla bateri und steinextraktion aus dem ductus choledochus. *Dtsch Med Wochenschr* 1974; **99**: 496–7.
3. Kullman E, Borch K, Lindstrom E, Ansehn S, Ihse I, Anderberg B. Bacteremia following diagnostic and therapeutic ERCP. *Gastrointest Endosc* 1992; **38**: 444–9.
4. Rossos PG, Kortan P, Haber G. Selective common bile duct cannulation can be simplified by the use of a standard papillotome. *Gastrointest Endosc* 1993; **39**: 67–9.
5. Siegel JH, Pullano W. Two new methods for selective bile duct cannulation and sphincterotomy. *Gastrointest Endosc* 1987; **33**: 438–40.
6. Shakoor T, Geenen JE. Pre-cut papillotomy. *Gastrointest Endosc* 1992; **38**: 623–7.
7. Dowsett JF, Vaira D, Hatfield RW *et al.* Endoscopic biliary therapy using the combined percutaneous and endoscopic technique. *Gastroenterology* 1989; **96**: 1180–6.
8. Tweedle DEF, Martin KF. Needle knife papillotomy for endoscopic sphincterotomy and cholangiography. *Gastrointest Endosc* 1991; **37**: 518–21.
9. Siegel JH, Ben-Zvi JS, Pullano W. The needle knife: a valuable tool in diagnostic and therapeutic ERCP. *Gastrointest Endosc* 1989; **35**: 499–503.
10. Leung JWC, Banez VP, Chung SCS. Precut (needle knife) papillotomy for impacted common bile duct stone at the ampulla. *Am J Gastroenterol* 1990; **85**: 991–3.
11. Leese T, Neoptolemos JP, Carr-Locke DL. Successes, failures, early complications and their management following endoscopic sphincterotomy: results in 394 consecutive patients from a single center. *Br J Surg* 1985; **72**: 215–19.
12. Nakajima M, Kizu M, Akasaka Y, Kawai K. Five year experience of endoscopic sphincterotomy in Japan. *Endoscopy* 1979; **2**: 138–41.
13. Reiter JJ, Bayer HB, Mennicken C, Manegold PC. Results of endoscopic papillotomy: a collective experience from 9 endoscopic centers in West Germany. *World J Surg* 1978; **2**: 505–7.
14. Safrany L. Endoscopic treatment of biliary tract diseases. *Lancet* 1978; **2**: 983–5.
15. Siegel JH. Endoscopic papillotomy in the treatment of biliary tract disease: 258 procedures and results. *Dig Dis Sci* 1981; **26**: 1057–64.
16. Cotton PB, Vallon AG. British experience with duodenoscopic sphincterotomy for removal of bile duct stones. *Br J Surg* 1981; **68**: 373–5.
17. Lambert ME, Betts CD, Hill J, Faragher EB, Martin DF, Tweedle DEF. Endoscopic sphincterotomy: the whole truth. *Br J Surg* 1991; **78**: 473–6.
18. Vaira D, Ainley C, Williams S *et al.* Endoscopic sphincterotomy in 1000 consecutive patients. *Lancet* 1989; **2**: 431–3.

19. Despland M, Clavien PA, Mentha G, Rohner A. Gallstone ileus and bowel perforation after endoscopic sphincterotomy. *Am J Gastroenterol* 1992; **87**: 886–7.
20. Lewis FW, Moloo N, Steigmann GV, Goff JS. Splenic injury complicating therapeutic upper gastrointestinal endoscopy and ERCP. *Gastrointest Endosc* 1991; **37**: 632–3.
21. Tam F, Prindiville T, Wolfe B. Subcutaneous emphysema as a complication of endoscopic sphincterotomy of the ampulla of Vater. *Gastrointest Endosc* 1989; **35**: 447–9.
22. Cotton PB, Lehman G, Vennes J *et al.* Endoscopic sphincterotomy complications and their management: an attempt at consensus. *Gastrointest Endosc* 1991; **37**: 383–93.
23. Sherman S, Ruffolo TA, Hawes RH, Lehman GA. Complications of endoscopic sphincterotomy. A prospective series with emphasis on the increased risk associated with sphincter of Oddi dysfunction and nondilated bile ducts. *Gastroenterology* 1991; **101**: 1068–75.
24. Vaira D, Dowsett JF, Hatfield ARW *et al.* Is duodenal diverticulum a risk factor for sphincterotomy? *Gut* 1989; **30**: 939–42.
25. Shemesh E, Klein E, Czerniak A, Coret A, Bat L. Endoscopic sphincterotomy in patients with gallbladder in situ: the influence of periampullary duodenal diverticula. *Surgery* 1990; **107**: 163–6.
26. Spach DH, Silverstein FE, Stamm WE. Transmission of infection by gastrointestinal endoscopy and bronchoscopy. *Ann Intern Med* 1993; **118**: 117–28.
27. Moreira VF, Arribas R, Sanroman AL *et al.* Choledocholithiasis in cirrhotic patients: is endoscopic sphincterotomy the safest choice? *Am J Gastroenterol* 1991; **86**: 1006–9.
28. Sherman S, Hawes RH, Nisi R, Lehman GA. Endoscopic sphincterotomy-induced hemorrhage: treatment with multipolar electrocoagulation. *Gastrointest Endosc* 1992; **38**: 123–6.
29. Sherman S, Lehman GA. ERCP- and endoscopic sphincterotomy-induced pancreatitis. *Pancreas* 1991; **6**: 350–67.
30. Bedford RA, Johnson GK, Geenen JE *et al.* Does the use of non-ionic contrast prevent post-ERCP pancreatitis? Results of a prospective multicenter study. *Gastrointest Endosc* 1993; **39**: 315.
31. Barkin JS, Casal GL, Reiner DK, Goldberg RI, Phillips RS, Kaplan S. A comparative study of contrast agents for endoscopic retrograde pancreatography. *Am J Gastroenterol* 1991; **86**: 1437–41.
32. Persson B, Slezak P, Efendic S, Haggmark A. Can somatostatin prevent injection pancreatitis after ERCP? *Hepatogastroenterol* 1992; **39**: 259–61.
33. Binmoeller KF, Harris AG, Dumas R, Grimaldi C, Delmont JP. Does the somatostatin analogue octreotide protect against ERCP induced pancreatitis? *Gut* 1992; **33**: 1129–33.
34. Sternlieb JM, Aronchick CA, Retig JN *et al.* A multicenter, randomized, controlled trial to evaluate the effect of prophylactic octreotide on ERCP-induced pancreatitis. *Am J Gastroenterol* 1992; **87**: 1561–6.
35. Lai ECS, Lo CM, Choi TK, Cheng WK, Fan ST, Wong J. Urgent biliary decompression after endoscopic retrograde cholangiopancreatography. *Am J Surg* 1989; **157**: 121–5.
36. Hawes RH, Cotton PB, Vallon AG. Follow-up 6 to 11 years after duodenoscopic sphincterotomy for stones in patients with prior cholecystectomy. *Gastroenterology* 1990; **98**: 1008–12.
37. Ikeda S, Tanaka M, Matsumoto S, Yoshimoto H, Itoh H. Endoscopic sphincterotomy: long-term results in 408 patients with complete follow-up. *Endoscopy* 1988; **20**: 13–17.

38. Lygidakis NJ. Surgical approaches to recurrent choledocholithiasis:choledochoduodenostomy versus T-tube drainage after choledochotomy. *Am J Surg* 1983; **145**: 636–9.
39. Baker AR, Neoptolemos JP, Leese T, James DC, Fossard DP. Long-term followup of patients with side to side choledochoduodenostomy and transduodenal sphincteroplasty. *Ann Royal Coll Surg* 1987; **69**: 253–7.
40. Ricci E, Bertoni G, Conigliaro R, Contini S, Mortilla MG, Bedogni G. Endoscopic sphincterotomy in Billroth II patients: an improved method using a diathermic needle as sphincterotomy and a nasobiliary drain as guide. *Gastrointest Endosc* 1989; **35**: 47–50.
41. Shaw MJ, Dorsher PJ, Vennes JA. A new mechanical lithotripter for the treatment of large common duct stones. *Am J Gastroenterol* 1990; **85**: 796–8.
42. Siegel JH, Ben-Zvi JS, Pullano WE. Mechanical lithotripsy of common duct stones. *Gastrointest Endosc* 1990; **36**: 351–6.
43. Chung SCS, Leung JWC, Leong HT, Li AKC. Mechanical lithotripsy of large common bile duct stones using a basket. *Br J Surg* 1991; **78**: 1448–50.
44. Van Dam J, Sivak MV. Mechanical lithotripsy of large common bile duct stones. *Cleve Clin J Med* 1993; **60**: 38–42.
45. Shaw MJ, Mackie RD, Moore JP *et al.* Results of a multicenter trial using a mechanical lithotripter for the treatment of large bile duct stones. *Am J Gastroenterol* 1993; **88**: 730–3.
46. Birkett DH. Biliary laser lithotripsy. *Surg Clin N Am* 1992; **72**: 641–54.
47. Ell C, Lux G, Hochberger J, Muller D, Demling L. Laser lithotripsy of common bile duct stones. *Gut* 1988; **29**: 746–51.
48. Cotton P, Kozarek RA, Schapiro RH *et al.* Endoscopic laser lithotripsy of large bile duct stones. *Gastroenterology* 1990; **99**: 1128–33.
49. Ponchon T, Gagnon P, Valette PJ, Henry L, Chavaillon A, Thieulin F. Pulsed dye laser lithotripsy of bile duct stones. *Gastroenterology* 1991; **100**: 1730–6.
50. Picus D. Intracorporeal biliary lithotripsy. *Rad Clin N Am* 1990; **28**: 1241–9.
51. Siegel J, Ben-Zvi J, Pullano W. Endoscopic electrohydraulic lithotripsy. *Gastrointest Endosc* 1990; **36**: 134–6.
52. Hixson LJ, Fennerty MB, Jaffee PE, Pulju JH, Palley SL. Peroral cholangioscopy with intracorporeal electrohydraulic lithotripsy for choledocholithiasis. *Am J Gastroenterol* 1992; **87**: 296–9.
53. Leung JWC, Chung SSC. Electrohydraulic lithotripsy with peroral choledochoscopy. *Br Med J* 1989; **299**: 595–8.
54. Bonnel DH, Liquory CE, Cornud FE, Lefebvre JF. Common bile duct and intrahepatic stones: results of transhepatic electrohydraulic lithotripsy in 50 patients. *Radiology* 1991; **180**: 345–8.
55. Gordon SJ, Stampfl DA, Grimm IS, Dahnert W, Goldberg BB, Taglienti G. Successful shock-wave lithotripsy of bile duct stones using ultrasound guidance. *Dig Dis Sci* 1991; **36**: 1102–9.
56. Ponchon T, Martin X, Barkun A, Mestas JL, Chavaillon A, Boustiere C. Extracorporeal lithotripsy of bile duct stones using ultrasonography for stone localization. *Gastroenterology* 1990; **98**: 726–32.
57. Bland KI, Jones RS, Maher JW *et al.* Extracorporeal shock-wave lithotripsy of bile duct calculi. *Ann Surg* 1989; **209**: 743–55.
58. Sauerbruch T, Stern M. Fragmentation of bile duct stones by extracorporeal shock waves. A new approach to biliary calculi after failure of routine endoscopic measures. *Gastroenterology* 1989; **96**: 146–52.
59. Weber J, Ademek HE, Riemann JF. Extracorporeal piezoelectric lithotripsy for retained bile duct stones. *Endoscopy* 1992; **24**: 239–43.
60. Palmer KR, Hofmann AF. Intraductal mono-octanoin for the direct dissolution of bile duct stones: experience in 343 patients. *Gut* 1986; **27**: 196–202.

61. Neoptolemos JP, Hall C, O'Connor, Murray WR, Carr-Locke DL. Methyl-tert-butyl-ether for treating bile duct stones: the British experience. *Brit J Surg* 1990; **77**: 32–5.
62. Kaye GL, Summerfield JA, McIntyre N, Dooley JS. Methyl tert butyl ether dissolution therapy for common bile duct stones. *J. Hepatol* 1990; **10**: 337–40.
63. Brandon JC, Teplick SK, Hasking PH *et al.* Common bile duct calculi: updated experience with dissolution with methyl tertiary butyl ether. *Radiology* 1988; **166**: 665–7.
64. Murray WR, Laferla G, Fullarton GM. Choledocholithiasis – *in vivo* stone dissolution using methyl tertiary butyl ether (MTBE). *Gut* 1988; **29**: 143–5.
65. Swobodnik W, Baumgaertel H, Janowitz P, Fuchs S, Ditschuneit H. Dissolution of calcified gallbladder stones by treatment with methyl-hexyl ether and urea-EDTA. *Lancet* 1988; **2**: 216.
66. Neoptolemos JP, Hofmann AF, Moossa AR. Chemical treatment of stones in the biliary tree. *Br J Surg* 1986; **73**: 515–24.
67. Leung JWC, Cotton PB. Endoscopic nasobiliary catheter drainage in biliary and pancreatic disease. *Am J Gastroenterol* 1991; **86**: 389–94.
68. Kiil J, Kruse A, Rokkjaer M. Large bile duct stones treated by endoscopic biliary drainage. *Surgery* 1989; **105**: 51–6.
69. Rustgi AK, Schapiro RH. Biliary stents for common bile duct stones. *Gastrointest Endosc Clin N Am* 1991; **1**: 79–91.
70. Nordback I. Management of unextractable bile duct stones by endoscopic stenting. *Anneles Chirugiae et Gynaecologiae* 1989; **78**: 290–2.
71. Cotton PB, Forbes A, Leung JWC, Dineen L. Endoscopic stenting for long-term treatment of large bile duct stones: 2- to 5-year follow-up. *Gastrointest Endosc* 1987; **33**: 411–12.
72. Soomers AJ, Nagengast FM, Yap SH. Endoscopic placement of biliary endoprostheses in patients with endoscopically unextractable common bile duct stones. *Endoscopy* 1990; **22**: 24–6.
73. Foutch PG, Harlan J, Sanowski RA. Endoscopic placement of biliary stents for treatment of high risk geriatric patients with common duct stones. *Am J Gastroenterol* 1989; **84**: 527–9.
74. Johnson G, Geenen JE, Venu RP, Schmalz MJ, Hogan WJ. Treatment of non-extractable common bile duct stones with combination ursodeoxycholic acid (UDCA) plus endoprosthesis. *Gastrointest Endosc* 1991; **37**: 253.
75. Tritapepe R, di Padova C, di Padova F. Non-invasive treatment for retained common bile duct stones in patients with T tube in situ: saline washout after intravenous ceruletide. *Br J Surg* 1988; **75**: 144–6.
76. Josephs LF, Birkett DH. Laser lithotripsy for the management of retained stones. *Arch Surg* 1992; **127**: 603–5.
77. Burhenne JH. Percutaneous extraction of retained biliary tract stones. *Am J Radiol* 1980; **134**: 888–98.
78. Cotton PB. Retained bile duct stones: T-tube in place, percutaneous or endoscopic management? *Am J Gastroenterol* 1990; **85**: 1075–8.
79. Caprini JA. Biliary stone extraction. *Am Surg* 1988; **54**: 343–6.
80. Nussinson E, Cairns SR, Vaira D, Dowsett JF, Mason RR. A 10 year single centre experience of percutaneous and endoscopic extraction of bile duct stones with T tube in situ. *Gut* 1991; **32**: 1040–3.
81. Tandon RK, Nijhawan S, Arora A. Management of retained common bile duct stones in patients with T-tube in situ: role of endodoscopic sphincterotomy. *Am J Gastroenterol* 1990; **85**: 1126–31.
82. Bickerstaff KI, Berry AR, Chapman RW, Britton J. Early postoperative endoscopic sphincterotomy for retained biliary stones. *Ann R Coll Surg Engl* 1988; **70**: 350–1.

83. Soehendra N, Kempeneers I, Eichfuss HP, Reynders-Frederix V. Early postoperative endoscopy after biliary tract surgery. *Endoscopy* 1981; **13**: 113–17.
84. Simpson CJ, Gray GR, Gillespie G. Early endoscopic sphincterotomy for retained common bile duct stones. *J R Coll Surg Edinburgh* 1985; **30**: 288–9.
85. O'Doherty DP, Neoptolemos JP, Carr-Locke DL. Endoscopic sphincterotomy for retained common bile duct stones in patients with T-tube in situ in the early postoperative period. *Br J Surg* 1986; **73**: 454–6.
86. Danilewitz MD. Early postoperative endoscopic sphincterotomy for retained common bile duct stones. *Gastrointest Endosc* 1989; **35**: 298–9.
87. Lambert ME, Martin DF, Tweedle DEF. Endoscopic removal of retained stones after biliary surgery. *Br J Surg* 1988; **75**: 896–8.
88. Baillie J, Cairns S, Cotton P. Endoscopic management of choledocholithiasis during pregnancy. *Surgery* 1990; **171**: 1–4.
89. Binmoeller KF, Katon RM. Needle knife papillotomy for an impacted common bile duct stone during pregnancy. *Gastrointest Endosc* 1990; **36**: 607–9.
90. Beck G, Brodmekel G. Choledocholithiasis in pregnancy: treatment by endoscopic sphincterotomy. *Gastrointest Endosc* 1991; **100**: A252.
91. Brolin RE, Siemons GO, Fynan TM. Critical analysis of retained and residual common duct stones. *Am Surg* 1986; **52**: 588–93.
92. Danilewitz MD. Early postoperative endoscopic sphincterotomy for retained common bile duct stones. *Gastrointest Endosc* 1989; **35**: 298–9.
93. Cranley B, Logan H. Exploration of the common bile duct – the relevance of the clinical picture and the importance of preoperative cholangiography. *Br J Surg* 1980; **67**: 869–72.
94. Sheridan WG, Williams HOL, Lewis MH. Morbidity and mortality of common bile duct exploration. *Br J Surg* 1987; **74**: 1095–9.
95. Hill J, Martin F, Tweedle DEF. Risks of leaving the gallbladder in situ after endoscopic sphincterotomy for bile duct stones. *Br J Surg* 1991; **78**: 554–7.
96. Siegel JH, Safrany L, Ben-Zvi JS *et al.* Duodenoscopic sphincterotomy in patients with gallbladders in situ: report of a series of 1272 patients. *Am J Gastroenterol* 1988; **83**: 1255–8.
97. Escourrou J, Cordova JA, Lazorthes F, Frexinos J, Ribet A. Early and late complications after endoscopic sphincterotomy for biliary lithiasis with and without the gallbladder in situ. *Gut* 1984; **25**: 598–602.
98. Davidson BR, Neoptolemos JP, Carr-Locke DL. Endoscopic sphincterotomy for common bile duct calculi in patients with gallbladder in situ considered unfit for surgery. *Gut* 1988; **29**: 114–20.
99. Rosseland AR, Solhaug JH. Primary endoscopic papillotomy (EPT) in patients with stones in the common bile duct and the gallbladder in situ: a 5–8 year follow-up study. *World J Surg* 1988; **12**: 111–16.
100. Tanaka M, Ikeda S, Yoshimoto H, Matsumoto S. The long-term fate of the gallbladder after endoscopic sphincterotomy . *Am J Surg* 1987; **154**: 505–9.
101. Gracie W, Ransohoff D. The natural history of silent gallstones. *New Eng J Med* 1982; **307**: 798–800.
102. Worthley CS, Toouli J. Gallbladder non-filling: an indication for cholecystectomy after endoscopic sphincterotomy. *Br J Surg* 1988; **75**: 796–8.
103. Holbrook RF, Jacobson FL, Pezzuti RT, Howell DA. Biliary patency imaging after endoscopic retrograde sphincterotomy with gallbladder in situ: clinical impact of nonvisualization. *Arch Surg* 1991; **126**: 738–42.
104. Neoptolemos JP, Carr-Locke DL, Fossard DP. Prospective randomized study of preoperative endoscopic sphincterotomy versus surgery alone for common bile duct stones. *Br Med J* 1987; **294**: 470–4.

105. Stiegmann GV, Goff JS, Mansour A, Pearlman N, Reveille RM. Precholecystectomy endoscopic cholangiography and stone removal is not superior to cholecystectomy, cholangiography, and common duct exploration. *Am J Surg* 1992; **163**: 227–30.
106. The Southern Surgeons Club. A prospective analysis of 1518 laparoscopic cholecystectomies. *New Eng J Med* 1991; **324**: 1073–8.
107. NIH Consensus Conference on Gallstones and Laparoscopic Cholecystectomy. *Am J Surg* 1993; **165**: 390–547.
108. Flowers JL, Zucker KA, Graham SM, Scovill WA, Imbembo AL, Bailey RW. Laparoscopic cholangiography: results and indications. *Ann Surg* 1992; **215**: 209–16.
109. Sackier JM, Berci G, Phillips E, Carroll B, Shapiro S, Paz-Partlow M. The role of cholangiography in laparoscopic cholecystectomy. *Arch Surg* 1991; **126**: 1021–6.
110. Hunter JG. Laparoscopic transcystic common bile duct exploration. *Am J Surg* 1992; **163**: 53–6.
111. Cotton PB, Baillie J, Pappas TN, Meyers WS. Laparoscopic cholecystectomy and the biliary endoscopist. *Gastrointest Endosc* 1991; **37**: 94–7.
112. Del Santo P, Kazarian KK, Rogers JF, Bevins PA, Hall JR. Prediction of operative cholangiography in patients undergoing elective cholecystectomy with routine liver function chemistries. *Surgery* 1985; **98**: 7–11.
113. Hauer-Jensen M, Karesen R, Nygaard K *et al.* Predictive ability of choledocholithiasis indicators. *Ann Surg* 1985; **202**: 64–8.
114. Lacaine F, Corlette MB, Bismuth H. Preoperative evaluation of the risk of common bile duct stones. *Arch Surg* 1980; **115**: 1114–16.
115. Neuhaus H, Feussner H, Ungeheuer A, Hoffmann W, Siewert JR, Classen M. Prospective evaluation of the use of endoscopic retrograde cholangiography prior to laparoscopic cholecystectomy. Endoscopy 1992; **24**: 745–9.
116. Aliperti G, Edmundowicz SA, Soper NJ, Ashley SW. Combined endoscopic sphincterotomy and laparoscopic cholecystectomy in patients with choledocholithiasis and cholecystolithiasis. *Ann Intern Med* 1991; **115**: 783–5.
117. Boulay J, Schellenberg R, Brady PG. Role of ERCP and therapeutic biliary endoscopy in association with laparoscopic cholecystectomy. *Am J Gastroenterol* 1992; **87**: 837–42.
118. Cotton PB. Removing duct stones without sphincterotomy. *Gastrointest Endsoc* 1993; **39**: 312.
119. Ibuki Y, Kudo M, Todo A. Endoscopic retrograde extraction of common bile duct stones with drip infusion of isosorbide dinitrate. *Gastrointest Endosc* 1992; **38**: 178–80.
120. Staritz M, Poralla T, Dormeyer HH, Buschenfelde MZ. Endoscopic removal of common bile duct stones through the intact papilla after medical sphincter dilation. *Gastroenterology* 1985; **88**: 1807–11.
121. Deslandres E, Gagner M, Pomp A *et al.* Intraoperative endoscopic sphincterotomy for common bile duct stones during laparosopic cholecystectomy. *Gastrointest Endosc* 1993; **39**: 54–8.
122. Opie EL. The etiology of acute hemorrhagic pancreatitis. *Bull Johns Hopkins Hosp* 1901; **12**: 182–8.
123. Moody FG, Senninger N, Runkel N. Another challenge to the Opie myth. *Gastroenterology* 1993; **104**: 927–31.
124. Acosta JM, Ledesma CL. Gallstone migration as a cause of acute pancreatitis. *New Eng J Med* 1974; **290**: 484–7.
125. Kelly TR. Gallstone pancreatitis: the timing of surgery. *Surgery* 1980; **88**: 345–350.
126. Stone HH, Fabian TC, Dunlop WE. Gallstone pancreatitis. Biliary tract pathology in relation to time of operation. *Ann Surg* 1981; **194**: 305–12.
127. Acosta JM, Rossi R, Galli OMR, Pellegrini CA, Skinner DB. Early surgery for acute gallstone pancreatitis: evaluation of a systematic approach. *Surgery* 1978; **83**: 367–70.

128. Leese T, Shaw D. Comparison of three Glasgow multifactor prognostic scoring systems in acute pancreatitis. *Br J Surg* 1988; **75**: 460–2.
129. Osborne DH, Imrie CW, Carter DC. Biliary surgery in the same admission for gallstone-associated pancreatitis. *Br J Surg* 1981; **68**: 758–61.
130. Ranson JHC. The timing of biliary surgery in acute pancreatitis. *Ann Surg* 1979; **189**: 654–62.
131. Kim U, Bosner B. Timing of surgery for acute gallstone pancreatitis. *Am J Surg* 1988; **156**: 393–6.
132. Kelly TR. Wagner DS. Gallstone pancreatitis: a prospective randomized trial of the timing of surgery. *Surgery* 1988; **104**: 600–5.
133. Safrany L, Cotton PB. A preliminary report: urgent duodenoscopic sphincterotomy for acute gallstone pancreatitis. *Surgery* 1981; **89**: 424–8.
134. Rosseland AR, Solhaug JH. Early or delayed endoscopic papillotomy (EPT) in gallstone pancreatitis. *Ann Surg* 1984; **199**: 165–7.
135. Shemesh E, Czerniak A, Schneabaum S, Nass S. Early endoscopic sphincterotomy in the management of acute gallstone pancreatitis in elderly patients. *Am Geriat Soc* 1990; **38**: 893–6.
136. Neoptolemos JP, Carr-Locke DL, London NJ, Bailey IA, James D, Fossard DP. Controlled trial of urgent endoscopic retrograde cholangiopancreatography and endoscopic sphincterotomy versus conservative treatment for acute pancreatitis due to gallstones. *Lancet* 1988; **2**: 979–83.
137. Fan ST, Lai ECS, Mok FPT, Lo CM, Zheng SS, Wong J. Early treatment of acute biliary pancreatitis by endoscopic papillotomy. *New Eng J Med* 1993; **328**: 228–32.
138. Ros E, Navarro S, Bru C, Garcia-Puges A, Valderrama R. Occult microlithiasis in "idiopathic" acute pancreatitis: prevention of relapses by cholecystectomy or ursodeoxycholic acid therapy. *Gastroenterology* 1991; **101**: 1701–9.
139. Lee SP, Nicholls JF, Park HZ. Biliary sludge as a cause of acute pancreatitis. *New Eng J Med* 1992; **326**: 589–93.
140. May GR, Shaffer EH. Should elective endoscopic sphincterotomy replace cholecystectomy for the treatment of high-risk patients with gallstone pancreatitis? *J Clin Gastroenterol* 1991; **13**: 125–8.
141. Csendes A, Sepulveda A, Burdiles P *et al.* Common bile duct pressure in patients with common bile duct stones with or without acute suppurative cholangitis. *Arch Surg* 1988; **123**: 697–9.
142. Reynolds BM, Dargan EI. Acute obstructive cholangitis – a distinct clinical syndrome. *Ann Surg* 1959; **150**: 299–303.
143. Boey JH, Way LW. Acute cholangitis. *Ann Surg* 1980; **191**: 264–70.
144. Gould RJ, Vogelzang, Neimen HL, Pearl JG, Politcha SM. Percutaneous biliary drainage as an initial therapy of the biliary tract. *Surg Gynecol Obstet* 1985; **160**: 523–7.
145. Kadir S, Baassiri A, Barth KH, Kaufman SL, Cameron JL, White RT. Percutaneous transhepatic biliary drainage in the management of biliary sepsis. *Am J Roentgenol* 1982; **138**: 25–9.
146. Pessa ME, Hawkins IF, Vogel SB. The treatment of acute cholangitis. Percutaneous transhepatic biliary drainage before definitive therapy. *Ann Surg* 1987; **205**: 389–92.
147. Ditzel H, Schaffalitzky DE, Muckadell OB. Endoscopic sphincterotomy in acute cholangitis due to choledocholithiasis. *Hepatogastroenterol* 1990; **37**: 204–7.
148. Leese T, Neoptolemos JP, Baker AR, Carr-Locke DL. Management of acute cholangitis and the impact of endoscopic sphincterotomy. *Br J Surg* 1986; **73**: 988–92.
149. Leung JW, Chung SCS, Sung JJY, Banez VP, Li AKC. Urgent endoscopic drainage for acute suppurative cholangitis. *Lancet* 1989; **1**: 1307–9.

150. Gogel HK, Runyon BA, Volpicelli NA, Palmer RC. Acute suppurative obstructive cholangitis due to stones: treatment by urgent endoscopic sphincterotomy. *Gastrointest Endosc* 1987; **33**: 210–13.
151. Nunez D, Guerra JJ, Al-Sheikh WA, Russell E, Mendez G Jr. Percutaneous biliary drainage in acute suppurative cholangitis. *Gastrointest Radiol* 1986; **11**: 85–9.
152. Ikeda S, Tanaka M, Itoh H, Kishikawa H, Nakayama F. Emergency decompression of bile duct in acute obstructive suppurative cholangitis by duodenoscopic cannulation: a lifesaving procedure. *World J Surg* 1981; **5**: 587–93.
153. Lai ECS, Mok FPT, Tan ESY *et al.* Endoscopic biliary drainage for severe acute cholangitis. *New Eng J Med* 1992; **326**: 1582–6.
154. Lai ECS, Paterson IA, Tam PC, Choi TK, Fan ST, Wong J. Severe acute cholangitis: the role of emergency nasobiliary drainage. *Surgery* 1990; **107**: 268–72.

6.3

Laparoscopic Management of Choledocholithiasis

J. PETELIN

INTRODUCTION

The telescopic approach to cholecystectomy, which has become the gold standard for surgical treatment of cholelithiasis, solved many problems for physicians, surgeons and patients alike.[1,2] As of the early 1990s, physicians and surgeons no longer had to expect the morbidity of pulmonary and deep venous complications and other associated medical problems that had previously accompanied referral of their patients for open cholecystectomy. Patients, too, benefited from decreased pain, better cosmesis and a much quicker return to preoperative lifestyle. However, along with these solutions came new problems.

One of the most notable of these new concerns is the management of abnormalities of the biliary ductal system. Choledocholithiasis is present in approximately 10% of patients who present with symptomatic gall bladder disease.[3,4] Whereas in the era of open cholecystectomy, 1888–1988, preoperative, intraoperative and postoperative diagnosis and treatment protocols for choledocholithiasis became firmly established, the biliary tract surgeon of the 1990s and beyond is faced with a variety of modalities and options for handling this issue. Initially, because of unfamiliarity with equipment and lack of technical skill, surgeons pursued an "avoidance" approach. Common duct stones suspected preoperatively were either considered a contraindication to laparoscopic cholecystectomy or were treated with preoperative endoscopic retrograde retrieval techniques. Selective rather than routine intraoperative cholangiography helped ensure that the surgeon wouldn't have to deal with common duct stones found intraoperatively. Nevertheless, as experienced leaders in the field demonstrated the importance of the other reasons to perform intraoperative cholangiograms, namely for accurate anatomical definition and for development of proficiency, methods to perform them efficiently developed quickly. Similarly, a variety of manoeuvres to clear the common duct during laparoscopic cholecystectomy were relatively rapidly established.

The addition of these techniques to the surgical armamentarium is seen as a positive step towards integrating a multimodal or multidisciplinary approach for management of choledocholithiasis. Preoperative evaluation and treatment of common duct abnormalities still has a place in this protocol, as does postoperative management of retained stones. Nevertheless, the degree of dependence on such "non-surgical" modalities decreases as experience and technical skill with laparoscopic methods is achieved by the biliary tract surgeon. The surgeon is advised to incorporate these techniques into his or her own protocol.

PATIENT MANAGEMENT

Patients with biliary tract symptoms may or may not present with signs or symptoms suggestive of choledocholithiasis. The routine preoperative work-up includes history, physical examination, evaluation of liver and pancreatic chemistries, sonography of the abdomen and, in Europe, intravenous cholangiography. Nuclear imaging may be useful in some cases.

Choledocholithiasis may be suspected in patients who describe or exhibit jaundice. Elevated bilirubin, alkaline phosphatase, transaminase and amylase levels increase the suspicion of common duct stones. Sonographic detection of ductal stones is not usually very accurate, but nuclear imaging may be helpful by revealing no flow of nucleotide into the duodenum. In Europe, intravenous cholangiography is often helpful in documenting the status of the common bile duct in patients suspected of harbouring common duct calculi; its use in the United States has been limited because of governmental concerns regarding the contrast agent.

When the preoperative presentation suggests choledocholithiasis, the clinician must decide whether to attempt clearance of the duct before, during or after laparoscopic cholecystectomy. Endoscopic retrograde clearance (ERC) techniques have been shown to be effective in over 90% of cases.[5–10] There is, however, an indisputable failure rate and the procedure is not without recognized morbidity. Intraoperative laparoscopic common duct exploration has also been shown to be an effective method of clearing the duct, with success rates in experienced hands of over 90%.[11–14] The approach chosen will depend on local expertise in the various procedures, the availability of equipment and the condition of the patient. Figure 6.3.1 depicts a logical framework that may be applied to the management of suspected choledocholithiasis. It should be modified by the surgeon based on the factors listed above.

When stones are found at the time of laparoscopic cholecystectomy, the decision making process is similar to that mentioned above. The surgeon may proceed with laparoscopic common duct exploration (CDE), convert to open common duct exploration or leave the ductal stones in place for subsequent treatment with ERC, lithotripsy, dissolution or observation. Each of these alternatives has its proponents and its own potential benefits and drawbacks.

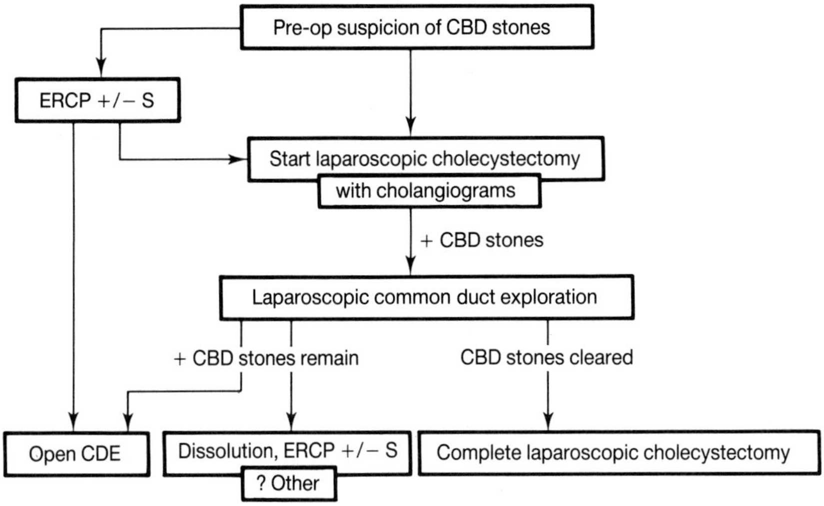

Figure 6.3.1 Protocol for management of common bile duct stones.

The surgeon should decide which is most surgically appropriate, efficient and cost effective for each patient.

EQUIPMENT

It is assumed that standard laparoscopic equipment is available to perform laparoscopic cholecystectomy. In addition to that, cholangiography hardware, including a fluoroscopic unit, is considered state of the art in the 1990s. A variety of devices may be used to obtain access for cholangiograms, but the author prefers a relatively low technology set which includes a 2″ long 14 gauge intravenous catheter, a standard cholangiography catheter and a laparoscopic clip.

Embolectomy balloon-type catheters are also often useful. A 4 French vascular embolectomy catheter fits nicely through the 14 gauge sleeve and the balloon is large enough to be effective in most common ducts. The open surgery biliary balloon catheter is not long enough to be of use here.

Stone retrieval baskets, available in helical (Dormia-type) or straight wire (Segura-type) configurations, are essential elements of a laparoscopic common duct exploration kit. Each surgeon will develop a preference regarding basket type. The author prefers a 4-wire straight configuration for most common duct work because its shape expands to dilate the duct for excellent exposure and because the interstices are large enough to capture most stones. Most of these baskets are less than or equal to 1 mm maximum outside diameter so that they will fit into the working channel of the newer small diameter flexible choledochoscopes.

Choledochoscopes have undergone dramatic changes in the past five years. In order to accommodate minimal access techniques, such as transcystic common duct exploration, the outside diameter of these devices has shrunk to less than 3 mm. Despite this miniaturization, the optical quality remains excellent. The light-delivering capacity is adequate to illuminate all but the most dramatically dilated ducts. Flexibility is generally increased over larger models because of the smaller outside diameter of the scope itself. The only major limitation of the smaller diameter scope is that the working channel is almost completely filled when a basket is in place. This limits saline instillation since basket and saline introduction occur through the same channel. This factor becomes significant when trying to locate a stone in a convoluted duct with the basket in place.

Most choledochoscopes are suited to coupling with a video camera. While a second camera set-up is not essential, it certainly facilitates choledochoscopic manipulations. With a second camera system, the surgeon's non-dominant hand is free to manoeuvre the scope and/or basket instead of being used to support the eyepiece for direct visual contact. Additionally, the surgeon's view of the laparoscopic field is not eliminated by having to concentrate on the choledochoscopic image alone. The surgeon and team members may view both the laparoscopic and choledochoscopic images on the video monitors connected to the cameras.

A significantly more efficient system of video display may be obtained by employing a video mixer to render both images on the same monitor (Fig. 6.3.2). This still requires a second camera system, but a second monitor system is not necessary. Using this arrangement, clutter is reduced in the operating theatre. Visual fatigue is also significantly decreased, since the surgeon isn't required to alternate from one monitor to the other during the exploration.

In order to employ a transcystic approach, cystic duct dilators are often necessary. Two basic types are available: graduated, over-the-wire dilators and pneumatic balloon dilators. The former have the advantage of being relatively inexpensive and can be found in most urology departments. The latter are thought to have an added degree of safety, since the mechanism of dilation is uniform radial force rather than shearing force. When using the graduated type, successively larger diameter dilators are advanced over a guide wire. Pneumatic dilators are also advanced over a guide wire, but are actuated with a screw-type syringe. An attached gauge allows accurate measurement of the amount of pressure being exerted on the dilatation balloon.

Initial reports of laparoscopic common duct intervention suggested that lithotripters might play a large role in the minimal access approach to choledocholithiasis.[14] Electrohydraulic, mechanical and laser models have been used, but have not become the mainstay of laparoscopic common duct exploration that some thought they might. Both the electrohydraulic and laser models have the added potential of duct injury associated with their use. Additionally, laser models are prohibitively expensive.

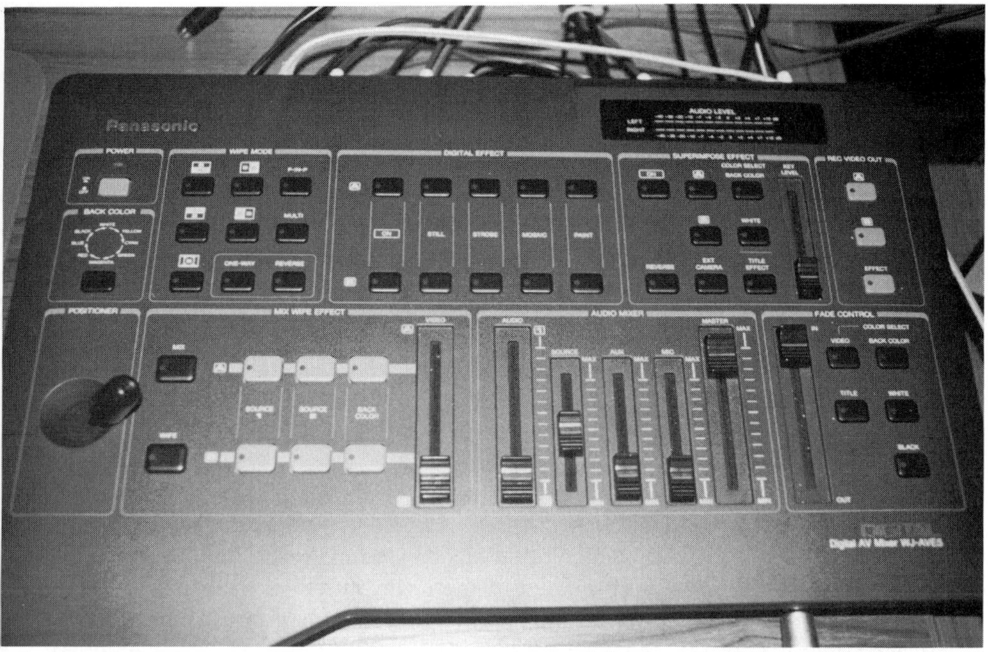

(a) Video mixer (switcher). (Model: Panasonic WJ AVE5.)

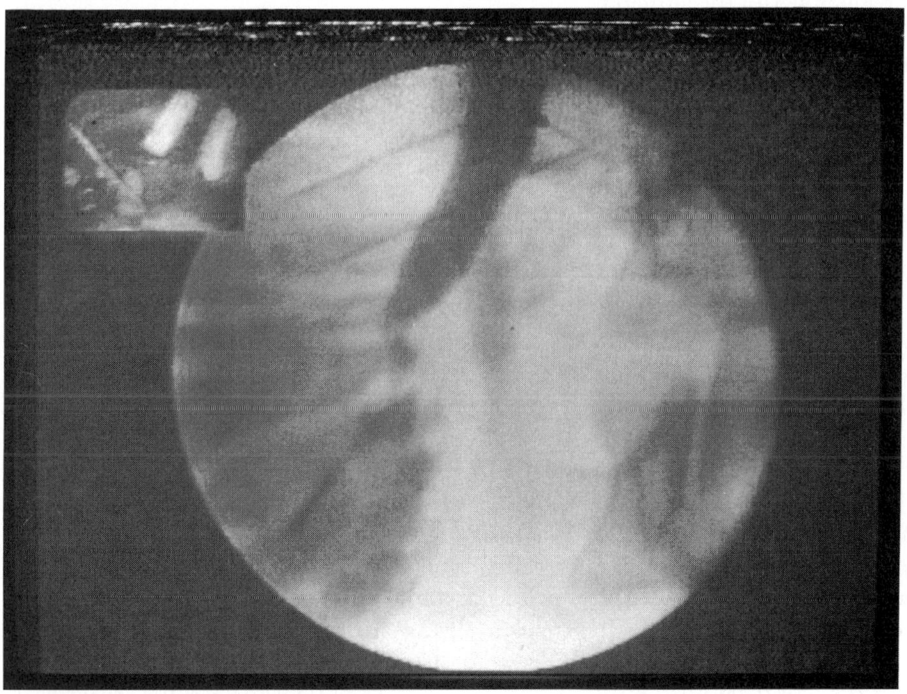

(b) Video mixing effect. Two full images displayed on the same monitor, one maximized and one minimized.

Figure 6.3.2

Additional equipment, which is usually present in the theatre already, includes a laparoscopic scalpel or scissors, T-tubes and laparoscopic needle holders. Attempts at common duct exploration without the necessary equipment neatly organized on a separate trolley is fraught with chaos and frustration and commonly an unsuccessful outcome. The surgeon should communicate these needs to the administrator of the operating suites so that the experience of common duct exploration is a positive one for all involved.

OPERATIVE TECHNIQUE

Overview

Laparoscopic common duct exploration involves the application of a number of techniques in a rational protocol that evolves from lesser to more invasive manoeuvres. These will be discussed in the order in which the author usually employs them. In most situations, only a few of the manoeuvres will be required to clear the duct. In others (e.g. intrahepatic or impacted stones), not only will all of the known techniques be needed, but their effective application may tax the ingenuity of the surgeon.

The following considerations are included in the current approach to common duct exploration:

Porta hepatis exposure
Cholangiography
Balloon and/or basket manoeuvres
Dilatation of the cystic duct
Choledochotomy
Choledochoscopic manoeuvres
T-tube placement
Completion cholangiography
Cholecystectomy

Porta Hepatis Exposure

This discussion assumes that laparoscopic access for cholecystectomy, using a four port configuration, has already been achieved. With the patient in the supine position, the dissection in the porta hepatis is commenced in the usual fashion in order to expose the cystic artery, cystic duct and at least a portion of the common duct. Better visualization of this area may be obtained by using a reverse Trendelenburg position and rotating the patient toward the left lateral decubitus position. This displaces the hepatic flexure of the colon and the duodenal sweep inferiorly and medially away from the porta hepatis. In routine laparoscopic cholecystectomy, the dissection in the triangle of Calot is limited in order to avoid injury to the common duct. When common duct exploration is indicated, however, more detailed dissection is often necessary. Usually it is helpful to expose the common hepatic and common bile duct, unless inflammatory reaction in this area makes such dissection hazardous. Occasionally the cystic duct will enter the common duct posteriorly. This arrangement makes instrument and scope entry into the common duct from the cystic duct quite difficult. It may be improved by releasing the lateral attachments of the duodenum, i.e. Kocher's manoeuvre, as well as the lateral attachments of the cystic–common duct junction. This allows the junction to be "unwrapped" when gentle traction is applied on the cystic duct.

Cholangiography

Mirizzi introduced intraoperative cholangiography in 1932.[15] The procedure gained widespread acceptance until the last decade when a re-evaluation of its role in open surgery resulted in more selective, rather than routine application.[16–18] Laparoscopic cholangiography was first performed by Calamé in 1954.[19] At that time, however, the current arsenal of laparoscopic instrumentation was not available, so the films were of diagnostic value only. In the more recent era of laparoscopic surgery for biliary tract disease, however, many experts have encouraged a return to routine use of intraoperative cholangiography.[20–27] Three reasons are cited for this recommendation: to define accurately the anatomy, to establish proficiency with the technique and to identify common duct pathology.[11] Many of these experts believe that arguments opposed to this stance have their true basis in lack of familiarity with the technique and lack of proficiency in its application. Certainly the added anatomical information provided by a fluoroscopic evaluation of the ductal system is of tremendous benefit to those who have become proficient in its use. In experienced hands, the entire cholangiographic event, from cannulation of the duct to completion of the radiological evaluation, is usually accomplished in less than five minutes.

Two methods of laparoscopically directed cystic duct cholangiography have been developed: the portal method, advanced by Reddick and Olsen in 1989,[28] and the percutaneous method developed by the author in 1990.[29] In the former, a cholangiocatheter is loaded into a specialized clamp which is advanced through one of the ports in the right upper quadrant. The catheter is placed into the cystic duct and secured into position with the loading clamp. Since the initial reports of this technique, a number of other devices which use a portal approach have been manufactured to provide the surgeon with a wide selection from which to choose.

The percutaneous method is felt by the author to be much easier to learn and provides benefits not provided by the portal method. Here, a 14 gauge intravenous sheath is advanced through the abdominal wall approximately 3 cm medial to the midclavicular port. A cholangiocatheter is inserted through this sheath and advanced into the cystic duct with forceps introduced through the medial epigastric port. It is fixed into position with a clip partially applied at a right angle to its axis. Because the forceps controlling the gall bladder don't have to be removed to allow access for the catheter, better exposure is maintained during cannulation and more rapid resumption of the procedure is allowed after completion of the films. Additionally, the 14 gauge sheath may be used as an access route for balloon catheters and baskets during common duct exploration. When it is not in use, the sheath may be capped with a standard terminal cap.

With either method, a variety of cholangiocatheters may be used. In some cases, however, the cystic duct is difficult to cannulate. This may be secondary to scarring, inflammation, inherently small diameter or Heister valves. In these situations the author has found that an epidural catheter works very nicely; in fact, the author has not encountered a case in which the cystic duct cannot be accessed with it. Caution must be used when fixing it into position, however, since it may be easily occluded by an overly zealous clip or clamp application.

In the past, standard radiographs were used to record the cholangiogram. While this method has certainly proved its value, digital fluoroscopic cholangiography promises to supplant it by offering the advantages of real-time high resolution radiographic imaging of the entire ductal system. There is no delay in waiting for films to be developed and the surgeon may control the C-arm of the fluoroscope so that specific areas of the ductal system may be scanned and rescanned at his or her discretion. Magnification views and computerized image enhancement capabilities afforded by these units allow a highly detailed examination of the entire ductal system within minutes. The output of the unit may be routed to the video mixer so that both the laparoscopic and fluoroscopic signals may be displayed on the same video monitor. This enhances efficiency.

Initial Manoeuvres to Clear the Duct

When spasm is suspected to be the cause of distal ductal obstruction, relaxation may be achieved by administration of 1–2 mg of intravenous glucagon. When combined with flushing of the duct with saline, this technique quite often converts an abnormal cholangiogram into a normal one.

When this is not successful, a 4 French Fogarty balloon catheter is inserted through the 14 gauge sleeve, through the cystic duct and into the common duct. It is advanced into the duodenum and the balloon inflated. Gentle traction on the catheter, with forceps inserted through the medial epigastric port, produces movement of the duodenum at an intraductal catheter length of approximately 8 cm. At that point, the balloon is deflated and the catheter is withdrawn approximately 1 cm. The balloon is reinflated and the catheter withdrawn under the guidance of forceps inserted through the medial epigastric port. Not infrequently, stones and/or debris will be expressed through the cystic duct with this manoeuvre. Although the potential for displacement of stones into the proximal hepatic system is present, the author has not encountered this situation in over 100 laparoscopic common duct explorations. Obviously, in a number of cases this technique is not successful in clearing the duct. Nevertheless, it is a relatively harmless manoeuvre that may be employed while the surgeon awaits the preparation of the choledochoscopic equipment.

The next step in attempting to clear the duct involves the use of a stone retrieval basket. This is inserted through the 14 gauge sleeve, into the cystic duct and into the common duct. Its exact location in the bile duct may be monitored with the fluoroscope. Both the laparoscopic and fluoroscopic representations of the surgical manipulations may be displayed on the same video monitor using the video mixer. This greatly enhances the surgeon's efficiency. Accurate localization of ductal stones is facilitated by leaving some contrast material in the system. As basket manipulations are performed, however, the contrast naturally leaks from the duct. If visualization is poor, the basket may have to be removed and more contrast instilled with the cholangiocatheter. Once the stone is captured, the basket is guided out of the duct with the forceps inserted through the medial epigastric port. The stone is delivered onto the omentum and retrieved with forceps inserted through the medial epigastric port.

In some cases, the author has employed the basket technique without the use of a fluoroscope. This application requires prior calibration of the length of the duct and the basket so that precise localization of the wire frame of the basket is maintained and accidental capture of the papilla is avoided. Stone capture in this situation is heralded by failure of the control handle of the basket to close completely. When the surgeon recognizes this, the basket is guided out of the duct using forceps inserted through the medial epigastric port. Obviously the yield here is less than superb, but it is a safe technique that may be employed while the surgeon is otherwise just waiting for preparation of the choledochoscope.

Dilatation of the Cystic Duct

When neither of the methods above results in clearance of the duct, choledochoscopic intervention usually becomes necessary. Although some authors prefer to perform a choledochotomy here,[30–32] common duct access for the choledochoscope can be achieved through the cystic duct in most cases.[11–14] In some instances, the cystic duct will already be large enough to accept the newer generation of 9 and 10 French-sized choledochoscopes. In others, dilatation is necessary.

To accomplish this task, a guide wire (0.028 or 0.035″ diameter) is inserted through the midclavicular port into the cystic duct. It is advanced into the common duct with forceps inserted through the medial epigastric port. Over this wire, either mechanical-graduated or pneumatic dilators are advanced until the cystic duct is large enough to accept the choledochoscope. When graduated dilators are used, the author has found that if the cystic duct won't initially accept at least a 9 French size, it is unlikely that it will allow dilatation to the 11 or 12 French size necessary to provide for easy motion of the scope in and out of the duct. In these cases, the surgeon should consider choledochotomy or other techniques to clear the duct, rather than risk tearing the cystic–common duct junction. When pneumatic dilators are used, the surgeon should monitor not only the pressure in the dilatation balloon, but also the visual representation of the process on the video screen. In this way, accurate location of the balloon and avoidance of injury can be ensured.

Choledochotomy

When the cystic duct cannot be dilated enough to accept the scope or to allow removal of the largest stone in the common duct choledochotomy may be necessary. Intrahepatic stones present another situation in which direct common duct access is preferred. This may be accomplished with a laparoscopic scalpel, scissors or Nd.Yag contact tip laser. Electrocautery and other laser types should not be used for this manoeuvre.

The choledochotomy may be performed by cutting the cystic duct along its axis until a large enough opening in the common duct is produced. This technique is especially useful when a large stone has already been captured but defies attempts to remove it from the cystic duct. It has the disadvantage of making the closure of the choledochotomy somewhat more complicated.

Alternatively, the common duct may be opened longitudinally at a separate site on its anterior surface. This has the advantage of allowing the surgeon to select the best location for the choledochotomy. Additionally, closure of this defect is usually easier than that of the extended cystic duct choledochotomy.

Interestingly, "stay sutures", which are commonly used in open common duct exploration, are not necessary here. The choledochoscope can usually be easily advanced into the common duct without lateral retraction of the duct walls at the choledochotomy site. This avoids the potential complication of a ductal tear from excessively vigorous traction on such sutures.

Choledochoscopic manoeuvres

The choledochoscope is inserted through the midclavicular port. A guide wire left in place after cystic duct dilatation sometimes facilitates introduction into the ductal system. The scope is controlled laparoscopically with atraumatic forceps inserted through the medial epigastric port. Once the common duct is entered, saline is instilled through the working port of the scope in order to gently distend the duct; without this, visualization is limited. Further manipulations usually require the surgeon to place both hands on the choledochoscope.

One hand controls the deflection lever on the head piece, while the other provides torque on the body of the scope at its trocar insertion site at the level of the skin. The surgeon then negotiates the duct until the stone is identified.

These manoeuvres require that both the laparoscopic and choledochoscopic images be monitored simultaneously. This is most efficiently accomplished by placing both of the images on the same video screen using the video mixer described above. The author conceived the use of this technology in 1991 and has employed it extensively since then.[33] Laparoscopic choledochoscopy without this mixer is time-consuming, arduous and inefficient.

After the stone is located, the surgeon transfers control of the body of the choledochoscope to the assistant who must provide the same amount of torque on it in order keep the stone in view. The saline instillation through the working channel of the scope is temporarily interrupted, and a stone retrieval basket is inserted until its tip is seen protruding from the end of the scope. It is advanced past the stone, opened and withdrawn to the level of the stone. If immediate capture is not achieved, the surgeon must apply an oscillating motion to the basket in order to allow the stone to fall within its interstices. The basket is closed around the stone. The entire ensemble, stone, basket and choledochoscope, is then guided out of the duct with forceps from the medial epigastric port. The stone is delivered onto the omentum, where it is retrieved with forceps from the medial epigastric port. Alternatively, it may be placed in a small bag (the amputated finger of a size 8 glove serves well for this purpose) and temporarily stored in the abdomen for final removal with the gall bladder later in the case.

In some cases, the size or configuration of the stone(s) makes their entrapment seemingly impossible. Here, insertion of the balloon-tipped catheter (e.g. Fogarty) through the 14 gauge sleeve, through the cystic duct and alongside the choledochoscope may be useful. The balloon is advanced past the stone, inflated and withdrawn back toward the choledochoscope. Once the stone is trapped in this position, the entire scope–stone–balloon aggregate may be removed as a unit.[11]

Stones impacted in the distal duct may initially be fragmented with a lithotripter in order to more easily displace them off the wall. Great caution and accurate localization of the lithotripter probe tip is essential here, however, to ensure that duct wall damage is avoided. While lithotripsy may be invaluable in this situation, its routine use for any common duct stones is discouraged because of the amount of debris that is generated. This clouds the fluid in the duct and limits visualization of stones and debris.

The author has also found that irrigation with a pulsatile saline jet (e.g. Waterpik (R)) is useful to remove diffusely adherent minute particles from the duct wall. Since there are no commercially made adapters for this application, the surgeon will need to fashion a connection to his or her particular choledochoscope.

Intrahepatic stones are usually approached through a choledochotomy unless the cystic duct is short and oriented perpendicular to the common duct. Stone capture is accomplished in the same fashion as for distal stones. The small size of

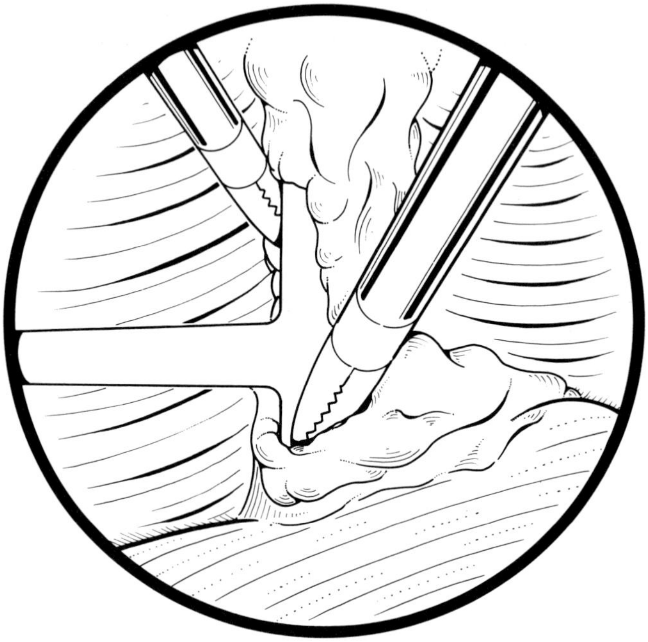

Figure 6.3.3 Laparoscopic T-tube placement.

these ducts sometimes limits full deployment of the basket, making stone capture difficult. The balloon trapping technique is useful in this situation.

If a drainage procedure is indicated, it may be accomplished at the time of laparoscopic common duct exploration. De Paula has demonstrated that antegrade sphincterotomy is safe and effective.[34] The sphincterotome is advanced alongside the choledochoscope through the common duct into the duodenum. Its position is accurately determined by simultaneous duodenal inspection with a side-viewing duodenoscope. Gagner also advocates intraoperative sphincterotomy, but he prefers insertion of the sphincterotome through the duodenoscope.[35] With either method, care must be taken to limit the amount of air instilled into the duodenum so that laparoscopic visualization of the porta hepatis is not compromised.

T-tube Placement

If a choledochotomy is used to access the common duct, it is usually closed around a T-tube (Fig. 6.3.3). The T-tube is prepared in the standard fashion, loaded into an 8 mm sheath and introduced into the abdomen through the medial epigastric port.[11,36] The duct is then closed with interrupted or continuous sutures of 4-0 Vicryl®. It is important for the surgeon to take advantage of the magnification afforded by the choledochoscope and camera so that accurate approximation of the duct walls may be accomplished without injury or stricture. Intracorporeal knot tying techniques are preferred here, since they are inherently more delicate than the extracorporeal method.

Completion Cholangiography

After the ductal exploration is completed, cholangiograms are repeated. If the transcystic method was employed, the cholangiocatheter must be reinserted through the 14 gauge sleeve and secured in the cystic duct. If a T-tube has been placed, contrast may be injected through it. If the films demonstrate residual stones, the surgeon must decide whether to proceed with further laparoscopic attempts to clear the duct, whether to convert to open exploration or whether to leave the stones in place for subsequent treatment with ERCP, lithotripsy or dissolution agents.

Cholecystectomy

After completion of the cholangiograms, the cystic duct is clipped or ligated. In cases where a T-tube has been inserted, this will already have been done. It is important to ensure that the cystic duct is secure. In cases where it is >5–6 mm in diameter, or where subsequent ERCP is possible, it is best to use a ligature and clips rather than to depend on clips alone.

If a T-tube has been placed, it is usually best to withdraw it back into the abdomen temporarily and occlude its tip with a clip. This provides better exposure of the porta hepatis and decreases the likelihood of accidental displacement from the common duct during gall bladder dissection. After the gall bladder has been separated from the liver, the T-tube may be passed out of one of the 5 mm ports in the right upper quadrant prior to closure. A closed-system drain is also placed in this area and brought out through the other 5 mm port site in the right upper quadrant.

The gall bladder is then removed through the umbilicus while the process is monitored with the camera in the medial epigastric port. The fascia at the umbilicus is closed with O-Vicryl® with the camera still in place in the epigastrium. The posterior aspect of the umbilical closure is checked for haemostasis. If it is not secure, one of the 5 mm ports (usually the drain site) is re-established and the electrocautery is used to control the bleeding. The drain is then replaced through the 5 mm site. The medial epigastric port is removed, the abdomen is deflated and the fascia at that site is closed with O-Vicryl® suture. The skin is closed at each site with subcuticular suture of 4-0 Vicryl®.

RESULTS

The author has employed these techniques of common duct exploration since first undertaking laparoscopic cholecystectomy in 1989. Up to January 1993,

1128 patients have undergone laparoscopic cholecystectomy. Twenty-nine patients with suspected choledocholithiasis underwent preoperative endoscopic retrograde cholangiography. Operative cholangiography was performed in 1027 patients (89%) and abnormal films were observed in 104. Eighteen of these patients underwent postoperative endoscopic retrograde cholangiography which confirmed stones in the common bile duct of five patients. In all five of these patients, the stones were successfully removed following endoscopic sphincterotomy. Laparoscopic duct exploration (LCDE) was attempted in the remaining 86 patients.

LCDE was performed successfully in 83 of 86 patients (97%), three patients going on to open cholecystectomy and duct exploration due to failure of LCDE. Fogarty balloon extraction of stones or dilation of the cystic duct was successful in 28 (34%) patients. Basket extraction techniques were successful in five further patients. Choledochoscopic duct clearance was successfully accomplished in 50 (60%) patients.

LCDE increased the operating time from a mean of 83 minutes for laparoscopic cholecystectomy alone to 146 minutes. The mean postoperative stay in hospital was also increased from 24 hours to 46 hours. There were seven complications in patients undergoing LCDE. Two patients went on to postoperative ERC for retained stones. One 89 year old female who underwent successful removal of two unsuspected common duct stones suffered a myocardial infarction on the first postoperative day and died. Another 96 year old patient suffered a cerebrovascular accident but recovered without significant neurological deficit. One patient developed transient right upper quadrant pain and underwent a normal postoperative endoscopic retrograde cholangiogram. Two patients required further treatment for urinary retention.

DISCUSSION

Laparoscopic cholecystectomy is now established as the treatment of choice for symptomatic gallstone disease and surgeons worldwide have become increasingly proficient in its technique. There remain several options for the management of common duct stones, ranging from preoperative endoscopic retrograde cholangiography through laparoscopic common duct exploration to postoperative endoscopic retrograde cholangiography. All of these procedures have major roles to play and the emphasis placed on each of these will depend upon the availability of local expertise. However, the ability to perform successful laparoscopic common duct exploration with low morbidity, as has been reported here and in other studies,[12–14] makes this technique an attractive option for the management of both suspected and unsuspected ductal stones. As more surgeons become experienced in advanced laparoscopic techniques, laparoscopic common duct exploration will undoubtedly become more popular. This, in turn, will permit the surgeon to offer the same spectrum of surgical procedures laparoscopically to the patient with symptomatic gallstone disease as has, until now, only been possible at open surgery.

REFERENCES

1. Dubois F, Icard P, Berthelot G, Levard H. Coelioscopic cholecystectomy. Preliminary report of 36 Cases. *Ann Surg* 1990, 211: 60–2.
2. Reddick E, Olsen D, Daniell J *et al.* Laparoscopic cholecystectomy. *Laser Med Surg News Adv* 1989; February: 38–40
3. Way LW, Admirand WJ, Dunphy JE. Management of choledocholithiasis. *Ann Surg* 1972; **176**: 347–59.
4. DenBesten L, Doty JE. Choledocholithiasis. *Surg Clin North Am* 1981; **61**: 893–907.
5. Aliperti G, Edmundowicz SA, Soper NJ, Ashley SW. Combined endoscopic sphincterotomy and laparoscopic cholecystectomy in patients with choledocholithiasis and cholecystolithiasis. *Ann Int Med* 1991; **115**: 783–5.
6. Cronin KJ, Kerin MJ, Williams NN *et al.* Endoscopic management of common duct stones with laparoscopic cholecystectomy. *I.J.M.S.* 1991: **160**: 265–97.
7. Cotton PB. Endoscopic management of bile duct stones (apples and oranges). *Gut* 1984; **25**: 587–97.
8. Carr-Locke DL. Acute gallstone pancreatitis and endoscopic therapy. *Endoscopy* 1990; **22**: 180–3.
9. Traverso L, Kozarek R, Ball T *et al.* Endoscopic retrograde cholangiopancreatography after laparoscopic cholecystectomy. *Am J Surg* 1993; **165**: 581–6.
10. Arregui ME, Davis CJ, Arkush AM, Nagan RF. Laparoscopic cholecystectomy combined with endoscopic sphincterotomy and stone extraction or laparoscopic choledochoscopy and electrohydraulic lithotripsy for management of cholelithiasis with choledocholithiasis. *Surg Endos* 1992; **6**: 10–15.
11. Petelin J. Laparoscopic approach to common duct pathology. *Surg Lap & Endosc* 1991; **1**: 33–41.
12. Hunter JG. Laparoscopic transcystic common bile duct exploration. *Am J Surg* 1992; **163**: 53–8.
13. Carroll BJ, Phillips EH, Daykhovsky L *et al.* Laparoscopic choledochoscopy: an effective approach to the common duct. *J Laparoendosc Surg* 1992; **2**: 15–21.
14. Birkett D. Technique of cholangiography and cystic duct choledochoscopy at the time of laparoscopic cholecystectomy for laser lithotripsy. *Surg Endosc* 1992; **6**: 252–4.
15. Mirizzi P. Operative cholangiography. *Surg, Gynecol & Obstet* 1937, **65**. 701–10.
16. Grogono JL, Woods W. Selective use of operative cholangiography. *World J Surg* 1986; **10**: 1009–13.
17. Del Santo P, Kazarian K, Rogers F, Bevins P, Hall J. Prediction of operative cholangiography in patients undergoing elective cholecystectomy with routine liver function chemistries. *Surgery* 1985; **98**: 7–11.
18. Gregg R. The case for selective cholangiography. *Am J Surg* 1988; **155**: 540–5.
19. Calame A, Montant R. La cholangiographie laparoscopique son interet diagnostique preoperatoire. *Helv Chir Acta* 1954; **21**: 438–40.
20. Hunter J. Avoidance of bile duct injury during laparoscopic cholecystectomy. *Am J Surg* 1991; **162**: 71–6.
21. Phillips E, Berci G, Carroll B, Daykhovsky L, Sackier J, Paz-Partlow M. The importance of intraoperative cholangiography during laparoscopic cholecystectomy. *Am Surg* 1990; **56**: 792–5.

22. Handy J, Rose S, Nieves A, Johnson R, Hunter J, Miller F. Intraoperative cholangiography: use of portable fluoroscopy and transmitted images. *Radiology* 1991; **181**: 205–7.
23. Blatner M, Wittgen C, Andrus C, Kaminiski D. Cystic duct cholangiography during laparoscopic cholecystectomy. *Arch Surg* 1991; **126**: 646–9.
24. Pietrafitta J, Schultz L, Graber J, Josephs L, Hickok D. Cholecystcholangiography during laparoscopic cholecystectomy: cholecystcholangiography or cystic duct cholangiography. *J Laparoendosc Surg* 1991; **1**: 197–206.
25. Sackier J, Berci G, Phillips E, Carroll B, Shapiro S, Paz-Partlow M. The role of cholangiography in laparoscopic cholecystectomy. *Arch Surg* 1991; **126**: 1021–6.
26. Gompertz R, Rhodes M, Lennard T. Laparoscopic cholangiography: an effective and inexpensive technique. *Br J Surg* 1992; **79**: 233–4.
27. Cantwell D. Routine cholangiography during laparoscopic cholecystectomy. *Arch Surg* 1992; **127**: 483–4.
28. Reddick EJ, Olsen DO. Personal communication, 1989.
29. Petelin J. The argument for contact laser laparoscopic cholecystectomy. *Clin Laser Monthly* 1990; 71–4.
30. Ferzli GS, Massaad A, Ozuner G, Worth MH. Laparoscopic exploration of the common bile duct. *Surg, Gynecol & Obstet* 1992; **174**: 419–21.
31. Franklin ME, Pharand D. *Laparoscopic Common Bile Duct Exploration.* Proceedings of the III International Congress of Laparoscopic Surgery, Brazil, 1993, 100–3.
32. Stoker ME, Leveillee RJ, McCann JC, Maini BS. Laparoscopic common bile duct exploration. *J Laparoendosc Surg* 1991; **1**: 287–93.
33. Petelin J. Laparoscopic approach to common duct pathology. *Am J Surg* 1993; **165**: 487–91.
34. DePaula A, Hashiba K, Bafutto M, Zago R, Machado M. Laparoscopic antegrade sphincterotomy. *Surg Lap & Endosc* 1993; **3**: 157–60.
35. Gagner M, Deslandres E, Pomp A, Rheault M, Potvin C, Leduc R. *Double Endoscopy: The Role of Intraoperative ERCP during Laparoscopic Cholecystectomy for Choledocholithiasis.* Proceedings of the III International Congress of Laparoscopic Surgery, Brazil, 1993, 126–7.
36. Kitano S, Iso Y, Moriyama M, Sugimachi K. A rapid and simple technique for insertion of a T-tube into the minimally incised common bile duct at laparoscopic surgery. *Surg Endosc* 1993; **7**: 104–5.

Overview

Choledocholithiasis

As surgeons become experienced in laparoscopic surgery it is only natural that they will turn their attention to the laparoscopic management of common bile duct stones. As can be seen from Petelin's data, this can be performed successfully with excellent results. However, we must not ignore the tremendous advances made over the last two decades in the endoscopic management of choledocholithiasis. For patients who present with obstructive jaundice and whose initial investigations confirm the presence of common bile duct stones, endoscopic retrograde cholangiography (ERC), for many clinicians, will remain the first line treatment of choice. It remains to be seen whether concerns regarding the long-term sequelae of performing a sphincterotomy in the younger patient will be realized.

It is in the management of common bile duct stones detected during laparoscopic cholangiography that laparoscopic exploration of the choledochus has the greatest potential. Surgeons should be prepared to learn the lessons regarding choledochoscopy and open exploration described by Motson and Menzies, and incorporate, where possible, the flexible choledochoscope into the laparoscopic exploration as described by Petelin. These stones should be easier to remove laparoscopically than larger stones, which may be more likely to be detected pre-operatively.

If laparoscopic exploration of the common bile duct fails, the surgeon has two options: convert to open operation, or close the cystic duct and perform post-operative ERC. The size and number of the stones, the clinical expertise in the institution and the general condition of the patient will influence this decision.

7.1

Bypass Surgery for Malignant Low Bile Duct Obstruction

R. C. G. RUSSELL

INTRODUCTION

Malignant obstruction of the lower bile duct can be caused by a carcinoma of the pancreas, a carcinoma of the bile duct and a carcinoma of the ampulla of Vater. Occasionally, duodenal tumours cause obstruction of the lower end of the bile duct and rarely tumours, either primary or secondary, involving the lymphatic glands may obstruct the lower end of the biliary tree. The type of tumour is important both prognostically and from the alternatives available in the therapeutic management of the tumour; hence an exact diagnosis is essential.

The frequency of low biliary tree obstruction has been increasing over the past three decades but there is a suggestion that the incidence of cancer of the pancreas is levelling off. Over the past 40 years the incidence of carcinoma of the exocrine pancreas has doubled in western Europe, has trebled in the USA and has more than quadrupled in Japan.[1,2] In the United States in 1989, 27 000 new cases were diagnosed and about the same number died of the disease.[3] In the experience of most pancreatic surgeons only 10–15% of patients with pancreatic cancer have disease suitable for resection and possible cure by the time the diagnosis is made. Such figures however, are taken from series of patients presented to large specialist centres and almost certainly overestimate the resectability rate in the community at large.[4] It is almost certain that a more common community based figure of 3–5% resectability is the more usual.

From a major review of 5650 patients presenting with pancreatic cancer between 1981 and 1990, it was estimated that 49% of patients were submitted to surgical bypass, 15% to resection, 22% to laparotomy alone, 10% to non-operative biliary decompression and 12% to no definitive treatment.[4] The authors of the 17 articles reviewed had a specialist interest in pancreatic cancer and these data present a more optimistic picture of the management of pancreatic cancer than probably occurs in the community at large. The survey of Ubhi and Doran[5] reviewed 98 patients treated in the Nottingham area and found that only one patient was resected, 82 underwent surgical bypass and 15 laparotomy alone. Indeed, with the median age of patients with malignant low bile duct obstruction being 72 years, large numbers of patients do not reach the surgeon and are merely managed without biliary drainage and receive palliative therapy under the care of geriatric physicians.

It is this group of elderly patients that provide the real challenge to minimal access surgery to determine a better alternative to laparotomy or laparotomy and surgical bypass. This challenge led to the introduction of percutaneous transhepatic stenting[6] and endoscopic stenting.[7] Considerable advances have been made in the management of bile duct obstruction by non-surgical methods such that decompression of the biliary tree can be undertaken with low morbidity and low mortality. The disadvantage of these techniques is that they rely on the insertion of an endoprosthesis to relieve the obstruction. This stent may block, leading to cholangitis and the need for a further hospital admission or outpatient episode to replace the stent. Until recently, these techniques have been limited to specialist centres and surgeons have been slow to grasp the potential of this aspect of minimal access therapy, leaving the developments to physician endoscopists and radiologists.

In the management of patients with malignant low bile duct obstruction it is essential to determine first whether the tumour is operable and suitable for resection with a view to cure and second, if it is not amenable to curative therapy, how best to relieve the jaundice. Obstructive jaundice occurs in about 70% of patients with pancreatic cancer at some time. It is present at diagnosis in as many as 90% of patients with carcinoma of the head of the pancreas, most commonly at the site where the tumour directly compresses the common bile duct as it passes through the pancreatic tissue, but in a smaller proportion of patients the duct is obstructed by metastatic nodes which compress the bile duct along the free edge of the lesser omentum or within the porta hepatis. Jaundice is less common in cancers of the body and tail, occurring in only 6% of these patients; in these patients it is almost always caused by compression of the common bile duct by involved nodes at the porta hepatis or by impaired liver function secondary to liver metastases.

Painless jaundice, often said in the past to be the cardinal symptom of pancreatic cancer, actually occurs in about one third of the patients. In more than 60% of patients with low bile duct obstruction jaundice is accompanied by pain.[8] There are a variety of reasons why the jaundice should be relieved. First, prolonged jaundice impairs liver function and this may culminate in liver failure. Second, although more common with obstructive jaundice from calculous biliary disease, cholangitis develops in about 10% of patients with unrelieved biliary obstruction from malignant disease. Anorexia and malabsorption may ensue, leading to malnutrition. Third, about 25% of patients with jaundice are distressed by pruritis which is well nigh impossible to manage effectively with drugs. Fourth, the jaundice is a constant reminder to the patient and the family of the uncontrolled disease within. Additionally, there is some evidence that the relief of jaundice prolongs survival. Sarr and his associates[9] reviewed 10 000 patients who underwent palliative procedures for pancreatic cancer and found that the mean survival time of those who underwent biliary bypass was 5.4 months compared with 3.5 months in those who did not. Of course, those who did not have the operation may have had more advanced disease. Nevertheless, the relief given to the patient by the decompression of the biliary tree has only to be seen to leave no doubt that this manoeuvre provides useful palliation; the instantaneous improvement achieved by the simple insertion of an endoscopic stent convinces even the sceptic of the value of minimal access therapy in palliative treatment.

The majority of patients with malignant low bile duct obstruction require palliative treatment. Optimal palliation must strive to alleviate symptoms effectively, thereby improving the quality of life and extending the period of useful survival while minimising the duration of hospital stay.

The principle of optimal palliation which stresses minimal intervention and minimal duration of hospital stay demands that the techniques of minimal access therapy are considered as a route to improved outcome. Indeed, this is an area where minimal access therapy by the insertion of stents either percutaneously or transhepatically has proved to be outstandingly successful. The advent of laparoscopic surgery calls into question whether a laparoscopically performed bypass of the bile duct will provide an alternative approach to the techniques already available and give to the patient optimal palliation not achieved by other methods. Laparoscopic biliary surgery, apart from cholecystectomy, is in its infancy and thus comparisons with established techniques are not yet possible. Nevertheless, it is important to establish the basis on which such comparisons can be made and indeed to consider whether further development of these techniques will prove fruitful in the light of developments occurring in the relief of jaundice by stenting and traditional surgery.

In order to establish these guidelines it is important to consider the management of low bile duct obstruction. This chapter will review the diagnosis of low bile duct obstruction, the assessment of operability, the assessment of the patient and the alternative techniques available in the management of malignant low bile duct obstruction.

DIAGNOSIS OF LOW BILE DUCT OBSTRUCTION

It is important to emphasize the gravity of making the diagnosis of low bile obstruction due to a malignant process; such a diagnosis commits the patient to a median survival of 20 weeks. Rarely will patients survive beyond one year and by the end of two years nearly all patients will be dead if the diagnosis is correct. The ease with which biliary obstruction can be relieved by the percutaneous insertion of a stent often neglects the fact that certain tumours of the lower biliary tree are operable and such curative operations can provide a 40% five year survival.

The first step in the diagnosis of the cause of malignant low bile duct obstruction is a haematological screen and a biochemical profile to assess whether coagulation defects are present and ensure that the liver function tests are compatible with a diagnosis of bile duct obstruction. Ultrasound invariably reveals a grossly dilated extrahepatic biliary tree with or without intrahepatic dilatation and a dilated gall bladder, if the gall bladder is present and not previously diseased. Good ultrasound will frequently delineate the nature of the obstruction within the pancreas and alert the surgeon to the rarer causes of obstruction or even the presence of a benign disease such as a stone in the common bile duct.

The next stage in diagnosis is an endoscopy to exclude a tumour of the ampulla of Vater. Contrast studies of the pancreatic and biliary duct will frequently show the characteristic 'double-duct' sign (Fig. 7.1.1). Brushing for cytology or even biopsy can confirm the histological diagnosis and the nature of the malignancy. A decision at this point whether to stent or not is made. On the whole, it is useful to insert a stent at this stage to relieve the jaundice and the itching which accompanies the jaundice. Nevertheless, such an action does increase the risk of infection and sepsis associated with stenting remains a major problem. If stenting is not undertaken at this procedure it is essential to avoid the injection of contrast into the upper biliary tree as the combination of stasis and injection of contrast into a column of static bile can give rise to infection even if prophylactic antibiotics are given and a meticulous aseptic technique observed during endoscopy.

At endoscopy it is important to determine whether or not the tumour encroaches on the duodenum and if it does an assessment is made whether that tumour will cause gastric outlet obstruction during the course of the disease. Tumour involvement of the duodenum causing gastric outlet obstruction occurs in approximately 15% of patients but in many instances is a preterminal event. Often, vomiting associated with pancreatic cancer is not due to tumour compressing the duodenum but to involvement of the coeliac axis and incoordination of gastroduodenal motility as a result of the involvement of the nerves to the stomach and duodenum.

During this stage of the procedure it is essential to exclude benign disease. It is rare for gallstones to mimic pancreatic cancer but it can happen and this is adequately excluded by a proper endoscopy and imaging of the biliary tree. Similarly, chronic pancreatitis can occasionally confuse and this should be rigorously pursued as the prognosis and management are entirely different.

ASSESSMENT OF RESECTABILITY

Since pancreatic resection is of benefit in patients with localized disease, the aim of preoperative evaluation should be not only to assess resectability of the

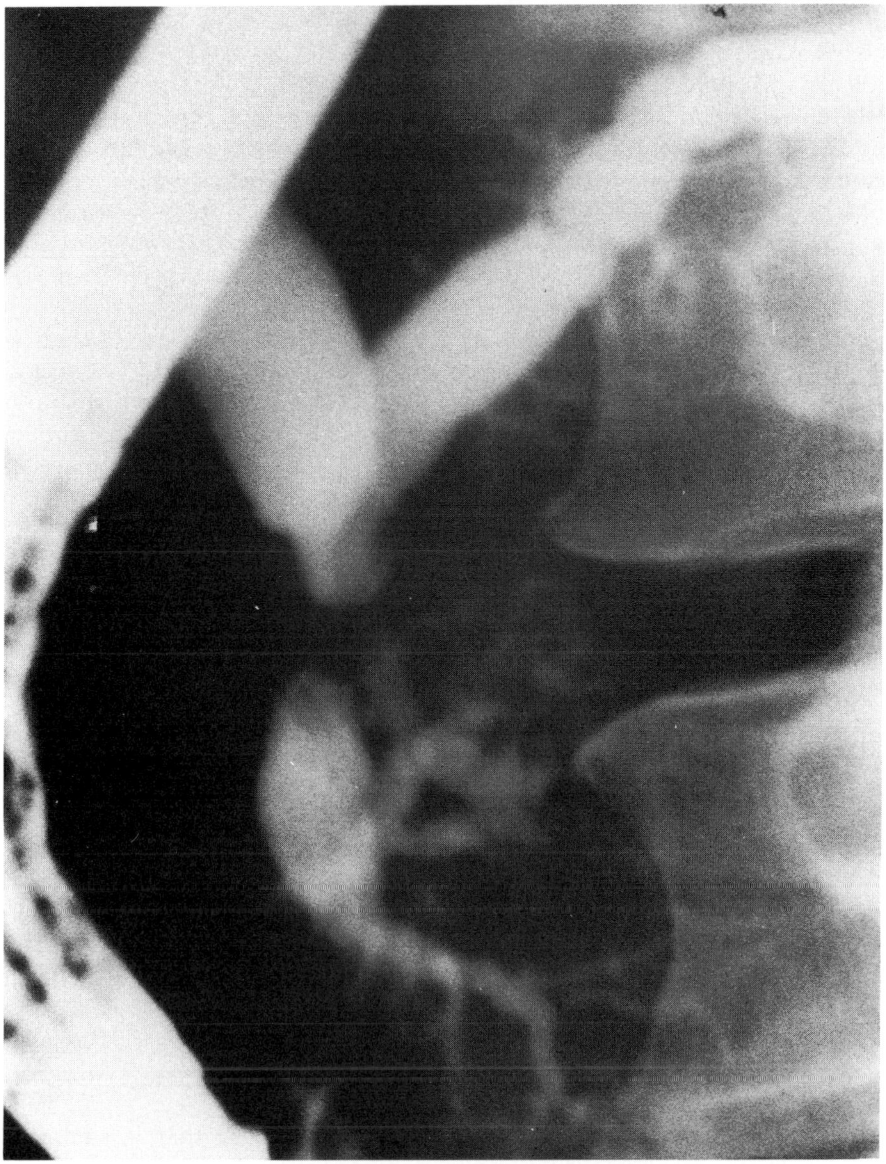

Figure 7.1.1 Radiograph obtained at ERCP showing narrowing of both the biliary and pancreatic ducts, with tenting of both towards the tumour.

primary tumour but also to search for metastases. The extent of the cancer can be sometimes gauged on clinical grounds. Back pain, which is present in about a quarter of patients with cancer of the pancreatic head, is a sombre symptom; in one series 20 of 33 such tumours were irresectable.[10] Likewise, back pain occurs frequently in patients with cancer of the body and tail of the pancreas and in such instances no patient is resectable. Data from 393 patients have been carefully analysed to relate prognosis to clinical presentation; 46% of those patients with irresectable but localized tumours and 47% of those with advanced disease had back pain, while only 5% of those with resectable tumours had this symptom.[11] Physical signs inconsistent with resectability include cervical adenopathy, ascites, a rectal shelf and an umbilical nodule.

Many imaging studies are now available for preoperative evaluation of patients with pancreatic carcinoma and the order in which these are used must relate to the experience within the local imaging department. Nevertheless, simple investigations should be used first. Carcinoma of the pancreas rarely metastasizes to the lung but any abnormality on a chest X-ray should alert the surgeon to problems that may occur if the pancreatic tumour is resected. Detailed ultrasound with colour flow Doppler is commonly the first line of investigation. Indeed, the experienced ultrasonographer can more accurately define the tumour by ultrasound than is frequently possible by computed tomography scanning. Careful examination of the surrounding pancreatic tissue for lymph node involvement is essential and in particular it is vital to examine the porta hepatis, involvement of which may prevent biliary decompression by an operative approach. Involvement of the portal vein should be seen on ultrasound and spread posteriorly to involve the vena cava can be defined clearly; involvement of either of these major vessels or of the superior mesenteric artery indicates inoperability.

A computed tomography scan with a specific protocol for the pancreas will define the tumour (Fig. 7.1.2). Pictures should be taken at 4 mm intervals with and without oral and intravenous contrast with enhanced views of the head of the pancreas and superior mesenteric artery (Fig. 7.1.3). Lymphatic spread around the origin of the superior mesenteric artery is invariably associated with inoperability as is tumour spread to the liver. Among 66 patients with pancreatic cancer who were potential surgical candidates, computed tomography predicted resectability with a sensitivity of 75% and a positive predictive value of 38% using the absence of local extension or distant metastases as the criteria for resectability.[12] Irresectability was predicted with a sensitivity of 72% and a positive predictive value of 93%. Thus, computed tomography was better at predicting irresectability than resectability, especially when hepatic or distant metastases were present.

Ultrasonography can achieve a sensitivity approaching that of computed tomography in detecting pancreatic carcinoma and assessing inoperability. Nevertheless, resectability is indicated with much less accuracy and in one study only seven of 19 'resectable' lesions were successfully removed. Ultrasound, however, does determine accurately the size of the lesion and it may well be that this is as good a predictor as any to determine the appropriateness of resection. The advent of improved endoscopic ultrasound may enable a better determination of operability particularly in the periampullary region. Tio and Tytgat[13] accurately predicted resectability in seven of eight patients and suggested irresectability in five of six because of deep infiltration of the tumour around

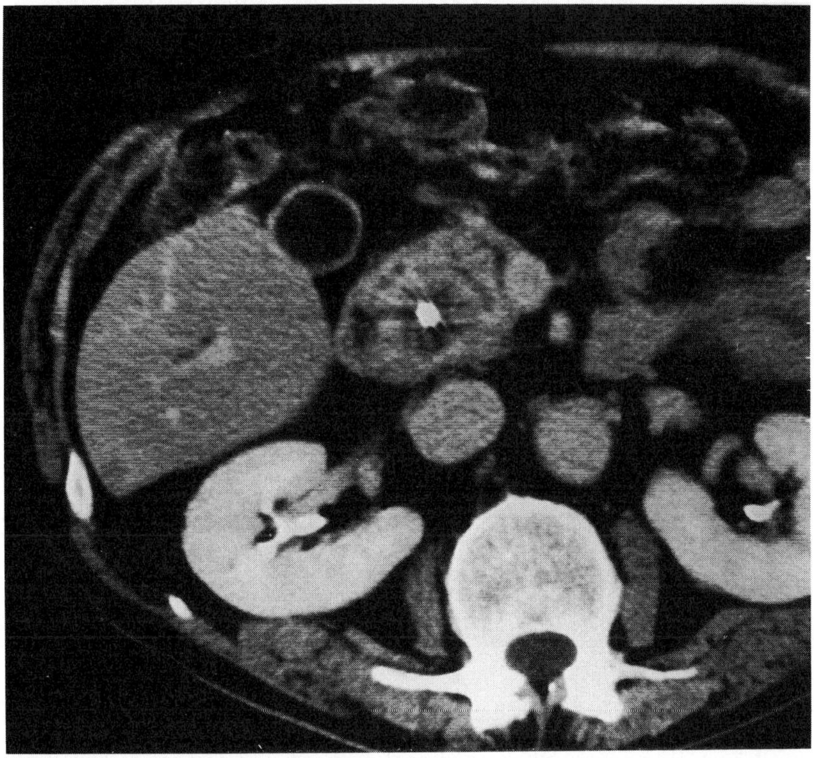

Figure 7.1.2 CT scan of the pancreatic head with oral and intravenous contrast, and a tumour around a stent in the common bile duct.

major blood vessels and adjacent organs. In a Japanese study of 42 patients with pancreatic cancer and eight with chronic pancreatitis[14] endoscopic ultrasound detected all tumours, even those smaller than 20 mm diameter. Among 12 patients with small cancers (less than 30 mm) malignant invasion of the portal vein was correctly diagnosed in all but one case. Our own experience with the latest available instruments is that tumours less than a centimetre in size can be adequately imaged provided that an expert ultrasonographer and endoscopist are working together. These tumours can be clearly seen on the ultrasound image and their extent mapped with accuracy. It is anticipated that with further improvement in the technology, endoscopic ultrasound will prove the preferred method of assessment of operability.

In the preoperative evaluation of pancreatic cancer, some believe that visceral angiography provides two pieces of crucial information: detail of anatomical anomalies of the blood vessels which will be encountered at operation and vascular invasion of the tumour. Atypical arterial patterns, notably a right hepatic artery arising from the superior mesenteric artery, can be anticipated in 25% of patients considered for pancreatectomy and this information is useful

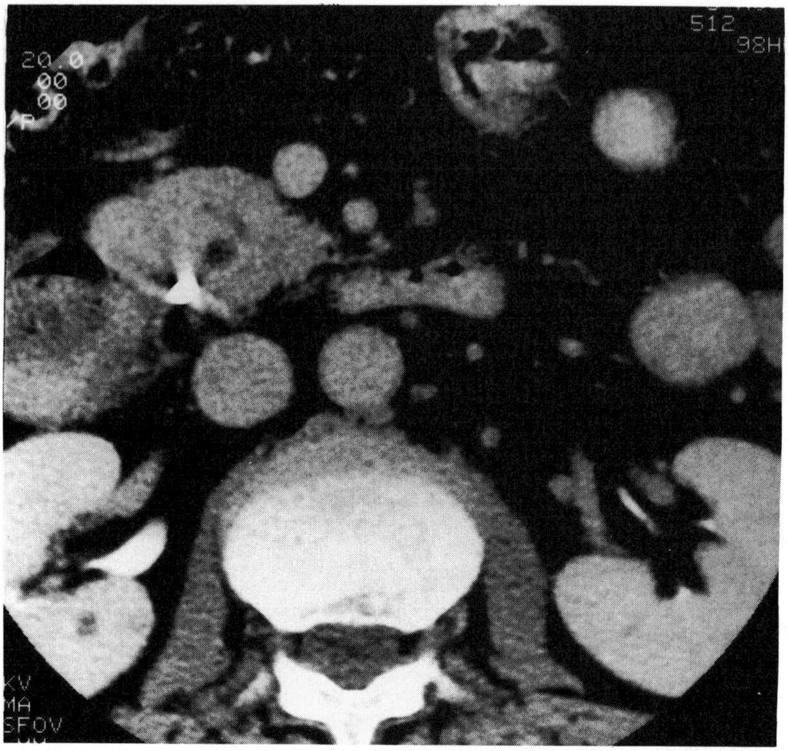

Figure 7.1.3 CT scan with enhanced view of the head of the pancreas, delineating the superior mesenteric artery.

during mobilization of the head of the pancreas.[15] The most reliable angiographic sign of irresectability is clear cut invasion or obstruction of the portal or superior mesenteric vein, especially when the presence of collaterals shows that this finding is not an imaging artefact. Arterial encasement is a less reliable criterion, although total inclusion of one of the major arteries nearly always denotes irresectability.[16] Modern ultrasound should, however, define this problem with equal ease, particularly if colour Doppler is used.

Despite the advances in conventional imaging, Warshaw and colleagues found that nearly half the patients who came to laparotomy with apparently localized pancreatic cancers had unsuspected intra-abdominal metastases.[17] They therefore evaluated laparoscopy as a further staging modality in 40 pancreatic cancers. Laparoscopic assessment was accurate in 93% overall and altered the treatment plan in 35%, usually by avoiding open operation. Cuschieri undertook laparoscopy in 73 patients with pancreatic cancer as an immediate prelude to laparotomy in 51 cases.[18] Forty-two of 47 patients were accurately staged as having incurable lesions but only four of nine judged to be resectable at laparoscopy had truly resectable tumours at laparotomy. Although most hepatic deposits visualized by laparoscopy had been detected preoperatively, peritoneal and omental deposits were only identified endoscopically.

Warshaw prospectively evaluated four different imaging techniques for detecting resectability in 88 patients with pancreatic and ampullary tumours.[19] Computed tomography was 92% accurate for predicting irresectability but only 56% sensitive; by contrast, it was only 45% accurate in predicting resectability. Magnetic resonance had no advantage over computed tomography. Visceral angiography was 95% accurate at predicting irresectability but only 66% sensitive. Laparoscopy detected liver or peritoneal seedlings in 22 of 23 patients and was 100% accurate concerning their absence. When computed tomography, angiography and laparoscopy were combined, 51 of 57 irresectable tumours (89%) and 28 of 31 resectable tumours (90%) were correctly identified.

The concensus view is that no single preoperative test is sufficiently reliable to determine the resectability of every pancreatic cancer. Nevertheless, the problem is not as great as it at first appears. First, most patients over the age of 72 are not suitable for resection of a pancreatic cancer. There are studies showing that in certain very fit patients resection can be undertaken with a low mortality, but such patients require most careful selection and thought to determine whether submitting an elderly patient to a major pancreatic resection is appropriate and, in particular, whether such surgery will produce good palliation. If it is accepted that most patients over 72 do not require resection then detailed investigation is limited to the younger patient. In many instances, it is apparent that there is disseminated disease on ultrasound or computed tomography scanning. Such patients do not require detailed consideration of operability. If the tumour is of small size on computed tomography and ultrasound scanning, that is less than 3 cm in size, and without evidence of distant spread, then careful assessment should be undertaken. It is suggested that in the first instance these patients require endoscopic stenting to relieve the jaundice. My own practice is to allow such patients out of hospital to recover from their jaundice during a three week period. The patient is then readmitted for further assessment with detailed ultrasound using colour Doppler imaging and dynamic contrast-enhanced computed tomography scanning with a special pancreatic protocol; if these investigations suggest that the tumour is resectable the patient then proceeds to endoscopic ultrasound and is only submitted to resection at that stage.

The final assessment for such patients could well be laparoscopy and this is suggested as appropriate on the experience of Warshaw and colleagues.[17] If the tumour is found to be inoperable at this stage with seedling metastases in the liver, diaphragm or omentum then some form of laparoscopic treatment would seem appropriate. However, such patients who have been so carefully assessed are shown to have minimal morbidity with a surgical bypass. A study of highly selected patients from the Johns Hopkins Medical Institution, Baltimore, suggests that such patients have a mortality of 2.5%, postoperative morbidity rate of 37% and a mean hospital stay of 14 days (range 4–46 days). The survival in this highly selected group was 7.7 months.[20]

ASSESSMENT OF PATIENT

Before embarking on the management of the patient with low bile duct obstruction it is essential to determine their general fitness regardless of whether the patient is being considered for curative or palliative therapy. With many alternatives available in the palliation of jaundice, the presence of significant coexistent disease can alter the management of the patient from curative to palliative therapy and then influence the decision whether the palliation should be surgical, endoscopic or radiological. Thus a full assessment of the respiratory and cardiovascular system is necessary. The renal function should be ascertained to determine that this is normal. It is advisable to check the coagulation immediately preoperatively as this can change during the course of a period of investigation. Preferably, such patients should be given vitamin K in the days before an operation. Patients with significant associated diseases which may prejudice survival from the operation should be excluded from consideration for resection; these patients are ideal candidates for the palliative relief of jaundice by minimal access surgery.

If the assessment of operability suggests that the patient is unsuitable for resection then the question of tissue diagnosis must be considered. With the improvement in cytology and endoscopic biopsy[21] more than half the patients will have evidence of malignancy from their preliminary assessment. In those who are unsuitable for resection but who require some palliative intervention and at this stage have no cytological or histological evidence of the diagnosis, histological confirmation of the diagnosis must be achieved before the patient's assessment has been completed. The preferred technique, and one that is even better than a blind approach, is a percutaneous biopsy with ultrasound or computed tomography guidance using for example a Biopty spring-loaded Trucut needle (Radiplast Biopty, Uppsala), which obtains slivers of tissue suitable for detailed histological assessment. Such biopsies can be achieved with safety and be a guidance as to the prognosis.[22] Further, there are patients who present with jaundice who have chronic pancreatitis; such patients should not be given a definitive prognosis until malignancy is confirmed or rejected. Patients with rare pancreatic tumours such as non-functioning neuroendocrine tumours tend to live longer (median survival four years) than those with ductal adenocarcinoma and patients with cystadenocarcinomas, either of the serous or mucinous variety, have a much better prognosis than ductal carcinoma, often living for ten years.

ALTERNATIVES IN THE MANAGEMENT OF LOW BILE DUCT OBSTRUCTION

Endoscopic and Percutaneous Techniques

Several non-operative methods have been developed to relieve jaundice due to malignant low bile duct obstruction. Initially, external drainage was accomplished by percutaneous transhepatic insertion of a catheter; later manipulation of a guide wire and drainage catheter through the obstructing lesions allowed both internal and external bile flow.[6,23] The disadvantages of external biliary drainage include the risk of spontaneous catheter dislodgement, inflammation and pain at the puncture site, leaks of ascitic fluid and bile around the catheter and loss of fluid and electrolytes.[24]

The use of non-operative techniques was advanced by the description of a percutaneous transhepatic insertion of an indwelling stent without an external catheter.[25] The technique for endoscopic insertion of a biliary stent through the papilla was established in 1980.[7] Small stents were used initially but wider channel endoscopes became available that allowed the use of stents with an external diameter of more than 3.2 mm. The endoscopic approach is technically more difficult than the percutaneous transhepatic method but is less traumatic for the patients and has the advantage that blocked stents can be removed and changed easily. A variety of different types of endoprosthesis are now available with lumens ranging from 9 to 14 French in external diameter. Stent materials include Teflon, polyethylene and percuflex. Nevertheless, whatever the stent material, the major problem has proven to be sludge within the stent occurring at a mean time of 20 weeks following initial insertion.[26]

It was hoped that the advent of self-expanding metallic endoprostheses would open a new era in the management of such patients.[27] These can be placed either percutaneously or endoscopically. Unfortunately, tumour grows through the web of the expandable stent (Fig. 7.1.4) causing obstruction later in the course of the disease. Modified silicone covered Gianturco expandable metal stents and silicone covered Wallstents (Medivent SA, Lausanne, Switzerland) have now been introduced; however, their cost is high and as 60% of patients do not require replacement of a polyethylene stent, remaining jaundice-free with their initial stent at the time of death, it is debatable whether such expense is justified.

Despite the advances in stent design and the use of the more complex expandable stents, the insertion of a Teflon 10 French stent appears the preferred method of relieving malignant low bile duct obstruction.[28,29] For high bile duct obstruction there is advantage in the use of percutaneous transhepatic stenting primarily and in these instances, the use of silicone covered expandable stents may be of advantage because of the difficulty in replacing such stents and in clearing the stent if it becomes clogged with debris.

Surgical Biliary Bypass

The most common biliary–enteric bypass carried out for irresectable low bile duct malignant obstruction is still cholecystjejunostomy. The relative frequency of cholecystjejunostomy has increased from 50% in the 1970s to 62% in the 1980s. Choledochojejunostomy has also increased from 7% to 22% during this time.[4] Some centres, notably the Cleveland Clinic[30] still prefer the use of the duodenum for biliary–enteric bypass, but the choice of either duodenum or jejunum is generally decreasing because of the potential which is largely

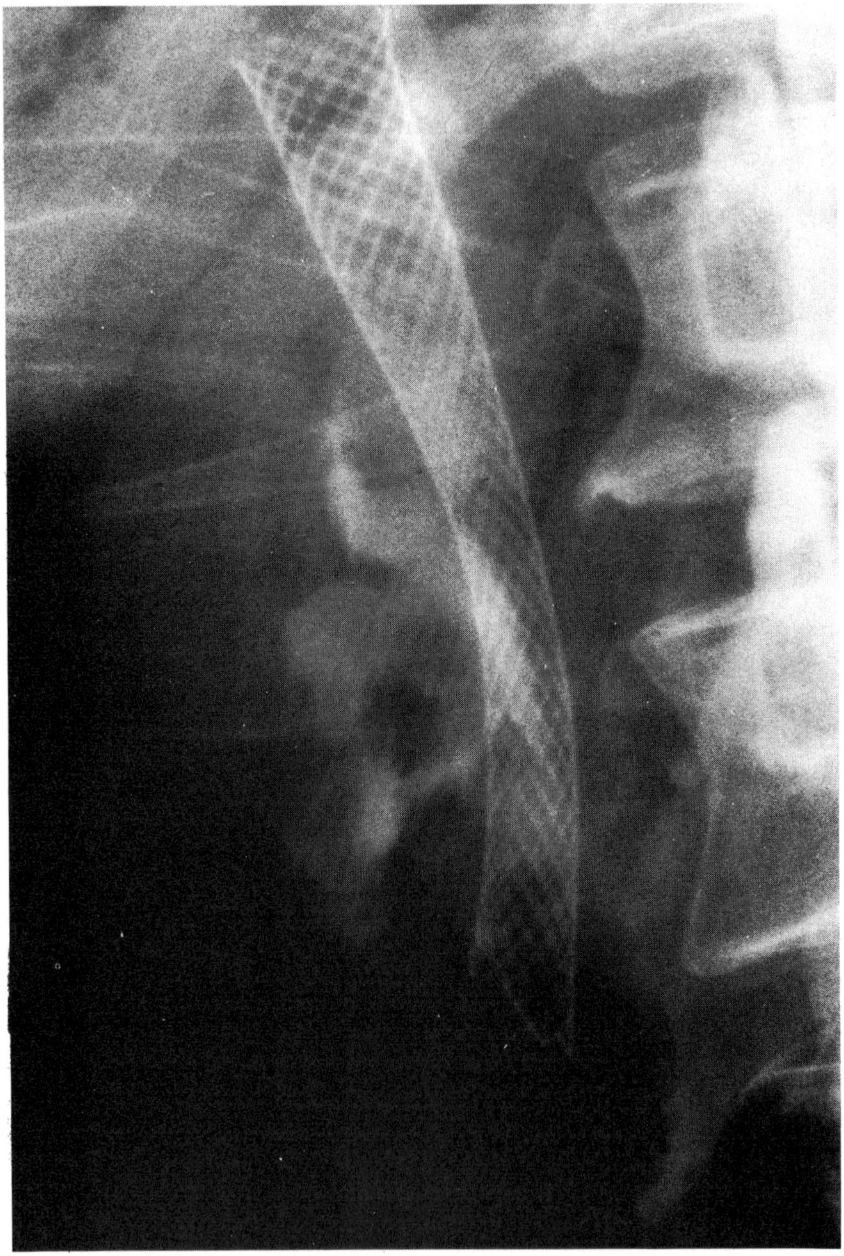

Figure 7.1.4 A Wallstent which has been placed endoscopically to relieve obstruction at the lower end of the bile duct.

theoretical for duodenal obstruction and bile gastritis. Use of the distended gall bladder on the biliary side of the anastomosis is certainly the simplest option and it is associated with a shorter operative time than using the common bile duct.

The operative mortality rate of cholecystjejunostomy has decreased from 17% before 1980 to 10% since that time. Choledochojejunostomy used to carry a much higher operative mortality (34% during 1971–80), but this is no longer the case (7% since 1981). The greater technical difficulty of choledochojejunostomy may be balanced by the modern trend to reserve cholecystjejunostomy for the patients with advanced cancer who are expected to survive for only a few weeks. In a well-matched study by Rosemurgy[31] 22 patients underwent cholecystjejunostomy and 15 patients underwent choledochojejunostomy. The operative mortality rate was 23% for gall bladder–enteric bypass and only 7% for common duct–enteric anastomosis; the morbidity rates were similar (59 and 53% respectively). In a meta-analysis of eight articles comparing these two procedures, cholecystenterostomy carries an 89% success rate while that of choledochoenterostomy is 97%. An important finding from this review is the 20% incidence of recurrent jaundice or cholangitis following gall bladder bypass compared with only 8% after common bile duct anastomosis.[4] In general, choledochoenterostomy should therefore be preferred in patients with a reasonable expectation of survival. If the gall bladder is selected for the anastomosis it is essential to ensure that the cystic duct is patent and that it enters the common duct at least 2–3 cm above the tumour mass. Intraoperative cholangiography is essential to establish these facts. Mere observation is fallible since the cystic duct may merge with the common duct and join lower down the bile duct.

A continuing debate is whether the additional anastomosis required to create a defunctional (Roux) loop is justifiable in the palliation of pancreatic cancer. Experimentally, the Roux loop is associated with a lower incidence of cholangitis than simple anastomosis to a functioning loop of jejunum. However, in clinical practice when a biliary–enteric bypass is performed and a long survival anticipated a Roux loop is essential but in patients whose median survival is only five months such complex surgery is unnecessary and indeed, Sarr and Cameron found no advantage for a Roux-en-Y anastomosis over a simple loop in a review of 1100 patients.[9] Brooks[32] confirmed no superiority for the one procedure over the other and recently Potts[30] reported a similar incidence of biliary sepsis followed each technique of anastomosis. The infrequency of ascending cholangitis when functioning jejunum is used is probably due to the short survival of these patients. In consequence, the added operative time associated with the formation of a Roux loop is not justified in patients with the short survival associated with pancreatic cancer; for even a group which has been carefully selected for resection, and found inoperable, the median survival was only 7.7 months.[20] In view of the minimal differences between procedures, it is preferable to undertake the simplest, safest and least invasive surgical procedure in order to reduce mortality and morbidity.

My own preference is for a choledochoduodenostomy. Like the experience of the Cleveland Clinic, I can find no evidence that duodenal obstruction or reflux gastritis affects these patients disadvantageously during their short life expectancy. The advantage of the choledochoduodenostomy is that it is a simple procedure and can be performed by minimal access techniques.

My technique is an extension of the minicholecystectomy procedure;[33] a 5–6 cm transverse right upper abdominal incision lateral to the rectus muscle is performed. A muscle-splitting incision is used and the rectus muscle is deflected medially to gain access to the bile duct. The size of opening (5 cm) is not large enough to undertake a full assessment of the tumour. In my own practice this has invariably been performed prior to surgery by radiological methods and the tumour considered as inoperable. A stabilized ring retractor is then used with one blade underneath the liver to display the porta hepatis and a second malleable blade inferiorly to deflect the hepatic flexure of the colon inferiorly. Minimal dissection of the duodenum is undertaken. The bile duct is then dissected out by dividing the peritoneum longitudinally over the free edge of the lesser omentum to display the common hepatic and common bile ducts. A point on the anterior surface of the common bile duct is then chosen at least 2–3 cm above the upper border of the carcinoma and a disc 1 cm in diameter removed from the front of the bile duct. If an endoprosthesis has been inserted this is removed. A disc of duodenum of similar size is then removed and an anastomosis performed using interrupted 3/0 Vicryl sutures between the bile duct and the duodenum. It is frequently possible to test the integrity of this anastomosis by compressing the gall bladder. The gall bladder is only removed if the cystic duct merges with the bile duct low down and is likely to obstruct. Obstruction of the gall bladder can cause local sepsis and lead to pain and discomfort later in the course of the disease. If there is evidence of duodenal obstruction either at operation or at endoscopy a gastroenterostomy can be undertaken through this small incision between a loop of jejunum and the front of the stomach.

The wound is closed with interrupted number 1 PDS and a 3/0 subcuticular suture to the skin. Before the end of the operation the wound is infiltrated with bupivacaine and adrenaline 0.25% to relieve postoperative discomfort. Such a minimally invasive procedure has the advantages of minicholecystectomy. The postoperative recovery is rapid, the mortality 5% and the complication rate 20%.

RELIEF OF DUODENAL OBSTRUCTION

Nausea and vomiting are a presenting symptom in 30–45% of patients with pancreatic cancer, although actual gastric outflow obstruction occurs in only 5% at the time of diagnosis.[34] As the tumour enlarges there is a further risk of duodenal invasion and obstruction. Tumours of the head of the gland normally obstruct the second part of the duodenum although tumours within the uncinate process will obstruct the fourth part of the duodenum and may be missed unless the endoscopist or surgeon is aware of this entity.

A review of more than 1600 cases of pancreatic cancer from 15 articles published between 1973 and 1990 showed that the mortality rate of biliary bypass was not increased by adding gastrojejunostomy.[4] The mean survival time for patients without initial gastroenterostomy was slightly longer than for those with initial gastroenterostomy(7.4 vs. 6.7 months), probably because those with more advanced disease were chosen for the extra procedure. Seventeen percent of patients who underwent biliary bypass alone developed duodenal obstruction at a mean of 8.6 months later and required subsequent gastric bypass. Nevertheless, it has been my experience that many patients have an inappropriate gastric bypass because the vomiting associated with their advancing carcinoma is due to infiltration of the neural plexuses around the coeliac axis rather than direct obstruction of the duodenum. Such patients can be well managed by the use of drugs such as cisapride to improve gastric emptying. Because of the advanced stage of the disease the mortality of a second operation is high (mean 22%) and the mean survival thereafter is only three months.

The disadvantage of undertaking a routine gastroenterostomy is that delayed gastric emptying occurs after operation in 20% (range 6–29%) of patients undergoing gastroenterostomy at the time of the biliary bypass. Doberneck and Berndt[35] found that delayed gastric emptying complicated recovery in seven of the 43 patients who had no preoperative evidence of duodenal obstruction and in eight of 14 patients who did. Two of the 12 patients with gastroenterostomy proximal to the biliary–enteric anastomosis had delayed gastric emptying compared with six of 22 patients with a gastroenterostomy distal to the biliary bypass. Jacobs[36] described a 29% incidence of delayed gastric emptying in patients who underwent both biliary and gastric bypass, while no delayed gastric emptying occurred in the group with biliary bypass alone. Barkin[37] showed that nine of the 15 patients with pancreatic cancer without duodenal obstruction or electrolyte imbalance had gastric emptying curves more than two standard deviations below the normal mean values. Nausea and vomiting were present in three of nine with abnormal gastric emptying but in none of those with a normal test. The mechanism of the delayed gastric emptying remains uncertain. Some patients may have partial obstruction at or close to the stoma whereas others with extensive nodal secondaries may have a degree of autonomic gastric denervation. Fortunately, the condition usually settles spontaneously after varying periods of nasogastric intubation.

Upper gastrointestinal bleeding occurs in 0–17% of patients with double bypass and 2–6% in those with biliary bypass alone. Sarr[38] reported bleeding from stomal ulcers in three of 100 patients; others may have duodenogastric reflux and alkaline gastritis. Vagotomy is probably not justified because of the low incidence of stomal ulcer and it may further complicate delayed gastric emptying after operation. The routine use of histamine receptor antagonists seems, however, a useful precaution after operation.

My own practice is not to undertake a gastroenterostomy unless it is essential as the increase in morbidity around the time of the operation, particularly in those patients who develop delayed gastric emptying, can be distressing to the patient and detract from the quality of palliation. If obstruction occurs late in the disease, this is invariably managed conservatively.

COMPARISON OF TECHNIQUES

Endoscopic Versus Percutaneous Stent Insertion

The major trial to define whether one treatment was better than the other was undertaken by Speer *et al.* at the Middlesex Hospital.[39] In this trial, which was the first prospective randomized comparison of percutaneous and endoscopic methods for insertion of biliary stents in malignant obstructive jaundice, it was shown that endoscopic insertion was more likely to succeed and was safer than the percutaneous technique. The higher 30 day mortality associated with the percutaneous technique was due to complications resulting from the puncture of the liver with large bore tubes. The higher mortality in patients with successful insertion of a percutaneous stent was a cause for concern and has been reported in other series.[40,41] Further, obstruction of the percutaneous stent by clot or debris resulted in a higher incidence of leakage of bile into the peritoneal cavity with local complications. The percutaneous technique carried a substantial risk even when the stent insertion failed whereas failed insertion of an endoscopic stent seldom gives rise to complications. Another disadvantage of the percutaneous approach is the difficulty in quantifying the pain and discomfort caused by the procedure and the presence of an external drain which is left in situ for a short time after insertion. For low bile duct strictures the difficulty in the endoscopic technique is no greater than in the percutaneous technique, although this is not true for high bile duct strictures. Interestingly, in that study the median survival of patients who had an endoscopic stent was longer than those who had a percutaneous stent although this was not statistically significant.

In the seven years since Speer and colleagues reported their results, there has been considerable improvement in the technique for percutaneous transhepatic stent placement. Nevertheless, for the low bile duct stricture the endoscopic approach still has considerable advantage in that the stent can be placed at the same time as the diagnostic study is undertaken and can be combined with histological diagnosis by biopsy or cytological diagnosis by brushing of the biliary tree. It should be emphasized that for obstruction of the common hepatic duct or the right and left hepatic ducts, a percutaneous approach remains preferable.

Endoscopic Versus Bypass Surgery

A prospective randomized controlled trial was established at the Middlesex Hospital in 1985 to determine whether an endoscopically placed stent was preferable to a surgical bypass. After determining that the patient was inoperable and did not have duodenal obstruction, the patient was entered into the trial and randomly allocated for endoscopic or surgical treatment. Two hundred and four patients were recruited, 103 patients were randomized to surgery and 101 to stenting. Three patients, one in the stented group and two in the surgical group, were later found to have benign disease and excluded. The groups were well matched for factors known to affect outcome such as age, haemoglobin, white cell count, urea, albumin and tumour size. At the time of randomization all patients had a bilirubin greater than 100 $mmol\,l^{-1}$. The procedure was successful in 93% in the surgical group and in 95% in the stent group. Therapeutic success in those that had a successful bypass (defined by a 20% fall in bilirubin at five days) was achieved in 98% of the surgical group and 97% of those patients who had a stent.

There was a significant difference between the surgical and stenting groups in the procedure related mortality. Procedure related deaths occurred in 14 surgical patients compared with only three stented patients. However, there was no significant statistical difference in the 30 day mortality which was documented in 15 out of 101 surgical patients and eight of 100 stented patients. There was a significant difference in major complications in the stented group (11/100) compared with the surgical group (29/101). Of the 11 stented patients with major complications, seven had severe cholangitis, four had acute renal failure, two experienced severe gastrointestinal bleeding, one had acute pulmonary oedema and one patient developed gastric stasis after stent failure and required subsequent bypass surgery. In the surgical group ten patients had gastrointestinal bleeding, nine developed gastric stasis (defined as persistent postoperative vomiting greater than ten days), nine had acute renal failure, seven experienced severe pneumonia, seven severe cholangitis, five had a bile leak resulting in peritonitis, three developed acute liver failure, two had a fatal pulmonary embolus, two had wounds leaking ascites and two had severe pulmonary oedema. Minor complications occurred in 23 of the stented patients and 28 of the surgical patients. The median length of stay in hospital was significantly longer in the surgery group following randomization and following the actual procedure. Even the total hospital stay, that is the time of diagnosis to death and including all readmissions for subsequent treatment, was still longer in the surgical group than in those treated with stents (26 vs. 20 days).

Recurrent jaundice was defined as the development of clinical jaundice after the patient had been initially rendered anicteric by either biliary bypass or stenting. Recurrent jaundice was documented in 34 patients due to stent blockage, while in the surgical group only six patients redeveloped jaundice.

Overall survival was significantly longer in the surgical patients than in the stented group. The median survival was 26 weeks for surgery and 21 weeks for stenting despite the initial lower morbidity and procedure related mortality in the stenting group.

This carefully documented trial thus showed that there were advantages for surgery, the longer survival and the lower incidence of recurrent jaundice, but major initial advantages for stent placement such as the lower initial mortality and the shorter hospital stay. However, these differences are surprisingly small and it is undoubtedly true that both techniques are suitable in the management of low bile duct obstruction.

CONCLUSION

It is difficult to determine the advantage that laparoscopic surgery will offer to the patient with malignant low bile duct obstruction. Undoubtedly, as a diagnostic tool Warshaw and colleagues have shown that this technique is of value in defining the extent of disease once a full radiological assessment has been undertaken. It is logical to suggest that a laparoscopic bypass procedure is appropriate for the patient who is found to be inoperable at laparoscopy; in such circumstances a cholecyst jejunostomy without Roux-en-Y formation appears to be entirely adequate. Such a procedure should be able to be performed relatively rapidly and without great morbidity or mortality. Thus, it would be an appropriate alternative to open surgery or endoscopic stenting.

To determine whether in selected patients laparoscopic bypass would be preferable to either endoscopic or surgical approaches will be difficult, as the differences even in comparison to open surgery, are likely to be slight. A trial with 100 patients in each arm would be necessary to show significant differences and would be difficult to achieve. Further, the open surgical approach has the ability to add a gastroenterostomy with comparative ease and no additional mortality. To undertake a gastroenterostomy laparoscopically would be a major undertaking even using stapling devices.

It is suggested that endoscopic stenting will be the major minimally invasive therapy for the treatment of all elderly patients who present with malignant low bile duct obstruction. For the younger patient or those with a better prognosis, a surgical approach is warranted but, with minimal access surgical techniques, the advantages of the laparoscopic approach are likely to be modest.

REFERENCES

1. Gordis L, Gold EB. Epidemiology of pancreatic cancer. *World J Surg* 1984; **8**: 808–21.
2. Hirayama T. Epidemiology of pancreatic cancer in Japan. *J Clin Oncol* 1989; **19**: 208–15.
3. American Cancer Society. *Cancer Facts and Figures – 1987*. New York, American Cancer Society, 1987.
4. Watanapa P, Williamson RCN. Surgical palliation for pancreatic cancer: developments during the last two decades. *Br J Surg* 1992; **79**: 8–20.

5. Ubhi CS, Doran J. Palliation for carcinoma of the head of the pancreas. *Ann R Coll Surg Engl* 1986; **68**: 159–62.
6. Kaude JV, Weidermier L, Agee CF. Decompression of the bile ducts with the percutaneous technique. *Radiology* 1969; **93**: 69–71.
7. Soehendra N, Reynders-Frederick V. Palliative bile duct drainage: a new endoscopic method of introducing a transpapillary drain. *Endoscopy* 1980; **12**: 8–11.
8. Singh SM, Reber HA. Surgical palliation for pancreatic cancer. *Surg Clin N Am* 1989; **69**: 599–611.
9. Sarr HG, Cameron JL. Palliation of pancreatic cancer. *World J Surg* 1984; **8**: 906–18.
10. Richards AB, Sosin H. Cancer of the pancreas: the value of radical and palliative surgery. *Ann Surg* 1973; **177**: 325–31.
11. Kalser MH, Barkin J, Macintyre JH. Pancreatic cancer: assessment of prognosis by clinical presentation. *Cancer* 1985; **56**: 397–402.
12. Ross CB, Sharp KW, Kaufman AJ, Andrews T, Williams LF. Efficacy of computed tomography in the pre-operative staging of pancreatic carcinoma. *Am Surg* 1988; **54**: 221–6.
13. Tio TL, Tytgat GNJ. Endoscopic ultrasonography in the staging local resectability of pancreatic and periampullary malignancy. *Scand J Gastroenterol* 1986; **21**(suppl 123): 135–42.
14. Yasuda K, Mukai H, Fujimoto S, Nakajima M, Kawai K. The diagnosis of pancreatic cancer by endoscopic ultrasonography. *Gastrointest Endosc* 1988; **34**: 1–8.
15. Appleton GUN, Bathurst NCG, Virjee J. Cooper MJ, Williamson RCN. The value of angiography in the surgical management of pancreatic disease. *Ann R Col Surg Engl* 1989; **71**: 92–6.
16. Mackie CR, Lu CT, Noble HG *et al.* Prospective evaluation of angiography in the diagnosis and management of patients suspected of having pancreatic cancer. *Ann Surg* 1978; **189**: 11–17.
17. Warshaw AL, Tepper JE, Shipley WU. Laparoscopy in the staging and planning of therapy for pancreatic cancer. *Am J Surg* 1986; **151**: 76–80.
18. Cuschieri A. Laparoscopy for pancreatic cancer. Does it benefit the patient? *Eur J Surg Clin Oncol* 1988; **14**: 41–4.
19. Warshaw AL, Gu Z, Wittenburg J, Waltman AC. Pre-operative staging and assessment of resectability of pancreatic cancer. *Arch Surg* 1990; **125**: 230–3.
20. Lillemoe KD, Sauter PK, Pitt HA, Yeo CJ, Cameron JL. Current status of surgical palliation of periampullary carcinoma. *Surg Gynecol Obstet* 1993; **176**: 1–10.
21. Kurzawinski T, Deery A, Davidson BR. Diagnostic value of cytology for biliary stricture. *Br J Surg* 1993; **80**: 414–21.
22. Hall-Craggs MA, Lees WR. Fine needle aspiration biopsy: pancreatic and biliary tumours. *Am J Roentgenol* 1986; **147**: 399–403.
23. Nakayama T, Ikeda A, Okuda K. Percutaneous transhepatic drainage of the biliary tract. *Gastroenterology* 1978; **74**: 554–9.
24. Hoevels J, Lunderquist A. Results of percutaneous internal–external drainage. In: *Non-surgical Biliary Drainage* (eds Classen M, Geenen J, Kawai K), pp. 43–6. Berlin, Springer-Verlag, 1984.
25. Burcharth F. A new endoprosthesis for non-operative intubation of the biliary tract in malignant obstructive jaundice. *Surg Gynecol Obstet* 1978; **146**: 76.
26. Speer AG, Cotton PB, Rode J *et al.* Biliary stent blockage with biofilm. *Ann Intern Med* 1988; **108**: 546–53.
27. Adam A, Chetty N, Roddie M, Young E, Benjamin IS. Self expandable stainless steel endoprostheses for treatment of malignant bile duct obstruction. *Am J Roentgenol* 1991; **156**: 321–5.
28. Dowsett JF, Russell RCG, Hatfield ARW *et al.* Malignant obstructive jaundice: what is the best management? A prospective randomised trial of surgery versus endoscopic stenting. *Gut* 1988; **29**: A1493.

29. Speer AG, Cotton PB, MacRae KD. Endoscopic management of malignant biliary obstruction: stents of 10 French gauge are preferable to stents of 8 French gauge. *Gastrointest Endosc* 1988; **34**: 412–17.
30. Potts JR III, Broughan TA, Hermann RE. Palliative operations for pancreatic carcinoma. *Am J Surg* 1990; **159**: 72–8.
31. Rosemurgy AS, Burnett CM, Waselle JA. A comparison of choledochoenteric bypass and cholecystoenteric bypass in patients with biliary obstruction due to pancreatic cancer. *Am Surg* 1989; **55**: 55–60.
32. Brooks DC, Osteen RT, Gray EB Jr, Steel GDJ, Wilson RE. Evaluation of palliative procedures for pancreatic cancer. *Am J Surg* 1981; **141**: 430–3.
33. Cheslyn-Curtis S, Russell RCG. New trends in gallstone management. *Br J Surg* 1991; **78**: 143–9.
34. Andersson A, Bergdahl L. Carcinoma of the pancreas. *Am Surg* 1976; **42**: 173–7.
35. Doberneck RC, Berndt GA. Delayed gastric emptying after palliative gastrojejunostomy for carcinoma of the pancreas. *Arch Surg* 1987: **122**: 827–9.
36. Jacobs PPM, van der Sluis RF, Wobbes T. Role of gastroenterostomy in the palliative surgical treatment of pancreatic cancer. *J Surg Oncol* 1989; **42**: 145–9.
37. Barkin JS, Goldberg RI, Sfakianakis GN, Levi J. Pancreatic carcinoma is associated with delayed gastric emptying. *Dig Dis Sci* 1986; **31**: 265–7.
38. Sarr MG, Gladen HF, Beart RWJ, van Heerden JA. Role of gastroenterostomy in patients with unresectable pancreatic carcinoma. *Surg Gynecol Obstet* 1981; **152**: 597–600.
39. Speer AG, Cotton PB, Russel RCG *et al.* Randomised trial of endoscopic versus percutaneous insertion in malignant obstructive jaundice. *Lancet* 1987; **ii**: 57–62.
40. Dooley JS, Dick R, George P *et al.* Percutaneous transhepatic endoprosthesis for bile duct obstruction. *Gastroenterol* 1984; **86**: 905–9.
41. Coons HG, Carey PH. Large bore long biliary endoprosthesis (biliary stents) for improved drainage. *Radiology* 1983; **148**: 89–94.

7.2

Laparoscopic Biliary–Enteric Bypass

N. O'ROURKE and L. NATHANSON

The clinical application of the endoluminal approach to the biliary tree and pancreatic ducts has expanded rapidly using sphincterotomy, palliative stenting techniques and stricture dilation.[1] These choices have lead to a substantial decrease in patients undergoing the standard open surgical treatments of potentially curative resection, palliative resection and palliative bypass.

The minimal access laparoscopic approach adds to the complexity of the treatment options available, with the attraction of accelerated recovery postoperatively. The techniques will be outlined below and an attempt made to evaluate their particular place in management with our experience accumulated to date.

PATIENT SELECTION

The vast majority of patients requiring biliary bypass are for pancreatic adenocarcinoma. Small numbers of patients with primary duct calculi will require drainage. Most of these will have this achieved by endoscopic papillotomy. Occasionally choledochoduodenostomy is indicated for those unable to achieve drainage by papillotomy. This can be performed laparoscopically but remains in the experimental phase of our experience. For this reason only the simpler cholecystjejunostomy and gastrojejunostomy techniques will be described.

Curative resection for pancreatic adenocarcinoma is undertaken on the basis of disease localized within the organ and a patient with sufficient physiological reserve to survive the operation. Surprisingly histological confirmation of the nature of a tumour within the pancreas remains challenging.[2,3] In the absence of a successful biopsy under imaging guidance, laparoscopic exposure will allow rapid assessment of the peritoneal surface throughout the entire abdomen.[4] By use of at least two accessory ports, head up/down and lateral tilt of the patient combined within organ displacement, most of the peritoneum can be visualized.

The presence of any metastatic disease confirms the diagnosis and renders biopsy of the primary tumour unnecessary.

Physiologically compromised individuals and those with disseminated tumour precluding cure may be offered palliation with endoscopic stenting of the common bile duct, cholecystjejunostomy, choledochojejunostomy, gastrojejunostomy, sympathetic coeliac ganglion block or, occasionally, no treatment at all. Crucial to the choice of management is an accurate assessment of the extent of infiltration of the cystic duct, common bile duct and duodenum. Diagnostic laparoscopy can proceed to definitve laparoscopic bypass if unresectable disease is established or can be deferred until paraffin sections of biopsies confirm the diagnosis.

Laparoscopy at the commencement of planned open curative resection will allow thorough inspection of the peritoneum and if metastases are confirmed, palliative laparoscopic bypass can then proceed.

PALLIATIVE BYPASS

With small tumours not leading to incipient duodenal obstruction simple passage of an endoscopic stent at the time of diagnostic ERCP is often justified by its simplicity and low mortality. The risks of encrustation, obstruction and recurring cholangitis are higher than for surgical bypass. However, the ease of stent placement under sedation, results in mortality less than 5%. Subsequent replacement of the stent for encrustation does entail repeated admission to hospital but is becoming less problematical as techniques and stent designs improve.[1] Those patients who subsequently develop duodenal obstruction can be submitted to surgical bypass when this complication arises. Laparoscopic bypass to the gall bladder is planned for patients in whom stent placement is considered inappropriate and where this is not possible for technical reasons. At open surgery, bypass of the duodenum by gastroenterostomy is often combined with a biliary bypass to anticipate duodenal obstruction, which will occur in approximately 50% of patients. When such palliation is undertaken at laparotomy, prophylactic duodenal bypass would appear to be appropriate since a second laparotomy in a frail patient with limited duration of survival would constitute poor palliation.

The case for the prophylactic combination of gastroenterostomy and biliary bypass using laparoscopic exposure would seem far more tenuous. The morbidity related to a second laparoscopic procedure is minor, the ileus induced minimal and any subsequent gastroenteric bypass usually functions within three days. It therefore seems reasonable, although no data at present validate this approach, for gastroenterostomy to be reserved for those with existing or incipient duodenal obstruction. This approach will minimize the morbidity which might result from unnecessary gastroenterostomy.

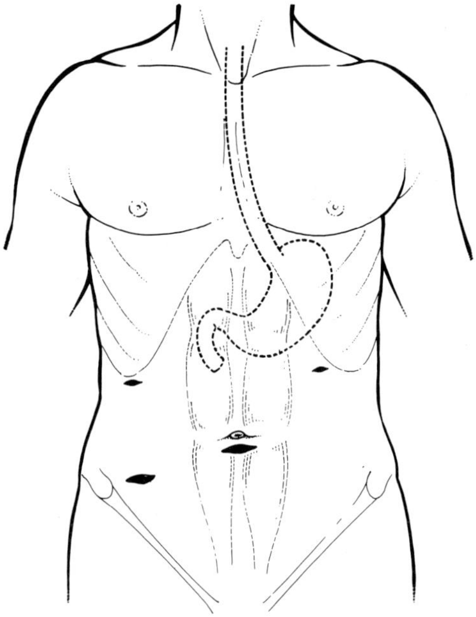

Figure 7.2.1 Port placement for biliary and duodenal bypass. A 10 mm port conveys the laparoscope at the umbilicus, a 12 mm for the stapler in the right iliac fossa and two 5 mm ports.

In patients with incipient or established duodenal obstruction surgical bypass of the bile duct and duodenum as a single procedure is in the best interests of the patient. However if the insertion of the cystic duct is low down the bile duct, or clearly near enough to the tumour to require bypass to the common hepatic duct, then consideration should be given to placing a stent. Bypass of any subsequent duodenal obstruction could be undertaken by a laparoscopic gastroenterostomy.

Physicians performing ERCP should be aware of this dilemma, attempt to document the anatomy of the cystic duct and be willing to discuss the treatment options available with a surgeon at the time.

CHOLECYSTJEJUNOSTOMY

The patient is placed supine with appropriate preparation for operative cholangiography. The surgeon stands on the patient's right with the ancillary instrument stand and video monitor placed at the head of the table opposite the patient's left shoulder. The assistant stands opposite the surgeon with the scrub nurse on the same side as the surgeon. Port placement is illustrated in Fig. 7.2.1. The right iliac fossa port is 12 mm in diameter to accommodate the linear

Table 7.2.1 Instrumentation required

Bowel grasping forceps
Atraumatic grasping forceps
Needle holder
External anchoring suture
Linear cutter/stapler
Endoscopic measuring device

stapler/cutter. The two ports used by the surgeon must be anchored to the skin to prevent displacement and have flapper or silicone valve mechanisms, which improve instrument manipulation, an important factor during suturing.

Cholangiography

Unless accurate preoperative information concerning the site of cystic duct entry to the common hepatic duct is available, cholangiography is achieved by introducing contrast into the gall bladder as the first step of the procedure. The Veress needle is introduced through the abdominal wall under visual control for this purpose and bile is aspirated until the gall bladder is at least half empty. Difficulty caused by thick inspissated bile can be overcome by the introduction of saline into the gall bladder, mixing it with the bile by gentle agitation followed by aspiration. Contrast is introduced under fluoroscopic control to observe filling of the gall bladder, to note the precise point of entry of the cystic duct to the common bile duct and the relative position of the carcinoma obstructing the duct distally. Early visualization of the flow of the contrast is important, as most accurate information regarding the course of the cystic duct is often available on initial flow into the common bile duct. Once larger volumes of contrast are injected, large dilated ducts overlap the image, leading to uncertainty in some instances as to the site of cystic duct entry relative to the tumour. Successful mapping of the cystic duct course allows a decision to be taken early in the operation on whether the patient is suitable for laparoscopic cholecystjejunostomy or if an alternative open bypass to the common hepatic duct should be performed.

The anastomosis can be fashioned using sutures entirely, mechanical stapling devices entirely or a combination of the two. The technique found to be most useful with currently available equipment uses the linear cutter/stapler to complete the main part of the anastomosis with closure of the residual defect using sutures. Table 7.2.1 lists the instrumentation required.

Stapled and Sutured Anastomosis

On completion of the cholangiogram the contrast fluid is aspirated, the needle withdrawn and a suitable segment of jejunum selected for the anastomosis. This is achieved as follows. The duodenojejunal flexure is identified by carefully grasping the transverse colon and omentum with two atraumatic forceps and elevating these structures anterior and cephalad to the stomach. The assistant is then able to maintain this position with one atraumatic grasper while the surgeon, using two atraumatic graspers, follows the small bowel up in a "hand over hand" manner until the flexure is reached. The small bowel is followed down and a suitable point chosen for the anastomosis by allowing the transverse colon to fall back into position and bringing the small bowel around it up to the gall bladder and anterior wall of stomach (in those cases where a combined bypass is required). This is important as there is a tendency to underestimate the length of proximal small bowel required when viewing and handling it endoscopically. The small bowel is then held by the assistant using atraumatic grasping forceps. An 8 mm opening in the gall bladder is made and bile aspirated before a slightly smaller incision is made on the antimesenteric aspect of the jejunum. Support of the gall bladder and bowel may be improved by using an external anchoring suture on a straight needle. This is inserted through and then back out of the abdominal wall laterally after anchoring the gall bladder and jejunum and provides countertraction for insertion of the stapler. The 30 mm Endo GIA (United States Surgical Corporation, Norwalk, CT) loaded with the bowel stapling cartridge is introduced as illustrated in Figure 7.2.2, its position checked and then fired. Closure of the residual defect is with a 15 cm 3/O polyglactin suture with a pretied jamming loop knot (Fig. 7.2.3). This is commenced with care to include the apex and includes bites of tissue 5 mm apart incorporating the full thickness of the gall bladder wall and extra mucosal layers of the jejunum. Completion of the suture line is by internally tied reef knot.

This combination of stapled anastomosis with closure of the defect by sutures is in our hands the most practical method of creating a cholecystjejunostomy at present. It has been found to be easier than closing the residual defect by triangulation using a second firing of staples. The difficulty experienced arises from inability to precisely apply the second firing of the Endo GIA, so on the one hand ensuring complete closure of the defect and on the other avoiding stenosis of the efferent jejunal lumen. The main reason for this is that the presently available stapling devices are not able to angulate correctly to adjust to the required plane of staple application.

Sutured Cholecystjejunostomy

An alternative to the use of the mechanical linear cutter/stapler is an entirely sutured anastomosis. The principal difference in technique here is to open the gall bladder and jejunal lumen only after the posterior suture line is complete. After selection of the suitable anastomotic site of jejunum (as described above), a 25 mm length of the antimesenteric border and of serosa of the gall bladder fundus is marked with light diathermy. These lines identify the incision site, ensure that an adequate size of anastomosis is planned and maintain the surgeon's orientation during suturing.

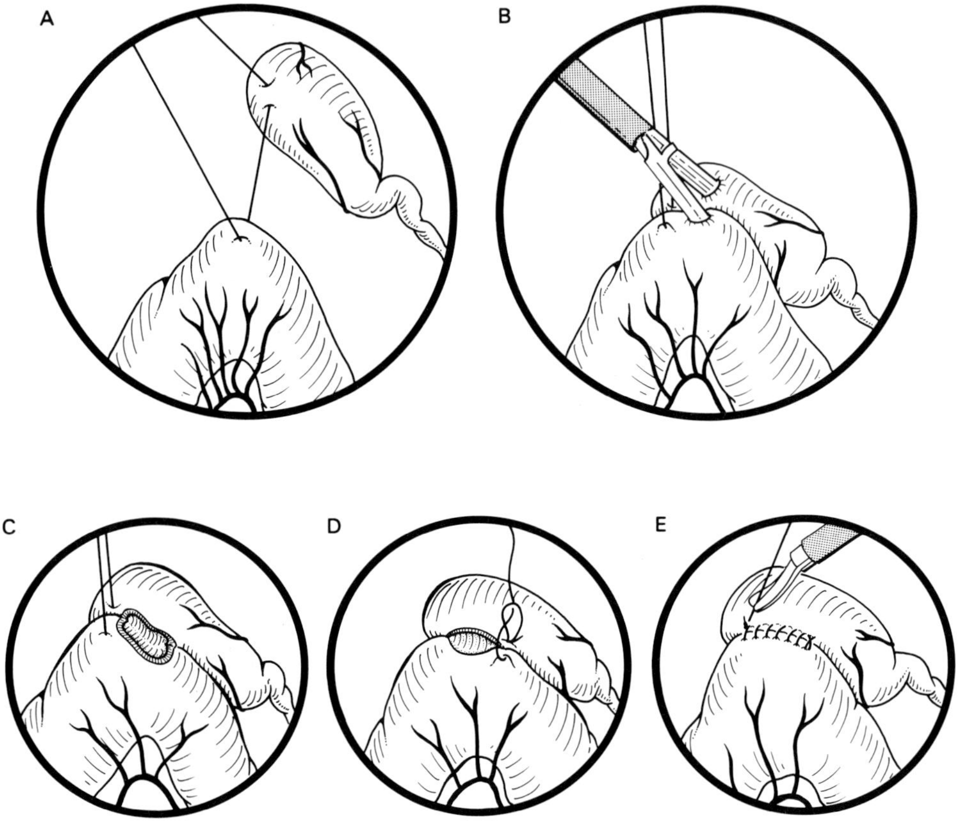

Figure 7.2.2 The stapled and sutured cholecystjejunostomy. A: A polypropelene suture sling is inserted through the abdominal wall and anchored externally. B: Small cholecystotomy and enterotomy incisions are made and a linear cutter stapler fired to approximate the gall bladder and jejunum. C: The staple line is inspected through the defect left by the stapler. D: The enterotomy is closed with a running suture. E: A reef or Aberdeen knot finishes the suture line and excess suture is removed.

The suture is prepared by fashioning a loop at the tail of the suture with a jamming loop knot (Fig. 7.2.3). The suture is introduced into the peritoneum with care to prevent inadvertent closure of the loop. The needle is passed through the tissue and through the loop, which is closed by traction on the body of the suture. In this way the suture line is commenced quickly and easily. The suture used is 3/O polyglactin with a standard 26 mm semicircular taper needle about 15 cm in length. Sutures are placed taking the full thickness of the gall bladder wall and extramucosal bites of bowel wall. After each suture is placed tension for correct tissue approximation is maintained by the assistant grasping the suture with rubber-shod or atraumatic grasping forceps some 2 cm away from the suture line. This "following" of the suture by the assistant is repeated after each pass of the needle.

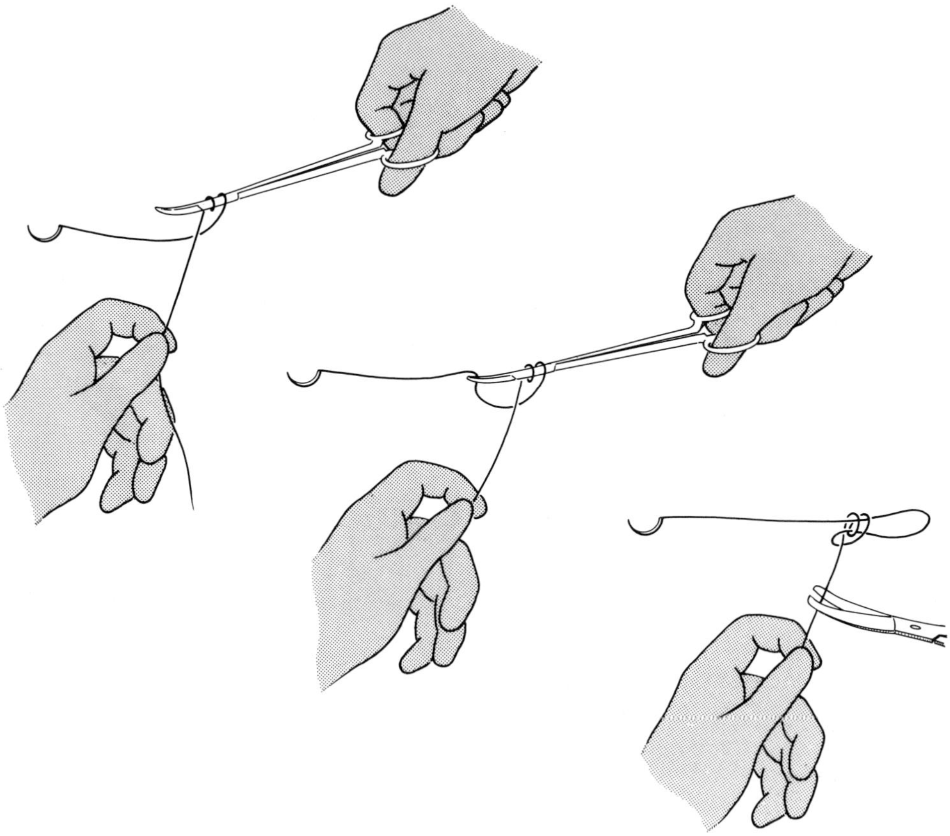

Figure 7.2.3 A jamming loop knot made outside the abdomen. The knot is started by wrapping the tail around a needle holder. The body of the suture is grasped and pulled back through the initial wrap to create a loop and the tail is then trimmed.

On completion of the posterior layer the suture is tied with a reef knot and the tail left about 3 cm long. The gall bladder is opened along the diathermy line and aspirated dry to minimize bile spillage. The bowel is similarly opened over a 25 mm length. A second suture 15 cm in length with a pretied jamming loop knot is introduced, the apex identified and the continuous suture line fashioned. Extramucosal or full thickness bites of 5 mm intervals complete the anastomosis.

STAPLED AND SUTURED GASTROJEJUNOSTOMY

The combination of stapling combined with suture closure of the residual defect is attractive for this 6 cm long anastomosis. It allows rapid creation of the stoma and its only drawback lies with the expense of the disposable stapler and refill cartridge.

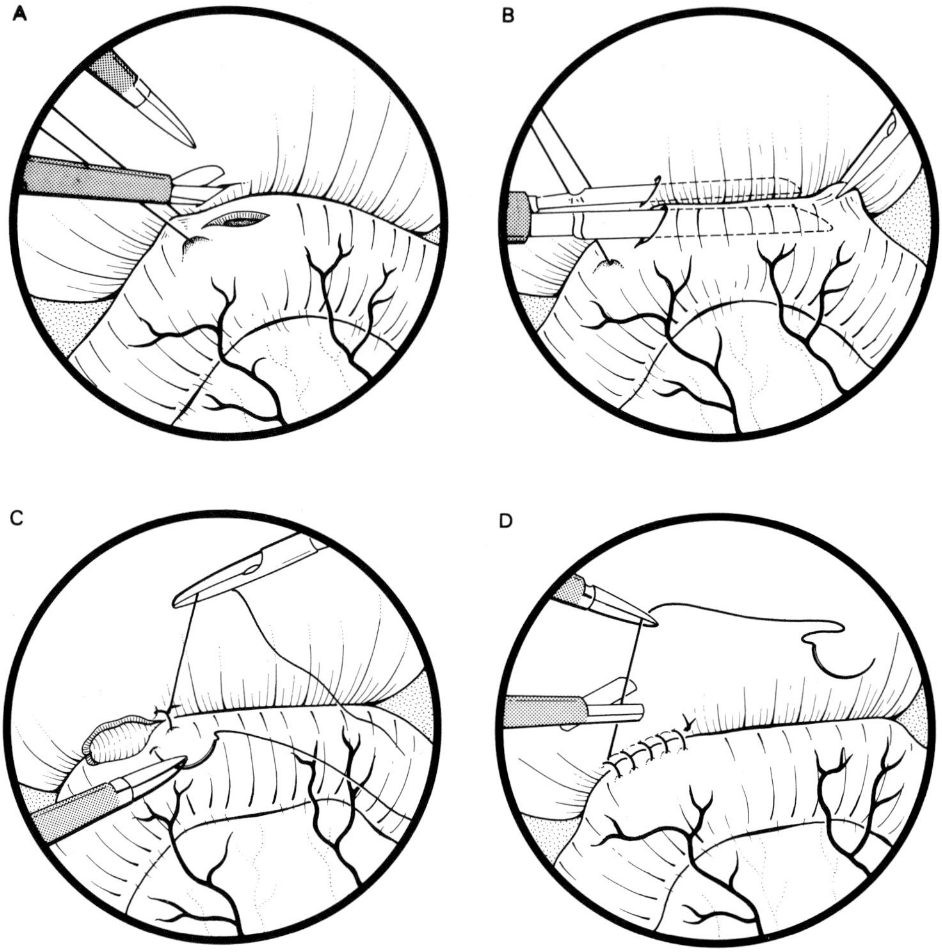

Figure 7.2.4 Stapled and sutured anterior gastroenterostomy. A: A polypropelene suture sling is inserted through the abdominal wall and anchored externally, the stomach aspirated via the nasogastric tube and small enterotomy and gastrotomy incisions made. B: A 60 mm linear cutter stapler is applied (or two 30 mm cartridges) to approximate the stomach and jejunum. C: The staple line is inspected through the defect left by the stapler and the enterotomy closed with a running suture. D: A reef or Aberdeen knot finishes the suture line and excess suture is removed.

The selected portion of jejunum is grasped by the assistant and an 8 mm enterotomy made using diathermy and scissors, followed by a similar enterotomy in the antrum of the stomach at the distal end of the proposed anastomosis. An external anchoring suture placed through the stomach and jejunum at the efferent aspect of the anastomosis facilitates retraction and approximation of the jejunum and stomach (Fig. 7.2.4). The 60 mm Endo GIA is introduced and inserted into jejunum and the stomach parallel to the greater curve. The stapler is clamped, its position checked and fired. After removal the suture line is inspected but diathermy should not be applied to the staple line for haemostasis.

If the 30 mm Endo GIA is used two firings will be required. The first is completed as described for the larger stapler. The stapler is removed and a fresh bowel cartridge inserted. The reapplication of the stapler to extend the suture line takes care by the surgeon as the apex of the previous two rows of staples must be accurately found and the second firing must continue from this point if a devascularized segment of bowel is to be avoided. Once the stapling has been completed the defect in the stomach and jejunum is closed with a continuous 3/O polyglactin suture on a standard curved needle.

Routine peritoneal drainage is not employed.

Sutured Gastrojejunostomy

A sutured anastomosis of the stomach to the jejunum using the technique as described for cholecystjejunostomy can be safely achieved, with some precautions. Care must be taken to empty the stomach using the nasogastric tube prior to opening the stomach. The 6 cm long anastomosis should be fashioned again as a simple continuous layer suture, but the suture tied at intervals. This maintains the approximation of the suture line on the tissue which may otherwise slacken as bowel shortening and relaxation occur during peristalsis. The stomach is very vascular and bleeding vessels must be clearly identified and controlled with diathermy to maintain a clear field for precise suture placement.

The major disadvantage of the entirely sutured techniques is that the long suture line is tedious to fashion and this may result in a shorter anastomosis being fashioned. All such anastomoses scar down to some extent but the thick walled stomach is especially likely to do so. There is a risk that anastomosis significantly shorter than 6 cm will result in stenosis at a later stage. It is for these reasons that the stapled anastomosis is preferred for the gastrojejunostomy.

Measures to minimize the risk of stomal ulceration are taken in all patients who have not undergone concomitant vagotomy. These usually entail the long term use of alginates or H_2 receptor blockers. Alternatively truncal vagotomy (see Chapter 10) can simply be performed at the same time as gastrojejunostomy. If this is planned, it should be the first step of the operation prior to opening the bowel or gall bladder to minimize the contamination of the oesophagogastric junction and posterior mediastinum.

CONVERSION TO LAPAROTOMY

The most common reason for conversion to open bypass to the bile ducts would be tumour encroachment on or near to the cystic duct. Laparotomy will also be required where the identification of the duodenojejunal flexure has not been achieved, with the attendant risk of siting of the anastomosis incorrectly along the jejunum. Uncontrollable bleeding has not been a problem to date. Bile contamination is common but easily controlled by aspiration and lavage with warm Ringers lactate solution. The presence of cholangitis and spillage of contaminated bile have not resulted in complications, but all patients receive broad spectrum prophylactic antibiotic cover intraoperatively.

Technical breakdown of equipment may well abort an otherwise successful operation but can be minimized by having back-up equipment.

POSTOPERATIVE RECOVERY

Patients are encouraged to mobilize and take oral fluids as soon as they have recovered from anaesthesia. Experience has shown in the experimental[8] and clinical situation that these anastomoses can function immediately with minimal apparent alteration of motility in most patients. All wounds are infiltrated with 0.25% bupivacaine in combination with 1/200 000 adrenaline and indomethacin suppository 100 mg given twice daily. Decreased postoperative narcotic administration resulting from this regimen markedly decreases the unwanted side effect of impaired bowel function and patients are usually tolerating food by the first or second day after the operation and request discharge by the third postoperative day.

CONCLUSION

Palliative bypass offered to patients without duodenal obstruction will most often be by endoscopic stent placement. In those where this is not achieved laparoscopic bypass to the gall bladder offers accelerated recovery compared to open techniques. In those with duodenal obstruction a gastrojejunostomy can be combined with this. In some situations a stent will have been placed prior to surgery for duodenal obstruction. A subsequent laparoscopic gastroenterostomy will provide palliation but the advantage of avoiding a general anaesthetic is lost and recurring stent obstruction and cholangitis may reduce the quality of the remaining months of life.

It is possible to fashion a choledochoduodenostomy laparoscopically but this type of bypass is prone to obstruction as tumour encroachment ensues and is not advocated for palliation for pancreatic adenocarcinoma.

Data allowing objective assessment of the outcome of this laparoscopic approach compared to stenting and open surgery remain anecdotal due to the short duration the techniques have been used and the small numbers of patients reported.[5,6,7] In this group of nine patients and a further five in our institution, no mortality occurred, no anastomotic leakage was noted and only one stoma required subsequent clearance due to blockage by blood clot and debris. However, careful documentation of postoperative pain, recovery of bowel function and mobility in a substantial number of patients is required to validate our initial impression that selected patients will indeed benefit from minimal access bypass palliative surgery.

REFERENCES

1. Vitale GC. Interventional endoscopic retrograde cholangiopancreatography: state of the art (part 1). *J Roy Coll Surg Edinb* 1992; **37**: 289–97.
2. Coupland GAE, Townend DM, Martin CJ. Peritoneoscopy – use in assessment of intra-abdominal malignancy. *Surgery* 1981; **86**: 645–9.
3. Warshaw AL. Trepper JE, Shipley WU. Laparoscopy in the staging and planning of therapy for pancreatic cancer. *Am J Surg* 1986; **151**: 76–80.
4. Cuschieri A, Hall AW, Clark J. Value of laparoscopy in the diagnosis and management of pancreatic carcinoma. *Gut* 1978; **19**: 672–7.
5. Shimi S, Banting S, Cuschieri A. Laparoscopy in the management of pancreatic cancer: endoscopic cholecysto-jejunostomy for advanced disease. *Br J Surg* 1992; **79**: 317–19.
6. Fletcher DR, Jones RM. Laparoscopic cholecystjejunostomy as palliation for obstructive jaundice in inoperable carcinoma of pancreas. *Surg Endosc* 1992; **6**: 147–9.
7. Hawasli A. Laparoscopic cholecysto-jejunostomy for obstructing pancreatic cancer: technique and report of two cases. *J Laparoendosc Surg* 1992; **2**: 351–5.
8. Nathanson LK, Shimi S, Cuschieri A. Sutured laparoscopic cholecysto-jejunostomy evolved in an animal model. *J Roy Coll Surg Edinb* 1992; **37**: 215–20.

Overview

Bypass surgery

Many hepatobiliary surgeons insist that hepaticojejunostomy is the most appropriate bypass procedure for malignant distal bile duct obstruction, but, as Russell has suggested, this is not always true and many patients gain good palliation from either cholecystjejunostomy or choledochoduodenostomy. The size of the tumour and its relationship to the insertion of the cystic duct is important in the former, and encroachment on the duodenum in the latter. Thus circumstances may exist where laparoscopic cholecystjejunostomy (with or without gastroenterostomy) is appropriate. Although the long-term palliation may be inferior to hepaticojejunostomy, patients may succumb to the disease before recurrent obstruction occurs, at which time the patient could be considered for open surgical bypass. The main question is whether the frail patient with limited life expectancy is best served by laparoscopic bypass (assuming cystic duct patency) or ERCP and stent insertion. Although the latter is less invasive, the recurrence of jaundice from the former may be less, and results of prospective studies are awaited with interest.

8.1

Expectations of Colorectal Surgery (Benign and Malignant)

R. K. S. PHILLIPS

INTRODUCTION

This chapter is divided into two parts. The first part will address the various tenets of good operative colorectal surgical practice, such as exposure, mobilization, anastomosis and such like and will highlight areas where some of the advantages of a laparoscopic approach might be won back by the "conventional" surgeon. The second part will consider a number of pathological processes and will describe, and where necessary challenge, these orthodox objectives.

Today's colorectal surgeon is driven by many competing forces: economics, leading to shortened hospital stay and more efficient use of resources; short term and long term outcome; and patient desires – usually for a painless uncomplicated procedure with the smallest possible scar. But none of these forces should be allowed to dominate the ultimate assessment of what should now constitute best surgical practice.

Length of stay for colorectal surgery has been much too long in the United Kingdom. In the United States of America third party insurers have specified how many days they are prepared to fund for a patient undergoing a straightforward conventional operation: for example, five days for a right hemicolectomy and six days for a left hemicolectomy. This has meant that patients are often prepared for surgery as outpatients, sometimes even being admitted for major surgery on the day of operation itself. The cost of overnight accommodation close to the hospital both immediately before surgery and while still only partially ambulant after surgery may be the patient's own personal responsibility.

The situation in the United Kingdom is very different. Firstly, there has not been the same urgency to maximize the use of beds. This has meant that there has not been the same infrastructural development that permits rapid patient turnover: high quality secretarial support that can troubleshoot and sort out administrative problems; sufficient support services to allow rapid medical and laboratory assessment and thereby allow admission and limited rapid work-up on the day of surgery; and guaranteed beds for elective surgery. Indeed, empty beds are essential for efficient practice; for as bed occupancy rises above 90% so cancellations become more and more necessary, patient and medical frustration increases and efficiency falls. Secondly, there is little that can be done by the medical staff when confronted by a patient who simply will not go home because it is not convenient. No charges can be levied; so nobody is prepared to move out into an adjacent hotel at their own expense, nor are many prepared to make any domestic arrangements at their own expense that would facilitate an earlier discharge.

All of this means that there are inherent underlying flaws that will act against efficiencies being achieved by a more minimalist approach to colorectal surgery. These flaws will act both for and against laparoscopic surgery.

At the moment, the ultimate determinant of medical discharge from hospital after major gastrointestinal surgery is the return of gut function. This allows oral nutrition to be commenced and the intravenous infusion to be discontinued. After major conventional surgery on the large intestine this interval is on average 4–5 days, by which time most patients who are not extremely old or frail are sufficiently ambulant that the immediate need for them to be in hospital has passed. Many would be suitable to be looked after, either in the community by primary health care workers or in an adjacent hostel visited by the clinical team, were either available and adequately funded. It may yet prove to be the case that laparoscopically assisted surgery leads to an earlier return of gut function and thereby an opportunity for earlier discharge, but any gain here is at best going to be marginal and must be offset in economic terms by the massively increased cost in the operating theatre. This cost is not just in terms of the expensive equipment that is necessary nor just in terms of the longer time spent in the operating theatre. If such longer operating times remain after the initial learning period, then more operating theatres are going to need to be built, and more surgical teams trained, in order to achieve a similar throughput of cases; and all of this means borrowing large sums of capital and repaying the interest, the capital and the increased numbers of salaries.

Thereafter, the patient is still at risk of short term complications, such as wound infection, anastomotic dehiscence and deep vein thrombosis and pulmonary embolism. Whereas some of these complications, for example, wound infection, may prove less likely after laparoscopically assisted surgery, others, such as thromboembolic complications, might prove more likely, because of the extra length of time under anaesthesia. Furthermore, those most at risk will surely be those attempted laparoscopically who are then converted to a conventional operation.

One is then left with longer term complications, such as disease recurrence or adhesional obstruction, and economics. Any gain in return to work for a laparoscopically assisted operation by the average patient (which might conceivably be anything from two to four weeks) is unlikely to earn for the Exchequer any sum that remotely approaches the costs mentioned above. Since so many patients undergoing major colorectal surgery are already retired and therefore no longer making such an economic return, and as the increased costs of unsuccessful attempts will also need to be recovered, it is unlikely that an economic argument for laparoscopically assisted colorectal surgery will ever win the day.

Which leaves medical contraindications to a long abdominal incision – in particular, severe pulmonary disease – and patient preference, which certainly should not be ignored and which will largely be centred on postoperative pain, early return to full mobility and a smaller incision.

THE SICK PATIENT

For most patients with severe concomitant illness and a large bowel pathology, there are already conventional alternatives that may help militate against a large, conventional abdominal incision. Examples include perineal operations for rectal prolapse (such as Delorme's and Altmeier's operations)[1] and posterior parasacral approaches to the rectum that are derived from the old Kraske operation. Such posterior approaches permit mobilization of the rectum under direct vision and intestinal anastomosis, but they are limited in the length of intestine and the amount of lymph nodes that can be removed. The limitation is caused by an inability to deal with the inferior mesenteric artery near its origin through a posterior approach, which in turn limits the amount of length that can be gained on the proximal colonic end; but this limitation can be overcome through the addition either of a Rutherford–Morrison left iliac fossa incision (Localio operation)[2] or through a laparoscopically assisted abdominal phase, which would also allow splenic flexure mobilization.

There of course remain other circumstances, such as carcinoma of the colon, where an abdominal incision sufficient to perform an appropriate resection will need to be employed; but even here most surgeons adapt their incision to the special circumstances of the case, often adopting quite a small transverse incision sited over the lesion.

THE CONVENTIONAL INCISION

This achieves ready access to the extremes of the abdomen and does not compromise potential future stoma sites. When operating on the left colon, it is necessary to mobilize the splenic flexure and often to dissect the rectum also. The simplest and speediest way to achieve these aims is by a long midline incision, but it is also possible to perform a rather slower and bloodier infraumbilical transverse incision which curls up towards the relevant flexure. Some believe such an incision to be more cosmetic, perhaps to be less painful and to heal better.

The length of the incision in the abdominal wall is dictated often by the need to exert traction from a previously inaccessible quarter. All surgeons will be familiar with the improved ease of an operation simply by extending the incision. Laparoscopic surgery has now taught us that traction can be brought to bear simply by inserting a fresh port in an appropriate place and there is nothing to prevent the surgeon operating conventionally similarly inserting one or more grasping instruments through laterally placed stab wounds rather than extending the incision. Such an approach would go some of the way towards reducing one of the claimed advantages of a laparoscopically assisted operation.

The length of the skin incision conventionally matches the length of the incision in the abdominal wall. But there is nothing to stop a surgeon from undercutting the skin at the level of the abdominal wall in order to achieve a high degree of mobility of the skin and subcutaneous fat on the abdominal wall. This would then allow a much smaller (and, for the patient, more cosmetic) skin incision, while at the same time permitting many of the advantages of a much larger incision in the abdominal wall itself. The outer wound would simply be retracted appropriately in order to supply the relevant view. Up until now, surgeons have not seen a need to make an operation even the slightest bit more awkward when the same exposure can be achieved more simply by extending the whole incision. But now that many surgeons are adopting much more complicated laparoscopic methods of, among other things, achieving a smaller skin incision, it is possible to see that the same effect might be achieved very much more simply and at a fraction of the time and cost in a manner similar to the one outlined above.

Postoperative pain control has improved dramatically in recent years with patient operated and continuous infusion devices. Nonetheless, pain control relies heavily either on opiate analgesics given systemically, with all the attendant risks of sedation and respiratory depression, or on epidural analgesia, which suffers from the need to have skilled personnel available out of hours to top them up. Local incisional analgesics have largely been employed on a "one-off" basis and rely on the half life of bupivacaine which is much too short to have a realistic effect on postoperative recovery. However, were there to be an investment into implantable local anaesthetic wound infiltration devices that was but a fraction of the size of the investment into laparoscopic surgical equipment, then yet another of the perceived disadvantages of a conventional surgical wound might be abated.

THE ASSESSMENT

After gaining access to the abdomen, the relevant pathology needs to be evaluated, as do more remote sites that might influence the management of the case. For example, in cancer, the liver and the rest of the large intestine need to be evaluated, whereas in inflammatory bowel disease the small intestine needs careful assessment, in case a previously unsuspected area of Crohn's disease should be overlooked; and when dealing with a known case of Crohn's disease, it helps to measure the length of the small intestine before deciding on one long resection or a bowel length conserving combination of minimal resections and stricturoplasties.

Much more information can be acquired preoperatively now than ever used to be the case, in particular with regard to the state of the liver and the rest of the large bowel. However, it is not always possible to image proximal to an obstructing or partially obstructing tumour and even when such evaluation does prove possible, either preoperatively or indeed intraoperatively, the result may be far from accurate. Furthermore, preoperative evaluation of the small intestine remains quite limited and often overlooks significant extra pathology.

Preoperative assessment of the relevant local pathology can be very poor indeed and may fail to show important lymph node and urinary tract involvement in cancer cases. In cases of Crohn's disease the junction between macroscopically involved bowel and adjacent uninvolved bowel can be very difficult to identify. Indeed, the only sign that Crohn's disease is still present at the proposed site of resection may be thickening of the mesenteric wall of the bowel when it is rolled between thumb and forefinger.

It is this very important tactile assessment that is missing when operating laparoscopically and despite the potential for developing other modalities such as ultrasound it will very likely remain one of the major drawbacks of laparoscopic colorectal surgery. For another example, when dissecting posteriorly in the pelvis in the plane behind the mesorectum in a case of cancer, it is the tactile sensation that the tumour is encroaching on this plane that leads the surgeon to abandon this anatomical approach and to excise more widely, even if this is at the risk of sacrificing the presacral nerves.

THE DISSECTION

There are essentially two ways of achieving a dissection. One is the conventional way of *touch* dissection, usually performed with a combination of blunt dissection and sharp dissection using scissors. This technique relies very much on continually feeling the boundaries between relevant structures and then cutting along these boundaries. It is not essential to have an absolutely bloodless field as the surgeon is guided as much by feel; neither is it important to set up each step – the operation proceeds as a continuous process, like the running of a cine film, rather than as a number of still scenes.

The second way is by "*see*" dissection. That is, the surgeon relies much more on being able to see and very little, if at all, on touch. Such dissection is usually performed with an energy source, such as a diathermy instrument or a laser, but the method is the same when dissecting intra-abdominally with a scalpel. The essential steps are: set up a static scene; rely on quite firm traction to identify the "tension points" that need division; dissect precisely, layer by layer; ensure absolute haemostatis all the time; and then set up the next scene. The operation thus proceeds like a succession of still shots, rather than as a cine film.

Touch dissection is unsuited to laparoscopic assisted surgery for obvious reasons. However, "see" dissection can just as easily be used when operating conventionally as it can be when operating laparoscopically. And it is "see" dissection that is to a very large extent responsible for the claims by surgeons operating laparoscopically that the view is very much better than when they operate conventionally. There are, of course, other reasons: for example, the ability to get good lighting into inaccessible places and the superb close-up views that can be obtained. However, these must be offset by the lack of stereoscopic vision, the lack of the large scale "strategic" view and the potential to improve lighting during conventional surgery.

ANASTOMOSIS

Anastomosis is often the critical part of a colorectal operation. It must be performed without tension, with well-vascularized bowel and preferably on a well-prepared intestine (although there is some evidence that this last is not so important as it was once thought).[3] The surgeon who performs the anastomosis is probably more important than the actual technique used,[4] the best results being claimed by interrupted serosubmucosal hand suturing in one layer,[5] but good results being reported by all manner of handsewn and stapled end-to-end and side-to-end and even side-to-side techniques.[6] Handsewn anastomoses are difficult, if not well nigh impossible, to achieve intracorporeally with the laparoscope and although they can be performed during a laparoscopically assisted procedure, it is often more convenient to staple.

There are some concerns that disease may recur more readily at an anastomosis and this applies particularly to Crohn's disease and cancer.[7] Viable colorectal cancer cells can be recovered from the cut ends of bowel at the time of bowel cancer resection and this has persuaded many English surgeons to irrigate the cut ends of bowel with a cytocidal solution, such as povidone iodine or chlorhexidine/cetrimide, before anastomosis.[8] North American surgeons have, on the whole, not been so persuaded. Both sutures and staples seem worse experimentally than a sutureless technique in promoting new tumour formation at anastomoses.[9] In practice, insofar as disease recurrence is concerned, neither conventional nor laparoscopically assisted colorectal anastomoses can on *a priori* principles claim the intellectual high ground.

SPECIFIC CONDITIONS

Colorectal Cancer

The other issues that remain to be addressed are the extent of lymphatic clearance; high versus low ligation of the inferior mesenteric artery; whether early vascular ligation or the use of occluding tapes proximal and distal to a tumour have an advantage; and the amount of colon that needs to be removed.

The Extent of Lymphatic Clearance

The lymphatic drainage of a tumour follows its arterial blood supply. In the left colon, and particularly at the splenic flexure, it is not always easy to know in advance what that arterial supply is going to be. This is because there are quite large variations between individuals in their vascular anatomy. For example, 6% of patients have no left colic artery, the splenic flexure being supplied by an enlarged middle colic artery; and in 22% of patients the middle colic artery is absent and the blood supply of the splenic flexure is shared between the left colic and right colic arteries.[10] This means that lymphatic clearance when operating on a case of splenic flexure carcinoma may need to encompass as far as the right and left colic arteries; the simplest operation is thus an extended right hemicolectomy, although in the elderly preservation of the ileocolic artery will permit a caecodescending anastomosis instead, which may have a functional advantage.[11]

When it comes to dissection of the rectum, so long as the whole mesorectum is removed by a skilled surgeon and a cytocidal lumenal wash-out is performed, the conventional view is that local recurrence is uncommon.[12] However, there is evidence that lymphatic involvement outside these boundaries along the internal iliac chain of lymph nodes is really quite common. Such lymph node involvement has been described in as many as 18% of curative cases overall and in 36% of Dukes' C cases.[13] Furthermore, in 6% of cases lateral pelvic side wall lymph node involvement is the *only* lymph node involvement and this is outside the boundaries of a conventional dissection.

It follows from the above that the expected local recurrence rate after conventional surgery that removes the mesorectum but not the internal iliac group of lymph nodes should be of the order of 18% overall for curative cases. Reasons for a lower local recurrence rate than this must include case selection; concentrating on local recurrence that causes a clinical problem (the clinical rate of local recurrence) and overlooking local recurrence that is an insignificant component of more generalized recurrence in an otherwise dying patient (the biological rate of local recurrence); and the use of adjuvant radiotherapy to sterilize involved lymph nodes left behind on the pelvic side walls.

Extending the lymphadenectomy to include the pelvic side wall lymph nodes is not without its own major disadvantages. In a study of 232 cases treated by extended pelvic lymphadenectomy, 50% were ultimately found not to have needed the operation as they did not have any lymph node involvement at all;

the average operating time was five and a half hours (despite the fact that the patients were smaller and thinner than an equivalent western group of patients); blood loss averaged 1.6 litres and 100% had sexual and urinary disturbance afterwards (10% needing permanent urinary catheterization).[13]

High Versus Low Ligation of the Inferior Mesenteric Artery

There have now been a number of careful retrospective studies in which the outcome of cases where the inferior mesenteric artery has been ligated flush with the aorta (high ligation) has been compared with cases where the left colic artery has been preserved and the ligature has been placed at the level of the aortic bifurcation (low ligation).[14,15] There is no doubt that about 19% of cases with lymph node involvement at the level of the apical ligature are ultimately cured of their cancer,[16] so one might expect that a higher ligation should be reflected in a small but detectable improvement in survival. However, this has not proved to be the case. One explanation may be that the dissection is extended only in the plane along the axis of the inferior mesenteric artery without at the same time extending the dissection laterally towards the pelvic side wall. As a greater lymph node burden imparts an increased risk of pelvic side wall lymph node involvement, it is perhaps not surprising after all that high ligation alone has not shown a cancer specific advantage.

In practical terms, high ligation is a necessary part of a low anastomosis, because without it the proximal colon is tethered by the left colic artery and will not reach the distal rectum or anus without tension. Conversely, for a high anastomosis a low ligation will allow anastomosis without tension.

Tumour Isolation

Viable cancer cells may be shed from the lumen of the bowel and may be incorporated by stitches into the anastomisis and thereby lead to anastomotic recurrence.[17] Because of this theoretical risk, Cole used occluding tapes proximal and distal to the cancer before starting tumour mobilization.[18] However, most surgeons consider such practice to be outdated, particularly as povidone iodine or chlorhexidine/cetrimide can be used more simply to wash out the freshly cut bowel ends, thus killing any residual cells.[8]

Cancer cells may be shed from the serosal surface of the bowel or from cut lymphatics and potentially seed into the raw operative site or into the wound, particularly if the tumour is forcibly dragged through a small wound without adequate wound protection. Cytocidal agents that are safe to use in the lumen of the bowel are by no means as safe to use in the peritoneal cavity: mercuric perchloride will be absorbed by the peritoneum and lead to renal damage; and povidone iodine and chlorhexidine/cetrimide in undiluted form cause dense adhesions experimentally in rats (unpublished observations).

Cancer cells can also be found both in the portal and in the systemic circulation.[19] Their precise relevance is unknown; they are certainly not equivalent to *de facto* distant metastases. Nonetheless, early evidence for this persuaded

Rupert Turnbull at the Cleveland Clinic to adopt a policy of dissection characterized by early vascular ligation in order to prevent intraoperative tumour cell embolization to the liver. At first sight, his results were very much better than those of the five other staff surgeons at the Cleveland Clinic who continued to use a conventional approach with vascular ligation after tumour mobilization. However, these staff surgeons also removed only the immediately involved segment of bowel, whereas Turnbull performed a more extensive excision of bowel with its associated lymphatics.[20]

The question of early vascular ligation seems finally to have been answered by a randomized controlled clinical trial from the Netherlands. In a study of 236 cases, the extent of mesenteric clearance and the length of bowel removed were similar and survival at five years was not statistically significantly different, being 60% for the "no-touch" technique and 56% for conventional dissection.[21]

The Amount of Colon that Needs to be Removed

The length of bowel that is removed is ultimately decided by the position of the arterial ligature, as this determines what length of bowel might become ischaemic. Clearly, a good marginal blood supply will allow a shorter length to be removed, but the marginal is absent in the sigmoid and tenuous in the ascending colon and at the splenic flexure. This is why sigmoid colon should never be used for anastomosis and why left colon operations should invariably have the splenic flexure mobilized so that the descending colon, which has a good marginal blood supply, can be used for anastomosis. Similarly, the potential weakness of the marginal blood supply at the splenic flexure means that the two terminal branches of the left colic artery should be preserved in order to support the marginal artery at this point.

The other issue that determines the extent of bowel removed is the degree to which colorectal cancer has a potential to spread within the bowel wall beyond the macroscopic edge of the tumour. For poorly differentiated tumours this distance may be up to 5 cm, but tumours with other differentiation very rarely spread for more than 1.5 cm, which means that a 2 cm margin is usually safe. The issue has recently been extensively reviewed elsewhere.[22]

It is probably the case that too short a clearance of bowel and mesentery should be avoided. Indeed, any advantage claimed by Turnbull from his "no-touch" technique might instead be lain at the door of his more extensive clearance of bowel and mesentery, although there is no direct evidence to show that such is indeed the case.

Inflammatory Bowel Disease

Ulcerative Colitis

Abdominal operations for ulcerative colitis are performed for three main indications: an acutely ill patient whose life is in imminent danger; chronic ill health (so-called failed medical treatment); and for the risk or actuality of cancer.

Operations in acute circumstances. These operations are usually conducted on a frail, sick patient, who is malnourished and on steroids. The bowel is extremely fragile and may already have perforated. The surgical options are colectomy and ileostomy with mucous fistula; proctocolectomy and ileostomy; loop ileostomy with multiple "blowhole" colostomies;[23] and a definitive procedure, such as colectomy and ileorectal anastomosis (IRA) or proctocolectomy and pouch.

For many reasons, the vast weight of knowledgeable surgical opinion has swung firmly behind colectomy and ileostomy with mucous fistula as *the* operation to be done in these circumstances. Earlier series showed that proctocolectomy and ileostomy was attended by a significant morbidity and mortality.[24] Proctocolectomy also now deprives a sick patient, who can never be in full command of his or her faculties and can thus hardly be in a position to give informed consent, from the future option of a pouch. Perhaps the only indication in the very acute situation would be for massive haemorrhage, which does occur rarely and for which proctocolectomy would still be the first choice.

The Cleveland Clinic approach of loop ileostomy and multiple "blowhole" colostomies is rarely used now, even at that institute. Nonetheless, there can be special circumstances when such an approach might be the best way forward.[25]

A more definitive approach is fraught with danger. The complication rate for elective pouch surgery is high enough as it is and pouches constructed in patients who are already on steroids have a higher complication rate still; to which must be added the effects of starvation and endotoxaemia.

The conduct of a colectomy and ileostomy with mucous fistula in the acute stage differs from the elective operation largely through fear of perforating the "wet blotting paper" fragile colon or through fear of uncovering a spontaneous perforation before the operation has proceeded far enough that the specimen can be rapidly removed and any contamination limited. The steps are: mobilize the bowel without pulling on it (particularly with any grasping instruments); leave any "stuck areas" until last, as there may be a sealed perforation at that site; and do not try to detach omentum from areas where it has become attached. If there is an area stuck to the lateral abdominal wall (and this is usually in the region of the splenic flexure), then leave that area until last. Divide all relevant blood vessels, including the blood supply to the unmobilized segment of bowel, and divide the bowel proximally and distally, so that the stuck area is all that remains before the specimen can be removed and contamination ceases. For many reasons, such an operation is unlikely to be safely attempted laparoscopically.

The question of how to complete the operation is largely outside the remit of this chapter, but suffice it to say that the options are: a matured mucous fistula; a subcutaneous closed mucous fistula; and an intraperitoneal closed rectal stump. The first is the safest, but the mucous fistula is very smelly. The second is tremendous when it works, but the patient can be very demoralized by the "complication" of the closure breaking down and a wound infection developing, even if they have been warned that this might happen. The third is unsafe, as the distal bowel is usually the most fragile and any closure that breaks down will result in a pelvic abscess, an increased mortality and, perhaps in the female patient, sterility.

Failed medical treatment. A definitive operation is to be preferred, the choice lying between proctocolectomy and ileostomy, proctocolectomy and pouch, and colectomy and IRA. The decision should take into account the quality of the anal sphincter, the amount of rectal inflammation and the patient's ability to withstand complications, as well as the natural desires of the patient. Colectomy and IRA has a low complication rate, a reasonable functional result and a low risk of cancer developing later in the rectal stump; but not many patients have a suitable rectum for it.[26] Proctocolectomy and ileostomy and the pouch operation have similar rates of complication (30–40%) and readmission even after a permanent ileostomy is not infrequent (being 45% at six years).[27] However, most surgeons would accept that morbidity after pouch surgery, if not more frequent, is nonetheless more severe and this usually persuades them to avoid pouch surgery in older and frailer patients.

In the absence of a cancer, there is no need to excise widely, particularly during the pelvic phase of the operation. Great care should be taken to preserve bladder and sexual function and orthodox opinion is that this means that a close rectal dissection should be employed.[28] A close rectal dissection is particularly characterized by a posterior dissection within the fatty mesorectum, away from the conventional plane, which can be quite tedious and bloody. Such a dissection avoids damage to the presacral nerves posteriorly, which in the male subserve ejaculation. The nervi erigentes, that subserve erection, and the nerves to the bladder are most at risk when dissecting anterolaterally.

It is a simple matter to identify the presacral nerves lying in the plane immediately posterior to the conventional plane at the level of the sacral promontory and, staying in this anterior anatomical plane, to preserve them as a thyroidectomy surgeon might similarly identify and preserve the recurrent laryngeal nerve. Another advantage of not performing a close rectal dissection is the possibility of there being a missed rectal cancer. This is not so very far-fetched, as cancer in ulcerative colitis may have very little to show for it from the mucosal surface. Indeed, it is because of the difficulty of detecting cancer in ulcerative colitis that surgery is often undertaken for high grade dysplasia; not infrequently a cancer is then found by the pathologist. A further advantage of avoiding a close rectal dissection when constructing a pouch is that removal of the whole mesorectum allows the pouch to sit more comfortably in the pelvis instead of sitting perched at the entrance of the pelvis with a long "snout" pulled down for the anal anastomosis.

It is clear that a close rectal dissection would be hard, if not impossible, to achieve laparoscopically, but from the above discussion it is equally clear that the intellectual argument is not entirely on the side of close rectal dissection and some surgeons operating conventionally no longer favour it – including this author.

The cancer risk. This must still be considered unknown. Some specialist centres have quoted quite high risks, but some community reports have found hardly any increase in risk. Any increased risk seems confined to those with barium enema evidence of ulcerative colitis at least as far as the hepatic flexure of more than eight years. Patients who on barium enema have less extensive colitis do not seem to be at an increased risk. Some patients with less extensive colitis on barium enema may nonetheless have a total colitis when examined by colonoscopy and some may just have biopsy evidence of a total colitis. It might be assumed that these patients are also at an increased risk, but such an assumption is similar to considering all patients with inflammation of whatever extent to be at risk and this does not seem to be the case.

The risk is higher when there is dysplasia present; particularly high grade dysplasia or dysplasia associated with a lesion or mass (DALM). But dysplasia is patchy and may itself be absent from a colon that already harbours a malignancy. All this uncertainty means that the following clinical choices are possible: ignore the risk; perform prophylactic surgery at eight years; or embark on some form of colonoscopic screening programme and operate on those with high grade dysplasia or actual cancer.[29] The actual choice of operation and its conduct would be similar to that for failed medical treatment, except a close rectal dissection would be unwise.

Crohn's Disease

Abdominal surgery for Crohn's disease is dominated by the knowledge that surgery is only a part of the lifetime management of the patient and that future surgery is highly likely. Operations that result in a stoma have a much lower incidence of recurrence than when an anastomosis is performed: for example, after proctocolectomy and ileostomy 20% have recurrence by ten years, which compares favourably with the 60% after colectomy and IRA.[30]

Ileocolic disease. Almost all patients will come to surgery and as attempts to delay are not infrequently met by complications such as internal fistulae when surgery finally does become inevitable, many gastroenterologists and surgeons have a fairly low threshold for offering early surgery. Recurrence can be detected endoscopically in at least 80% within one year[31] and by ten years 50% have had to have further surgery. Patients with a long segment of Crohn's disease are at greater risk of recurrence, but otherwise there is little that will predict recurrence.[7] Certainly, the resection margin does not seem to be important, and there does not seem to be a place for frozen section assessment of it. In addition, there is no evidence that removal of the associated lymph nodes prevents recurrence. This is important, as in Crohn's disease the mesentery is often very thick because of these enlarged lymph nodes and it is often difficult to dissect out the origins of the arterial blood supply without either losing vascular control or creating a large intramesenteric haematoma.

Most recurrence is in the neoterminal ileum. Whether this is because the anastomosis acts as a functional obstruction or because there is reflux of colonic contents or because the constituents of the anastomosis in some way favour recurrence is unknown. There is at present no evidence that side-to-side anastomosis has any advantage over end-to-end anastomosis, nor that an antireflux nipple valve is useful, nor indeed that a sutureless technique results in fewer recurrences; but it is tempting to speculate that some such avenues might be worth exploring.

Large bowel disease. In the rare case of purely anorectal disease without any colonic disease, proctectomy and end colostomy is reasonable but once there is also some colonic Crohn's disease, recurrence in the retained colon is sufficiently frequent to recommend proctocolectomy and ileostomy, which has a recurrence rate at 10 years of 20%.[30]

As with pelvic dissection in ulcerative colitis, the orthodox view is that a close rectal dissection should be performed and the anus should be removed through an intersphincteric approach. However, the same arguments can be marshalled in support of an anatomical approach in the natural plane of dissection as have been presented above for ulcerative colitis. Furthermore, proctectomy in Crohn's disease may result in a perineal wound that is extremely slow to heal and it is by no means certain that this problem does not arise from continuing Crohn's disease in the retained lymph nodes of the mesorectum when a close rectal dissection has been performed.

Less extensive large bowel Crohn's disease that spares the anorectum may be treated by colectomy and IRA but recurrence occurs just as frequently as after right hemicolectomy.[7]

Small bowel disease. This is the rarest, if terminal ileal disease is excluded. The preoperative assessment of the small bowel remains suboptimal and it is particularly with small bowel disease that touch is so important in determining disease extent. It is also here that intraoperative measurement of small bowel length helps the surgeon decide whether resection alone can be performed or whether bowel preserving stricturoplasties and minimal resections might not be better.

Recurrent and complex disease. This surgery can be very exacting. Other organs such as the duodenum, bladder and ureter can be densely adherent, if not the site of an actual fistula, and there can often be an associated abscess. It is unlikely that a laparoscopic assisted operation will have any place here.

Rectal Prolapse

Until the last decade, abdominal rectopexy was considered the operation of choice for rectal prolapse. Most patients could be offered the operation and the results in terms of operative mortality and morbidity and subsequent recurrence were impressive. In the United Kingdom the Wells operation was favoured, which entailed a full rectal mobilization down to the pelvic floor with division of the lateral ligaments followed by posterior placement of prosthetic material, either Ivalon sponge or Marlex mesh.[32]

In recent times, it has become apparent that up to 50% of patients so treated will develop severe postoperative constipation.[33] Some have wondered whether the extensive rectal mobilization, particularly with lateral ligament division, might not render the rectum insensitive and thereby cause the constipation, but a randomized trial of abdominal rectopexy with and without lateral ligament division failed to support such a view.[34] Others have wondered whether the redundant loop of sigmoid left after returning the prolapsed rectum to the abdomen might not in some way contribute to the constipation and have argued for a sutured rectopexy with sigmoid resection (the Frykman–Goldberg operation).[35] There is some evidence that such an operation not only has a low rate of recurrence but also is associated with less postoperative constipation, so there is much to recommend it for the rare young patient in their twenties and thirties with rectal prolapse. However, there is increasing interest in perineal operations.

The two main perineal operations are Delorme's and Altmeier's operations, or modifications of them. Delorme's operation consists of a mucosal proctectomy performed on the prolapsed rectum, followed by imbricating sutures that concertina the bowel wall and completed by a mucosal reanastomosis.[1,36] Altmeier's operation consists of a perineal amputation of the prolapse (rectosigmoidectomy), followed by coloanal reanastomosis. There is the opportunity more easily to perform a pelvic floor repair at the same time than with Delorme's operation.

Results of perineal surgery are reasonable: recurrence is higher than after an abdominal rectopexy (about 16% as against less than 10%, being often as little as 1 or 2%[1]), but the operations are easily repeatable, constipation does not seem to be a postoperative complication and the operations are more minor than their abdominal counterparts. It is unlikely that laparoscopically assisted operations for rectal prolapse will be able to compete either with the low recurrence rates of the abdominal procedures or the absence of postoperative constipation and the minimal morbidity and the inherent repeatability of the perineal operations.

Stoma Formation

There are times when an abdominal stoma may be useful, either in the temporary management of an anal problem, such as a troublesome fistula, or permanently in a patient with idiopathic faecal incontinence – particularly when there has been a background element of obstructive defaecation, because operations to improve continence simply make the obstructive defaection worse and vice versa.

The most conventional approach has been by a midline laparotomy ending in an end sigmoid colostomy. It is possible, however, to perform an end sigmoid colostomy through a left iliac fossa trephine[37,38] without recourse to laparotomy. The difficulties relate to identifying correctly the proximal from the distal end of colon and to gaining enough length when the sigmoid colon is stuck down in the left iliac fossa, as it can be on some occasions.

A laparoscopically assisted operation would help confirm the orientation, although it is just as simple to confirm it by intraoperative air insufflation via the anus or by intraoperative flexible sigmoidoscopy, and there would be the added benefit of allowing sigmoid mobilization. However, it is usually possible to perform some sigmoid mobilization directly through the trephine and failure to achieve a conventional trephine colostomy because of sigmoid tethering occurs but is uncommon. Added to this, a laparoscopically assisted end sigmoid colostomy takes substantially longer to set up and to perform, it results in more abdominal scarring and the cost is very much greater. Postoperative length of stay depends upon the reason for the colostomy (for example, the operation may be part of the treatment of a complex anal condition) and on stoma care education.

Diverticular Disease

Operations for diverticular disease are usually for its complications. It is hard to know whether there is a difference between irritable bowel syndrome and painful diverticular disease, which might explain the longer term lack of success of operations such as sigmoid myotomy for uncomplicated diverticular disease.

Urgent complications of diverticular disease, such as acute inflammation, abscess formation, purulent peritonitis, faecal peritonitis and haemorrhage, are managed acutely. If the diagnosis can be made, then acute diverticulitis is best managed without an operation by antibiotics. After just one acute attack, the chance of further trouble is not unduly high and elective surgery to remove the involved segment is unnecessary; although it does become wise after more frequent attacks.[39] Abscess formation can be treated by percutaneous drainage, followed later by a definitive resection but purulent, and particularly faecal, peritonitis is best treated by Hartmann's operation.[40]

Hartmann's reversal usually follows acute surgery for diverticular disease or cancer, but quite a number of patients are deemed unfit and end up with a permanent stoma (in some series as many as 40%).[41] Furthermore, Hartmann's reversal can be a challenging operation: there are adhesions from the previous surgery; the patients are often obese and the splenic flexure needs to be mobilized; small bowel may be densely adherent to the oversewn rectal stump and may be injured while freeing it; and the bladder and vagina may fall back over the rectal stump and become inadvertently incorporated in a stapled reanastomosis unless great care is taken to prevent it. It remains controversial whether a laparoscopic Hartmann's reversal (an operation that could be completed with intracorporeal anastomosis and without laparotomy) should be attempted in patients otherwise thought too frail for conventional reversal and whether the operation might be attended by any fewer complications.

Other Conditions

Operations for other conditions such as constipation, volvulus and even polyposis syndromes from a technical point of view are similar to the operations previously described of segmental colectomy, colectomy and IRA, and restorative proctocolectomy with the advantage that, certainly in polyposis and constipation, the patients are usually young and fit. Benign caecal villous tumours that cannot be removed endoscopically are rare and can be removed conventionally through a small grid-iron incision as for appendicectomy.

REFERENCES

1. Senapati A, Nicholls RJ, Thomson JPS, Phillips RKS. Delorme's operation – the St Mark's experience. In: *Modern Coloproctology. Surgical Grand Rounds From St Mark's Hospital* (eds Phillips RKS, Northover JMA), pp. 57–68. London, Edward Arnold, 1993.
2. Localio SA, Eng K, Coppa GF. Abdominosacral resection for mid-rectal cancer. A 15 year experience. *Ann Surg* 1983; **198**: 320–4.
3. Irving AD, Scrimgeour D. Mechanical bowel preparation for colonic resection and anastomosis. *Br J Surg* 1987; **74**: 580–1.
4. Fielding LP, Stewart-Brown S, Blesovsky L, Kearney G. Anastomotic integrity after operations for large bowel cancer: a multicentre study. *Br Med J* 1980; **281**: 411–14.
5. Matheson NA, Irving AD. Single layer anastomosis after rectosigmoid resection. *Br J Surg* 1975; **62**: 239–42.
6. Nicholls RJ, Phillips RKS. Surgical therapy for colorectal tumors. In: *The Large Intestine: Physiology, Pathophysiology and Disease* (eds Phillips SF, Pemberton JH, Shorter RG), pp. 657–85. New York, Raven Press, 1991.
7. Scott ADN, Phillips RKS. The postoperative recurrence of Crohn's disease. In: *Modern Coloproctology Surgical Grand Rounds From St Mark's Hospital* (eds Phillips RKS, Northover JMA), pp. 123–39. London, Edward Arnold, 1993.
8. Umpleby HC, Williamson RCN. The efficacy of agents employed to prevent anastomotic recurrence in colorectal carcinoma. *Ann R Coll Surg Engl* 1984; **66**: 192–4.
9. McCue JL, Sheffield JP, Uff CR, Phillips RKS. Experimental carcinogenesis at sutured and sutureless colonic anastomoses. *Dis Colon Rectum* 1992; **35**: 902–9.
10. Griffiths JD. Surgical anatomy of the blood supply of the distal colon. *Ann R Coll Surg Engl* 1956; **19**: 241–56.
11. Aldridge MC, Phillips RKS, Hittinger R, Fry JS, Fielding LP. Influence of tumour site on presentation, management and subsequent outcome in large bowel cancer. *Br J Surg* 1986; **73**: 663–70.
12. Heald RJ, Ryall RDH. Recurrence and survival after total mesorectal excision for rectal cancer. *Lancet* 1986; **2**: 1479–82.
13. Moriya Y, Hojo K, Sawada T, Doyama Y. Significance of lateral node dissection for advanced rectal carcinoma at or below the peritoneal reflection. *Dis Colon Rectum* 1989; **32**: 307–15.
14. Pezim MF, Nicholls RJ. Survival after high and low ligation of the inferior mesenteric artery during curative surgery for rectal cancer. *Ann Surg* 1984; **200**: 729–33.
15. Surtees P, Ritchie J, Phillips RKS. High versus low ligation of the inferior mesenteric artery in rectal cancer. *Br J Surg* 1990; **77**: 618–21.
16. Phillips RKS, Hittinger R, Blesovsky L, Fry JS, Fielding LP. Large bowel cancer: surgical pathology and its relationship to survival. *Br J Surg* 1984; **71**: 604–10.
17. Umpleby HC, Fermor B, Symes MO, Williamson RCN. Viability of exfoliated colorectal cancer cells. *Br J Surg* 1984; **71**: 659–63.
18. Cole WH, Packard D, Southwick HW. Carcinoma of the colon, with special reference to the prevention of recurrence. *JAMA* 1954; **155**: 1549–53.

19. Engell HC. Cancer cells in the blood: a five year follow-up study. *Am Surg* 1959; **149**: 457–61.
20. Turnbull RB, Kyle K, Watson FR, Spratt J. Cancer of the colon; the influence of the no-touch technique on survival rates. *Ann Surg* 1967; **166**: 420–7.
21. Wiggers T, Jeekel J, Arends JW *et al.* No-touch isolation technique in colon cancer: a controlled prospective trial. *Br J Surg* 1988; **75**: 409–15.
22. Phillips RKS. Adequate distal margin of resection for adenocarcinoma of the rectum. *World J Surg* 1992; **16**: 463–6.
23. Turnbull RB, Hawks WA, Weakley FL. Surgical treatment of toxic megacolon: ileostomy and colostomy to prepare patients for colectomy. *Am J Surg* 1971; **122**: 325–31.
24. Ritchie JK. Ileostomy and excisional surgery for chronic inflammatory disease of the colon. A survey of one hospital region. *Gut* 1971; **12**: 528–46.
25. Fazio VW, Lavery IC. Loop ileostomy and "blow-hole" transverse colostomy for toxic megacolon. In: *Rob and Smith's Operative Surgery*, 4th edition (eds Todd IP and Fielding LP), pp. 421–8. London, Butterworths, 1983.
26. Hawley PR. Ileorectal anastomosis. *Br J Surg* 1985; **72**: S75–S76.
27. Phillips RKS, Ritchie J, Hawley PR. Proctocolectomy and ileostomy for ulcerative colitis: the longer term story. *J Roy Soc Med* 1989; **82**: 386–7.
28. Lee ECG, Dowling BL. Perimuscular excision of the rectum for Crohn's disease and ulcerative colitis. *Br J Surg* 1972; **59**: 29–32.
29. Collins RH, Feldman M, Fordtran JS. Colon cancer, dysplasia, and surveillance in patients with ulcerative colitis. *New Eng J Med* 1987; **316**: 1654–8.
30. Ritchie JK. The results of surgery for large bowel Crohn's disease. *Ann R Coll Surg Engl* 1990; **72**: 155–7.
31. Rutgeerts P, Geboes K, Vantrappen G, Kerremans R, Coenegrachts JL, Coremans G. Natural history of recurrent Crohn's disease at the ileocolonic anastomosis after curative surgery. *Gut* 1984; **25**: 665–72.
32. Porter NH. Complete rectal prolapse: posterior wrap (Wells operation). In: *Rob and Smith's Operative Surgery*, 4th edition (eds Todd IP and Fielding LP), pp. 412–8. London, Butterworths, 1983.
33. Mann CV, Hoffman C. Complete rectal prolapse: the anatomical and functional results of treatment by an extended abdominal rectopexy. *Br J Surg* 1988; **75**: 34–7.
34. Madden MV, Kamm MA, Nicholls RJ, Santhenam AM, Cabot R, Speakman CTM. Abdominal rectopexy for complete rectal prolapse: a prospective study evaluating changes in symptoms and anorectal function. *Dis Colon Rectum* 1992; **35**: 48–55.
35. Watts JD, Rothenberger DA, Buls JG, Goldberg SM, Nivatvongs S. The management of procidentia. 30 years' experience. *Dis Colon Rectum* 1985; **28**: 96–102.
36. Monson JRT, Jones NAG, Vowden P, Brennan TG. Delorme's operation: the first choice in complete rectal prolapse? *Ann R Coll Surg Engl* 1986; **68**: 143–6.
37. Senapati A, Phillips RKS. The trephine colostomy: a permanent left iliac fossa end colostomy without recourse to laparotomy. *Ann R Coll Surg Engl* 1991; **73**: 305–6.
38. Anderson ID, Hill J, Vohra H, Schofield VF, Kiff ES. An improved means of faecal diversion: the trephine stoma. *Br J Surg* 1992; **79**: 1080–1.
39. Rodkey GV, Welch CE. Colonic diverticular disease with surgical management. A study of 338 cases. *Surg Clin N Am* 1974; **54**: 655–74.
40. Goldman S, Ihre T. Treatment of acute diverticulitis of the colon. In: *Modern Coloproctology. Surgical Grand Rounds From St Mark's Hospital* (eds Phillips RKS, Northover JMA), pp. 57–68. London, Edward Arnold, 1993.
41. Haas PA, Haas PG. A critical evaluation of the Hartmann procedure. *Am Surg* 1988; **54**: 380–5.

8.2

Laparoscopic Colorectal Surgery

G. A. FIELDING and R. W. STITZ

As expertise has increased in laparoscopic surgery, it has become apparent that laparoscopic colonic mobilization and resection can be performed safely and adequately.[1–4]

After the rapid and almost universal acceptance of laparoscopic cholecystectomy many procedures in the general surgeon's armamentarium have been performed by laparoscopic techniques. Unlike other procedures that have so far been performed via the laparoscope a large proportion of colorectal cases will be performed for the treatment of malignancy. There are well-established survival rates and local recurrence rates which depend very heavily on the surgical skill of the operator, especially with carcinoma of the rectum. These skills have to be transposed into the laparoscopic arena to ensure that no patient is disadvantaged by inadequate cancer clearance.

Fundamental long-standing principles of colorectal surgery such as a tension-free anastomosis, wide resection including the draining lymphatics, resection of the mesorectum for carcinoma of the rectum and luminal lavage and avoidance of spillage of bowel contents adjacent to a tumour must all be observed. It is vital in the current wave of enthusiasm for laparoscopic surgery that these principles are not forgotten and that surgeons proceed to laparoscopic colorectal surgery only when they have mastered the techniques that are necessary for other laparoscopic procedures such as laparoscopic cholecystectomy, inguinal hernia repair and appendicectomy. All colorectal procedures which are performed at open surgery can and have been performed via the laparoscope, either completely or with laparoscopic assistance.

Management of benign disease such as idiopathic megacolon, diverticulitis, inflammatory bowel disease and carcinoma are all suited to laparoscopic approaches. Procedures requiring development of a stoma such as Hartmann's procedure for perforated diverticular disease, carcinoma, abdominoperineal resection and defunctioning ileostomy or colostomy are also suitable.

The procedures that will be discussed in this chapter are right hemicolectomy, left hemicolectomy, anterior resection, abdominoperineal resection, stoma formation and total colectomy.

INSTRUMENTS REQUIRED

As with all laparoscopic surgery, the success of the procedure depends on three fundamentals, namely the skill of the surgeon, the skill of the assistant and the quality of the equipment.

There is no doubt that operating times and the ease of the procedure will be greatly reduced by the availability of skilled assistants, both for the camera and also for the traction, countertraction and presentation of the bowel to the operator.

It is my belief that all laparoscopic procedures should be performed after an open insertion of the umbilical port to avoid injury to underlying bowel or vascular structures. This requires the use of a blunt tipped trocar and cannula after direct dissection into the peritoneal cavity through the umbilicus (see Chapter 4). The majority of colorectal procedures require the umbilical port, one and sometimes two 12 mm ports for insertion of stapling devices and usually two 5 mm ports for the insertion of graspers.

The decision to use disposable or non-disposable ports is made by the individual surgeon and may often be based on cost. Certainly the advent of disposable stapling devices for both bowel and vasculature has greatly increased the speed of laparoscopic surgery and these instruments currently require the use of 12 mm, and more recently, 15 mm and 18 mm disposable ports.

Adequate scissors, preferably with a diathermy capability and good suction and irrigation, are essential, as is an instrument for retraction of the small bowel. There are numerous fan-shaped retraction devices currently available that are of particular benefit when operating in the pelvis to hold the small bowel out of the pelvis and allow adequate dissection.

Both the 0° and 30° telescopes can be used. The 30° telescope is particularly helpful with mobilization of the hepatic and splenic flexures and with mobilization of the distal rectum. Various atraumatic bowel grasping forceps are used, mainly of the Debakey or Duval type, which allow safe and easy manipulation of large and small bowel. My preference is for the Debakey type which seems to be the least traumatic as they apply the force over a broad area. Babcock type grasping instruments have a tendency to tear serosa and potentially result in bowel perforations which may initially be silent and present later as a bowel leak.

GENERAL TECHNIQUE

Traction and countertraction are the foundation for safe and time effective laparoscopic colorectal surgery. By elevation of the bowel and triangulation, the incision of the peritoneum and subsequent dissection is made much easier. This requires an assistant who is able to use graspers to elevate the bowel, and is greatly facilitated by a two-handed operating technique by the surgeon using graspers in one hand and scissors in the other. This exposure is enhanced by placing the ports for the graspers, which are used to expose the bowel, a significant distance away from the part of the bowel that is to be removed. This increases the possible range of movement of the graspers and scissors and allows more direct movement of the bowel rather than leverage which has a tendency to tear the serosa.

Strict haemostatis is important to ensure a good view of the operating site. Furthermore, pooling of blood absorbs light and reduces the light available to the operator. It is easiest to have a suction and irrigation device in the peritoneal cavity to rapidly remove blood as necessary. However, if the surgeon enters the correct plane after exposure with traction and countertraction, there should be minimal bleeding. Any small vessels can be coagulated as the procedure develops. Patients should be fixed to the table so that they can be rotated either into Trendelenburg or reverse Trendelenburg positions and also with right and left side down rotation to increase exposure, particularly of the splenic flexure.

SURGICAL PROCEDURES

The use of laparoscopic techniques is aimed primarily at reducing the patient's pain postoperatively, thereby improving their well-being, reducing the hospital stay and hopefully making their return to normal life more rapid than if they had had open surgery. It does not, however, have any effect at all on the type of procedure that is performed and that is perhaps the most important aspect of the discussion of laparoscopic colectomy. Therefore the procedures that will be discussed here are those that are performed at open surgery, the only real modifications being that they are performed with the use of long instruments guided by laparoscopy and that the specimen is removed through a small incision. The dissection and exposure are just as for open surgery. The only limiting factors, therefore, are large bulky tumours that cannot be removed through a small incision, since it is vital that they are removed without shedding cells. For a large bulky tumour, for example of the caecum, there is no real advantage in mobilizing the bowel via the laparoscope since this can be adequately done through a reasonably sized right iliac fossa transverse incision which would be required with laparoscopy to remove such a large specimen. On the left side, it is probably still an advantage to perform the mobilization of the left colon and splenic flexure laparoscopically, and then proceed to an open resection through an infraumbilical incision.

If, at laparoscopy, there is invasion from the colonic lesion into contiguous organs then the procedure should be converted to an open resection.

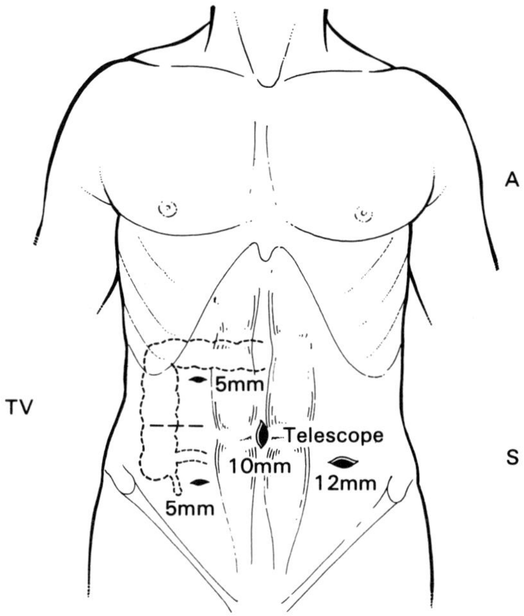

Figure 8.2.1 Right hemicolectomy. A: assistant; S: surgeon. 5 mm: graspers and scissors. 12 mm: scissors and Endo GIA.

At the time of laparoscopic colectomy for carcinoma, full laparoscopic evaluation of the peritoneal cavity must be made. There have been recent advances in laparoscopic ultrasonology of the liver and this will provide an even more detailed staging of the patient at the time of surgery (see Chapter 15.3).

Right Hemicolectomy

The aim of this procedure is to mobilize the terminal ileum and the right colon around to the right branch of the middle colic vessels. This will involve exposure of the right ureter and the duodenum after division of the lateral attachments of the colon and of any adhesions to the liver. This is best performed with the patient supine on the operating table and there is no advantage in placing the legs in stirrups. The surgeon, the camera operator and preferably the second assistant stand on the patient's left side facing the area to be dissected and the monitor which is usually placed level with the umbilicus on the patient's right side (Fig. 8.2.1.).

The procedure starts with mobilization of the colon along the white line, mobilization of the subhepatic peritoneum and division of any adhesions. This exposes the right ureter and the duodenum. The ileocolic vessels are dissected free and divided with the Endo GIA (US Surgical) at the junction of the superior mesenteric vessels. The ileum is then divided with the Endo GIA and a 5 cm incision is made in the right iliac fossa at the level of the umbilicus; this is a muscle-splitting incision. The cut end of the ileum is withdrawn; sometimes this can be facilitated by placing an Endo loop around the ileum and withdrawing it through the wound first, as a guide to the colon. The colon is then withdrawn and divided with an Endo GIA or linear cutter (Ethicon). The wound is protected by Betadine soaked swabs or by small plastic wound drapes through which the specimen is drawn.

The proximal end of the ileum is then brought to the wound and a side-to-side anastomosis or an end-to-end handsewn anastomosis is fashioned. The decision as to whether to staple or handsew the anastomosis is based on the ease with which the specimen can be adequately withdrawn through the wound. The mesentery is closed, the anastomosis returned to the peritoneal cavity and the wound closed.

Left Hemicolectomy

Left hemicolectomy is performed usually for large polyps or carcinomas of the sigmoid, descending colon or splenic flexure. It is advantageous to have the patient's legs elevated in stirrups. The surgeon stands on the patient's right side as does the camera operator, the second assistant stands between the legs and the theatre nurse stands on the patient's left side (Fig. 8.2.2). A 12 mm port is placed low in the iliac fossa. Two and sometimes three 5 mm ports are placed for insertion of graspers and scissors, one in the right iliac fossa, one in the left iliac fossa and one in the upper midline. In a particularly large patient the port in the right iliac fossa may be better placed in the right upper quadrant, just to the right of the midline to allow easy access to the splenic flexure.

The patient is rotated right side down and head up and the colon is dissected along the white line with triangulation of the splenic flexure. The attachments to the spleen are divided and the omentum is divided along the embryological cleavage plane. The colon is mobilized forward to expose the ureter and the gonadal vessels are mobilized completely to allow full mobility of the splenic flexure. The Endo GIA is then used to divide the vascular pedicle; this will usually require up to four firings of the Endo GIA with vascular cartridges. The distal side of division is chosen usually at the upper rectum and the rectum is then divided with the Endo GIA. With the original instrument this has required sometimes two and three firings but with the newer generation of 6 cm instruments from US Surgical and Ethicon, this will now be achieved by one firing of the instrument.

A left iliac fossa 5 cm transverse muscle-splitting incision is made and the proximal divided end of the bowel is withdrawn to the level of the proposed

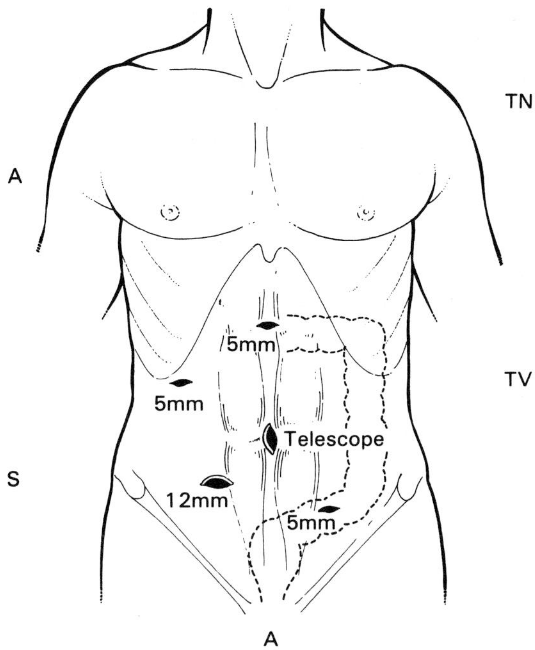

Figure 8.2.2 Left hemicolectomy. A: assistant; S: surgeon; TN: theatre nurse.

upper transection. It is surprising, initially, just how much bowel can actually be removed through this small incision after it has been adequately mobilized. The bowel is transected and the anvil of a stapling device, either the curved premium EEA or the curved ILS stapler (Ethicon), is inserted into the open end of the exteriorized bowel and secured with a pursestring suture. The bowel and anvil are then returned to the peritoneal cavity, the wound closed and pneumoperitoneum re-established. The stapler is then inserted via the rectum and the spike advanced through the stapled upper rectum. This is connected to the anvil using a grasper.

My preferred grasper is a heavy toothed grasper which seems to grasp the neck of the anvil most easily. This is then guided into the stapler and the anastomosis completed. This same heavy toothed grasper is also most appropriate for removal of the spike which can sometimes be quite difficult. If there is any difficulty at all in removing the spike from the port, then it is best to encircle the spike with an Endo loop to manipulate this pointed smooth object into the end of the port in the correct alignment.

It is vital to identify correctly small tumours perioperatively. Techniques of marking with India ink have been tried but I have personally found this to be not particularly helpful. To be completely sure, it is necessary to visualize the lesion at operation using the colonoscope and then mark the lesion externally on the bowel with a clip, prior to performing the resection.

Anterior Resection

This is the most difficult of all laparoscopic procedures and it is here that technique is paramount, especially when operating on cases for malignancy. While it is possibly the most demanding procedure in laparoscopic surgery, it is also one which I believe is greatly enhanced by the improved vision of the operative field that is afforded via the laparoscope.

Once one enters Heald's "holy plane" in front of the sacrum[5] by careful manipulation of the rectum and haemostasis as one proceeds, the dissection continues to Waldeyer's fascia. The rectum is resected with the attached mesorectum, with minimal blood loss and full vision of the procedure as one proceeds.

This is perhaps the one procedure which has a truly technical advantage over the open standard procedure which was hampered by poor vision and difficult retraction, and subsequently inadequate resection of tumour. These factors may have resulted in increased local recurrence of carcinoma.

For this procedure, the legs are again elevated. It is important that they are not elevated too high, and should preferably be kept almost level with the patient's torso. If the knees are too high, the thighs can interfere with the mobility of graspers and actually make the procedure more difficult. The set-up is similar to that of a left hemicolectomy except on this occasion the second assistant should stand on the patient's lefthand side and the scrubbed nurse between the legs to pass instruments to either the surgeon or the second assistant (Fig. 8.2.3). Once again the patient is rotated with right side down but for an anterior resection, once the mobilization of the lateral attachments and splenic flexure have been completed, the patient should be tipped into a Trendelenburg position to facilitate removal of the small bowel from the pelvis. This is still an extremely difficult part of laparoscopic anterior resection. Recently, however, fanshaped retraction devices have made a big impact on this problem and I believe they should be used routinely.

Mobilization is as for a left hemicolectomy. Once the patient is tipped down, the pedicle is divided well above the pelvic brim using the Endo GIA. Attention then turns to the pelvis. Lateral division of the peritoneum around the pelvic brim is completed with exposure of both ureters. A grasper is used to elevate the rectum towards the anterior abdominal wall and another to elevate the peritoneum. A plane is created in front of the sacrum and the pelvic autonomic nerves are well seen at this time. Dissection then continues down along the curve of the sacrum and if one is in the correct plane this is usually almost bloodless. Any small vessels can be easily managed with diathermy. Bipolar diathermy is used to divide the lateral ligaments. It is useful to have a suction and irrigation device present in the peritoneal cavity for rapid aspiration of any blood as the dissection proceeds.

If the procedure has been performed for severe diverticular disease, anastomosis will be into the more proximal rectum which is divided by the Endo GIA and the procedure carried out as already described for a left hemicolectomy.

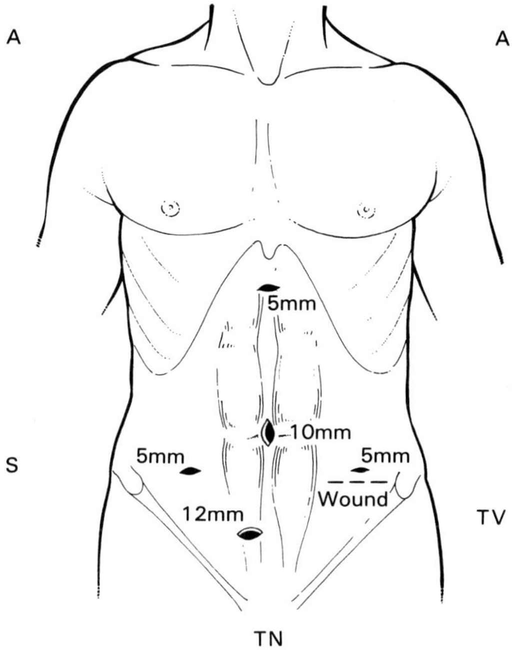

Figure 8.2.3 Anterior resection. A: assistant; S: surgeon; TN: theatre nurse.

For tumours of the upper rectum, well above the dentate line, dissection continues past the tumour down towards Waldeyer's fascia. Once the distal dissection is complete the distal colon is lavaged with Betadine solution and the bowel is divided with the Endo GIA. Where a low division is anticipated, as in the majority of cases of carcinoma of the rectum, the port for the Endo GIA should be placed as low as possible in the abdomen just to the right of the midline so that it can be placed in an almost vertical fashion over the rectum (Fig. 8.2.3).

With the current instrumentation that is available I believe that real difficulty still exists for resection of low rectal tumours. It is this particular group of patients which must not be compromised in any way. At present it is virtually impossible to get below low tumours and obtain adequate clearance prior to application of the stapling devices. This is due purely to the bulky nature of these tumours, which prevents adequate application of the stapling devices. It is anticipated that very soon roticulated devices and laparoscopic TA instruments will change this.

It is, however, possible to resect very low lesions which are not bulky externally such as large polyps that are unsuitable for local intraluminal resection, since good vision can be obtained and the level of transection can be aided by sigmoidoscopic examination of the lesion after the application of clamps. With low anterior resection, especially if there have been any technical difficulties or the patient is obese, then the covering ileostomy is fashioned in the right iliac fossa laparoscopically.

Once the distal rectum has been divided, a stapled anastomosis is performed with very low anastomoses. Splenic flexure mobilization is imperative to ensure a tension-free anastomosis. A drain is inserted into the pelvis.

Stoma Formation

Stoma formation is usually performed either for a Hartmann's operation for perforated diverticular disease or as a defunctioning procedure.

For Hartmann's procedure, dissection is as already described for a left hemicolectomy and is exactly as at open surgery. The proximal end of the bowel is then withdrawn through the preplanned stoma site and the stoma fashioned. Where an already functioning colostomy/ileostomy is performed, a suitable segment of bowel is chosen, the stoma incision made and the bowel removed through the wound and the stoma fashioned.

Abdominoperineal Resection

The great advantage of abdominoperineal resection performed with the aid of the laparoscope is the removal of the midline incision. The dissection is identical to that for low anterior resection and the abdominal surgeon meets the perineal operator at Waldeyer's fascia as in the open procedure. Once the abdominal operator has dissected down to this level, the stoma is then created, usually through the left iliac fossa port site and the perineal operator completes the procedure.

Total Colectomy

The most common indication for total colectomy is dysfunctional megacolon. These patients have had full work-up of colorectal function including transit studies, anorectal manometry, gastric and small bowel emptying times and proctography. Many of the patients are young women and certainly the laparoscopic method offers them a much more acceptable cosmetic result.

Patients are placed supine in a lithotomy position with the thighs level on the same plane as the trunk to minimize interference with instruments. For this, the longest colorectal procedure, either a long-acting antibiotic or a second dose of antibiotics should be given during the procedure. Since tilting of the operating table is vital, the patient must be strapped carefully to the table.

For this procedure it is best for the surgeon to stand between the legs with a monitor at either side level with the patient's shoulders (Fig. 8.2.4). Mobilization proceeds initially with the right colon to the hepatic flexure, and the left

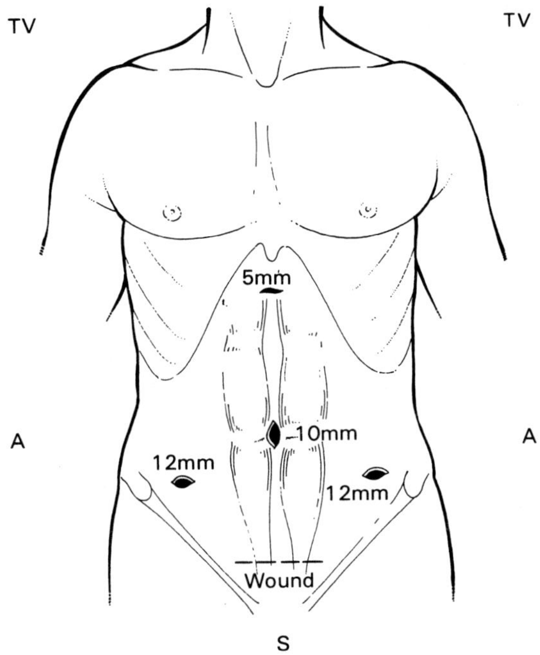

Figure 8.2.4 Total colectomy. A: assistant; S: surgeon.

colon around the splenic flexure. The omentum is removed from the transverse colon along the embryological cleavage plane such that the entire colon down to the upper rectum is mobilized. The vascular pedicles of the ileocolic, right, middle and left colic arteries are divided with the Endo GIA. The terminal ileum is divided and a Pfannensteil or small left iliac fossa incision is made. The colon is withdrawn and the rectum divided. Ileorectal anastomosis is then completed.

It is this procedure in particular which benefits from skilled assistants. There is obviously an extensive amount of dissection required which can be very time consuming unless two surgeons can work in tandem with graspers and scissors, progressing sequentially around the bowel.

RESULTS

At this stage there are very few published series of results for laparoscopic colectomy as the procedure is still in its infancy.

Jacobs *et al.*[6] first published a series of 20 cases of laparoscopic assisted colon resection for a combination of benign and malignant diseases. These were all procedures performed above the peritoneal reflection. They had a mean operating time of 170 minutes (range 95–255 minutes) for sigmoid colectomy and

Table 8.2.1 Laparoscopic procedures

	Procedure	**Malignancy**
Total colectomy	18	
Anterior resection	44	15
Right hemicolectomy	22	15
Left hemicolectomy	1	
Abdominoperineal resection	12	12
Colostomy/ileostomy	3	2
Total	100	44

155 minutes (range 110–260 minutes) for right hemicolectomy. Fourteen to 20 patients were discharged within four days of surgery. They had three major complications and no operative mortality.

Monson *et al.*[7] recently published a series of 40 cases, mainly for malignant disease, which included six anterior resections and two abdominoperineal resections. Seven of the 40 cases were converted to an open resection, three due to difficulty with defining anatomy, one because of inability to see due to distended loops of bowel, two due to fixity of tumour in the pelvis and one because of multiple adenomatous polyps. For leftsided lesions the mean operating time was 240 minutes (range 150–330 minutes) and for right lesions was 210 minutes (range 120–310 minutes). Mean postoperative stay was eight days (range 5–14 days) and there was one perioperative death due to myocardial infarction.

At the Royal Brisbane Hospital we have recently collated our results for the first laparoscopic colorectal resections performed between June 1991 and October 1992. Procedures performed are listed in Tables 8.2.1–3. Forty-four patients had operations for malignancy including anterior resection (15), right hemicolectomy (15), abdominoperineal resection (12) and colostomy (2).

We have looked at the operating time in the first 50 patients compared with the second 50 patients and there has been a reduction in operating time as our experience has improved. Operation times are tabulated in Table 8.2.4. These operating times are similar to our times for open surgery.

We have had to convert four patients to open procedures: two patients had impenetrable adhesions from previous pelvic surgery, one had bleeding from an inferior epigastric artery which had been penetrated by a port and the fourth patient was severely obese with a very bulky mesentery and it was impossible to gain adequate retraction of the small bowel from the pelvis.

Postoperative complications occurred in several patients (Table 8.2.5). Our wound infection rate was 8%. We have tried to improve this by giving second doses of intraoperative antibiotics for longer procedures such as total colectomy, by use of small Betadine soaked swabs in the wounds and also the use of plastic wound protectors when the anastomosis is performed at the level of the wound. Five patients had an anastomotic leak, four after anterior resection and one after

Table 8.2.2 Laparoscopic procedures

	Colectomy & IRA	APR	Anterior & L colon resection	Right colon resection
First fifty patients				
Number	9	5	22	12
Number discharged 7 days or less	5	1	11	9
Percent discharged 7 days or less	56%	20%	50%	75%
Second fifty patients				
Number	9	7	23	10
Number discharged 7 days or less	5	4	16	6
Percent discharged 7 days or less	56%	57%	70%	60%

Table 8.2.3 Laparoscopic procedures

	Colectomy & IRA	APR	Anterior & L colon resection	Right colon resection
Total number of operations				
Number	18	12	45	22
Number discharged 7 days or less	10	5	28	15
Percent discharged 7 days or less	56%	42%	62%	68%

Table 8.2.4 Operating Time (second 50 patients)

	Hours (mean)	Range
Total colectomy	4.5	(4.0–5.5)
Anterior resection	3	(2.5–5.0)
Right hemicolectomy	3	(1.25–4.0)
Abdominoperineal resection	3.5	(2.0–4.5)

Table 8.2.5 Complications

Wound infection	8%
Bowel obstruction	3%
Anastomotic leak	5%
Mortality	3%

Table 8.2.6 Discharge (days)

	Mean	**Range**
Total colectomy	7	(6–13)
Anterior resection	5	(2–33)
Right hemicolectomy	6	(3–31)
Abdominoperineal resection	7	(5–21)

a right hemicolectomy. Three were managed conservatively with a drain and total parenteral nutrition and settled without problem. Two patients required laparotomy and both made a full recovery. Three patients developed bowel obstruction requiring surgery. One was a simple adhesive band after a total colectomy, the second resulted from a suction drain which had become adherent to small bowel, and the third was a hernia through a 12 mm port hole. Subsequent to this last complication we now close all 10 and 12 mm port holes. The best suture for this is a strong non-absorbent suture on a J-shaped needle to allow access in a very small wound.

We had three deaths within a 30 day period, one being a myocardial infarction postoperatively and two patients who died from disseminated malignancy. Both of these patients had had laparoscopic assisted colostomies for palliation of disseminated malignancy.

Our discharge times were similar to those of Monson and colleagues[7] (Table 8.2.6).

The greatest advantage has been for patients having anterior resection and right hemicolectomy, where many patients are discharged on the third postoperative day. One patient was discharged on the second postoperative day after an anterior resection.

Patients having a total colectomy for megacolon had a mean time of discharge of seven days (range 6–13). It is likely that this will not be much reduced as these patients often have an ileus postoperatively due to dysfunction of the small bowel and from the extent of the required dissection.

Patients who have abdominoperineal resection had a mean time of discharge of seven days and this has been due to the healing of the perineal wound.

CONCLUSIONS

There is no doubt that laparoscopic colonic resection can be achieved safely and expeditiously. It is important that surgeons contemplating laparoscopic colectomy tread cautiously and this is particularly so when contemplating anterior resection for carcinoma of the rectum. It is beneficial for surgeons commencing laparoscopic colorectal surgery to visit other surgeons who have already performed the technique and if possible have experienced assistants with the first cases attempted.

Possession of the correct equipment will greatly enhance one's ability to perform this surgery and the overriding guideline must be to perform an adequate cancer operation, namely, performing the same operation that the surgeon would have chosen to do at open surgery, using laparoscopic techniques.

As time passes, the results for resection for colorectal carcinoma will become available and allow full assessment of the place of laparoscopic colectomy for colorectal carcinoma.

REFERENCES

1. Wexner SD, Johansen UB. Laparoscopic bowel resection: advantages and limitations. *Ann Med* 1922; **24**(2): 105–10.
2. Corbitt JD. Preliminary experience with laparoscopic guided colectomy. *Surg Laparosc Endosc* 1992; **2**(1): 79–81.
3. Peters WR. Laparoscopic total proctocolectomy with creation of ileostomy for ulcerative colitis. *J Laparo-Endosc Surg* 1992; **2**(3): 175–8.
4. Ballantyne GM. Laparoscopically assisted anterior resection for rectal prolapse. *Surg Laparosc Endosc* 1992; **3**: 230–6.
5. Heald RJ, Ryall RDH. Recurrence and survival after total mesorectal excision for rectal cancer. *Lancet* 1986; **2**: 1479–82.
6. Jacobs M, Verdeja JC, Goldstein HS. Minimally invasive colon resection (laparoscopic colectomy). *Surg Laparosc Endosc* 1991; **1**(3): 144–50.
7. Monson JRT, Darzi A, Carey PD, Guillou PJ. Prospective evaluation of laparoscopic assisted colectomy in an unselected group of patients. *Lancet* 1992; **340**: 831–3.

Overview

Colorectal surgery

Many surgeons remain uneasy about the role of laparoscopic surgery in the management of colorectal cancer. There are already reports of early local and port site recurrences following laparoscopic and laparoscopic-assisted procedures for patients with colorectal cancer. First and foremost, the objective in these patients must be directed at achieving a cure, with return to normal activities being of less importance. However, for frailer patients and for those with proven metastases, this may no longer be a consideration, and perhaps it is in these patients that current attention should be focused. Until the long-term results from these studies are available, the jury will remain out regarding the surgeon's ability to undertake a satisfactory curative resection of colorectal cancer using laparoscopic dissection. The exception to this rule may be in cases of abdomino–perineal resection for low rectal and anal tumours where much of the cancer resection is performed by the perineal operator.

Of course, the arguments related to colorectal cancer do not hold true when benign conditions of the colon and rectum are considered. Laparoscopic techniques would appear to have real advantages over conventional surgery, and Fielding's vast experience in this field would support this. Nonetheless, surgeons should be cautious in lowering the threshold for surgical intervention in the treatment of benign colonic disease.

9.1

Expectations of Surgery for Benign Oesophageal Disease

A. WATSON

The principal benign conditions of the oesophagus which may be treated surgically, either by a conventional open approach or an endoscopic approach, are gastro-oesophageal reflux disease and achalasia. Both of these conditions are functional disorders and therefore the end point of treatment of these conditions, whether by open surgery or laparoscopy, is a functional one, in contradistinction to cholecystectomy where the end point is purely anatomical. Functional evaluation over a prolonged period of time is necessary to assess whether the expectations of treatment have been fulfilled and the fact that a procedure for the correction of these conditions is technically feasible by a laparoscopic approach does not necessarily imply that the functional results are the same as those obtained by open surgery.

In outlining the expectations of surgical treatment, it is important to discuss the indications for surgical treatment, the techniques available, the perceived aims of surgical treatment, the means of assessing whether these aims have been met and finally the results of established surgical techniques in the management of each condition.

GASTRO-OESOPHAGEAL REFLUX DISEASE

Indications for Surgery

The vast majority of patients with gastro-oesophageal reflux disease (approximately 80%) have mild disease which can be controlled satisfactorily by a combination of lifestyle changes and pharmacological agents including antacids, H_2 receptor antagonists, prokinetic drugs and the proton pump inhibitor, omeprazole. However, despite advances in pharmacological treatment, it is not always successful firstly in producing symptomatic relief and healing of endoscopic oesophagitis and secondly in maintaining that situation once healing has taken place. While omeprazole has been shown to result in healing of endoscopic oesophagitis in 90% of cases,[1,2] most series fail to stratify between the various grades of oesophagitis and as the milder grades are the most common, it is most likely that these grades comprise the majority of patients in published series. One series which has stratified between various grades of oesophagitis has shown that the healing rate is less than 67% with the more severe grades of oesophagitis.[3] Eighty-two percent of all cases relapse within six months of cessation of treatment,[3] but this proportion can be reduced to 33% at the end of one year if full dosage omeprazole is maintained.[4] Data do not exist regarding recurrence rate within the different grades of oesophagitis, but it is likely that the more severe grades have a higher recurrence rate and it can be predicted on the basis of available data that approximately 50% of patients with Savary and Miller grade 3 oesophagitis will be unhealed at the end of one year of treatment with omeprazole.

Failure of medical treatment, therefore, still remains a significant indication for surgery. By looking at various characteristics of reflux patients who have been followed longitudinally, initially treated on medical therapy with surgery being reserved for failure, predictive factors can be identified in those patients unlikely to respond to medical treatment, which include manometric evidence of lower oesophageal sphincter failure, severe "pump" function impairment, grade 3 oesophagitis and the presence of alkaline reflux.[5] Of the patients who may respond to medical treatment, some may be intolerant of the medication. Intolerance due to side effects is unusual, particularly with ranitidine and omeprazole, but it does occur. Many younger patients do not wish to commit themselves to a lifetime of continued medication, knowing that safe and effective alternatives exist, and many patients and indeed some gastroenterologists remain concerned that the long term effects of taking omeprazole for up to 40–50 years remain unknown.

Complications of gastro-oesophageal reflux disease, such as Barrett's ulcer, reflux stricture or Barrett's columnar-lined oesophagus, are relative indications for surgery. Because these patients represent the most severe end of the spectrum of pathophysiological defects in gastro-oesophageal reflux disease, with a high proportion of the predictive factors mentioned above, medical treatment is less likely to be successful in this group. While many patients with reflux stricture are elderly and surgical treatment would be inappropriate, in young patients, antireflux surgery has proved superior to H_2 receptor antagonists in terms of reducing dilatation requirements and resolution of strictures;[6] however, a similar study using omeprazole has not been reported. The ideal management of uncomplicated Barrett's columnar-lined oesophagus is controversial, although antireflux surgery has been shown to be effective in arresting progression of columnarization,[7] in controlling symptoms and reducing the incidence of complications.[8] It has been the only form of treatment repeatedly to show regression of the columnarization, although this appears to be only in a minority of patients.[8–10]

Surgical Techniques

A wide variety of antireflux procedures have been described over the years but those in current use can be divided into total fundoplication procedures, partial fundoplication procedures, fixation procedures and prosthetic insertion.

Total Fundoplication Procedures

Nissen Fundoplication. This procedure, first described by Rudolph Nissen in Basel in 1956, remains the most widely practised antireflux procedure. The essential principle of this procedure is a 360° wrap, whereby the anterior and posterior walls of the stomach are passed behind the oesophagus and the posterior wall is then sutured to the anterior wall of the stomach in front of the oesophagus. Nissen's original description involved four or five such sutures, which included a bite of the oesophagus, such that the fundoplication was 4–6 cm in length. The perceived mode of action was the augmentation of resting lower oesophageal sphincter pressure and the avoidance of distraction of the lower oesophageal sphincter during gastric distension and raised intragastric pressure, in which circumstances, by virtue of the wrap, lower oesophageal sphincter pressure would be increased even further. While the initial short term results for this procedure were good in terms of symptomatic improvement, it became apparent that a series of mechanical side effects detracted from the success, notably the gas bloat syndrome and inability to belch or vomit, which occurred in over 50% of patients and remained troublesome in over 20%.[12] This was felt to relate to the fact that the standard Nissen fundoplication acted as a very effective one-way valve. In order to overcome these problems, a modification of Nissen's original technique was described by Donohue and Bombeck in 1977, known as the "floppy" Nissen fundoplication, as it described a loose wrap conducted around a 50FG bougie, such that the index finger could be insinuated between the wrap and the oesophagus.[13]

Other modifications of the Nissen fundoplication have been described, largely in an attempt to reduce the incidence of complications. These include the modifications by Thal,[14] in which there is little fundal dissection and a short, less bulky wrap is produced, and the Rossetti Hell modification in which only the anterior portion of the gastric fundus is used for the wrap, being placed around the posterior aspect of the oesophagus in front of which it is sutured to an adjacent part of the anterior aspect of the gastric fundus.[15]

Some workers now feel that in order to reduce the mechanical complications of Nissen fundoplication to an acceptable level, all the short gastric vessels should be divided in order to ensure the gastric fundus is sufficiently mobile to produce a loose wrap and the wrap itself must be no longer than 1–2 cm, having been performed over a bougie at least 56FG in diameter.[16] Thus, there are many modifications of the Nissen fundoplication in current use and apart from the major modifications described above, there remains considerable variability as to the degree of mobilization of the gastric fundus, the length of the wrap, whether the wrap is sutured to the oesophagus and whether a crural repair is performed.

Partial Fundoplication Procedures

Several partial fundoplication procedures have been devised with the aim of enabling eructation to occur by avoiding total fundoplication but maintaining reflux control, usually by adding one or more additional procedures which result in a valvuloplasty, rather than sole reliance on the production of a supracompetent lower oesophageal sphincter.

Belsey Mark IV Procedure. The Belsey procedure was devised as an attempt to overcorrect the normal spatial relationships of the oesophagus, stomach and diaphragm, with restoration of an intra-abdominal segment of oesophagus that was exposed to positive intra-abdominal pressure.[17] Several modifications of Belsey's original procedure to fulfil these objectives resulted in the Belsey Mark IV procedure, which incorporates a crural repair, accentuation of the angle of His and two layers of sutures between the oesophagus and gastric fundus to produce a 270° partial fundoplication. Good results have been obtained with few mechanical complications but the procedure is technically demanding and requires a thoracotomy.

Hill Repair. This procedure was described by Hill in 1967 as a transabdominal partial fundoplication procedure.[18] The principle of this procedure is the fixation of an intra-abdominal segment of oesophagus to the median arcuate ligament, with a second layer of imbricating sutures to fix the gastric fundus immediately adjacent to the oesophagus to the median arcuate ligament, resulting in a 180° anterior wrap. The tension of the wrap is judged individually by the use of intraoperative manometry.

Good results have been claimed by Hill and other advocates for this procedure, the main disadvantages being the relative inaccessibility of the median arcuate ligament and the reliance on intraoperative manometry.

Toupet Procedure. This procedure was described in 1963 and comprises a posterior partial fundoplication of between 180–240°.[19] The posterior part of the fundus is passed behind the oesophagus and sutured initially to the right crus and subsequently to the right lateral side of the oesophagus. The anterior part of the stomach is similarly sutured to the left anterolateral portion of the oesophagus for a length of 4–5 cm. Good results have been obtained, particularly in avoidance of mechanical complications.

Lind Procedure. The Lind procedure described in 1965 is similar to the Toupet, but involves a crural repair and only a 180° posterolateral fundoplication, the anterolateral aspects of the oesophagus remaining unbuttressed.[20] Once more, good results have been obtained, particularly in the low incidence of mechanical complications (see section on results).

"Physiological" Antireflux Procedure. This procedure was described by Watson and colleagues in 1991 following clinical and objective evaluation over a 15 year

period involving more than 450 patients.[21] The aim was to provide effective reflux control whilst avoiding the mechanical complications of Nissen fundoplication by a relatively simple transabdominal procedure, by restoring and accentuating normal anatomical relationships and by retaining normal physiological lower oesophageal sphincter characteristics.

The procedure involves creation of a long intra-abdominal segment of oesophagus by blunt transhiatal dissection and fixture of this segment to a posterior crural repair. The angle of His is accentuated by suturing the superomedial aspect of the fundus to the under-surface of the diaphragm and studies have shown that a 120° anterolateral fundoplication is all that is required to complement these other factors to produce effective reflux control similar to the Nissen fundoplication, whilst avoiding the complications of gas bloat or inability to belch or vomit. The procedure is easier to perform than Nissen fundoplication, not requiring division of the short gastric vessels, and manometric studies have shown that a supracompetent LOS is not produced and normal relaxation on swallowing is preserved.

Prosthetic Insertion. The concept of prosthetic insertion to repair hiatal hernias and correct gastro-oesophageal reflux began in the 1960s with several descriptions of the use of Ivalon sponge in this situation, with encouraging early results but the potential for considerable perioesophageal fibrosis. However, prosthetic insertion achieved a resurgence of interest following the description in 1979 by Angelchik and Cohen[22] of a silicone-filled prosthetic collar which was placed around the lower oesophagus. This relatively simple procedure proved effective in controlling reflux symptoms and gained considerable popularity, initially in the United States and subsequently in the United Kingdom. However, there were several mechanical complications associated with its use, including migration within the peritoneal cavity and occasionally within the gastrointestinal tract and particularly the development of dysphagia in up to 30% of patients, which led to an unacceptable reoperation rate for removal of the prosthesis in over 10% of patients,[23] as a result of which the technique largely fell into disrepute.

Other Procedures

Round Ligament Gastropexy. The use of the round ligament to form a sling around the lower oesophagus to fix the oesophagogastric junction within the abdomen was initially described by Rampal *et al.*,[24] in 1964 and subsequently used more extensively by Narbona,[25] who added a gastropexy, which involved fixation of the medial aspect of the fundus of the stomach to the round ligament which accentuates the angle of His. The procedure is relatively easy to perform and good clinical results have been achieved by Narbona, but little objective evaluation has been performed.

Composite Procedures. Some workers, notably Henderson and colleagues,[26] have advocated the combined use of a Collis gastroplasty with a Nissen fundoplication performed over the neo-oesophagus, the principal objectives being to secure a long intra-abdominal "oesophageal segment" and to avoid slippage of the wrap. Excellent results have been claimed, although the procedure is quite difficult and is mostly performed via a thoracotomy.

The issue of whether to add a vagotomy to an antireflux procedure has aroused controversy over many years. The more physiological nature of highly selective vagotomy led to its advocation at the time of antireflux surgery by some workers[27,28] but a high incidence of lesser curve gastric necrosis has been reported when combining these procedures.[29] In fact, as the majority of patients with gastro-oesophageal reflux in the absence of a duodenal ulcer diathesis are normosecretors,[30] it would appear illogical to add vagotomy routinely, but to reserve this for those who have a proven ulcer diathesis and possibly those who are hypersecretors.

Aims of Treatment

The primary aim of treatment of symptomatic gastro-oesophageal reflux disease is to relieve symptoms. However, as with peptic ulcer disease, there is an imperfect relationship between symptoms and endoscopic findings.[31] Indeed, patients with the more severe degrees of gastro-oesophageal reflux resulting in complications such as reflux-induced stricture and Barrett's columnar-lined oesophagus often have fewer symptoms than those with erosive oesophagitis,[32] which is likely to be due to a diminished sensitivity to oesophageal acidification in these patients.[33] As the presence of significant erosive oesophagitis may lead to such complications as ulceration and stricture formation, it is clearly of paramount importance that successful antireflux surgery enables oesophagitis to heal, as well as relieving symptoms, in those patients who have endoscopic oesophagitis. As a counsel of perfection, it would appear appropriate also to restore the intraoesophageal pH profile to physiological levels, although few studies have addressed this aim. In patients with complications of gastro-oesophageal reflux disease, successful antireflux surgery has been associated with healing of strictures in 75% of patients[34] and, in Barrett's columnar-lined oesophagus, with arrest of progression[7] and regression of the columnar-lined oesophagus in 10–40% of cases.[8–10,35,36]

The assessment of success in antireflux surgery should be directed towards measurement of the degree of attainment of these objectives. Assessment of symptomatic success should ideally be done objectively by a scoring system or at the very least by Visick grading. This must be conducted by personal interview rather than questionnaire and in order to avoid bias either on the part of the patient or the observer, it is best that such assessment should be performed by someone not associated with the operating team. Because of the imperfect relationship between symptoms and endoscopic findings, those patients with endoscopic oesophagitis preoperatively should be re-endoscoped postoperatively to document endoscopic healing. It is unfortunate that so few series describing the efficacy of various anti-reflux procedures include endoscopic assessment. Clearly, objective assessment is necessary in order to avoid overestimating the degree of success, either by overlooking patients with residual asymptomatic oesophagitis or those who may experience a placebo effect from surgery.

The relevance of more complex oesophageal investigations, such as oesophageal manometry and pH monitoring, is more debatable. While the relief of symptoms and healing of endoscopic oesophagitis should be the primary aims of treatment and achievement of both of these objectives in a high proportion of patients is a good indicator of success, it would appear prudent in the evaluatory stages of new procedures to obtain as much objective evidence of success as possible. In this context laparoscopic antireflux surgery should be viewed in the same way as a new antireflux procedure, until it has been proved that existing procedures can be performed laparoscopically with equivalent objective as well as subjective success as achieved by open procedures. While manometric resting lower oesophageal sphincter pressure does not correlate precisely with the correction of reflux,[37,38] very low values of resting LOSP less than 5 mmHg are likely to result in failure and very high levels, greater than 20 mmHg, are more likely to result in mechanical complications. However, a simple manometric measurement which correlates very well with the incidence of mechanical complications is the ability of the LOS to relax on swallowing and it is advised that this is measured in the evaluation of any new antireflux procedure or laparoscopic adaptation of an existing procedure. Twenty-four hour ambulatory pH monitoring is an extremely reliable indicator of oesophageal acid exposure and in the evaluation of the success of laparoscopic antireflux surgery, the ability to restore intraoesophageal acid exposure to physiological levels, principally reduction of the percentage total time the pH is less than 4 to below 5%, should be documented.

Durability is an important quality of successful antireflux surgery and several series are now beginning to emerge with good ten year follow-up. This mostly relates to symptomatic assessment but it is the practice of our own and several other units prospectively to evaluate patients annually with endoscopy and pH monitoring where patient compliance allows for this. With the greater difficulty in suturing and knot tying in laparoscopic surgery, at least until considerable experience has been acquired, it would appear important that objective studies are continued for at least five years. It is our own practice to perform symptom assessment, endoscopy, manometry and 24-hour ambulatory pH monitoring preoperatively, three months postoperatively and annually thereafter on all our patients undergoing laparoscopic antireflux surgery. We believe it is only by making such a detailed assessment that we will be able to say with confidence whether or not our laparoscopic antireflux surgery measures up to the results we have obtained at open operation from the standpoint of symptomatic benefit, objective success and durability.

Results of Antireflux Surgery

Considerable data are now accumulating relating to the success of various antireflux procedures and fortunately an increasing number of series are reporting objective as well as subjective data and are looking at side effects of surgery as well as efficacy in control of reflux. Some prospective randomized controlled trials have also been performed comparing various antireflux procedures against each other.

The Nissen fundoplication has been shown to be extremely effective in the control of gastro-oesophageal reflux. Symptomatic control of reflux occurs in up to 91% of patients, this effect being maintained for up to ten years.[16] It is less effective in symptomatic control of patients with severe oesophagitis, with reports of 65% Visick 1 and 2 in these circumstances and as low as 32% Visick 1.[39] Objective data in the form of restoration to physiological pH profile have only been reported in more recent series, with 83–85% restoration to physiological acid exposure.[16,40] One series has reported endoscopic oesophagitis to be abolished in 93% of patients, although neither the proportion with no endoscopic oesophagitis preoperatively nor the grade of oesophagitis in the remainder is stated in this series.[41] However, these excellent results of the Nissen fundoplication in reflux control are detracted from somewhat by the mechanical complications of total fundoplication including slippage, disruption, the gas bloat syndrome and inability to belch or vomit. Many publications have attested to these problems[42–44] and the overall incidence of postfundoplication problems has been shown to be 28%.[45] It is generally believed that the genesis of these complications is the production of a supracompetent LOS which relaxes imperfectly on swallowing.[46,47] Attempts to modify the floppy Nissen fundoplication devised by Donohue and Bombeck to reduce even further the incidence of mechanical complications have involved full mobilization of the gastric fundus by taking down the short gastric vessels and performing a very short 1 cm wrap.[16] While this resulted in the reduction of the incidence of troublesome dysphagia from 21% to 3% in this series, the incidence of gas bloat remained at 11%, inability to belch 36% and inability to vomit 63%. Other workers have expressed the view that greater mobilization of the gastric fundus may result in its denervation,[48,49] which may make it difficult totally to resolve the problem of mechanical complications with the Nissen fundoplication.

The efficacy of other antireflux procedures has been studied with varying degrees of sophistication. The largest series of Belsey Mark IV procedures reported was from Frenchay Hospital, Bristol, in 1972.[50] A retrospective review of almost 900 patients followed up clinically showed symptomatic reflux control in 88% of patients at three years and 85% at ten years. The relevance of technical difficulty of this procedure was illustrated by the differing failure rate of 6% in patients operated on by Belsey compared with the 15% of those operated on by trainees. A more recent independent study of long term results of the Belsey Mark IV procedure illustrates the importance of quoting the degree of oesophagitis when documenting results.[51] Overall, 75% of patients had good to excellent clinical results to a mean follow-up period of 6.5 years. Stratified for degree of oesophagitis, 92% of those without oesophagitis had good results, falling to 67% with grade 3 and 50% with grade 4 oesophagitis. When grades 0–2 were combined, the overall success rate was 82%. A comparative, but non-randomized study comparing one surgeon's experience of the Belsey Mark IV procedure with Nissen fundoplication was reported by Stipa and colleagues in 1989.[52] Clinical results of excellent to good approached 90% in both groups. However, when side effects including dysphagia and gas bloat were taken into account, overall patient satisfaction was 82% in the Belsey group compared with 73% in the Nissen group.

The Hill repair has been shown to be effective at clinical follow-up to 15 years with large numbers of patients, with good or excellent results in 82%. The operative mortality was 1.3% and perioperative complications 8.3%, the commonest being incidental splenectomy. Postoperative dysphagia occurred in 6.3%.[53] An independent study by Maher *et al.*[54] also showed good results in 82% of patients, but with a 4.6% mortality. As with the Belsey procedure, only clinical data are available in the large series. However, a small prospective randomized study published in 1974[55] compared the Nissen fundoplication with the Hill and Belsey procedures from the standpoint of clinical improvement, but also included data on lower oesophageal sphincter characteristics and pH data by standard acid reflux test and 24-hour stationary pH monitoring in some patients. Considering the procedures were performed by surgical residents in this series, the Nissen fundoplication did amazingly well, with restoration to normality from a clinical and pH standpoint in 100% of cases, which has not been maintained in subsequent publications from the same centre. The Hill procedure was only 47% effective in controlling reflux symptoms, despite restoration to normal pH profile in 73%, and the Belsey strangely produced a reverse phenomenon, with 80% having abolition of reflux symptoms although only 46% were restored to normality on pH monitoring. When the postoperative sequelae were combined, including inability to belch or vomit, dysphagia and bloating, the Nissen fundoplication was associated with the highest incidence. It is difficult to draw many conclusions from this study, as the numbers in each group were very small, the procedures were performed by inexperienced operators, two of the procedures not being routinely performed in that institution, and the great disparity between symptoms and pH findings and the results of the Hill procedure compared with other studies beg several questions.

Both the Toupet and the Lind partial fundoplications have been the subject of prospective randomized controlled studies against the Nissen fundoplication. Thal and colleagues compared the floppy Nissen fundoplication against a modified Toupet hemifundoplication with clinical assessment, endoscopy and oesophageal manometry before and five years after surgery. The Toupet procedure showed significantly better clinical results, with good or excellent ratings in 95% of patients at five years compared to 67% with the Nissen fundoplication.[56] Their symptomatic rating included side effects, which were higher in the Nissen group, particularly from the standpoint of troublesome dysphagia and the gas bloat syndrome. These authors have subsequently conducted more than 300 Toupet procedures with a recurrence rate less than 5% at a mean follow-up of 3.5 years. A similar study was performed by Lundell *et al.*,[57] which included 24-hour pH monitoring. It concluded that both procedures were highly effective in reflux control both from a clinical and pH standpoint, the only difference being a greater incidence of dysphagia in the Nissen group at three months, although this difference was no longer present at six months. A similar study comparing the floppy Nissen fundoplication and the Lind procedure[58] showed no difference in reflux control, but a higher proportion of patients in Visick groups 3 and 4 in the Nissen group because of mechanical complications.

The "physiological" composite partial fundoplication procedure of Watson was studied in 100 patients by pre- and postoperative clinical symptom scoring, endoscopy, manometry and 24-hour ambulatory pH monitoring, the clinical and endoscopic assessments being performed by authors not associated with the operating team.[21] Ninety-four percent of patients were Visick 1 and 2, 82% being Visick 1. Healing of oesophagitis occurred in 86% of patients at six months and restoration to physiological pH profile in 84%. There was no incidence of gas bloat syndrome or inability to belch or vomit and a 2% incidence of troublesome dysphagia. The total reported experience of this procedure was 452 patients over a 15 year period with no incidence of splenic damage and 30 day hospital mortality of 0.2%. 3.8% had recurrent reflux requiring revisional surgery. An independent study of this procedure by Park and colleagues[59] showed similar results, but no randomized controlled study against the Nissen fundoplication has yet been reported.

The Angelchik prosthesis has attracted considerable evaluatory attention. Several series report clinical efficacy in around 80% of patients,[23,60,61] with restoration to physiological pH profile in 70%. However, mechanical complications have been significant, principally disruption and migration of the prosthesis and intractable dysphagia caused by angulation, necessitating reoperation to remove the prosthesis in 10–17% of patients.[17,60] Three prospective randomized studies comparing the Angelchik prosthesis with floppy Nissen fundoplication have been performed, one showing no difference in reflux control but more complications with the Angelchik prosthesis,[62] one showing superior reflux control by the Nissen fundoplication[63] and the third showing superior results with the Angelchik prosthesis.[39] This last series reported 23% of patients with persisting reflux after Nissen fundoplication, but 96% of patients in Visick grades 1 and 2 following Angelchik prosthesis insertion, which is a little surprising as four patients (15%) in this group had to be reoperated upon to remove the prosthesis for complications.

The round ligament gastropexy, which has considerable appeal to laparoscopic surgeons because of its relative ease of performance,[64] has been followed up in large numbers for a long period of time by Narbona[25] and has been shown to have a similar level of success to other antireflux procedures on clinical and radiological follow-up, but unfortunately these results as yet have not been supported by pre- and postoperative objective data or independent assessment in significant numbers.

The above discussion relates predominantly to uncomplicated gastro-oesophageal reflux disease about which most data exist. However, some data exist relating to the results of antireflux surgery in the management of complications of gastro-oesophageal reflux disease in comparison with those achieved by pharmacological therapy. In consideration of the expectations of laparoscopic antireflux surgery, it is important to be aware of the results achieved by conventional open procedures, although the role of laparoscopic surgery in complicated gastro-oesophageal disease has yet to be defined.

It is generally accepted that in patients with reflux-induced stricture, the results of antireflux surgery are not as good as in uncomplicated disease, largely because of oesophageal shortening. Furthermore, because of the severe motility disturbances frequently present in these patients,[34] many workers whose preferred procedure is the floppy Nissen fundoplication will perform one of the partial fundoplication procedures because of the greater risk of postoperative dysphagia.[65] Success rates of 71–75% in stricture patients are reported,[66,67] antireflux surgery being considerably more effective than pharmacological acid suppression in reduction of dilatation requirements.[8] In the management of patients with Barrett's columnar-lined oesophagus, antireflux surgery is the only modality which has been shown to arrest progression of columnarization[7] and regression in 11–40% of patients[8–10,35,36] Antireflux surgery is also considerably more effective in symptom control and prevention of complications of ulceration and stricture than pharmacological acid suppression,[8] but no series has yet demonstrated its ability to reduce the incidence of adenocarcinoma.

Conclusion

The principal objectives of antireflux surgery are control of symptoms, healing of oesophagitis, restoration to a physiological pH profile and prevention of complications. Other important factors contributing to efficacy are the incidence of side effects, durability and ease of performance. As with the evaluation of any antireflux procedure, these factors must be considered when assessing the efficacy of laparoscopic antireflux procedures, as well as saving of bed days and early return to work. In identifying the ideal antireflux procedure, whether it is performed by conventional open surgery or laparoscopically, there will always be a delicate balance between efficacy in reflux control, avoidance of troublesome mechanical complications and relative ease of performance. The natural prejudice of the author is towards the "physiological" antireflux procedure, which has been shown to be as effective as the floppy Nissen fundoplication in reflux control and durability, but with a significantly lower incidence of mechanical complications. This can be achieved without the necessity to divide the short gastric vessels, which makes it considerably easier than the Nissen fundoplication to perform both at open surgery and especially laparoscopically. However, it remains necessary to document carefully the above parameters preoperatively, postoperatively and in the long term, which is our practice both in laparoscopic and open procedures.

OESOPHAGEAL MOTILITY DISORDERS

Indications for Surgery

The only oesophageal motility disorders for which a laparoscopic or thoracoscopic approach may be appropriate are achalasia and diffuse oesophageal spasm. The principal indication for surgery in achalasia is currently failed conservative treatment. The conservative treatment of choice is pneumatic dilatation. Failure is a relative term, as dilatation is initially successful in up to 80% of patients.[67] However, recurrent dysphagia may occur after a varying interval following dilatation and the duration of remission and the age of the patient are major determinants as to the degree of success. In general terms, the necessity for dilatation more frequently than once a year, particularly in young patients, would signal the necessity for cardiomyotomy, assuming there was no contraindication. At the present time, there is little help from clinical features or manometric criteria as accurate predictors of response following dilatation, with the exception that elderly patients with gross oesophageal dilatation do less well after this procedure. In these circumstances, many workers would try the effect of one or even two pneumatic dilatations to see if a dramatic response could be obtained before recommending surgery in young patients and those with high dilatation requirements.

In diffuse oesophageal spasm, the situation is somewhat more complex. Medical treatment generally consists of nitrite compounds or calcium channel blockers. While total symptomatic control is difficult to achieve in this group of patients, in those with intractable symptoms, particularly those of severe incapacitating chest pain, a long myotomy may occasionally offer relief.[68] However, the success rate is considerably less than that achieved in the treatment of achalasia, which some have ascribed to the high incidence of psychiatric disease in these patients.[69] Long myotomy should, therefore, be considered with great care and only when symptoms are disabling, when other forms of treatment including balloon dilatation have been tried and when an associated psychiatric disorder has been excluded or treated.

Surgical Techniques

Cardiomyotomy

This operation was first described by Heller in 1913 and involved division in the longitudinal plane of both the circular and longitudinal muscle fibres overlying the lower oesophageal sphincter on both the anterior and posterior aspects of the oesophagus. However, the commonest operation now practised is a modification by Zaaiger, described in 1923, consisting of a single anterior myotomy. The lower oesophagus is approached either through an upper midline abdominal incision or by a thoracotomy through the 7th or 8th interspace and the lower 5–7 cm of the oesophagus are mobilized. This is easier through a transthoracic approach and the phreno-oesophageal ligament has to be divided if the transabdominal route is chosen, which may result in a higher incidence of postoperative gastro-oesophageal reflux.[70] The length of the myotomy is controversial, because of the opposing needs to relieve obstruction adequately and to prevent gastro-oesophageal reflux. Certain surgeons believe that a short myotomy of approximately 3 cm placed over the region of the lower oesophageal sphincter avoids reflux, but at the expense of a small incidence of residual obstruction.[71] Others believe that the myotomy should be up to 7 cm in length, extending over the oesophagogastric junction and gastric sling fibres. Whilst this invariably results in total relief of the obstruction, the incidence of postoperative reflux may approach 50%. In these circumstances, a concomitant antireflux procedure should be performed and some surgeons believe it is a wise precaution in all cases. Because of the relatively impaired peristalsis in achalasia, the antireflux operation should be one of the partial fundoplication procedures.[72]

Long Oesophageal Myotomy

In those cases of diffuse oesophageal spasm in which it is believed a long myotomy may be beneficial, the procedure is performed transthoracically through the 5th or 6th interspace. The length of the myotomy is variable and best tailored to the extent of the manometric abnormality. Many believe that the myotomy should traverse the lower oesophageal sphincter, in which case a prophylactic antireflux procedure is desirable.[71] In other respects, the principle of the procedure is similar to that of cardiomyotomy.

Aims of Treatment

The primary aim of treatment in achalasia and indeed in diffuse oesophageal spasm is relief of symptoms. Many patients with achalasia lose weight as a result of their dysphagia and a good symptomatic result comprises restoration of normal swallowing, regaining of any accompanying weight loss and avoidance of side effects, the principal one being gastro-oesophageal reflux. In achalasia, restoration of lower oesophageal sphincter characteristics is a desirable and achievable aim, with restoration of the normally hypertensive lower oesophageal sphincter to physiological values and, importantly, restoration of its ability to relax on swallowing. However, improvement in oesophageal body motility occurs in only approximately 30% of patients,[73] predominantly those with mild disease or the variant of "vigorous" achalasia where high amplitude contractions are present.[71]

The assessment of success therefore depends on clinical and manometric criteria, together with endoscopy or pH monitoring to exclude the complication of gastro-oesophageal reflux. Ideally, the dysphagia should be graded according to ability to swallow solids, semisolids or fluids by an objective scoring system and manometric criteria should include resting lower oesophageal sphincter pressure, ability of the LOS to relax on swallowing and oesophageal body characteristics measured pre- and postoperatively. In long myotomy for diffuse oesophageal spasm, any improvement is difficult to attain and most workers would be well satisfied by clinical improvement, although in some cases it is possible to show associated manometric improvement, particularly in the reduction of high-amplitude contractions which may produce the severe chest pain.

Results of Oesophageal Myotomy

There are far more data available on the results of cardiomyotomy for achalasia. The results are generally excellent, with a good clinical success rate in 90–95% of patients,[74,75] which is generally better than those reported following pneumatic dilatation, emphasizing the importance of consideration of surgical therapy in young patients. The only prospective randomized study between pneumatic dilatation and cardiomyotomy showed good long term results after cardiomyotomy in 95% of cases compared to 65% following pneumatic dilatation.[76] Cardiomyotomy is a safe procedure, no mortality being reported in the series quoted above. Morbidity is also infrequent and principally relates to the occurrence of gastro-oesophageal reflux and its complications. The incidence of gastro-oesophageal reflux varies depending on the extent of the myotomy and the degree of vigour with which such a diagnosis is sought and varies between 7–50%, with an incidence of reflux-induced stricture of approximately 5%.[71,77] While the incidence of gastro-oesophageal reflux may be less following pneumatic dilatation, varying from 0–17%, there is a risk of perforation of approximately 3% and a procedure related mortality of around 0.2%.[77] If a concomitant antireflux procedure is performed, this may result in dysphagia in up to 62% of patients if a Nissen fundoplication is used, emphasizing the importance of using one of the partial fundoplication procedures in these circumstances.[75]

The results of long myotomy for oesophageal spasm largely depend on how carefully patients are selected, the best results being achieved in those who have severe symptoms for prolonged periods, with radiographic and manometrically demonstrated abnormalities. In these patients, success rates of 50–62% of patients have been reported.[68,78] The disadvantage of long myotomy is that it has to be performed transthoracically, with a resulting morbidity of 5–10% and a procedure related mortality of up to 2%, and a prophylactic antireflux procedure is necessary if the myotomy includes the lower oesophageal sphincter.

Conclusions

The results of cardiomytomy for achalasia are excellent, the main disadvantage being the risk of gastro-oesophageal reflux, particularly in transabdominal cardiomyotomy, frequently necessitating a concomitant antireflux procedure. However, this may become less of a problem as minimally invasive cardiomyotomy develops, as it may be performed both thoracoscopically and transabdominally without the need to divide all phreno-oesophageal ligamentous attachments. However, it will be important to document not only clinical response but that measured manometrically, particularly resting lower oesophageal sphincter pressure, ability to relax on swallowing and recovery of motor function. It will be important to assess objectively the presence of gastro-oesophageal reflux as a complication, particularly if concomitant antireflux surgery is not performed for the reasons mentioned above, and it is our practice to perform 24-hour ambulatory pH monitoring as well as manometry following laparoscopic cardiomyotomy.

With regard to diffuse oesophageal spasm, the principal risk of the availability of minimally invasive surgery, which allows the replacement of thoracotomy by thoracoscopy, is that the same stringent selection criteria may not be applied. The fact that long myotomy can be performed less invasively should not alter the indications until new evidence emerges that myotomy is appropriate for patients other than those incapacitated by severe chest pain or dysphagia and who have been resistant to more conservative forms of treatment.

REFERENCES

1. Sandmark S, Carlsson R, Fausa O, Lundell L. Omeprazole or ranitidine in the treatment of reflux esophagitis. *Scand J Gastroenterol* 1988; **23**: 625–32.
2. Klinkenberg-Knol EC, Jansen JMBJ, Festen HPM *et al.* Double-blind multicentre comparison of omeprazole and ranitidine in the treatment of reflux oesophagitis. *Lancet* 1987; **1**: 349–51.
3. Hetzel DJ, Dent J, Reed WD *et al.* Healing and relapse of severe peptic oesophagitis after treatment with omeprazole. *Gastroenterology* 1988; **95**: 903–12.
4. Lundell L, Beckman L, Ekström P *et al.* Prevention of relapse of reflux esophagitis after endoscopic healing: the efficacy and safety of omeprazole compared with ranitidine. *Scand J Gastroenterol* 1991; **26**: 248–56.
5. Barlow AP, Norris TL, Watson A. Can failure of medical treatment be predicted in gastro-oesophageal reflux? *Gut* 1989; **30**: 730.
6. Watson A. Controlled trial of medical versus surgical reflux control in the management of peptic oesophageal stricture treated by intermittent dilatation. *Gut* 1985; **26**: 553–4.

7. Bremner CG. Barrett's oesophagus. *Br J Surg* 1989; **76**: 995–6.
8. Attwood SEA, Barlow AP, Norris TL, Watson A. Barrett's oesophagus: effects of anti-reflux surgery on symptom control and development of complications. *Br J Surg* 1992; **79**: 1050–3.
9. Bremner CG. The columnar-lined (Barrett's) oesophagus. *Surg Ann* 1977; **9**: 103–23.
10. Brand OL, Ylvisaker J, Gelfand M, Pope CE. Regression of columnar (Barrett's) epithelium after anti-reflux surgery. *New Eng J Med* 1980; **15**: 844–8.
11. Nissen R. Eine einfache Operation zut Beeinflussung der Reflux-oesophagitis. *Schweiz Med Wschr* 1956; **86**: 590–2.
12. Woodward ER. Surgical treatment of reflux peptic esophagitis. *Am Surg* 1982; **48**: 647–51.
13. Donohue PE, Bombeck C. The modified Nissen fundoplication – reflux prevention without gas bloat. *Chir Gastroenterol* 1977; **11**: 15–27.
14. Thal AP. A unified approach to surgical problems of the gastroesophageal junction. *Ann Surg* 1968; **168**: 246–8.
15. Rossetti N, Hell K. Fundoplication for treatment of gastro-esophageal reflux in hiatal hernia. *World J Surg* 1977; **1**: 439–43.
16. DeMeester TR, Bonavina L, Albertucci M. Nissen fundoplication for gastroesophageal reflux disease. *Ann Surg* 1986; **204**: 9–20.
17. Baue AE, Belsey RHR. The treatment of sliding hiatus hernia and reflux esophagitis by the Mark IV technique. *Surgery* 1967; **62**: 396–406.
18. Hill LD. An effective operation for hiatal hernia: an 8-year appraisal. *Ann Surg* 1967; **166**: 681–92.
19. Toupet A. Technique d'oesophago-gastroplastie avec phrenogastropexie appliquée dans la cure radicale des hernies hiatales et comme complément de l'operation d'Heller dans les cardiospasmes. *Mém Acad Chir Paris* 1963; **89**: 384–9.
20. Lind JF, Burns CM, MacDougall JT. "Physiological" repair for hiatus hernia – manometric study. *Arch Surg* 1965; **91**: 233–7.
21. Watson A, Jenkinson LR, Ball CS *et al.* A more physiological alternative to total fundoplication for the surgical correction of resistant gastro-oesophageal reflux. *Br J Surg* 1991; **78**: 1088–94.
22. Angelchik JP, Cohen R. A new surgical procedure for the treatment of gastroesophageal reflux and hiatal hernia. *Surg Gynecol Obstet* 1979; **148**: 246–8.
23. Wale RJ, Royston CMS, Bennett JR *et al.* Prospective study of the Angelchik anti-reflux prosthesis. *Br J Surg* 1985; **72**: 520–5.
24. Rampal M, Perillat PH, Ronzand R. Notes préliminaires sur une nouvelle technique de cure chirurgicale des hernies hiatales le cardiopexie par le ligament rond. *Marseille Chir* 1964; **16**: 488–91.
25. Narbona B, Olavarietta L, Iloris J. Hernia hiatal-reflux gastro-oesophagico. Rehabilitacion nofegica y resultados con la pexia del ligamento redondo (114 casos). *Cir Espanol* 1979; **33**: 487–91.
26. Henderson RD, Marryatt G. Total fundoplication gastroplasty. Long term follow-up of 500 patients. *J Thorac Cardiovasc Surg* 1983; **85**: 81–7.
27. Bahadorzadeth K, Jordan PH. Evaluation of the Nissen fundoplication for treatment of hiatal hernia: use of parietal cell vagotomy without drainage as an adjunctive procedure. *Ann Surg* 1975; **181**: 402–8.
28. Amdrup J. Should an antireflux procedure be used as a routine in surgical patients with duodenal ulcer? In: Vagotomy and Modern Surgical Practices (eds Baron JH, Williams JA, Allgo M, Muller G, Spencer J), p. 131. London, Butterworths, 1982.
29. Kennedy T, MacGill P, Johnston GW, Parks TG. Proximal gastric vagotomy, fundoplication and lesser curve necrosis. *Br Med J* 1979; **1**: 1455–6.

30. Barlow AP, Norris TL, Watson A. Does healing of oesophagitis depend solely on reducing acid exposure? *Gut* 1989; **30**: 1490.
31. Jenkinson LR, Norris TL, Watson A. Symptoms and endoscopic findings – can they predict abnormal nocturnal gastro-oesophageal reflux? *Ann Roy Coll Surg Eng* 1989; **71**: 117–19.
32. Watson A. A clinical study of the role of anti-reflux surgery combined with endoscopic dilatation in peptic esophageal stricture. *Am J Surg* 1984; **148**: 346–9.
33. Ball CS, Watson A. Acid sensitivity in reflux oesophagitis with and without complications. *Gut* 1988; **29**: 729.
34. Watson A. Reflux stricture of the oesophagus. *Br J Surg* 1987; **74**: 443–8.
35. Skinner DB, Walther BC, Riddell RH *et al.* Barrett's oesophagus. Comparison of benign and malignant cases. *Ann Surg* 1983; **198**: 546–54.
36. Fekete F, Paleron D. What is the place of antrectomy with Roux-en-Y in the treatment of severe reflux disease? *World J Surg* 1992; **16**: 349–52.
37. Higgs RH, Castell DO, Farrell RL. Evaluation of the effect of fundoplication on the incompetent lower esophageal sphincter. *Surg Gynecol Obstet* 1974; **141**: 571–5.
38. Fisher RS, Malmud LS, Lobis IF *et al.* Anti-reflux surgery for symptomatic gastro-esophageal reflux – mechanism of action. *Dig Dis* 1978; **23**: 152–60.
39. Washer GF, Gear MWL, Dowling BL *et al.* Randomised prospective trial of Roux-en-Y duodenal diversion versus fundoplication for severe reflux oesophagitis. *Br J Surg* 1984; **71**: 181–4.
40. Bancewicz J, Mughal M, Marples M. The lower oesophageal sphincter after floppy Nissen fundoplication. *Br J Surg* 1987; **974**: 162–4.
41. Mughal MM, Bancewicz J, Marples M. Oesophageal manometry and pH recording does not predict the bad results of Nissen fundoplication. *Br J Surg* 1990; **77**: 43–5.
42. Negre JB. Post fundoplication syndromes. Do they restrict the success of Nissen fundoplication? *Ann Surg* 1983; **198**: 698–700.
43. Dedinski GK, Vane DW, Black CT *et al.* Complications and re-operation after Nissen fundoplication in childhood. *Am J Surg* 1987; **153**: 177–82.
44. Leonardi HK, Corzier RE, Ellis FH. Re-operation for complications of the Nissen fundoplication. *J Thorac Cardiovasc Surg* 1981; **81**: 50–6.
45. Beauchamp G, Dube M, Perrault J. *The Post Nissen Fundoplication Syndrome.* Proceedings 4th World Congress International Society for Diseases of the Esophagus, 1989; 55.
46. DeMeester TR, Johnson LF. Evaluation of the Nissen anti-reflux procedure by esophageal manometry and 24 hour pH monitoring. *Am J Surg* 1975; **129**: 94–100.
47. Dent J, Toouli J, Sidey P, Barnes B. Incomplete relaxation of the lower esophageal high pressure zone – possible mechanism of action of fundoplication. *Gastroenterology* 1982; **82**: 1042–4.
48. Siewert JR, Feussner H. The options for surgical therapy of reflux oesophagitis. *Gullet* 1993; 3 (Suppl): 76–84.
49. Luostarinen MES, Koskinen MO, Isolauri JO. Effect of fundic mobilisation on oesophageal transit and dysphagia. *Br J Surg*; in press.
50. Orringer MB, Skinner DB, Belsey RHR. Long term results of the Mark IV operation for hiatal hernia and analysis of recurrences and their treatment. *J Thorac Cardiovasc Surg* 1972; **63**: 25–33.
51. Salama FL, Lamont G. Long term results of the Belsey Mark IV antireflux operation in relation to severity of oesophagitis. *J Thorac Cardiovasc Surg* 1990; **100**: 517–19.
52. Stipa S, Fegiz G, Iascone C *et al.* Belsey and Nissen operations for gastroesophageal reflux. *Ann Surg* 1989; **210**: 583–9.
53. Low DE, Anderson RP, Ilves R *et al.* Fifteen to twenty year results after the Hill antireflux operation. *J Thorac Cardiovasc Surg* 1989; **98**: 444–50.

54. Maher JW, Hollenbeck JI, Woodward ER. An analysis of recurrent esophagitis following posterior gastropexy. *Ann Surg* 1978; **187**: 227–30.
55. DeMeester TR, Johnson LF, Kent AH. Evaluation of current operations for the prevention of gastro-oesophageal reflux. *Ann Surg* 1974; **180**: 511–22.
56. Thor KBA, Silander I. A long-term randomized prospective trial of the Nissen procedure versus a modified Toupet technique. *Ann Surg* 1989; **210**: 719–24.
57. Lundell L, Abrahamsson H, Ruth M *et al.* Lower oesophageal sphincter characteristics and oesophageal acid exposure following partial or 360 degree fundoplication; results of a prospective randomized clinical study. *World J Surg* 1991; **15**: 115–21.
58. Walker SJ, Holt S, Sanderson CJ, Stoddard CJ. Comparison of Nissen total and Lind partial transabdominal fundoplication in the treatment of gastro-oesophageal reflux. *Br J Surg* 1992; **79**: 410–14.
59. Park K, Zentler-Munro P, Munro A. *An Evaluation of the Watson Fundoplication.* Proceedings Annual Meeting of the Association of Surgeons of Great Britain and Ireland 1992; 144.
60. Durrans D, Armstrong CP, Taylor TV. The Angelchik anti-reflux prosthesis – some reservations. *Br J Surg* 1985; **72**: 525–58.
61. deCaestecker JS, McLean Ross H, Heading RC, Macleod IB. Appraisal of the Angelchik anti-reflux prosthesis based on clinical and manometric data and pH monitoring. *J R Coll Surg Edinb* 1989; **34**: 9–12.
62. Deakin M, Mayer D, Temple JG. Surgery for gastro-oesophageal reflux: the Angelchik prosthesis compared to the floppy Nissen fundoplication. Two year follow up study and five year evaluation of the Angelchik prosthesis. *Ann Roy Coll Surg Eng* 1989; **71**: 249–52.
63. Stuart RC, Dawson K, Keeling P *et al.* A prospective randomized trial of Angelchik prosthesis versus Nissen fundoplication. *Br J Surg* 1989; **76**: 86–9.
64. Nathanson LK, Shimi S, Cuschieri A. Laparoscopic ligamentum teres (round ligament) cardiopexy. *Br J Surg* 1991; **78**: 947–50.
65. DeMeester TR. Management of benign esophageal strictures. In: *Medical and Surgical Problems of the Esophagus*, (eds Stipa S, Belsey RHR, Moraldi A), pp. 173–6. London Academic Press, 1981.
66. Hill LD, Gelfand M, Bauermeister D. Simplified management of reflux esophagitis with stricture. *Ann Surg* 1970; **172**: 638–46.
67. Barkin JS, Guelrud M, Renier DK *et al.* Forceful balloon dilatation: an outpatient procedure for achalasia. *Gastrointest Endosc* 1990; **36**: 123–6.
68. Henderson RD, Ryder D, Marryatt G. Reflux control following myotomy in diffuse esophageal spasm. *Ann Thorac Surg* 1982; **34**: 230–6.
69. Waterman DC, Dalton CB, Ott DJ *et al.* Hypertensive lower esophageal sphincter: what does it mean? *J Clin Gastroenterol* 1989; **11**: 139–46.
70. Andreollo NA, Earlam RJ. Heller's myotomy for achalasia: is an added anti-reflux procedure necessary? *Br J Surg* 1987; **74**: 765–9.
71. Ellis FH. Surgical management of oesophageal motility disturbances. In: *Disorders of the Oesophagus.* (eds Watson A, Celestin LR), pp. 53–62. London, Pitman, 1984.
72. DeMeester TR. Surgery for oesophageal motor disorders. *Ann Thorac Surg* 1982; **34**: 225–9.
73. Watson A. Oesophageal function and motility disorders. In: *Recent Advances in Surgery*, (eds Taylor I, Johnson CD), pp. 63–86. London, Longmans, 1993.
74. Paricio PP, Martinez DE, Haro L, Ortiz A, Aguyayo JL. Achalasia of the cardia: long-term results of oesophagomyotomy and posterior partial fundoplication. *Br J Surg* 1990; **77**: 1371–4.
75. Stipa S, Fegiz G, Iascone C *et al.* Heller–Belsey and Heller–Nissen operations for achalasia of the esophagus. *Surg Gynecol Obstet* 1990; **170**: 212–16.

76. Csendes A, Braghetto I, Henriquez A *et al.* Late results of a prospective randomized study comparing forceful dilatation and oesophagomyotomy in patients with achalasia. *Gut* 1989; **30**: 299–304.
77. O'Sullivan GC. Oesophageal mobility disorders. In: *Surgery of the Oesophagus*, (eds Hennessy TPJ, Cuschieri A), pp. 241–61. London, Baillière Tindall, 1986.
78. Orringer MB. Disorders of esophageal motility. In: *Textbook of Surgery*, (ed. Sabiston DC), pp. 705–25. London, WB Saunders, 1986.

9.2

The Laparoscopic Nissen Fundoplication

J. M. WEERTS, B. DALLEMAGNE, C. JEHAES, S. MARKIEWICZ and R. LOMBARD

Gastro-oesophageal reflux is a common condition and many patients can be quite debilitated by postural heartburn. This may be associated with flatulence, regurgitation of food and nocturnal coughing secondary to chronic pharyngitis. In a significant number of individuals, gastro-oesophageal reflux disease may progress, producing symptoms of severe oesophagitis, stenosis or metaplastic change (Barrett's oesophagus).

Conservative treatment is well established and may involve loss of weight or adequate control of diet, raising the head of the bed and the administration of prokinetic agents to improve lower oesophageal sphincter pressure.

Cost effective medical therapy comprises H_2 receptor antagonists and, more recently omeprazole, by reducing or eradicating gastric acid production. Unfortunately, none of these measures, apart from the administration of prokinetic drugs, attacks the root of the problem by correcting incompetence of the lower oesophageal sphincter.[1] As soon as treatment is discontinued by the patient, all of the symptoms usually recur.

General surgeons have always exhibited a great interest in the treatment of gastro-oesophageal reflux disease and the best results have been achieved by procedures which create a valve at the gastro-oesophageal junction.[2,3] Recently, DeMeester and his colleagues[4] have shown good long term control of gastro-oesophageal reflux disease by means of the Nissen fundoplication,[5] with over 90% of patients remaining symptom-free for a period in excess of ten years.

Critical evaluation of the results of such surgery has demonstrated not insignificant long term side effects, such as dysphagia, inability to belch, gas bloat syndrome, abdominal discomfort and increased flatus. Various modifications of the original surgical techniques have been described in an attempt to decrease these postoperative symptoms. One of the more important modifications involves the avoidance of too tight a wrap around the gastro-oesophageal reflux. This can be best achieved by fully mobilizing the gastric fundus through division of the short gastric vessels. The gastric wrap should not exceed 3 cm in length.

Surgical complications related to open surgery are not insignificant, with up to 20% incidence of accidental splenectomy having been reported,[6] in addition to infection of the chest and wound and subsequent development of incisional herniae. It is the European experience that recovery from laparotomy will take up to six weeks following surgery.[7,8]

It is important to bear in mind that gastro-oesophageal reflux is a functional disease and one which requires careful assessment before surgery is contemplated. An extensive evaluation is therefore mandatory and this will avoid intervention in patients who are unlikely to derive significant benefit from surgical treatment. Such individuals include those with oesophageal or gastric motility disorders.

It is the practice experience of our own unit to augment careful clinical examination with full preoperative assessment which will include the following:

Endoscopy to exclude malignancy and to assess the stage of oesophagitis according to the Savary–Miller classification. Biopsies are taken which provide histological confirmation of the degree of inflammation;

A *barium swallow* and *meal* undertaken to assess the reducibility of the hiatal hernia and to study gastric emptying;

Oesophageal manometry undertaken to identify any oesophageal dismotility and to measure the residual activity of the lower oesophageal sphincter. This latter evaluation may be of assistance in avoiding overcorrection of the gastro-oesophageal barrier;

A *24 hour pH study* performed to confirm the severity of reflux, which should be evaluated alongside the severity of the symptoms and the results of other investigations;

An *isotope gastric outlet study* undertaken as a matter of routine to identify potential gastric outlet obstruction.

We have reserved surgical intervention, whether open or laparoscopic, for patients with recurrent symptoms of gastro-oesophageal reflux after one full year of conservative treatment or for patients who remain symptomatic despite intensive medical therapy. Such patients will have positive endoscopic findings (at least stage II oeophagitis according to Savary–Miller), oesophageal manometry demonstrating absence of lower oesophageal sphincter pressure, positive 24 hour pH study and no elements of severe motility disorder.

Since January 1991, we have performed the Nissen fundoplication employing a laparoscopic technique[9] to avoid the more common complications reported for the open approach.

PROCEDURE

When the full preoperative assessment has been undertaken and the patient is confirmed fit for surgery, the procedure is undertaken under general anaes-

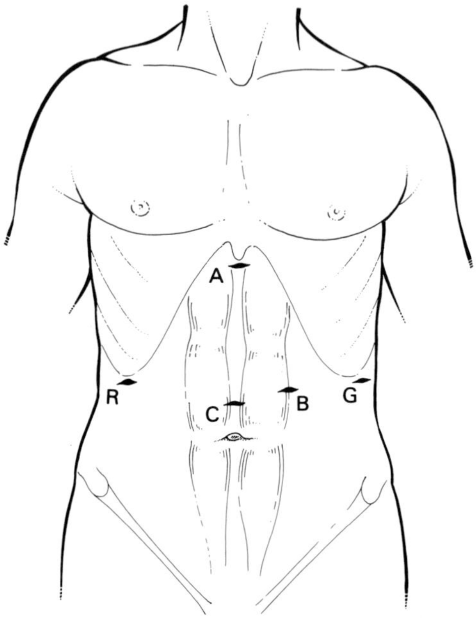

Figure 9.2.1 Positioning of trocars. A,B: working trocars; C: camera; R: liver retractor; G: gastric retractor.

thesia. All vital parameters are closely monitored and continuous assessment of expiratory PCO_2 level is undertaken. The patient is placed in the lithotomy position with the legs down. The surgeon stands between the legs with one assistant on the patient's left and a second assistant on the patient's right. The monitor(s) are placed at the head of the patient.

Once the pneumoperitoneum has been created, the first 10 mm port is inserted in the midline 5 cm or 6 cm above the umbilicus. The laparoscope is introduced and under direct vision four further 10 mm ports are inserted as depicted in Figure 9.2.1, with one port in the right hypochondrium, one beneath the xiphoid process, a further port in the left anterior axillary line and the remaining port in the left hypochondrium midway between the camera and the most distant left port.

The right port will enable the introduction of a 10 mm fanshaped retractor which will be used to lift the left lobe from the operating field. A Babcock-type forceps is introduced from the far left to maintain traction on the upper part of the stomach. The surgeon works through ports A and B using forceps and scissors with cautery.

Once display of anatomy is obtained, the initial step is to open the hiatus. The peritoneum is incised on the upper part of the hiatal triangle and the right and left crus muscles are exposed in turn. The oesophagus can be readily identified and is separated from the right crus. Dissection continues to mobilize the lower part of the thoracic oesophagus (Figure 9.2.2). Diffusion of CO_2 into the

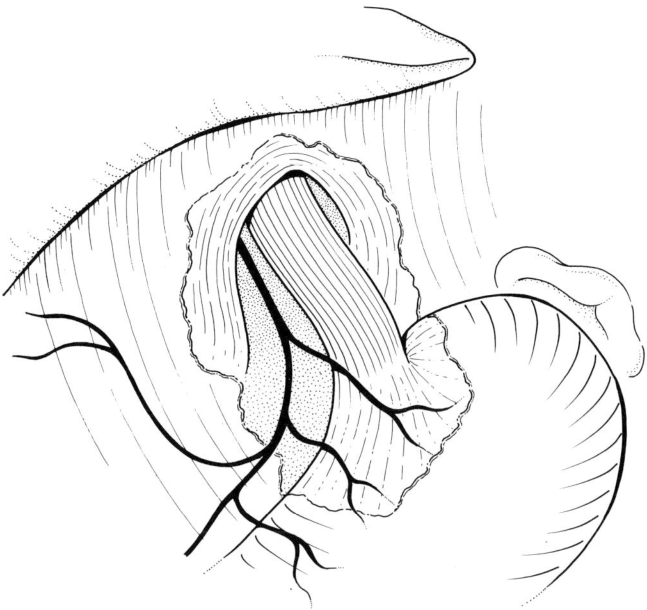

Figure 9.2.2 Exposure of the hiatus and dissection of the oesophagus.

mediastinum is generally well tolerated, although in some patients subcutaneous emphysema has been noted in the neck.

Once the dissection on the right side of the oesophagus is complete, the left crus muscle can be exposed. The Babcock forceps is used to maintain traction on the gastric fundus itself and so expose properly the lower part of the left crus. Display of the left side of the lower oesophagus can then be obtained.

The posterior wall of the oesophagus still requires mobilization and this is perhaps the most difficult part of the procedure. Dissection commences from the right side and requires that all the loose areolar tissue is separated from the oesophagus. The posterior vagal trunk can usually be easily identified and left behind by careful separation from the posterior wall of the oesophagus. Careful dissection is mandatory as the posterior wall can be easily traumatized at this stage. We have not found it helpful to pass a large size bougie into the oesophagus, since this produces a rigid tubular structure which is difficult to mobilize. Dissection with a blunt instrument is probably the safer way to create a posterior window which has to be large enough to accommodate the gastric wrap.

Once this window has been created, a rubber Penrose drain is passed around the oesophagus. This will facilitate handling and movement of the oesophagus without risk of damage. Fulminant mobilization of the lower oesophagus can be achieved, ensuring that the abdominal part of the oesophagus is at least 4–5 cm long. Good exposure of the crura can be obtained by lifting the encircled oesophagus anteriorly. Several non-absorbable sutures can be placed to

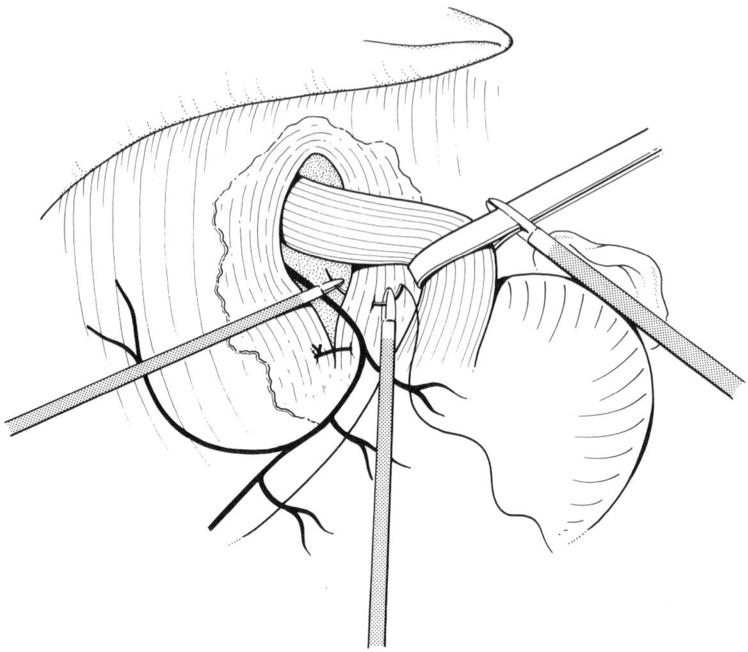

Figure 9.2.3 Narrowing of the hiatus. Rubber band around oesophagus.

approximate the two muscles and to provide a narrow enough hiatus (Figure 9.2.3). The surgeon may find it useful in early cases to introduce a large bougie (36 French gauge) to calibrate the hiatal narrowing. Suturing can be undertaken either with extracorporeal or intracorporeal knots.

Once the hiatus has been narrowed, the gastric pouch can be mobilized by dividing the short gastric vessels. The mobilization commences 4–5 cm below the first vessel so as to facilitate division of four or five arteries. We employ a clip applicator (Endoclip, USSC) and this transects the vessel between two clips. This stage of the operation is demanding, particularly if the gastric pouch lies close to the splenic hilum. A 30° laparoscope is of value at this stage of the operation. Mobilization of the gastric fundus is important for a variety of reasons. It is essential that the wrap be undertaken without any tension and must be able to be brought freely around the oesophagus. From the work of DeMeester and his colleagues,[4] it appears that relaxation of the lower oesophageal barrier will be improved once the short gastric vessels are free and the gastric fundus is well mobilized.

In certain cases, such as those involving large paraoesophageal hernias, this mobilization may be disregarded. The elongated short gastric vessels are often long enough to avoid any traction on the wrap. Similarly, in the elderly patient, the blood supply of the gastric fundus may be jeopardized if too many vessels are transected.

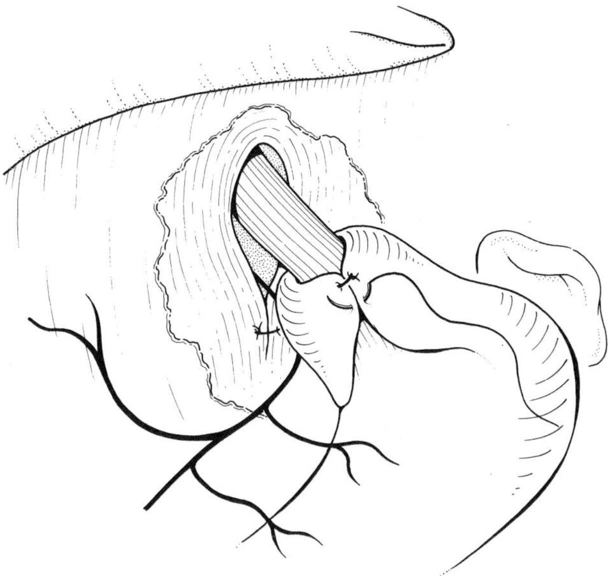

Figure 9.2.4 Suturing of the valve.

The final stage of the procedure involves the creation of the fundoplication. An atraumatic grasper is placed behind the oesophagus from the upper port in order to grasp the gastric fundus without any traction. The use of a roticulated instrument is particularly valuable for this manoeuvre. The righthand arm of the wrap can be passed behind the oesophagus and then grasped by the first assistant who can hold the structure in good position. Non-absorbable sutures (2/0) are placed continuously or in interrupted fashion (Figure 9.2.4). A good needle holder is mandatory at this stage and the first stitch will take the left arm of the pouch, the anterior oesophageal wall and the right arm of the pouch in turn. The fundoplication should be short (not more than 3–4 cm) and suturing can be undertaken in one or two layers. During this stage of the procedure it is useful to have a large bore nasogastric tube in the oesophagus (size 36 French or larger) in order to calibrate the fundoplication.

Once the fundoplication is completed, the abdominal cavity is rinsed with warm saline and the port sites inspected for any bleeding before removal of the laparoscope. Abdominal drainage is not undertaken routinely and the wounds are closed in standard fashion.

POSTOPERATIVE COURSE

A standard nasogastric tube which has usually been passed before the end of the operation is removed two to three hours following recovery. It is our practice to permit the patient to take free fluids within six hours of surgery. Normal feeding commences on the first postoperative day and the patient is normally discharged home two to three days following surgery. A soft diet is generally recommended for the first month following surgery. The patient is generally allowed to go back to work within two weeks to one month following surgery, depending upon their activity.

Almost all of our patients experience some sort of dysphagia within the first month following surgery and this is almost certainly related to the development of oesophageal oedema and dyskinesia at the lower oesophagus. These symptoms are normally transient.

RESULTS

Within a two year period from January 1991, 248 patients have been operated on for gastro-oesophageal reflux disease. All the patients had been on medical therapy for at least one year. The indication for surgical treatment was the failure of conservative therapy to control reflux symptoms or the development of recurrent symptoms when therapy was discontinued. All patients had stage II oesophagitis at endoscopy or persisting oesophagitis under treatment with omeprazole. All patients had evidence of lack of lower oesophageal sphincter pressure, with no more than mild dyskinesia of the lower oesophagus. Where there was doubt about the diagnosis, a 24-hour pH study was performed to assess the severity of reflux.

The mean operation time was 135 minutes (range 39–300 minutes). In those patients in whom an additional procedure was undertaken (i.e. cholecystectomy, proximal cell vagotomy), the duration of surgery was obviously longer. On five occasions the operation was converted to an open procedure. In one patient there was a breakdown of the light source, in a further patient there was a small perforation of the posterior wall of the cardia and in the remaining three patients, access to the cardia proved impossible and was associated in all three cases with hypertrophy of the left lobe of the liver. There was no major bleeding and no splenic trauma. All patients survived surgery.

On two further occasions, a small performation of the posterior wall of the cardia was noted but was repaired laparoscopically and covered by the wrap. All three perforations occurred at the beginning of our experience and were almost certainly due to the use of a 36 French gauge nasogastric tube which had been inserted to facilitate identification of the oesophagus. Because of this specific complication, we have now abandoned the use of large tubes *during dissection*.

The mean hospital stay for the laparoscopic approach was 2.8 days, while for the five "converted" patients, the mean hospital stay was 7.8 days.

In 12 patients intravenous fluids were prolonged for a mean period of 3.5 days because of the patients' inability to swallow properly. Only five patients experienced chest infections and these were all successfully managed by a combination of physiotherapy and antibiotics.

All the patients have been followed as outpatients by either the surgical team or the patients' own gastroenterologists. A controlled endoscopy is undertaken two to three months following the procedure and the patients are asked to volunteer for a control manometry and a 24-hour pH study.

Almost all of the patients experience some degree of dysphagia in the first month following surgery. In 11 patients endoscopy was required because of the development of acute dysphagia secondary to impaction of a food bolus. In all these patients endoscopy resolved this complication without further sequelae. Four patients experienced long term dysphagia. One underwent open surgery at another institution, it being apparent that the wrap had been undertaken too low down on the greater curvature, creating a situation analogous to a volvulus. One patient who had refused to undergo preoperative manometry presented with an akinetic oesophagus in the postoperative period and she responded to repeated oesophageal dilatation (five occasions) and is asymptomatic at the time of reporting. The remaining two patients responded to dilatations (two occasions) and are again asymptomatic on review.

One patient continues to complain of recurrent reflux six months following surgery. These symptoms are not related to position and a barium meal has demonstrated partial disruption of the wrap, although endoscopy and 24-hour pH monitoring have demonstrated no abnormality.

The majority of patients have been reviewed two to three months following surgery and on examination four individuals had developed small incisional hernias at the midline port site above the umbilicus. One hundred and ninety six patients agreed to a postoperative endoscopy. One patient was shown to have mild erythema (stage 1 oesophagitis), but was asymptomatic for reflux.

One hundred and thirty-two patients agreed to undergo control manometry and this demonstrated a rise in lower oesophageal pressure from a mean preoperative value of 3.2 mmHg (range 0–13 mmHg) to a postoperative value of 23.4 mmHg (range 12–56 mmHg). One patient presented ten months following surgery with chest pain thought to be due to diffuse oesophageal spasms which were confirmed on manometry. The preoperative manometry in this patient showed no abnormality and postoperative endoscopy and 24-hour pH studies were normal.

CONCLUSIONS

It is apparent that careful long term follow-up will be required to assess the quality of the fundoplication. Our early results are extremely encouraging and the low rates of conversion to an open procedure, along with the low associated morbidity, are arguments in favour of a laparoscopic approach. The lack of postoperative discomfort may result in a change in the surgical indications for the disease that is said to affect almost 20 million of the population in the United States of America.

It should be borne in mind, however, that the procedure is difficult to perform and more than basic experience in laparoscopic surgery is required before the procedure can be undertaken. Careful selection of patients, based on objective findings during preoperative work-up, is required. Careful surgical technique will be rewarded in the longer term.

REFERENCES

1. Skinner BD. Pathophysiology of gastro-oesophageal reflux. *Ann Surg* 1985; **206**: 546–56.
2. DeMeester TR, Stein HJ. Surgical treatment of gastro-oesophageal reflux disease. In: *The Esophagus* (ed. Castell), pp. 579–625. Boston, Little, Brown and Co, 1992.
3. DeMeester TR, Johnson LF, Kent AH. Evaluation of current operations for the prevention of gastro-oesophageal reflux. *Ann Surg* 1974; **108**: 511–22.
4. DeMeester TR, Bonavina L, Albertucci M. Nissen fundoplication for gastro-oesophageal reflux disease. Evaluation of primary repair in 100 consecutive patients. *Ann Surg* 1986; **204**: 9–20.
5. Nissen R. Eine einfache Operation zur Beeinflussung der Refluxoesophagitis. *Schweiz Med Wochenschr* 1956; **86**: 590–2.
6. Siewert JR, Feussner H. Treatment of peptic esophagitis Nissen repair. In: *Hernia*, 3rd edition (eds Nyhus LM, London RE), pp. 604–13. Philadelphia, J B Lippincott, 1989.
7. Gossot D, Sarjati E, Azoulaya D, Celerier M. Facteurs de Morbidité de l'intervention de Nissen. *J Chir* 1987; **124**: 367–71.
8. Saubier EC, Gouillat C, Teboul F. Traitement de reflux gastro-oesophagien par fundoplicature complete de Nissen. Resultats de 112 observations. *Chirurgie* 1986; **112**: 123–31.
9. Dallemagne B, Weerts JM, Jehaes C *et al.* Laparoscopic Nissen fundoplication – preliminary report. *Surg Laparosc Endosc* 1991; **1**: 138–43.

9.3

Laparoscopic Ligamentum Teres Cardiopexy

L. NATHANSON

The development of laparoscopic ligamentum teres cardiopexy occurred in 1990 shortly after the popularization of laparoscopic cholecystectomy. The adaptation of the sling procedure reported by Narbona-Arnau in 1965 was based on the belief that mobilization of the distal oesophagus and ligamentum teres could be easily achieved without the possible uncontrolled bleeding or splenic injury resulting from attempted division of the short gastric vessels. This did indeed prove to be true. The equivalent open operation reported by Narbona-Arnau has been well validated as an effective, low morbidity operation which lengthens the abdominal segment and increases the high pressure zone of the lower oesophageal sphincter without incurring the adverse effects of dysphagia and inability to belch.[1,2]

INDICATIONS AND PATIENT SELECTION

The patients are considered for surgery after evaluation including endoscopy, oesophageal manometry, 24-hour pH studies and a concerted attempt to control symptoms using histamine H_2 receptor antagonists, alginates and mechanical measures. Body habitus should not influence the choice of the laparoscopic approach although our experience to date has not been with excessively obese patients or those with large hiatal hernias.

Contraindications to the laparoscopic approach are previous surgery in the region of the oesophagogastric junction and documented shortening of the oesophagus precluding bringing it down into the abdomen. This may well only be established after a trial dissection. Acute presentation with incipient strangulation of the stomach within a large hiatal hernia would best be approached as an open procedure.

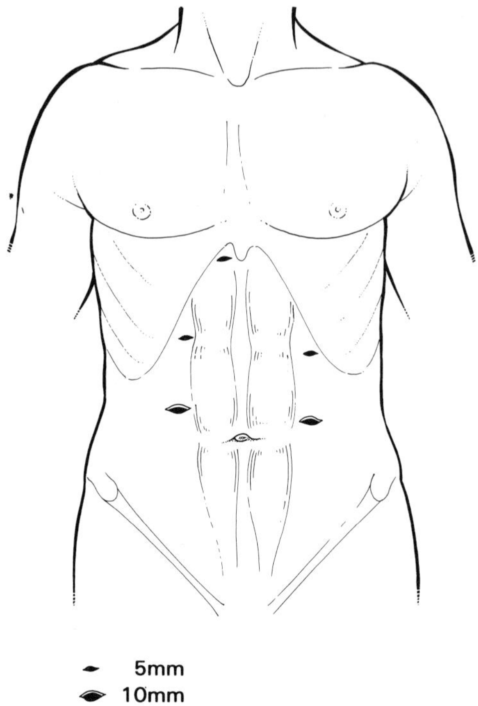

Figure 9.3.1 Port placement sites with the two operative fields requiring consideration.

OPERATIVE TECHNIQUE

Positioning

The patient is supine, 15–30° head-up, with the surgeon standing on the patient's left side and assistant standing opposite. A nasogastric tube is passed to decompress the stomach. Open laparoscopy is used to gain access at the 11 mm port site to the left of the midline. Placement of subsequent ports is illustrated in Figure 9.3.1.

Oesophageal Mobilization

The initial dissection may be mobilization of the ligamentum teres or the distal oesophagus but dissection of the oesophagus first will ensure that this critical phase of the dissection is successful prior to mobilizing the ligamentum teres.

The epigastric port is used for elevation of the left lobe of liver with a fan retractor or alternatively with a grasper anchored to the diaphragm. The assistant grasps the anterior wall of stomach with an atraumatic bowel grasper, the surgeon is equipped with a non-toothed grasper in the left hand and insulated curved dissecting scissors in the right hand. The hiatus is identified often by the crural outlines becoming prominent during the expiratory phase of ventilation and accentuated by downward traction on the stomach by the assistant. Horizontal peritoneal dissection is initiated high up at the junction of the fat pad and diaphragm, well superior to the nerve of Latarjet, with its clearly seen hepatic branches carefully preserved. The peritoneal incision is carried horizontally lateral to both crura. The plane is deepened revealing the reflection of the phreno-oesophageal membrane which is dissected off the anterior distal oesophagus. This dissection is extended around the oesophagus and allows entry into the posterior mediastinum and the two crura.

Of most importance at this point is to check that the carbon dioxide insufflation pressure is 10 mmHg or less. This prevents the development of mediastinal and cutaneous emphysema, which can occur to a dangerous degree at high pressures.

The anterior vagus is readily identified running closely applied to the anterior distal oesophagus. The distal oesophagus and stomach are dissected off the left crus taking care to clip a branch of the inferior phrenic artery often encountered at this time. A 6 cm length of oesophagus is cleared as far posteriorly as possible. Attention is turned to the right crus and by a combination of blunt and sharp scissor dissection the plane around the right side of the oesophagus is deepened. The confined space requires the careful use of the curved insulated scissors. Inadvertent electrosurgical contact with adjacent stomach and oesophagus, often out of the field of view, must be constantly guarded against. The posterior vagus is identified, the orogastric tube removed to improve the pliability of the oesophagus and with inferior and upward traction on the stomach by the assistant, the surgeon bluntly dissects behind the oesophagus under direct vision from the right side of the oesophagus to the left.

The next landmark to be identified is the left crus, to ensure the dissection remains below the diaphragm so preventing injury to parietal pleura. Once the left crus is on view gentle separation of remaining areolar tissue creates a window to the left upper quadrant as illustrated in Figure 9.3.3A. The use of the 30° forward oblique laparoscope greatly aids this process by allowing an angulated view of the operative field. This window behind the oesophagus is then enlarged sufficiently to allow easy passage of the round ligament and if desired a silicone sling may be placed around the oesophagus and brought back out through the skin to maintain oesophageal traction.

Ligamentum Teres Mobilization

Following successful mobilization of the distal oesophagus the next step is to mobilize the ligamentum teres with preservation of its blood supply which arises from the liver and peritoneal attachments (Figure 9.3.2A). A vascular arcade fed by hepatic branches runs parallel to the round ligament as far as the umbilicus

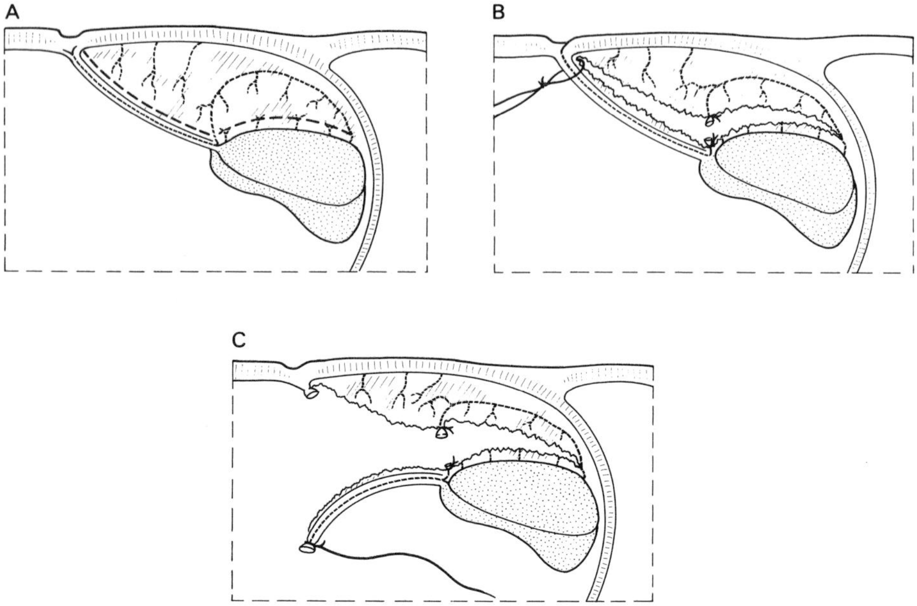

Figure 9.3.2 A: The longitudinal representation of the blood supply within the falciform ligament and the plane of dissection used to preserve the blood supply to the round ligament. B: The round ligament is detached from the umbilicus after ligation. C: Completed mobilization with the tail of the extracorporeal ligature left long to act as a "tow rope".

and must be preserved. Above the liver the two layers of peritoneum are closely apposed forming a translucent window which is outlined by a peripheral vascular suprahepatic arcade. Below the liver the peritoneal leaves are separated by a fatty layer of variable thickness which contains large veins.

Preservation of the blood supply to the ligamentum teres must be ensured by careful dissection. Dissection commences in the transparent window in the falciform ligament below the suprahepatic arcade. Insulated scissors and monopolar electrosurgery are well suited to this task. The distal limb of the arcade is next separated from the surrounding fat and ligated or clipped. The peritoneum on the left and right sides of the falciform ligament is divided by electrosurgery and scissors, keeping well away from the vascular arcade supplying the round ligament. This process is continued up to the umbilical insertion. A second telescope connected to another light source may be inserted from the opposite side and used to transilluminate the vessels running from the round ligament arcade to the anterior abdominal wall. The insertion of the ligamentum teres into the umbilicus is doubly ligated with catgut and divided. The proximal ligature tail is cut long to be used as a "tow rope" to pull the ligament around the oesophagus at a later stage and maintain traction on it prior to suture fixation. Final division of the remaining fat with small veins is accomplished by sequential bipolar coagulation and scissor division progressing from the umbilicus

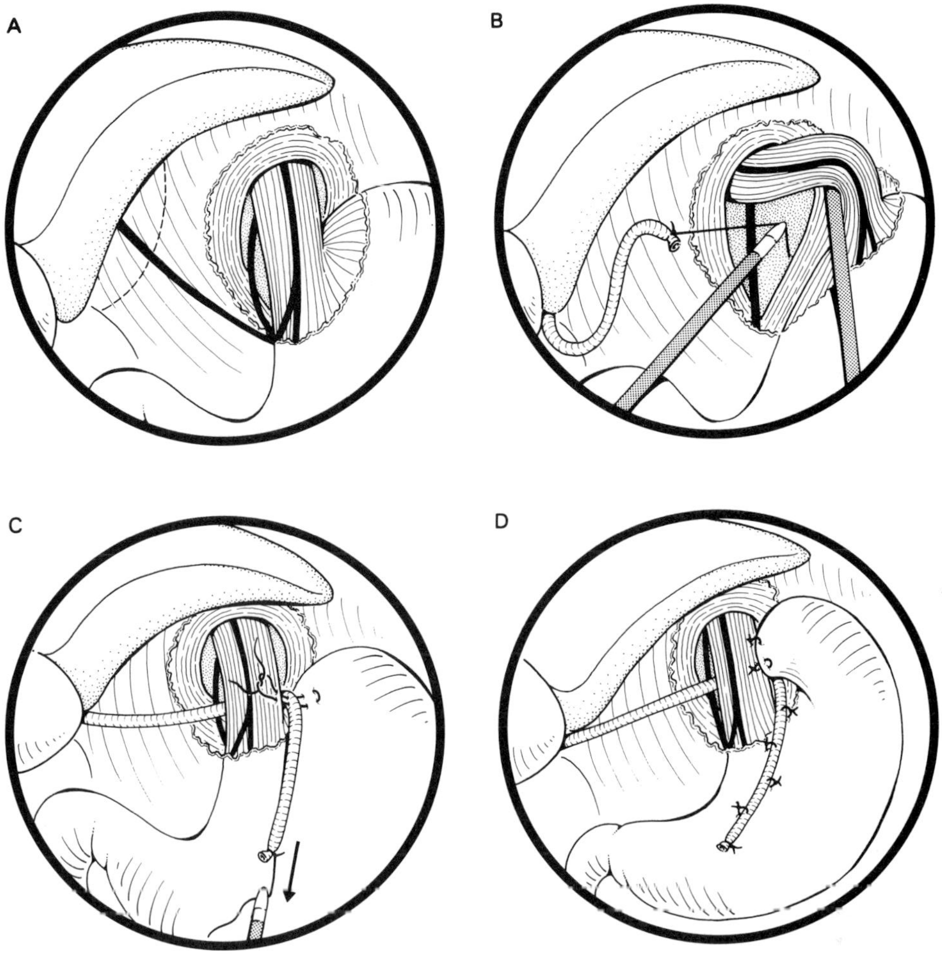

Figure 9.3.3 A: Completed mobilization of the distal oesophagus with preservation of the hepatic branches of the anterior vagus. B: Removal of the nasogastric tube and oesophageal mobilization with delivery of the "tow rope" behind the oesophagus from right to left. C: Downward traction on the sling is manometrically controlled to increase the distal sphincter pressure to 15–20 mmHg. The initial non-absorbable anchoring mattress suture is placed. D: Completed fixation with multiple interrupted sutures.

toward the window created in the suprahepatic region. Occasional larger vessels may require division between clips or ligatures (Figure 9.3.2B and C).

The left lobe of liver is retracted upward to reveal the hiatus, the assistant pulls down on the fat pad over the oesophagogastric junction and the window behind the oesophagus is displayed by an atraumatic grasper in the surgeon's right hand. The "tow rope" is grasped using atraumatic forceps in the surgeon's left hand and passed from right to left through the window to be picked up and pulled around the oesophagogastric junction (Figure 9.3.3B). Alternatively a curved instrument can be introduced into the abdomen, either using a flexible port or with the latest generation of memory metal graspers which are introduced straight and angulated while within the abdomen. The curved grasper is introduced behind the oesophagus from left to right and the "tow rope" grasped to pull the ligamentum teres around.

Manometrically controlled cardiopexy

The end of the ligament is then grasped and pulled down along the line of the oblique fibres of the stomach. The degree of traction influences both the length of the intra-abdominal segment and the pressure within the lower oesophageal sphincter. Simultaneous oesophageal manometry is commenced with zero calibration corresponding to the gastric pressure. Traction on the ligamentum teres is adjusted to achieve a pressure increment of 15–20 mmHg. Suturing is performed using interrupted 3/O silk sutures on a standard curved atraumatic needle with internal knotting. The first anchors the ligamentum teres to the oesophagogastric junction and is of the mattress type (Figure 9.3.3C). This fixes the apex of the sling in the intended position. The fundus of the stomach above the accentuated gastro-oesophageal angle (of His) is sutured to the adjacent oesophagus above the apex of the sling. Four sutures are used to fix the rest of the ligamentum teres to the anterior wall of the stomach along the line of the oblique fibres parallel to the lesser curve over a distance of 6 cm (Figure 9.3.3D). To maintain viability of the ligamentum teres these sutures should each only encompass a portion of the round ligament when tied down.

Approximation of the crura by suture has in our experience not been required, but is important if a large hiatal defect is encountered. The liver may well be folded down by the traction on the ligamentum teres but this has no apparent functional significance.

The peritoneum is lavaged clean with warm Ringer's lactate solution and aspirated dry. Peritoneal drainage is not routinely employed. The wounds are infiltrated with bupivacaine 0.25% and indomethacin 100 mg as a suppository given twice daily. Both these measures decrease postoperative narcotic analgesic requirements and hasten return of bowel function.

POSTOPERATIVE RECOVERY

Nasogastric tube decompression of the stomach is not generally necessary. Fluids and soft food are commenced the next day and discharge can be achieved between day 3 and 5 postoperatively.

RESULTS

Mild temporary dysphagia in the days following the operation settles down within three weeks and no long term cases of dysphagia or gas bloat have occurred. Barium contrast follow-up studies postoperatively are distinctive. There is lengthening of the intra-abdominal segment of the oesophagus owing to depression of the gastro-oesophageal junction equivalent to the length of two vertebral bodies and a marked accentuation of the angle of His.

The early experience has been with 16 patients since 1990 performed at a single institution. Twelve are free of symptoms of reflux and have normal endoscopic appearances of the distal oesophagus. Four patients have recurrent symptoms with recurrent oesophagitis present on endoscopy in two patients. No patients have required reoperative surgery for their reflux (A. Cuschieri, personal communication, March 1993).

COMMENT

The laparoscopic adaptation of the ligamentum teres cardiopexy of Narbona-Arnau[1] reproduces all the steps of the open operation except for the omission of the anchoring suture on the right side of the oesophagogastric junction. This was omitted to minimize the risk of devascularization of the round ligament.[3] The early results have been encouraging. However, the current place of this laparoscopic sling operation for the management of oesophageal reflux may well be limited. As experience with standard Nissen 360° and partial Toupet fundoplication has accumulated, the problem with controlling the short gastric vessels is less than initially anticipated. Combined with suture approximation of the crura, the steps of conventional fundoplication can be entirely duplicated laparoscopically.[4]

The place for laparoscopic ligamentum teres cardiopexy would seem to be limited therefore to patients without significant hiatal hernia and a small stomach unsuitable for fundoplication.

REFERENCES

1. Narbona-Arnau B. Pexy with the round ligament: the sling approach. In: *Diseases of the Esophagus* (eds Siewert JR, Holscher AH), pp. 1172–7. Berlin, Springer, 1988.
2. Narbona-Arnau B. The sling approach to the treatment of reflux peptic oesophagitis. In: *Hernia*, 3rd edition (eds Nyhus LIM, Condon RE), pp. 668–82. Philadelphia, JB Lippincott, 1989.
3. Nathanson LK, Shimi S, Cuschieri A. Laparoscopic ligamentum teres cardiopexy. *Br J Surg* 1991; **78**: 947–51.
4. Cuschieri A, Shimi S, Nathanson LK. Laparoscopic reduction, crural repair and fundoplication of large hiatal herniae. *Am J Surg* 1992; **163**: 425–30.

9.4

Laparoscopic Rossetti Fundoplication

J. MOUIEL and N. KATKHOUDA

The surgical treatment of incapacitating reflux oesophagitis is henceforth possible as a matter of routine and by laparoscopic means as a result of the experience gained from 1989 in the surgical approaches to the oesophageal hiatus for vagotomy.[1–4] It has been our approach to employ fundoplication adapted from the description of Rossetti[5] (Figure 9.4.1) which is a modification of the original technique described by Nissen[6,7] (Figure 9.4.2). This particular approach, which is well established at open surgery, has proved effective and reproducible when undertaken by laparoscopic means.[8]

PRINCIPLES

The principles of the operation which we propose have, as the main objective, the correction of the defects of the sphincter, the diaphragm and valvular

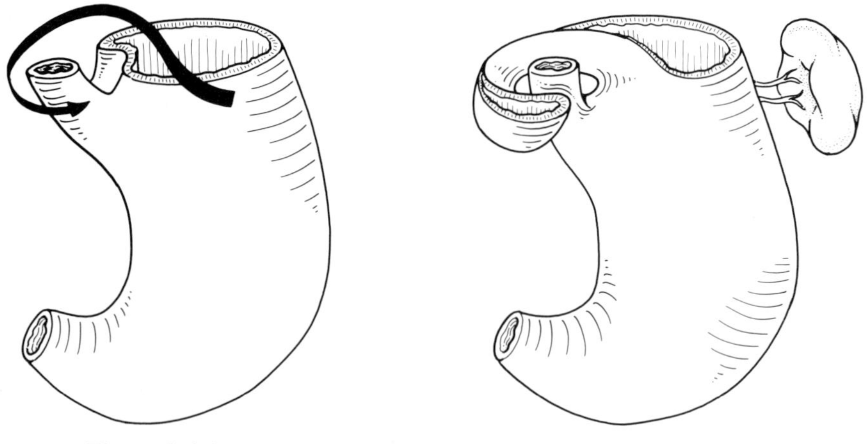

Figure 9.4.1 Author's modification of the Rossetti fundoplication.

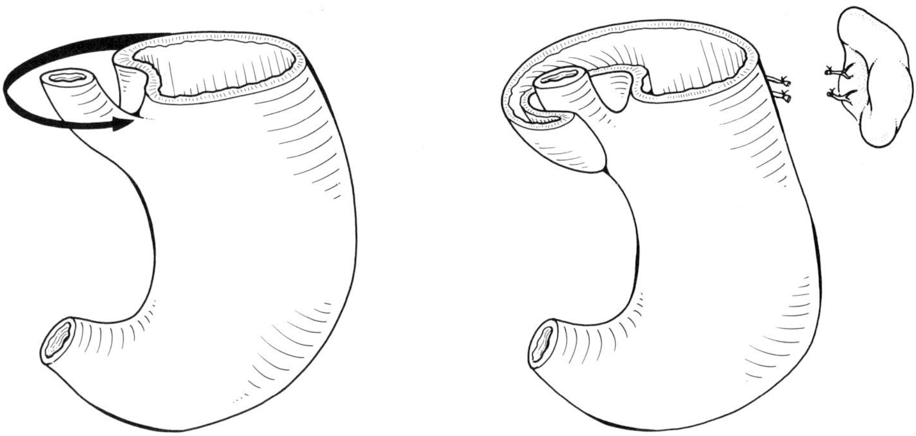

Figure 9.4.2 Nissen fundoplication requiring the dissection of the short gastric vessels.

mechanism in an attempt to produce gastro-oesophageal continence.[9–12] Firstly, by reducing the hernia, the lowering of the oesophagus allows the oesophageal sphincter to retain its tone and establishes a physiological pressure barrier. Secondly, closing the diaphragmatic crura behind the abdominal oesophagus reinforces the pressure barrier by closing down the hiatus. This avoids mechanical complications such as those involving the upward displacement of the abdominal oesophagus which, in turn, can result in impaction of the resultant repair in the mediastinum. Thirdly, a valve is created by a 360° fundoplication. This involves a complete wrap of the abdominal oesophagus using the entire fundus of the stomach on the entire length of the oesophageal sphincter. The ease with which the procedure can be undertaken if only the anterior surface of the fundus is used (Figure 9.4.3), as proposed by Rossetti, makes this procedure more attractive than the Nissen. By employing a large cuff of stomach, the Rossetti manoeuvre prevents overcorrection which is a potential source of postoperative dysphagia and therefore does not require freeing of the short gastric vessels at their origin which often results in incidental injury to the spleen. These three stages – the repositioning of the cardia, the tightening of the diaphragmatic crura and the fundoplication – are the keys to a successful repair.

SELECTION OF PATIENTS AND SURGICAL INDICATIONS

The preoperative evaluation of patients submitted for treatment of gastro-oesophageal reflux, with or without hiatus hernia and by laparoscopic means, is identical to the assessment employed for open surgery. This consists of an evaluation of the patient's general fitness for surgery and investigation of the reflux disease. Endoscopy is required to provide evidence of reflux, to grade the

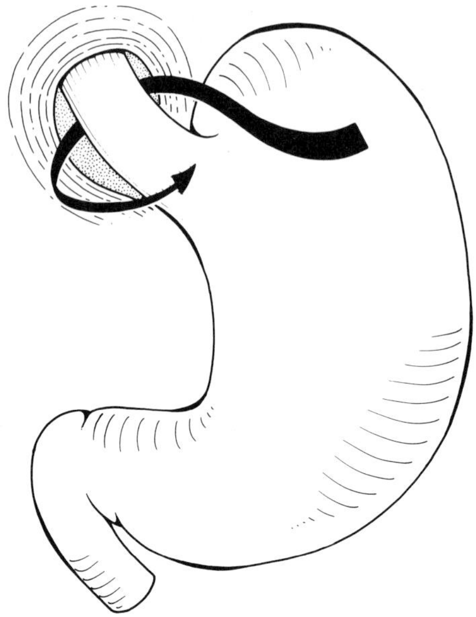

Figure 9.4.3 The Rossetti manoeuvre using the anterior surface of the fundus to fashion the fundoplication.

severity of oesophagitis and to detect the presence of associated lesions such as hiatus hernia and ulceration involving the oesophagus, the stomach or duodenum. A barium swallow and meal provides morphological information on the oesophagogastric junction and functional information on oesophageal clearance and gastric emptying, which can be better evaluated by isotope scanning. Functional tests are required and include 24-hour pH monitoring to assess the severity of preoperative reflux. Oesophageal manometry is required to specify the function of the lower oesophageal sphincter as pressure is generally less than 5 mmHg. This preoperative evaluation ensures that only patients with genuine reflux oesophagitis are submitted to operation and avoids unnecessary intervention on patients with motility disorders or delayed gastric emptying. It is only with this rigorous preoperative assessment that one will avoid therapeutic failures. In addition, these investigations need to be repeated in the postoperative period to assess the effectiveness of the repair. This process is demanding and often invasive for the patients but is nonetheless indispensable in this particular phase of evaluation of laparoscopic surgery.

The indications for laparoscopic repair are similar to those for open surgery. Only patients with incapacitating reflux oesophagitis are considered for surgical treatment and patients would generally have been expected to have undergone well-supervised medical treatment, including antacids, H_2 receptor antagonists and omeprazole for a period of at least six months.

The widening of these indications can be envisaged because of the introduction of laparoscopic treatment of what is basically a mechanical disorder of the oesophagus. The decision of the patient is therefore a new variable which has to be considered in therapy. Confronted by the distress of the illness, the patient must choose between a straightforward and effective medical treatment which is repetitive and prolonged, carrying with it the risk of complications and more invasive therapy, against a minimally invasive laparoscopic treatment which produces rapid healing of the oesophagus and is long-lasting without significant complication.

SURGICAL PROCEDURE

The preoperative evaluation of the patient, the use of general anaesthesia with endotracheal intubation and the peroperative monitoring are the same as those employed at open surgery. Similarly, the creation and maintenance of the pneumoperitoneum, the use of video laparoscopy, the techniques of suction and irrigation and the use of electrocoagulation and laser are similar to those employed in other laparoscopic surgical procedures and are described elsewhere in this book. We will, however, stress the specific problems of the abdominal fundoplication.

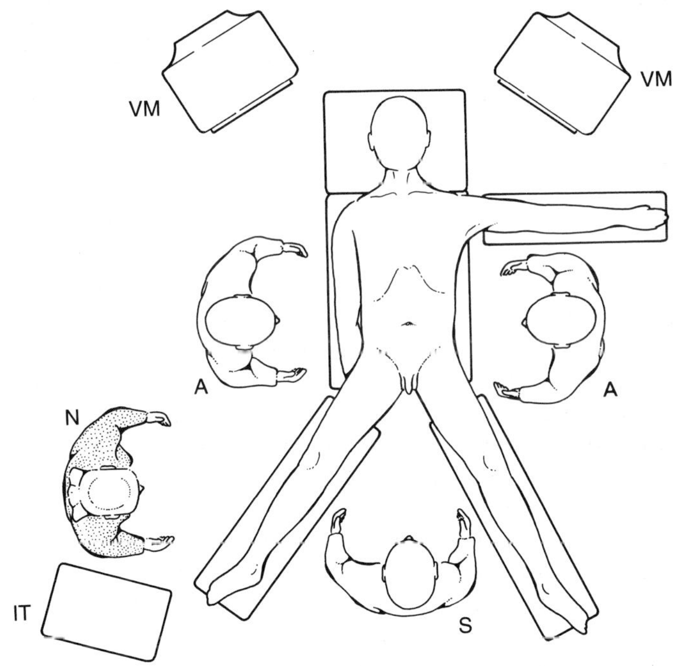

Figure 9.4.4 Operative positioning for laparoscopic fundoplication.

Positioning

The positioning of the patient for treatment of laparoscopic oesophageal reflux is similar to that for vagotomy. It is preferable to have a tilting operating table which allows a 15° reverse Trendelenburg and a left lateral tilt of 15°. We use a 10 cm rest which is positioned between the shoulder blades of the patient. With the patient under general anaesthesia and endotracheal intubation, a nasogastric tube is passed. The surgeon is positioned between the legs of the patient, the nursing assistant to the left with the laparoscopic equipment and suction apparatus and a second monitor is positioned to the right with the laser and the electrocoagulation (Figure 9.4.4). Two assistants, one on the left and one on the right, are required.

Instruments

In addition to standard laparoscopic instrumentation, we recommend that a 30° laparoscope or a laparoscopic endoretractor be employed to provide a good exposure of the operating field. As in laparoscopic vagotomy, we employ an abdominal wall retractor. A coagulating hook is used for dissection and it is useful if this has a channel which allows the escape of any smoke. A dissector used for holding small swabs, curved coagulating scissors and a dissecting forceps or a similar instrument with an articulated curve are useful. For haemostasis, we employ a clip applier or multiple disposable clip applier. For suturing, two needle holders are required and we employ roundbodied needles (32 mm and 26 mm), in addition to the ski-type needles which are mounted with non-absorbable 2/0 and 4/0 sutures.

Access

Five ports are inserted with CO_2 pneumoperitoneum controlled to a pressure of 14 mmHg (Figure 9.4.5). The first trocar which is used for the laparoscope is positioned at two fingers' breadth to the right and above the umbilicus and this allows controlled insertion of the remaining ports. The second, which is used for the palpating instrument, is placed in the epigastric region; the third in the right subcostal region and the fourth in the left subcostal region are used for grasping dissectors. The fifth trocar is placed at two fingers' breadth above and to the left of the umbilicus as an operating channel. It is useful to use 10 mm ports for the laparoscope, the operating channel, and for the left subcostal port which allows the laparoscope to be moved from one port to the other, so providing improved vision, particularly around the region of the oesophagogastric junction. We recommend the use of an abdominal wall retractor so that the pneumoperitoneum can be maintained at low pressure (8 mmHg), thereby avoiding the risk of pneumomediastinum and pneumothorax which can be seen following prolonged

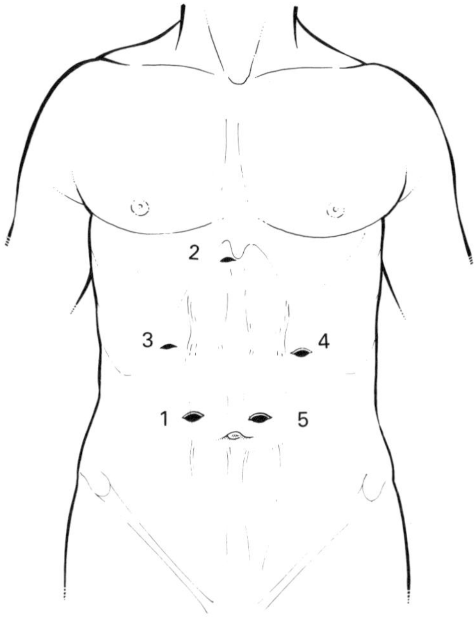

Figure 9.4.5 Sites of insertion of ports; 1, 4 and 5: 10–11 mm ports; 2 and 3: 5 mm ports.

dissection in obese patients or with complicated or large hernias. Similarly, in patients who have previously undergone surgical intervention, prolonged adhesiolysis will predispose these patients to hypercapnia and the risks of CO_2 leak into the mediastinum and chest.

EXPLORATION

The operation starts following the insertion of the laparoscopic port, allowing the diagnosis to be confirmed and, following mobilization of the intra-abdominal structures and in particular the left lobe of the liver, verifying that the operation can be undertaken safely by the laparoscopic approach. In cases of difficulty, open surgery is to be preferred, the patient having already agreed preoperatively that this may be required.

LAPAROSCOPIC DISSECTION

Sharp dissection is undertaken with the coagulating scissors and the coagulating hook, with the access to the hiatus. Blunt dissection is undertaken with a small dissecting swab to facilitate the mobilization of the oesophagus and in particular to locate the posterior vagal trunk. Haemostasis is achieved with electrocautery for small vessels and with clip or ligation for larger vessels. The approximation of tissues is undertaken by suturing. Interrupted sutures are inserted with the round curved needles or the ski needles, being knotted internally or externally; this must be well rehearsed by the operating surgeon. We do not recommend the use of clips for this procedure. The instruments available at the present time do not allow their accurate placement and, in particular, pose the risk of perforating the underlying mucosa.

Operative Technique

The procedure is undertaken in three parts and includes the access to the oesophageal hiatus, along with the reduction of the cardia, the closure of the diaphragmatic crura and the abdominal oesophageal wrap.

1. Access to the Hiatus and Reduction of the Cardia

The left lobe of the liver is displaced by the epigastric retractor and the surgeon gains access to the hiatal region above the pars nervosa of the lesser omentum. This direct approach respects the hepatic branches of the anterior vagal nerve and a possible accessory left hepatic artery. The essential landmark is represented by the right crus of the diaphragm, the prominent arch of which is grasped with the right grasping forceps to tent the peritoneum and expose the oesophagophrenic membrane. The peritoneal incision which begins along the length of the right crus follows the area of the hiatal arch and the anterior surface of the oesophagus and passes down along the length of the left crus. The peritoneal incision and the anterior phreno-oesophageal membrane which is adherent to it provide access to the potential perioesophageal space which is opened by the pneumoperitoneum and the displacement of the abdominal oesophagus to the left and right, with the help of the grasping forceps and the retractors which are advanced as the dissection progresses. This manoeuvre separates the anterior pneumogastric nerves which are adherent to the anterior surface of the abdominal oesophagus. The meso-oesophagus and the posterior aspect of the oesophagus are then freed by opening the oesophageal bed. The right grasping forceps is used to pull in the right crus. This is lifted anteriorly whilst the left grasping forceps is used as a retractor above and to the left of the abdominal oesophagus. This action opens the retro-oesophageal dihedral angle, at the summit of which the white cord of the posterior vagus can be recognized. Using blunt dissection, the posterior aspect of the oesophagus is dissected out, protecting the vagus nerve and avoiding freeing the tissues too superiorly, thereby causing pneumomediastinum from leaking CO_2 or a pneumothorax as a result of a pull or tear.

A tape is passed around the abdominal oesophagus which is almost completely freed using a dissector, a curved memory instrument or an active curved instrument. This manoeuvre allows the lowering of the abdominal oesophagus by placing moderate traction on the intubated oesophagus which completes the blunt dissection and freeing of all hiatal hernial attachments. At the same time the phreno-oesophageal membrane is pushed back and the loose areolar tissue is dissected out, freeing the oesophagogastric angle as far as the first few short gastric vessels. It is useful to use a 30° laparoscope at this stage or to place the 0° laparoscope in one of the ports to the left of the umbilicus. This manoeuvre is important, particularly where there is a large spleen adherent to the greater curvature and fundus of the stomach.

The removal of any loose fatty areolar tissue in the area of the hernia, which is often seen in mixed types of hernia, is essential to provide a substantial length of oesophagus and allows an easier construction of the valve. This resection of fatty tissue is undertaken using electrocautery but it may be necessary to complete haemostasis with clips or an Endoloop.

2. Closure of the Hiatus

Vertical traction on the oesophagus is exerted by means of the encircling tape and this presents the surgeon with the inverted V-shape of the diaphragmatic crura. The crura are exposed, the right by traction and the left by displacing the oesophagus to the left with the aid of the retractor. The hiatal orifice is reconstructed by suturing the crura, taking substantial bites of tissue with the help of a 32 mm curved needle or with a ski needle using a non-absorbable 2/0 suture. This manoeuvre is best undertaken with two needle holders. As soon as the sutures have been inserted, the ends of the needle holder and the needles themselves must always be kept under vision to avoid damaging the aorta behind and the caudate lobe of the liver to the right. The sutures are tied to ensure perfect tissue approximation, avoiding an unnecessarily tight suture which may produce muscle ischaemia. The knot can be further secured with an absorbable clip. One to three sutures are necessary, depending on the size of the defect, and overcorrection is avoided by the passage of a 60 F gauge oesophageal tube.

3. Fundoplication and Abdominal Oesophageal Wrap

With the oesophagus over a 45° traction on the tape, the right grasping forceps is passed behind to grasp the anterior aspect of the fundus, pulling its eminence to the right and behind, going to the superior border of the hiatus at its inferior border, no freeing of the lesser curve is necessary. This posterior right valve is matched with the anterior left valve and this completes the 360° fundoplication by rolling the anterior aspect of the fundus attached to the left and right. The bridging of these right and left valves is assured by an atraumatic grasping forceps or Babcock forceps which maintains the fitting. Three or four non-absorbable sutures are passed at a height of 1.5 cm to 2 cm with the use of the

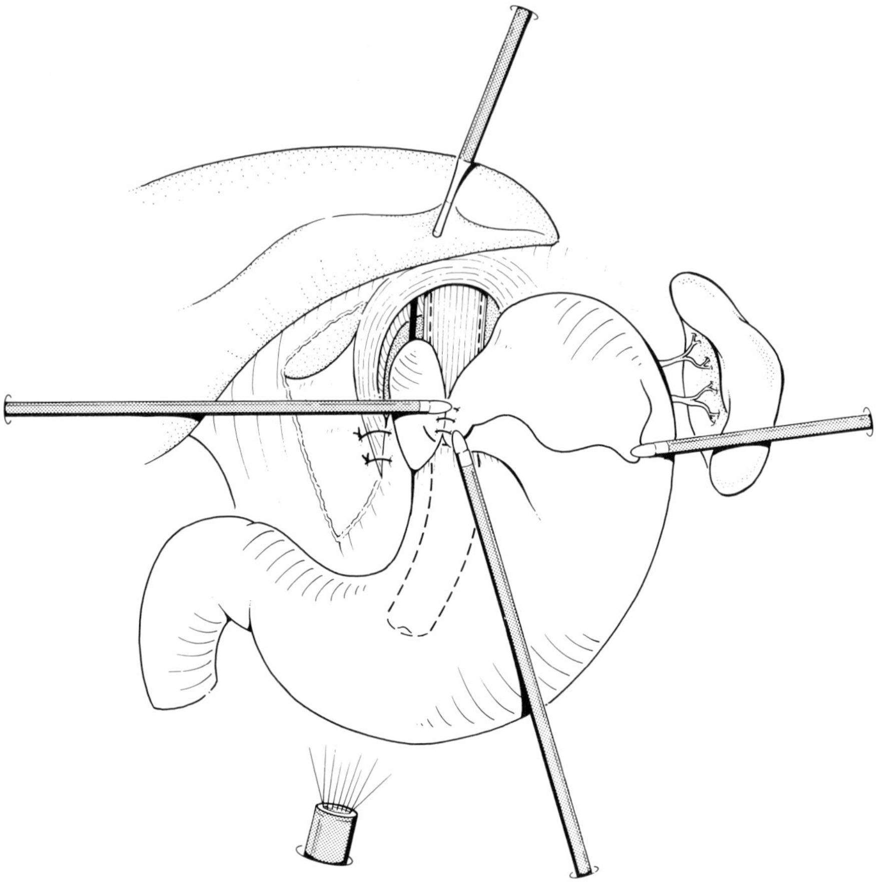

Figure 9.4.6 The fundoplication is fashioned over a 60 F gauge oesophageal tube. The anterior and posterior valves are opposed by three or four non-absorbable sutures.

26 mm round curved needles or the ski needles mounted with 4/0 non-absorbable sutures (Figure 9.4.6). Again, the sutures can be knotted either intra- or extracorporeally. It is sometimes recommended that when the fundus is weakened by haematoma formation or fraying of the tissues, small Teflon segments can be used to reinforce the sutures.[13] Overcorrection is again avoided with the use of the 60 F gauge oesophageal tube.

Having verified haemostasis following irrigation, the port sites are closed after evacuation of the pneumoperitoneum and infiltration of the wounds with bupivacaine.

Peroperative Monitoring

The integrity of the vagus nerves must be a constant source of concern and particularly in the dissection of the abdominal oesophagus.[5] In this area, they are situated in the perioesophageal space, covered with the phreno-oesophageal membrane. As soon as the hiatal peritoneum is opened, the displacement of the tissues by the pneumoperitoneum opens up this space, but the nerves at the anterior, more so than the posterior, remain adherent to the oesophagus and it seems to us dangerous to dissect them or to attempt to isolate them since damage to the posterior wall in particular seems to be associated with the gas bloat syndrome and with impaired gastric emptying.

Assessment of the wrap is essential to prevent overcorrection and this is achieved with the prior placement of a 60 F gauge oesophageal tube. In addition to this, the valvular laxity is verified by introducing between the body of the stomach and the wrap a small swab mounted on a dissector or with the aspirating suction device.

To avoid any loosening, sliding or displacement of the fundoplication, it is useful to inject 150 ml of fluid into the nasogastric tube, whilst at the same time palpating the antrum with a probe. This manoeuvre tends to distend the valves, avoiding any irregularity or pleating of the folds. Complementary fixation with one or two sutures can therefore be useful in this way in the area of the oesophagus at the upper part of the fundoplication, as recommended by Nissen,[7] or in the area of the lesser curve at the lower part of the fundoplication, as recommended by Rossetti.[5] A peroperative endoscopy completes the assessment by showing the good function of the valvular system on retroflexion of the endoscope.

The value of peroperative manometry is debatable, since the general anaesthetic uses muscle relaxants and the pneumoperitoneum itself may interfere with measurements.

Treatment of Associated Lesions

It is our practice to deal with any associated surgical pathology and these might include cholecystectomy for cholelithiasis, posterior vagotomy and anterior seromyotomy for duodenal ulceration, fenestration of hepatic cysts and adhesiolysis of adhesions. In these situations where prolonged pneumoperitoneum will be required, we have found it helpful to employ an anterior abdominal wall retractor, thereby allowing the use of CO_2 insufflation at low pressure.

POST-OPERATIVE COURSE

The post-operative course is generally uneventful and pain associated with the port sites is minimized by the infiltration of local anaesthesia. In our practice, it is unusual for patients to require any associated analgesics by injection. Post-operative mobilization can be achieved early and monitoring is usually limited to the first 24 hour period. The nasogastric tube is removed at this time and fluids and diet are gradually introduced from 24 hours with the patient being discharged generally between the fifth and seventh day.

We have now operated on 50 patients aged between 18–73 years using this technique alone. In all patients, the symptoms of gastro-oesophageal reflux have persisted from 2–20 years despite medical treatment, including dietary advice, antacids, H_2 receptor antagonists and treatment with omeprazole for at least six months. Thirty-nine patients had an associated sliding type hiatus hernia, three patients had large combined sliding and rolling type hiatus hernia and eight patients had isolated reflux oesophagitis. At endoscopy, seven patients had stage 2 oesophagitis, 38 stage 3 and five stage 4, one of which was associated with a large haemorrhagic ulcer. In nine cases, there was an associated pathology which required treatment at the same laparoscopy and these included two ulcers managed by seromyotomy, seven patients with cholelithiasis managed by cholecystectomy and one abdominal lymphoma which was submitted to laparoscopic staging.

The average duration of the procedure was 140 minutes (range 120–220). Three patients experienced severe hypercapnia which required conversion to an open procedure and there were no postoperative deaths. The postoperative course in these patients was relatively uneventful, limited to two episodes of pneumothorax which required chest drainage, two respiratory infections and seven patients who experienced transient dysphagia.

Forty patients have now been followed for between 3–30 months and have shown no evidence of recurrent reflux. Postoperative endoscopy in 25 patients has shown complete healing of the oesophagitis. Post-operative manometric assessment has been possible in only 12 patients and this has demonstrated a rise in lower oesophageal sphincter pressure from 6–15 mmHg. In one of the 12 cases, pH monitoring has shown isolated episodes of acid reflux without clinical symptoms.

Other authors using a laparoscopic Nissen fundoplication[14,15] or variations of the procedure[16–18] have also had equally favourable initial results. In all these reports, the immediate results are identical to those obtained at open surgery. One can therefore assume that the long term results of Nissen-type fundoplication will be similar, with an expected healing rate at ten years of the order of 90%. It will, however, be necessary to evaluate these techniques in analogous groups of patients with multicentre controlled studies using identical operative techniques and blind evaluation. This intensive endoscopic manometric and radiological evaluation would need to be undertaken preoperatively and in the postoperative period, explaining the need for this to the patient on a scientific and medicolegal basis.

DISCUSSION

The surgical correction of reflux oesophagitis is based on the restoration of a valvular system.[12,13,19] Three types of procedure have been described. The first consists of a simple reconstruction of the angle of His as proposed by Lortat-Jacob;[9] the second type involves a partial fundoplication of between 180° and 330° by creating an anterior valve, as suggested by Dor,[20] or a posterior valve as proposed by Toupet.[21] Hill[22] and Belsey[23–25] have proposed similar techniques. The third type of procedure involves a total 360° fundoplication of the Nissen type.[7,19,26] The effectiveness of these procedures depends on the more or less complete nature of the 0–360° valve.[26] It is in this way that Nissen's fundoplication has certainly been recognized as the most effective procedure,[11,13,19,27,28] but it is associated with complications.[29–33] In the peroperative period, perforation of the oesophagus or stomach can occur rarely, but more frequently the spleen is at risk at the time of the freeing of the fundus.

Postoperative complications include recurrence of reflux resulting from a dismantling of the wrap to correct dysphagia, arising from overcorrection of the initial defect. The gas bloat syndrome almost certainly arises as a result of trauma to the vagal nerves, producing a gastric dilatation with delayed gastric emptying. It is for this reason that several authors have looked to modify the procedure. Segol,[28] Cordiano[34] and Stoppa[35] emphasized the calibration of the wrap, whereas Donahue[36] has proposed a loose wrap, sometimes known as the floppy Nissen.

To improve the results of fundoplication, we had described a "neckline" procedure following stripping of the lesser curve, thereby allowing gastro-oesophageal competence to be restored, whilst preserving ability to belch.[37] Menguy has described a similar procedure.[38] De Meester[13] has remained faithful to the Nissen procedure and has stipulated the anatomical requirements for the preparation of the fundoplication in width and in height. The major advance came with Rossetti,[5] who proposed undertaking the fundoplication from the anterior surface of the fundus, which itself limits the gastro-oesophageal dissection. [This makes it unnecessary to divide the short gastric vessels to the left and to open widely the lesser to the right arc, preserving the gastrohepatic branches of the anterior vagal nerve.] Preservation of these structures, which are important points of anchorage for the wrap, contributes to the overall fixation and prevents its displacement.

Three technical points are worthy of further discussion. The fixation of the fundoplication at the anterior surface of the oesophagus, proposed by Nissen,[7] de Meester[13] and Siewert[33] at open surgery and by Dallemagne[14,39] at laparoscopy, has been judged, on the other hand, to be dangerous and inappropriate by Rossetti[5] at open surgery and Geagea[18] at laparoscopy. These last authors content themselves with fixing the lesser curve. For us, this fixation prevents the undoing of the wrap by preventing its displacement. At laparoscopy, these sutures can be undertaken with all security, the enlarging effect allowing the anterior vagal fibres to be recognized and avoided.

The position of the posterior valve also assumes importance. It can be passed behind the oesophagus and the vagal nerve or through the window between the nerve and the oesophagus, as has been proposed by Nissen[7] and de Meester[13] at open surgery and Hinder[15] at laparoscopy, to avoid damage to the nerve within the fundoplication. We personally believe that there is a risk of damaging the nerve through dissection and of producing a gas bloat syndrome. The same reservations have been expressed by Hinder,[15] who sutures the crura in front of the posterior vagal trunk. It seems to us more straightforward to leave the posterior nerve, with its associated vessels, adherent to the oesophagus in the same way as for the anterior branches and to incorporate them into a generous and well-calibrated fundoplication in such a way as to avoid compression of the nerve.

The closure of the hiatus by bringing together the crura behind the oesophagus has not been considered as an essential part of the procedure by Nissen.[7] We agree with other authors that this manoeuvre promotes the physiological function of the lower oesophageal sphincter in the surroundings of the abdominal pressure. Furthermore, this prevents the displacement upwards of the wrap and its impaction in the hiatal orifice being a source of ulceration and strangulation.[13,15,30,33,37]

CONCLUSIONS

The laparoscopic treatment of gastro-oesophageal reflux is an exemplary technical illustration of a straightforward, effective and reproducible procedure which carries the same guarantees as for conventional surgery with the advantages of a minimally invasive approach. The preoperative evaluation of the patients, confirmation of the technical procedures and postoperative audit of the results represent the challenge for progress in future years. Only in this way will patients suffering from poorly controlled gastro-oesophageal reflux be allowed to choose the most appropriate form of medical or laparoscopic treatment.

REFERENCES

1. Mouiel J, Katkhouda N, Gugenheim J. Traitement de l'ulcere duodenal par vagotomie tronculaire posterieure et seromyotomie anterieure sous video-laparoscopie. Note preliminaire avec presentation de film. Academie de Chirurgie, Paris, Seance due 6 juin 1990. *Chirurgie* 1990; **116**: 546–51.
2. Katkhouda N, Mouiel J. A new surgical technique of treatment of chronic duodenal ulcer without laparotomy by videocoelioscopy. *Am J Surg* 1991; **161**: 361–4.
3. Mouiel J, Katkhouda N. Traitement de l'ulcere duodenal non compliqué. In: *Chirurgie Digestive par Voie Coelioscopique* (eds Testas P, Delaitre B), pp. 137–45. Paris, Vigot, 1991.
4. Mouiel J, Katkhouda N. Laparoscopic posterior truncal vagotomy and anterior seromyotomy. In: *Operative Manual of Endoscopic Surgery* (eds Cuschieri A, Buess G, Perissat J), pp. 263–72. Berlin, Springer-Verlag, 1992.
5. Rossetti M, Hell K. Fundoplication for treatment of gastro-oesophageal reflux in hiatal hernia. *World J Surg* 1977; **1**: 439–44.

6. Nissen R. Eine enfache operation zur beeinflussung der reflux oesophagitis. *Schweitz Med Wochenschr* 1956; **86**: 590–2.
7. Nissen R. Gastropexy and fundoplication in surgical treatment of hiatal hernia. *Am J Dig Dis* 1961; **6**: 954–61.
8. Mouiel J, Katkhouda N. Reflux gastro-oesophagien: experience laparoscopique. In: *Actualites Digestives Medico-Chirurgicales*, 14e serie (ed. Mouiel, J), pp. 26–33. Paris, Masson, 1993.
9. Lortat-Jacob JL, Maillard JN, Mouiel J. Les oesophagites peptiques. In: *Encyclopedie Medico-Chirurgicale*, Paris 1966: 9202, **10**: 1–7.
10. Maillard JN, Conte-Marti J, Mouiel J. Etiopathogenie des ulceres de l'oesophage. In: *Les Ulceres de l'Oesophage*. Paris, Masson, 1965; 1–30.
11. Skinner DB. Pathophysiology of gastrooesophageal reflux. *Ann Surg* 1985; **202**: 546–56.
12. Jamieson GG, Duranceau A. *Gastrooesophageal Reflux*. London, WB Saunders, 1988.
13. De Meester TR, Bonavina L, Albertucci M. Nissen fundoplication for gastrooesophageal reflux disease. Evaluation of primary repair in 100 consecutive patients. *Ann Surg* 1986: **204**: 9–20.
14. Dallemagne B, Weerts JM, Jehaes C, Markiewicz S, Lombard R. Laparoscopic Nissen fundoplication: preliminary report. *Surg Laparosc Endosc* 1991; **1**: 138–43.
15. Hinder RA, Filipi CJ. The technique of laparoscopic Nissen fundoplication. *Surg Laparosc Endosc* 1992; **2**: 265–72.
16. Cuschieri A, Shimi S, Nathanson LK. Laparoscopic reduction, crural repair and fundoplication of large hiatal hernia. *Am J Surg* 1992; **163**: 425.
17. Bagnato VJ. Laparoscopic Nissen fundoplication. *Surg Laparosc Endosc* 1992; **3**: 188–90.
18. Geagea T. Laparoscopic Nissen's fundoplication: preliminary report of 10 cases. *Surg Endosc* 1991; **5**: 170–3.
19. Boutelier P, Chipponi J. *Le Traitement Chirurgical du Reflux Gastrooesophagien de l'Adulte*. Monographies de l'Association Francaise de Chirurgie. Paris, Masson, 1991.
20. Dor J, Monges H, Humbert P, Figarella JJ. *Reflexions sur 61 Observations de Hernies du Hiatus Oesophagien*. Congres Francais de Chirurgie, 64e session, Paris, 1962.
21. Toupet A. Technique d'oesophago-gastroplastie avec phrenogastropexie appliquée dans la cure radicale des hernies hiatales et comme complement de l'operation de Heller dans les cardiospasmes. *Mem Acad Chir* 1963; **89**: 394–8.
22. Hill LD. Surgery for hiatal hernia and esophagitis. In: The *Esophagus: Medical and Surgical Management* (ed. Hill LD) WB Saunders, pp. 139–47. London, 1988.
23. Belsey R. Surgical treatment of hiatus hernia and reflux esophagitis. *World J Surg* 1977; **11**: 421–3.
24. Orringer MB, Skinner DB, Belsey RH. Long term result of mark IV operation for hiatal hernia and analyses of recurrences and their treatment. *J Thorac Cardiovasc Surg* 1972; **63**: 25–33.
25. Skinner DB, Belsey RHR. Surgical management of gastroesophageal reflux and hiatus hernia; long term results with 1030 patients. *J Thorac Cardiovasc Surg* 1967; **53**: 33–54.
26. Ellis FH. Technique of fundoplication. In: *Medical and Surgical Problems of the Esophagus* (eds Stipa S, Belsey R), pp. 61–5. London, Academic Press, 1981.
27. Maillet P. Les hernies hiatales de l'adulte. Etude critique des techniques chirurgicales. In: *Actualites Digestives Medico-chirurgicales* (ed. Mouiel, J), pp. 1–16. Paris, Masson, 1980.
28. Segol PH, Ahkong MV, Marchand P. La fundoplicature complete calibree. *Presse Med* 1985; **14**: 99–101.
29. Negre JB, Markkulh HT, Keyrileinen O, Matikainen M. Nissen fundoplication results at ten years follow-up. *Am J Surg* 1983; **146**: 635–8.

30. Saubier EC, Gouillat C, Teboul F. Traitement du reflux gastro-oesophagien par fundoplicature complete de Nissen. Resultats de 112 observations. *Chirurgie* 1986; **112**: 123–31.
31. Gossot D, Sarfati E, Azoulay D, Celerier M. Facteurs de morbidite de l'intervention de Nissen. *J Chir* 1987; **124**: 367–71.
32. Henderson RD. Nissen hiatal hernia repair: problems of recurrence and continued symptoms. *Ann Thorac Surg* 1979; **28**: 587–93.
33. Siewert JR, Feussner H. Treatment of peptic esophagitis Nissen repair. In: *Hernia*, 3rd edition (eds Nyhus LM, London RE), pp. 604–13. Philadelphia, JB Lippincott, 1989.
34. Cordiano C, Quercy Della Rovere G, Agudario F, Mazzilli LG. Technical modification of fundoplication procedure. *Surg Gynecol Obstet* 1976; **143**: 977–80.
35. Stoppa R, Warlaumont C, Verhaeghe P, Henry X, Odimba BFK. Le manchonnage de l'oesophage distal dans le traitement du reflux gastro-oesophagien. *J Chir* 1985; **122**: 421–5.
36. Donahue PE, Samelson S, Nyhus LM, Bombeck T. The floppy Nissen fundoplication. Effective long term control of pathologic reflux. *Arch Surg* 1985; **120**: 663–8.
37. Mouiel J. Le traitement des hernies hiatales avec reflux gastro-oesophagien. Manchonnage de l'oesophage abdominal par plicature de la petite courbure apres vagotomie ultraselective. *La Nouvelle Presse Medicale* 1980; **9**: 2915–17.
38. Menguy R. Modified fundoplication with preserved ability to belch. *Surg* 1978; **894**: 301–7.
39. Dallemagne B, Weerts JM, Jehaes C, Markiewicz S, Lombard R. Laparoscopic management of gastrooesophageal reflux. In: *Surgical Laparoscopy Update* (ed. Zucker KA), pp. 217–39. St Louis, Missouri, QMP, 1993.

9.5

Laparoscopic Oesophageal Myotomy

M. MORINO

Oesophageal myotomy, first performed by Heller in 1913,[1] has been considered as the safest and most effective treatment for oesophageal achalasia since 1949;[2] only recently have its results been challenged by pneumatic dilatation.[3–4]

The Heller procedure is a simple but delicate surgical procedure that surgeons are used to performing through a large abdominal or thoracic incision, using strong retractors and thus gaining an otherwise difficult access to the operative field. Oesophageal myotomy appears to be a procedure well suited to the laparoscopic approach. A perfect view of the operative field is easily obtained, no large specimen needs to be extracted from the abdominal cavity and no difficult anastomosis has to be performed.

PATIENT'S POSITION AND LAYOUT

The operation is performed under general anaesthesia. The patient receives a mild laxative on the day before surgery and is required to fast overnight.

The patient is positioned supine on the operating table with the legs spread apart. A reverse Trendelenburg position of 20–30° is used, allowing the abdominal viscera to descend out of the operative field. Care must be taken to stabilize the patient on the table during any tilting away from the horizontal position. This can be obtained by a safety belt that anchors the pelvis to the table and by separately fixing each leg to its support on the table. The surgeon is situated between the patient's legs, with an assistant on each side of the patient (Fig. 9.5.1).

A nasogastric tube is routinely inserted at the very beginning of every laparoscopic procedure to ensure complete gastric deflation. It helps to avoid the risk of gastric perforation by the Veress needle and to obtain a clear operative field. In the presence of achalasia it is sometimes impossible to reach the stomach with a tube because of the stenosis of the distal oesophagus.

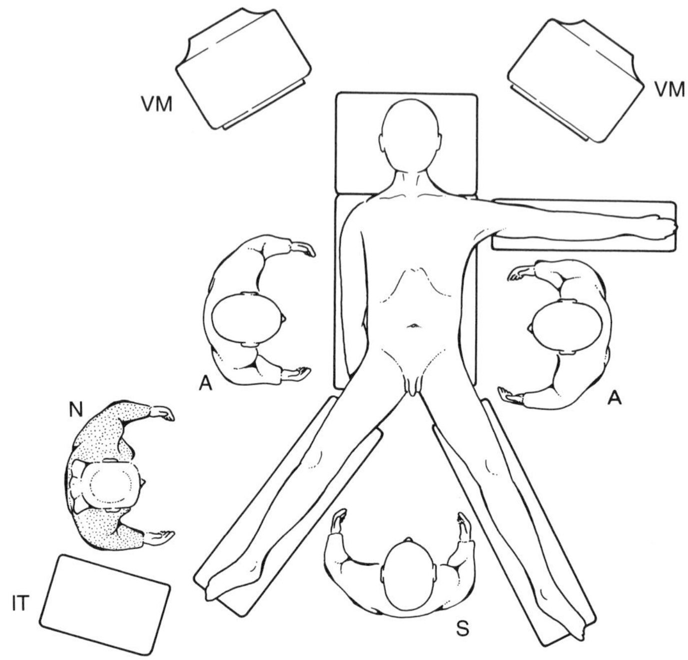

Figure 9.5.1 Layout of patient, staff and equipment. S: surgeon; A: assistant; N: scrub nurse; VM: video monitor; IT: instrument table.

Complete aspiration of oesophageal content preoperatively is of great importance to avoid the risk of regurgitation and bronchial inhalation during intubation manoeuvres. To avoid such a risk it would be useful to place a naso-oesophageal tube the evening before surgery and to leave it in place under continued aspiration overnight.[5]

We use routine catheterization of the urinary bladder prior to the insertion of the Veress needle for advanced laparoscopic procedures including oesophageal myotomy. The bladder catheter is removed at the end of the operation.

SURGICAL TECHNIQUE

Laparoscopy is a means of access, not a surgical procedure. Therefore laparoscopic oesophageal myotomy consists of performing the classical Heller procedure[5] without laparotomy, using endoscopic instruments.

A few steps are crucial to the success of the procedure:

1. the choice of insertion points for the ports;
2. the exposure of the oesophagogastric junction;
3. the dissection of the lower oesophagus;
4. a careful myotomy.

We usually perform an antireflux procedure with the myotomy, either the anterior hemi-Nissen fundoplication or Dor procedure, as we used to do in open myotomy. The rationale for this will be further discussed.

As far as the surgical technique is concerned, performing an antireflux procedure by laparoscopy will certainly and significantly prolong operative time and complicate the operation as laparoscopic suturing techniques are involved. It is our personal belief that the ability to suture under the laparoscopic approach is essential and that a surgeon should not undertake laparoscopic advanced procedures if he or she is not trained in laparoscopic suturing and knot tying.

Instrumentation

As in the vast majority of laparoscopic surgery, a 10 mm laparoscope is necessary to obtain an optimal view. The viewing angle of the laparoscope used depends on the preference of the surgeon, but we strongly suggest the use of a 30° forward oblique laparoscope for surgery on the oesophagogastric junction. The laparoscope introduced some centimetres above the umbilicus will reach the abdominal oesophagus at a very acute angle. Thus with a 0° forward-viewing laparoscope the surgeon will have a tangential view of this region, while the 30° laparoscope permits a more oblique view of the operative field, facilitating difficult dissections.

To carry out the surgical procedure we use standard laparoscopic instruments. A "laparoscopic cholecystectomy set" is in fact sufficient to perform the myotomy: electrosurgical hook knife, scissors, atraumatic grasping forceps, tissue retractor, suction/irrigation cannula. We will add only a laparoscopic needle holder to this standard set to enable an antireflux procedure to be performed at the end of the myotomy.

The standard procedure does not need any clip applier, but it is safer to have a disposable clip applier available in case of bleeding. It is important to remember that the control of bleeding during laparoscopic surgery is less easy to achieve than during open surgery. Therefore the surgical principle of preventing bleeding by controlling every vascular structure is particularly crucial in endoscopic surgery where active bleeding will obscure the visual field and sometimes blind the surgeon by splashing directly on the laparoscope. For haemostatic purposes we prefer disposable clip appliers because they are multiloaded and permit the application of more than one clip at a time without extracting the instrument from the abdomen.

Cannulae Insertion Sites (Fig. 9.5.2)

Five cannulae are used:

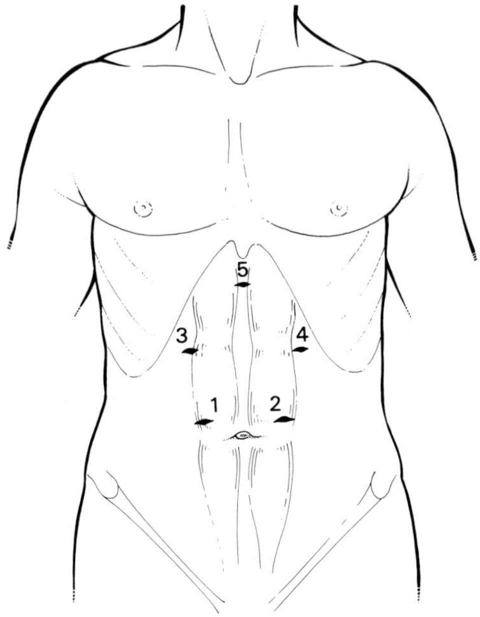

Figure 9.5.2 Sites of insertion of ports. 1 and 2: 10–11 mm ports; 3,4 and 5: 5 mm ports.

1. a 10–11 mm trocar/cannula is inserted 2–5 cm above the umbilicus and 1–2 cm to the right of the midline. A straightforward 0° or 30° forward oblique laparoscope is inserted through this port;
2. a 10–11 mm trocar/cannula 2–5 cm above the umbilicus and 2–3 cm to the left of the midline. The electrosurgical hook knife, scissors, endodissector, pledget swab and needle holder can be introduced through this operative port;
3. a 5 mm trocar/cannula in the right hypochondrium, 2–3 cm below the costal margin in the midclavicular line. The surgeon will use this port for grasping forceps using his or her left hand;
4. a 5 mm trocar/cannula in the left hypochondrium 2 cm below the costal margin in the midclavicular line. The assistant will introduce an atraumatic 5 mm grasping forceps;
5. a 5 mm trocar/cannula located in the midline just below the xiphoid process; this port will allow alternate introduction of tissue retractor and suction/irrigation cannula.

The surgeon stands between the patient's legs to hold instruments in port 2 in the right hand and port 3 in the left hand. The two instruments that the surgeon holds through ports 2 and 3 should reach the operative field at an approximate angle of 90°, ideal for dissecting and suturing in laparoscopy. The assistant surgeon standing on the patient's right holds the laparoscopic port 1 with the camera system. The assistant on the left retracts the liver with the tissue retractor or the suction/irrigation cannula port 5 in the right hand while the left hand holds the grasper that is inserted through port 4.

Access and Exposure

If the patient has not previously undergone upper abdominal surgery, the initial induction of pneumoperitoneum is performed with the Veress needle. Site of insertion will be the same as described for port 2, thus permitting the Veress needle to be left in place while port 1 is inserted.

When the patient has had previous upper abdominal surgery it is mandatory to perform an open laparoscopy using the Hasson cannula.[6]

In performing laparoscopic surgery on the gastro-oesophageal junction the position of ports 1 and 2 is important. The two ports are quite near each other (4–5 cm) and the instruments inserted through them converge. The two ports should penetrate in the abdomen perpendicular to the abdominal wall and should not be directed toward the midline (Fig. 9.5.3). In the latter case the extremities of the two ports inside the abdomen will get closer to each other and the operating instruments will be too close to the laparoscope. In such circumstances, control of dissection, electrocautery and suturing will be difficult.

Correct positioning of ports as previously described is crucial; 20–30° of reverse Trendelenburg allows the abdominal viscera to descend out of the

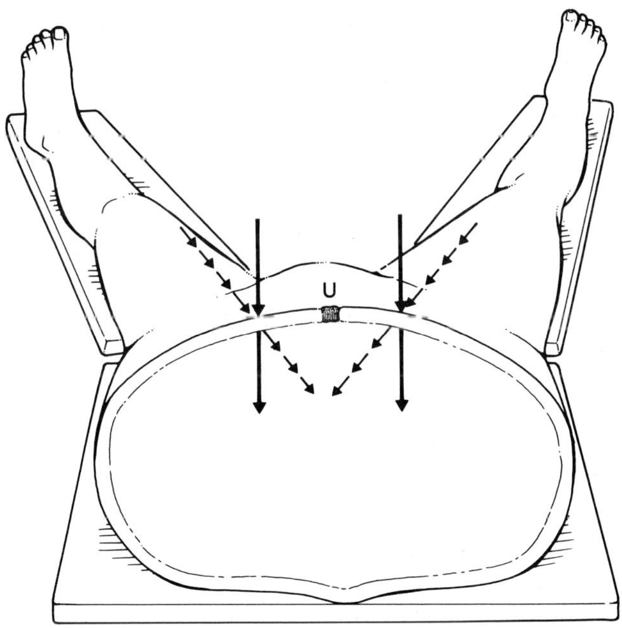

Figure 9.5.3 Correct (big arrows) and incorrect (small arrows) direction of insertion of ports 1 and 2. U: umbilicus.

operative field. The assistant has the most important role in exposing the region by lifting the left lobe of the liver away from the stomach with the instrument in the right hand through port 5 and by pulling down the stomach with the instrument in the left hand through port 4. When these two manoeuvres have been correctly performed the operative field is perfectly exposed and ready for dissection.

The left triangular ligament connecting the left lobe of the liver to the diaphragm should not be divided because it helps to retain the liver and to lift it.

We use the standard suction/irrigation cannula to retract the liver, with the advantage of rapidly cleaning the field by irrigation with Ringer's lactate and suction without any need to change instruments. New retractors are now available: they are characterized by the possibility to enlarge the retracting surface once in the abdomen; some of them are traumatic for the liver and it is important to use them very gently as bleeding from the liver will obscure the surgical field.

Dissection

Once good exposure is achieved, the surgeon will start dissecting the hiatal region by means of an atraumatic 5 mm grasping forceps in the left hand and an electrified hook or scissors in the right hand. The dissection needed to perform the myotomy by laparoscopy is less extensive than in open surgery because the exposure and the view obtained through the laparoscopic approach are of such a good quality and magnification. At the beginning of our experience we used to start the procedure by sectioning the pars flaccida of the lesser omentum in order to gain access to the oesophagus by the right lateral surface. However, this is unnecessary and can be dangerous when there is a left hepatic artery running through the pars flaccida of the lesser omentum.

Access to the lower oesophagus is obtained by a direct approach to the oesophageal hiatus. The phreno-oesophageal membrane is opened along the anterior surface of the oesophagus and, using a pledget swab, the oesophagus is progressively dissected and both crura exposed. It is not necessary to complete the dissection of the posterior oesophageal surface, but only to dissect the lower oesophagus on its anterior, right and left surfaces.

Meticulous care should be taken to dissect a consistent portion of the lower oesophagus by ascending along the thoracic oesophagus, as the failure of Heller's procedure may result from a short myotomy. The assistant surgeon allows the thoracic oesophagus to descend for some distance into the abdomen by pulling the stomach downward with an atraumatic grasper. The laparoscopic view is excellent and allows a blunt dissection above the hiatus of at least 5–7 cm. During this dissection care must be taken not to open the left pleura.

The dissection is completed when 12–15 cm of the anterior surface of the lower oesophagus have been dissected; the right and left vagus nerves are clearly visible and should be carefully identified and preserved.

During the dissection of the oesophagus we attempt to use as little electrocautery as possible. While dissecting during laparoscopy the surgeon must try to mediate between the need to have a completely bloodless operative field and the risks of monopolar coagulation. The region we are dealing with is not very vascularized and most of the time the hook can be used for blunt dissection without the need to coagulate. A pledget swab can be of great value to clean the field and advance the dissection.

Myotomy (Fig. 9.5.4)

The longitudinal oesophageal myotomy is started 2–3 cm above the cardia, to the left of the anterior vagus nerve, using the hook knife. Before starting the

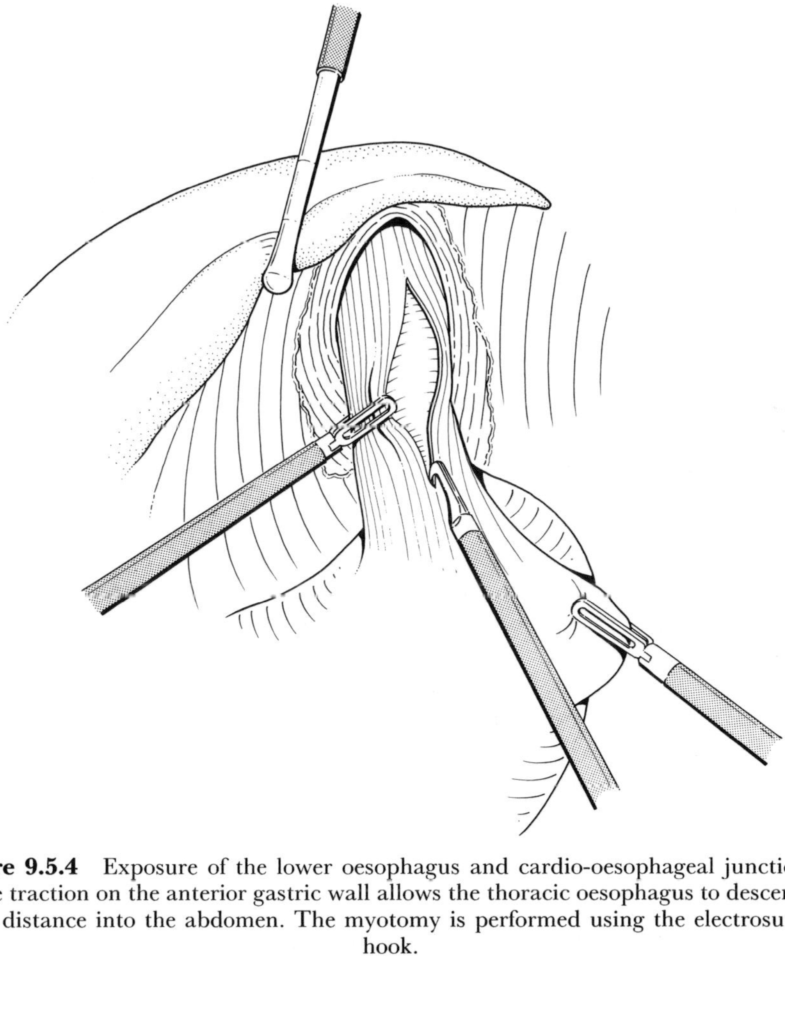

Figure 9.5.4 Exposure of the lower oesophagus and cardio-oesophageal junction. A gentle traction on the anterior gastric wall allows the thoracic oesophagus to descend for some distance into the abdomen. The myotomy is performed using the electrosurgical hook.

myotomy it is important to withdraw the nasogastric tube as it can represent a danger to the oesophageal mucosa which can be pushed toward the electrocautery.

The hook progressively dissects and sections the external and internal oesophageal muscular layers by lifting up small bites of tissue before the coagulating or cutting current is activated. When this manoeuvre is correctly and meticulously performed, risks of damaging the oesophageal mucosa are small. The method of avoiding thermal damage caused by the spread of electrical energy is to tent the tissues by the hook before the current is applied and use a voltage of less than 200 V.[7]

Once the correct plane between muscular layers and submucosa is identified, we prefer to carry on the myotomy proximally using scissors. Scissors are gently inserted between submucosa and circular muscle fibres and opened for dilatation, thus identifying the cleavage plane before cutting the muscle. Alternatively careful hook dissection by tenting and then coagulating is equally effective.

Myotomy must be extensive in length and complete in depth. It should ascend at least 5 cm along the thoracic oesophagus and include 1 cm of gastric muscular layers. The inferior part of the myotomy is the most awkward because of the difficulty in finding the correct surgical plane. Muscle fibres are densely adherent to the submucosa, particularly the helvetius muscle which is composed of oblique and circular fibres. This part of the myotomy should be done with the hook by progressively tenting muscular fibres, paying extreme attention to avoiding damage to the gastric mucosa.

The myotomy has two risks:

1. leaving some circular muscle fibres;
2. the opening of the mucosa.

In order to verify that the myotomy has been completed some authors[5] advocate the insertion of a Blakemore catheter followed by inflation in order to distend the oesophageal mucosa which will reveal any residual muscle fibres. This manoeuvre presents the risk of damaging the mucosa and we do not suggest its use, as the magnification of laparoscopic view is such that single circular muscle fibres are easily identified and sectioned. We use a pledget swab to clean the area of the myotomy and to verify its completeness.

We routinely use intraoperative manometry as a much more objective means of verifying the completeness of the myotomy. The manometric probe is inserted at the end of the myotomy before performing the antireflux procedure. The gradient of pressure between the stomach and the oesophagus is neutralized at the end of a complete myotomy. If this is not the case the operative field should be checked for persisting circular fibres.

The second risk is the opening of the mucosa. This can be verified by injecting methylene blue through the nasogastric tube. Furthermore the risk of such a lesion is one of the main reasons for performing an anterior antireflux valve that will in turn protect the oesophageal mucosa.

Antireflux Procedure

The recent literature[8–12] and our own experience suggest that the Heller myotomy should be completed by an antireflux procedure for three main reasons:[10]

1. protecting the oesophageal mucosa;
2. keeping both borders of the myotomy separated;
3. creating an antireflux mechanism.

Among the different antireflux procedures we prefer to perform an anterior hemi-Nissen or Dor technique because they allow all three of the abovementioned criteria to be achieved without any further dissection of the oesophagus being required. The antireflux Dor procedure is performed by suturing the anterior wall of the gastric fundus to the left muscular border of the oesophagomyotomy by means of three or four separate stitches. The oesophageal mucosa will be covered by the gastric serosa by suturing the anterior wall of the gastric fundus (4–5 cm further left of the previous sutures) to the right muscular border of the myotomy. Control of short gastric vessels is not necessary.

Standard laparoscopic suturing and knotting techniques are used. It is important, as mentioned previously, that ports 2 and 3 have been inserted correctly, thus obtaining an angle of 90° when suturing. We use standard non-absorbable monofilament sutures of 3/O gauge and we prefer extracorporeal knotting. Three stitches on both sides of the antireflux valve are sufficient.

At the end of the procedure the hiatal region is irrigated and suctioned dry. The peritoneal cavity is inspected and no drainage is needed. A nasogastric tube is inserted and left in place for 24 hours. This helps to prevent gastric distension and vomiting, as well as protecting the suture line. Oral feeding is permitted on the day after surgery.

COMPLICATIONS AND RESULTS

The most significant intraoperative or immediate postoperative complication of oesophageal myotomy is perforation of the oesophageal or gastric mucosa. This complication can occur intraoperatively during the open Heller operation as frequently as in 18% of cases.[8] The danger of perforation is higher at the level of the cardia where muscle fibres are densely adherent to the extremely fragile gastric mucosa.

A mucosal perforation may be caused by two different mechanisms: a primary direct mechanical perforation or a delayed perforation secondary to electrocoagulation.

The perfect view and magnification obtained by laparoscopy should lead to a more accurate myotomy, thus reducing the risk of primary direct perforation.

On the contrary, the use of the electrosurgical monopolar hook represents a specific risk of delayed perforation.

If a direct perforation should occur, it is crucial to identify it during surgery. Air insufflation or methylene blue injection through the nasogastric tube at the end of the myotomy can be useful. A perforation of the mucosa ignored during surgery will cause an acute abdomen in the early postoperative course and is an indication for immediate laparotomy.

A delayed perforation may occur a few days after surgery as a consequence of an inadvertent use of monopolar electrocautery. This may cause thermal damage of the mucosa, resulting in tissue necrosis and eventually delayed perforation.

Two long term complications may occur: recurrent dysphagia and gastro-oesophageal reflux. The dysphagia appears soon after surgery if the initial myotomy has been inadequate or the fibres cut by the myotomy have regrown. Dysphagia may be a late postoperative complication if the myotomy has been thorough, leading to reflux and peptic stricture.[13] Persistent severe dysphagia occurs in less than 5% of patients treated surgically.[3]

The most significant late complication of myotomy is gastro-oesophageal reflux. Overall incidence of symptomatic reflux reported after open myotomy is usually less than 10%,[14] but studies with longer follow-up have reported reflux rates as high as 52%.[9] The high frequency of late postoperative symptomatic gastro-oesophageal reflux is a strong argument in favour of performing an antireflux procedure as a complement to the myotomy.[8,10] However, Cuschieri[15] suggests that one of the major advantages of the laparoscopic myotomy is a reduced damage to the phreno-oesophageal attachments resulting in the avoidance of the gastro-oesophageal reflux. If this should be confirmed, the main argument for performing an antireflux procedure with the laparoscopic myotomy will cease.

At present it is very difficult to evaluate the complications of laparoscopic oesophageal myotomy. No long term results have been published and only a few recent abstracts report on postoperative complications.

In my personal series of 11 laparoscopic oesophageal myotomies for achalasia, mortality and morbidity were zero and none of the procedures had to be converted.

To my knowledge the largest series published is the one by de Paula presented at the 3rd World Congress of Endoscopic Surgery in Bordeaux in June 1992.[16] Twenty five patients with oesophageal achalasia secondary to Chagas' disease were treated by laparoscopic oesophageal myotomy with one perforation and no conversions.

Therefore, operative mortality and morbidity of laparoscopic myotomy would appear to be comparable to the results reported in the recent literature on traditional Heller's myotomy[8–12,17] where mortality rate varies from 0 to 4% and morbidity from 4 to 13%.

The major advantage of the laparoscopic operation compared to the open one is the postoperative course, which is characterized by all the benefits of minimal access surgery: minimum pain, no ileus, short hospital stay, optimum cosmetic results and early return to normal activity.

Our patients were all discharged from hospital between the third and fourth postoperative day, while in the de Paula series the average hospital stay was 64 hours.[16] Return to normal activities in our series was possible within ten days from surgery for four patients, between ten and 20 days for six patients and after more than 20 days for the last patient.

Long term results of the laparoscopic operation should reproduce those obtained by the open myotomy as the surgical techniques are the same.

At present, with a short follow-up ranging from one to 14 months, none of our patients complained of recurrent dysphagia and only one patient developed gastro-oesophageal reflux. Nine patients have been studied three months after surgery by manometric and pH monitoring. Manometric measurements revealed a significant decrease in gastro-oesophageal sphincter pressure when compared to preoperative data: mean preoperative pressure 38.1 mmHg, mean postoperative pressure 12.3 mmHg. No patients showed abolition of or zero sphincter pressure. Acid reflux tests were positive in two patients one of whom complained of mild heartburn.

DISCUSSION

Before the advent of laparoscopic surgery the choice of treatment for patients suffering from oesophageal achalasia lay between pneumatic dilatation and surgical myotomy. Csendes *et al.*[3] in 1989 reported the only randomized controlled trial comparing pneumatic dilatation and surgical myotomy. After a five year follow-up, 95% of the patients who underwent surgery were asymptomatic and 2% had mild heartburn, while 65% of the dilated patients were asymptomatic and none had heartburn.

Whilst these results suggest that surgery may be more efficacious than pneumatic dilatation in treating achalasia, gastroenterologists are still in favour of pneumatic dilatation because it has the advantage of requiring only an overnight hospitalization, the patients will recover in one week and the average cost of the procedure is evaluated as a quarter of the cost of surgery.[13]

Laparoscopic oesophageal myotomy appears to be the ideal treatment for oesophageal achalasia: it is as effective as traditional surgery in treating symptoms and has all the advantages of pneumatic dilatation in terms of short hospital stay, quick recovery and low cost. Therefore, even in the presence of only preliminary results, I believe that laparoscopic myotomy will rapidly become the treatment of choice for oesophageal achalasia for the majority of patients. Contraindications to the laparoscopic treatment of achalasia will essentially be those patients unfit for general anaesthesia.

Furthermore, the diffusion of the laparoscopic Heller operation will greatly benefit from future developments in laparoscopic instrumentation. In particular, the risk of injuring the oesophageal mucosa by using monopolar electrocoagulation will be consistently reduced by new means of cutting and coagulating such as bipolar electrocoagulation or the ultrasonically activated scalpel (Harmonic Scalpel, Ultracision, Smithfield, RI). We performed two cases of laparoscopic myotomy using this new device which cuts with haemostatic ability and minimum tissue injury and were impressed with the results.

Undoubtedly the full potential of minimal access surgery will be determined largely by technological advances, but laparoscopic functional operations, such as laparoscopic cardiomyotomy, already represent the most attractive option in the management of gastrointestinal disorders currently treated conservatively.

REFERENCES

1. Heller E. Extramukose Cardiaplastick beim chronischen Cardiospasmus mit Dilatation des Oesophagus. *Mitt Grenzgeb Med Chir* 1914; **27**: 141–9.
2. Barrett NR, Franklin RH. Concerning the unfavourable late results of certain operations performed in the treatment of cardiospasm. *Br J Surg* 1949; **37**: 194–202.
3. Csendes A, Braghetto I, Henriquez A, Cortes C. Late results of a prospective randomized study comparing forceful dilatation and oesophagomyotomy in patients with achalasia. *Gut* 1989; **30**: 229–304.
4. Richter JE. Achalasia: whether the knife or balloon? Not such a difficult question. *Am J Gastroenterol* 1991; **86**: 810–11.
5. Maillard JN, Hay JM. Les myotomies oesophagiennes. *Encyclopedie Medico Chirurgicale.* (Paris), Techniques Chirurgicales, Appareil Digestif, 1987; 40183, **11**: 1–8.
6. Hasson HM. Modified instrument and method for laparoscopy. *Am J Obstet Gynecol* 1971; **110**: 886–7.
7. Cuschieri A, Berci G. *Laparoscopic Biliary Surgery*, 2nd edition. London, Blackwell Scientific Publications 1992.
8. Black J, Vorbach AN, Collis JL. Results of Heller's operation for achalasia of the oesophagus. The importance of hiatal repair. *Br J Surg* 1976; **63**: 949–53.
9. Jara FM, Toledo-Pereira LH, Lewis JH, Mulligan DJ. Long-term results of oesophagomyotomy for achalasia of the oesophagus. *Arch Surg* 1979; **114**: 935–40.
10. Csendes A, Braghetto I, Mascaro J, Henriquez A. Late subjective and objective results of oesophagomyotomy in 100 patients with achalasia of the oesophagus. *Surgery* 1988; **104**: 469–75.
11. Stipa A, Fegiz G, Iascone C *et al.* Heller–Belsey and Heller–Nissen operations for achalasia of the oesophagus. *Surg Gynecol Obstet* 1990; **170**: 212–16.
12. Scotté M, Teniere P, Denis P, Testart J, Leblanc I, Michot F. Résultats à long terme du traitement chirurgical de l'achalasie de l'oesophage. *J Chir* 1991; **128**: 281–4.
13. Richter JE. Motility disorders of the oesophagus. In: *Textbook of Gastroenterology* (ed. Yamada T), pp. 1083–122. Philadelphia, JB Lippincott, 1991.
14. Vantrappen G, Hellemans J. Treatment of achalasia and related motor disorders. *Gastroenterology* 1980; **79**: 144–50.
15. Cuschieri A. The spectrum of laparoscopic surgery. *World J Surg* 1992; **16**: 1089–97.
16. de Paula AL, Hashiba K, Bafutto M, Zago R. *Laparoscopic Treatment of Oesophageal Achalasia.* Proceedings of the 3rd World Congress of Endoscopic Surgery, 1992, Bordeaux, p. 842.
17. Ellis FH, Drozier RE, Watkins E. The operation for oesophageal achalasia: results of oesophagomyotomy without antireflux operation. *J Thorac Cardiovasc Surg* 1984; **88**: 344–7.

Overview

Benign oesophageal surgery

The use of laparoscopic techniques and benign oesophageal conditions seems to be a 'marriage made in heaven', particularly in the case of achalasia. However, as in all forms of laparoscopic surgery, the lessons learnt from years and years of study at open surgery must not be abandoned just to simplify the laparoscopic approach. In Watson's chapter (9.1), the results from open surgery of a variety of anti-reflux repairs are clearly presented and the laparoscopic surgeon must aim to match, if not better, them. Rigorous pre-operative and post-operative assessment should be carried out, not just for clinical audit and subsequent publication, but as a quality control for the surgeon so that technique can be monitored constantly, and, if necessary, improved upon. The explosion of interest in laparoscopic treatment of reflux oesophagitis in some countries has been triggered by concerns regarding the long-term costs of medical anti-acid treatment. Such factors, however, should not be allowed to influence the clinical decision-making process as to whether laparoscopic treatment is more appropriate for the individual patient.

10.1

Expectations of Surgery for Chronic Peptic Ulcer Disease

T. V. TAYLOR

INTRODUCTION

The first half of the twentieth century witnessed a massive increase in the prevalence of peptic ulcer disease and consequently its complications and fatalities. The 1950s, however, heralded an abrupt interruption in this increase and over the last 30 years there has been a steady decline in the established overall prevalence of the condition, when expressed in terms of hospital admissions, outpatient attendances and time lost from work. This decline long preceded the introduction of the H_2 receptor antagonist drugs and other powerful acid secretory inhibitors. The decline in the prevalence of peptic ulcer disease does not, however, seem to have been influenced by the widespread use of these new drugs. In recent years there has, in fact, been an increase in overall ulcer associated mortality in England and Wales where there are some 4500 deaths per year.[1]

We tend to think of peptic ulcer as being a benign disease causing discomfort and perhaps economic dislocation for the patient and we tend not to think of it as a major killer. This is, in fact, far from the truth for the number of deaths from peptic ulcer disease remains equal to those from carcinoma of the pancreas and carcinoma of the oesophagus. There is one fundamental difference, however, between these conditions and that is that many deaths from peptic ulcer should be preventable by appropriate expert medical management, whereas it is hard to foresee any significant inroads being made into deaths from the above malignant conditions in the next few years.[2,3]

The widespread use of the H_2 receptor antagonist drugs has coincided with a dramatic decline in the use of elective peptic ulcer surgery.[4] These drugs are capable of healing the ulcers in some 90% of patients within two months of starting medication.[5,6] However, almost 90% of these will relapse within one year of stopping treatment as acid output returns to pretreatment level within a matter of days even after taking the drugs long term and the underlying ulcer diathesis still exists, leaving particularly the elderly patient vulnerable to the potentially fatal complications of perforation and bleeding.

The increase in ulcer associated mortality may be due to three factors. Firstly, the massive increase which has occurred in the use of non-steroidal anti-inflammatory drugs; there are now some 22 million prescriptions per annum for these drugs in the United Kingdom.[7] A second factor may be the impressive reduction in the number of elective ulcer operations performed in patients prior to the development of a potentially fatal ulcer complication.[8] A third and remote possibility may be the colonization of the stomach by increasingly aggressive strains of the organism *Helicobacter pylori*; such a hypothesis remains, however, entirely conjectural.[9]

The decline in peptic ulcer surgery has been physician-led in that most ulcer patients are now referred to an ever-increasing number of medical gastroenterologists who can provide a rapid and accurate diagnosis of peptic ulceration by endoscopy. The side effects of surgical treatment, chiefly dumping and diarrhoea which are untreatable, together with an escalating incidence of recurrence following highly selective vagotomy have significantly marred the reputations of surgery and surgeons in treating ulceration. Further disadvantages of surgery have been the risks, inconvenience and economic loss associated with an open operation which, when associated with a nine-day period of in-hospital treatment, can become prohibitively expensive. Now laparoscopic surgery is available for the treatment of peptic ulcer and with it the potential for greatly reduced periods of inpatient stay and thus cost saving. Truncal vagotomy, highly selective vagotomy and anterior lesser curve seromyotomy with posterior truncal vagotomy are all feasible laparoscopically and are being performed worldwide in increasing numbers.[10,11,12]

Never before has the debate relating to the optimal management of peptic ulcer disease been so open and certainly the choices of medication have never been so wide. Whilst efficacious ulcer healing drugs have been available now for some 15 years and are being developed in increasing numbers with greater potency, none has been shown to maintain ulcer healing in the long term with the possible exception of the use of triple therapy for the eradication of *Helicobacter pylori*.[13,14] In contrast we have available to us over a century's experience of ulcer surgery, its efficacy, safety, long and short term complications and we have knowledge from long term studies of longevity in relation to definitive acid-reducing operations.

MEDICAL TREATMENT

In assessing the optimal treatment for peptic ulceration and in considering the indications for any form of surgical intervention, attention must be given not only to the reduction of acid output and its undoubted healing properties, which have been expressed in both medical and surgical terms, but also to the role of *Helicobacter pylori* and its eradication. Indeed, it may be asked today whether helicobacter eradication therapy should be given to all patients with a peptic ulcer prior to consideration for surgery. Whilst definite scientific evidence is perhaps not completely available to answer this question, it is the author's feeling that eradication probably should first be carried out with appropriate medication. Whilst the aphorism of Schwartz, "no acid, no ulcer", is as true today as when pronounced some 80 years ago, levels of acid secretion are clearly not the only criteria which apply to the ulcer diathesis. There is a major overlap between levels of acid secretion recorded in normals, duodenal ulcer and gastric ulcer patients whether measured under basal or stimulated conditions by whatever stimulus.

From a scientific point of view, the data obtained from many thousands of scientific studies over the last century would suggest that there is no direct evidence that acid secretion is the only, indeed perhaps the major aetiological factor, in peptic ulcer; notwithstanding the clearly acid related Zollinger-Ellison syndrome.

Helicobacter pylori causes gastritis. It is extremely closely linked to the presence of ulcers, particularly duodenal, and its eradication results in ulcer healing, possibly in the long term.[15] Conversely, gastric colonization by the organism is common, increasingly so with age, so that one would have to say that the vast majority of people with *Helicobacter pylori* in their stomachs do not have and will never have an ulcer.[16] State of the art knowledge might probably suggest that the time honoured equation "acid + pepsin versus mucosal resistance" should be modified to "acid–pepsin + *Helicobacter pylori* infection versus mucosal resistance".

Successful eradication, rather than just suppression of the organism, can be achieved and some studies suggest that this may be maintained in the long term.[17] Eradication therapy results in ulcer healing with a much lower relapse and recurrence rate than can be achieved by temporary healing with acid secretory inhibitors. In the short term eradication therapy is as effective as the H_2 receptor antagonist and by virtue of the longer term healing rates it is probably the most important goal to be achieved therapeutically. There is as yet no definite evidence in the medical literature that eradication of *Helicobacter pylori* reduces the long term potentially fatal risks of bleeding and perforation though it clearly has the potential to do so and thereby to save lives. Although treatment does have side effects it is also very cost effective when compared with long term H_2 receptor antagonist maintenance therapy.

The choice of optimal agents used for the eradication of *Helicobacter pylori* remains controversial.[18] Colloidal bismuth subcitrate (CBS, DeNol) is effective alone in healing ulcers but has only a low incidence, probably about 30%, of efficacy in eradication. When combined with two antibiotics for two weeks eradication rates reach 80% or more.[19] Triple therapy, as it is referred to, consists of the combination of CBS with metronidazole and either tetracycline or amoxycillin. Tetracycline is probably superior to amoxycillin and is less likely to be complicated by side effects and allergies. It is also very inexpensive. Metronidazole is not always well tolerated and has the additional disadvantage of inducing the growth of resistant organisms which can occur in up to 30% of patients. The duration of triple therapy is also controversial. A two week period is probably best but effective clearance has been achieved with one week courses and even a one day course of quadruple therapy has been investigated with some success.

Before embarking on eradication therapy the patient should be endoscoped and the presence of *Helicobacter pylori* confirmed, usually by a CLO test on an endoscopic biopsy.[20] The urease producing properties of the organism produce a colour change in an indicator from yellow to purple, indicating colonization. Presence of the organism may also be confirmed by a "breath test" involving an isotope method or by a relatively simple ELISA antibody technique which can now be performed on a finger prick sample. Thus, before embarking on surgery, eradication of the organism can be checked.

Some dissatisfaction with triple therapy has led to the use of omeprazole and amoxycillin. Omeprazole has intrinsic bacteriostatic effects, though alone it will not eradicate the organism. By virtue of its profound acid secretory inhibitory properties, it does produce rapid symptomatic relief and the two agents have been reported to achieve eradication in 80% of patients. When combined with two antibiotics and CBS (quadruple therapy), eradication rates of 95% have been achieved.[21,22] Omeprazole is also effective when combined with a new macrolide antibiotic, 6-methyoxy-erythromycin.

By eradicating the organism from the stomach there is the potential to avoid surgery and also possibly, and entirely theoretically, to reduce the subsequent incidence of gastric cancer which seems to be closely associated with gastritis and the presence of the organism.

With regard to gastric ulcer, rather than duodenal ulcer per se, the role of *Helicobacter pylori* in the aetiology is perhaps a little less strong, though there remains an argument in favour of eradication of the organism from the stomach. The long term study of the efficacy of *Helicobacter pylori* eradication in duodenal ulcer disease will be of great importance in assessing which patients should undergo surgical treatment.[16] The author can see no strong argument for the prolonged use of H_2 receptor antagonist drugs in patients who have reached the age of 50 years with a strong and recurring ulcer diathesis. In these, helicobacter should be eradicated and if the diathesis persists, surgery should be carried out.[23]

SURGICAL TREATMENT

Gastroenterostomy

At the turn of the century ever increasing numbers of peptic ulcers were treated by gastroenterostomy.[24] The operation was shown to be simple and safe – the latter to an amazing degree as Moynihan and the Mayo Brothers had reported mortality rates as low as 1% in several thousand procedures performed before the First World War.[25,26] Between the wars, it became apparent, however, that despite achieving early healing of duodenal ulcers by diverting the flow of ulcerogenic gastric contents directly into the jejunum, there was an unacceptably high incidence of recurrent stomal ulcer, approaching 40% in some studies.[27] Knowledge of ulcer behaviour which has accrued over the recent years of the endoscopic era suggests that even these high figures may have been significant underestimates because of "silent" asymptomatic recurrences and the intermittent relapses and exacerbations which occur with the disease. Despite its shortcomings gastrojejunostomy alone continued to be used by a small number of surgeons with moderate success, in particular the Edinburgh surgeons who selected gastrojejunostomy for those patients with ulceration but a relatively low acid output. In considering the relative roles of acid secretion and *Helicobacter pylori* in producing peptic ulcers, gastrojejunostomy alone healed most ulcers but did nothing to reduce acid secretion, nor could it have affected helicobacter status. The operation may, however, depend for its success upon the diversion of acid pepsin and gastric contents from the duodenum through the stoma, thus bathing the ulcer with less acid than would otherwise have been the case.

Gastrectomy

Gastric resection for duodenal ulcer began to be carried out between the two world wars. The first resections essentially were pylorectomies and these were soon found to be unsatisfactory.[28,29] Farmer and Smithwick in 1952 developed the operation of antrectomy or hemigastrectomy and this operation appeared markedly to reduce the incidence of stomal ulceration at the cost of a somewhat higher mortality, in the region of 1–2%.[30] Dumping and diarrhoea occurred with gastric resection but were less of a problem than when vagotomy was performed as well. Weight loss and nutritional problems such as osteomalacia occurred in some patients and in the long term the incidence of recurrence increased.

The physiological basis for gastrectomy rests upon excision of the antral gastrin secreting area of the stomach and in addition, the removal of a significant part of the parietal cell mass. Compared with the more modern pylorus preserving types of vagotomy, recurrence rates are modest but few surgeons today would perform a gastric resection for duodenal ulcer disease without adding a vagotomy. In 1970, Farmer and Smithwick reported on 719 patients who had undergone vagotomy and antrectomy with an operative mortality of 1.9%.[31] Many of these procedures were carried out under emergency conditions for active bleeding. Dumping occurred in 20% but on the whole this was not severe. Significant weight loss occurred in only 3% and diarrhoea occurred in 15% but was only troublesome in 3%. The rate of recurrent ulcer was less than

1% as this operation represents the most aggressive form of acid secretory inhibition short of total gastrectomy. Vagotomy alone results in a 65% reduction of acid secretion, antrectomy alone likewise; together they produce in excess of 90% inhibition. Such profound secretory inhibition results in a very low incidence of recurrent ulcer.

The sustained ulcer healing properties of vagotomy and antrectomy are well documented, most impressively by the Nashville experience where 3771 patients underwent the procedure.[32,33] In 32% of these the major indication was massive bleeding though the surgery, on the whole, was not carried out on an actively bleeding haemodynamically unstable patient. Operative mortality was 1.5% and 98% were actively followed up. Most deaths occurred in those being treated for active bleeding. The overall ulcer recurrence rate was a strikingly low 0.5% and when the Zollinger–Ellison cases were extracted it was almost zero! Few would argue that this operation represents the most effective way of curing ulceration and maintaining healing in the long term. The price to be paid lies chiefly in the production of undesirable and usually incurable side effects such as dumping and diarrhoea. There are those who would still perform vagotomy and antrectomy in the emergency room situation because of active bleeding but they are becoming fewer, possibly because today few surgeons are, unlike those of the previous generation, getting sufficient experience and skill in gastric resection.

Vagotomy

For the elegant piece of work by which he showed that division of the vagus nerves abolished the cephalic phase of gastric secretion, Pavlov was awarded the Nobel Prize in 1904. Vagotomy, however, was rarely used in humans until it became strongly promulgated by Lester Dragstedt in the mid to late 1940s.[34,35] In fact, Dragstedt had been researching the effects of vagotomy since 1917. After operating upon his first case, a 35 year old with a repeated heavy bleeding from a duodenal ulcer, he stated, "There is now evidence to support the view that section of the vagus nerves to the stomach should favourably influence the clinical course of duodenal ulcer". Dragstedt emphasized the importance of acid secretion in the pathogenesis of peptic ulcer from two standpoints. Firstly, he showed that the isolated stomach in the dog with an occluded gastric outlet was very prone to form peptic ulcers; this ulceration was prevented by vagotomy. Secondly, he became interested in the nocturnal basal gastric secretory rate and showed that most duodenal ulcer patients had a high basal acid secretion.

It soon became apparent to Dragstedt that truncal vagotomy alone resulted in a profound degree of gastric stasis, leading to vomiting, foul eructations and gastric ulceration in many of these patients. Initially, gastrojejunostomy was used as a drainage procedure for the vagotomized stomach. The Heineke–Mikulicz pyloroplasty seemed not to empty the stomach as efficiently.[36] However, through the 1960s more surgeons used pyloroplasty and it became the more accepted drainage procedure, particularly in Europe.[37]

The incidence of dumping and diarrhoea does not seem to differ between the two drainage procedures. Pyloroplasty does have a significant advantage in emergency surgery carried out for uncontrollable bleeding in that it permits direct oversewing of the ulcer.

Operative mortality following truncal vagotomy and drainage was reported at about 0.8–1% in several large series, though higher levels in excess of 10% occurred in those undergoing surgery for active bleeding from their ulcers. Recurrence rates of 5–7% were recorded after five years follow-up; these rates depend to a considerable extent on the experience of the surgeon. The most common cause of recurrence was failure of the surgeon to divide the posterior vagus nerve trunk. This usually resulted in an early positive peak of acid secretion in response to an insulin stimulus and an inadequate degree of vagal denervation. It is almost true to say that in the absence of a significant delay in gastric emptying and of the rare Zollinger–Ellison syndrome, the aphorism "no vagus – no ulcer" pertains; there are occasional exceptions to this rule. Clearly, despite all of our subsequent knowledge that has accrued about the organism, *Helicobacter pylori* and its role in the pathogenesis of peptic ulcer, acid secretion and vagal drive are very important factors. Over 90% of people treated by truncal vagotomy and pyloroplasty remained ulcer-free for life.

Disillusionment surrounded the use of truncal vagotomy and drainage because of chronic morbidity in the form of dumping, diarrhoea, duodenogastric reflux of bile, distension, dysphagia and recurrent dyspepsia.

Dumping and diarrhoea are the major problems because these are on the whole incurable and can lead subsequently to more major surgery such as Roux-en-Y reconstruction which in itself, for vagotomized patients, may give a lot of trouble.[38,39] Dumping, the more treatable of the two problems, occurs in about 15% and when severe (3%) may respond to reconstruction of the pylorus. Persistent diarrhoea in about 5% is more of a problem. It can lead to incontinence and marked frequency of bowel action, particularly in the morning and after food. It is in part related to gastric incontinence or rapid early gastric emptying, though bacterial overgrowth and abnormalities of carbohydrate metabolism may play a role. Reflux alkaline gastritis may also be a problem.

A longer term problem following vagotomy and drainage which needs more detailed evaluation is gastric cancer which has been reported to occur in 5% of one long term study. There is also an increased incidence of gallstone formation after truncal vagotomy as a result of denervation of the gall bladder. Furthermore, the combination of truncal vagotomy and drainage with cholecystectomy is a bad one, resulting in an increased incidence of postvagotomy diarrhoea as a result of altered kinetics of bile acid secretion following cholecystectomy.[37,40,41]

Selective Vagotomy

Because of the problems of dumping and diarrhoea it was considered by Franksson[42] and Jackson[43] in 1948 that there would be some advantage in performing selective gastric vagotomy. Whilst preserving the extragastric parasympathetic nerve supply to the biliary tree, pancreas and small bowel, selective vagotomy completely denervates the stomach, hence the need for a drainage procedure. Diarrhoea seems to be less of a problem with selective vagotomy but the incidence of dumping remains unchanged. A further possible advantage for selective over truncal vagotomy is that of more complete vagal denervation of the stomach, there being less likelihood of the surgeon omitting to divide a major vagus nerve trunk. There remains a risk, however, of overlooking the "criminal nerve of Grassi" which veers over to the gastric fundus from behind the lower oesophagus.

Few large studies have been reported in the literature describing the results of selective vagotomy, but there is little doubt that despite the necessity for a drainage procedure, dumping and diarrhoea are uncommon and when they do occur they tend to be mild. Recurrent ulcer rates have also been low following this procedure for it has been argued that the technical performance of this operation is more likely to result in a complete gastric vagotomy than is the case with any other form of vagotomy. Tests of acid secretion would tend to support this. The operation also seems to be safe, Kennedy having reported no deaths in his series of 350 cases.[44]

Perhaps selective vagotomy has not been given an adequate test and it possibly should have received greater recognition and employed a greater role. It was surpassed, in theoretical terms at least, by proximal gastric vagotomy. In terms of the elimination of dumping and diarrhoea, surgeons were happier with this latter procedure but the high incidence of recurrent ulcer now being reported after highly selective vagotomy has put something of a question mark over its long term future. The other factor which led to the expression of some reservations in adopting selective gastric vagotomy was the more difficult nature of the technical procedure involved. One can certainly say, from the evidence available, that selective vagotomy, particularly when combined with a suprapyloric antrectomy, is a procedure which, as stated by Griffiths, "meets the old requirement of low recurrence and the new requirement of no dumping", albeit not as effectively as parietal cell vagotomy.[45–47]

Highly Selective Vagotomy

Highly selective vagotomy, the ultimate in conservative resection of the gastric vagi (hence the alternative names "proximal gastric vagotomy" and "parietal cell vagotomy"), restricts denervation to the acid–pepsin secreting part of the stomach, the fundus and corpus. The parietal cell area of the stomach is wholly denervated by this procedure whilst at the same time the innervation of the antrum and pylorus is completely preserved.[48,49] In order to achieve this the antral innervation is maintained by a careful preservation of the nerves of Latarjet as they run along the lesser curvature aspect of the anterior and posterior gastric walls. Preservation of the hepatic branches of the anterior vagus and the coeliac branches of the posterior vagus are maintained in order to save parasympathetic innervation of the extragastric structures within the abdomen.

The operation was promulgated to overcome three of the major side effects of the more radical forms of vagotomy: diarrhoea, dumping and duodenogastric reflux with bilious vomiting. These complications are unpredictable in their occurrence and frequently incurable. The concept underlying the operation of highly selective vagotomy originated in experimental work carried out by Griffiths in 1957.[50] Prior to that, back in the 1920s it is possible that Latarjet himself was performing a procedure not too dissimilar from this. It was Holle,[51] however, who introduced the technique in humans in 1967, though he performed a drainage procedure with it, usually a pyloroplasty. It was felt by those who wished to obtain as physiological a result as possible that the drainage procedure was not only unnecessary in the presence of an innervated antrum, but that it also might detract from the procedure by distorting the mechanism and rate of gastric emptying. Thus, Johnston in Leeds[49] and in Amdrup in Copenhagen[48] described the operation without a drainage procedure in 1970. Early results show little or no delay in gastric emptying in the vast majority of patients and thus a drainage procedure was abandoned by most of the investigators in Europe performing the procedure in the 1970s and early 1980s.

These early workers demonstrated the feasibility of complete parietal cell denervation, at least in the short term, by recording negative secretory responses to insulin induced hypoglycaemia. A disadvantage of the procedure is, however, that it is unquestionably more tedious to perform than truncal vagotomy and drainage and complete parietal cell denervation may not always be achieved by the less experienced operator. Arguments existed in the early days of the performance of the procedure about the preservation of the vagally innervated antrum which, when kept in continuity, seemed to offer potential, at least on theoretical grounds, of further protection against ulceration. The operation has now been shown to be very safe with a low incidence of dumping and diarrhoea, the former being virtually abolished; some longer term studies have, however, shown disturbingly high incidences of late recurrent ulceration, even of the order of 30%. Such figures, if the norm, would be unacceptable and are of the order of those which led to the abandonment of gastrojejunostomy alone in the treatment of peptic ulcer.

It was the Copenhagen group, founders of the procedure working in a centre of excellence, who experienced a high incidence of long term recurrent ulcer. One disturbing factor about this study has been the ever increasing incidence of ulceration which has continued to occur over periods in excess of ten years. Such observations can temporarily seem unique to this procedure. After all, other forms of vagotomy recurrence, if it does occur, tend to do so within two years of the operation and are directly attributable to incomplete vagotomy. The most likely conceivable explanation of recurrence is reinnervation of the parietal cell area of the stomach emanating from the sprouting of vagal fibres from the oesophagus above and the antrum below. There is no doubt that reinnervation, as expressed in terms of increasing acid output with time in response to an insulin stimulus, does occur. Following truncal vagotomy some 50% of insulin negative responses spontaneously convert to positive with time; after highly selective vagotomy the incidence is much higher, if not invariable.

If, however, the process of nerve sprouting was responsible for recurrence, why then do ulcers keep on recurring for up to at least 18 years after operation? Any process of reinnervation would be expected to be complete well before two years from the time of the operation. Joffe has suggested that reinnervation does occur and has produced evidence on electron microscopy that a "new set of parasympathetic nerves innervate the stomach".[52,53] Other factors responsible for late recurrence may relate either to hormonal events or possibly to varying degrees of colonization by *Helicobacter pylori*; both of these theories, the latter in particular, being entirely conjectural. It is particularly difficult to implicate *Helicobacter pylori* here as there is nothing in the sequence of events relating to the operation and subsequent years which is as yet known potentially to implicate the organism or its behaviour.

It is of interest and perhaps of major importance that Holle has not reported the high incidence of late ulcer recurrence that follows proximal gastric vagotomy when performed with a drainage procedure.[54] His reasons for performing pyloroplasty are to compensate for any reduction in antropyloric gastric motor function that may occur as a result of proximal gastric denervation. Vagotomy of the proximal stomach will result in loss of adaptive relaxation of the major reservoir capacity of the organ. This could in itself produce abnormalities of gastric emptying and contractility though it must be said those studies which report gastric emptying after highly selective vagotomy have been remarkably normal. By adding a pyloroplasty it is argued by Holle that inherent postprandial antral contractility can be lowered without impairment of gastric emptying. He states that this protective treatment is indispensable for the maintenance of adequate motility. His observations could turn out to be very important, if indeed he is right; if there is no significant price to pay for the pyloroplasty in terms of increased dumping and diarrhoea, then the reduced incidence of recurrent ulcer which follows the addition of a pyloroplasty could easily justify its more widespread use.

Abolition of dumping and diarrhoea must be regarded as important prerequisites to peptic ulcer surgery in the 1990s. The factors following truncal vagotomy which predisposed to these unpredictable, disabling and often incurable complications are: division of the hepatic branches of the anterior vagus nerve; division of the coeliac branches of the posterior vagus; and the gastric incontinence created by the drainage procedure. Drainage procedures alone or when combined with selective or highly selective vagotomy are accompanied by a low incidence of dumping and diarrhoea. Also when the posterior vagal trunk is divided but the hepatic branches of the anterior vagus and pylorus are preserved, as in the operation of anterior lesser curve seromyotomy with posterior truncal vagotomy, the incidence of dumping and diarrhoea has been shown consistently to be extremely low. Usually, therefore, perhaps at least two of these three factors are needed for the patient to be at significant risk of dumping and diarrhoea and when all these three factors are present, as after truncal vagotomy and drainage, the incidence is much higher than with two of them. It is likely, therefore, that the addition of a pyloroplasty to a highly selective vagotomy will not produce a significant problem with dumping and diarrhoea.

Writing in the 1990s about pyloroplasty instinctively creates an air of guilt, if not shame! In contrast, however, the long term, ever increasing rates of recurrence reported after highly selective vagotomy per se are worrying and inexplicable; in relation to acid secretion, they may relate to a motility disorder of the proximal stomach, which is exaggerated by the lack of a pyloroplasty. The loss of adaptive relaxation by the proximal stomach, which is a vagally mediated phenomenon inherent with all forms of vagotomy, affects reservoir capacity and fundus corpus motility. The effect of this loss is to lead firstly to the rapid early emptying of liquids from the stomach and later to the retention of solids in the atonic proximal part of the organ. Addition of a pyloroplasty might be expected to increase the rapid early emptying of liquids and hence early dumping but to militate also against the delay of emptying of solids which would be more likely to go through the wide open gastric outlet after pyloroplasty. Dumping is certainly abolished by pylorus preserving vagotomy; it is also rare after pyloroplasty is added, but it may occur and Holle quotes a 5% incidence of markedly increased gastric emptying but only a 1.5% incidence of clinical dumping. Retention of solids in the stomach might, however, be more of a long term problem, being conducive to gastritis and to bacterial overgrowth, possibly with *Helicobacter pylori*. Overall, Holle reports a 95.7% Visick grade 1 or 2 rating.[55] The argument relating to the use of a pyloroplasty with highly selective vagotomy is still open; though with so few ulcers being operated upon today, it might never be resolved.

The major argument in favour of highly selective vagotomy without pyloroplasty as the operation of choice for duodenal ulcer remains a low incidence of the untreatable side effects of dumping and diarrhoea which has been confirmed in all major studies. Highly selective vagotomy is also a very safe operation, Johnston having reported a 0.3% mortality in 5500 cases treated by 1975.[56] The major cause of death following the procedure was ischaemic necrosis of the lesser curvature of the stomach which is specific to this operation, unpredictable and uncommon but when it does occur, frequently fatal.

Perforation of the ischaemic segment may occur anywhere from the oesophagogastric junction down to the incisura angularis and may range in size from less than 1 cm to a 5–6 cm large defect. The condition occurs in less than 1% of highly selective vagotomies and is undeniably operator variable, being dependent upon operative technique. The technical points of excessive use of diathermy and ligature or clamping of the lesser curvature are importantly to be avoided. It has also been claimed that renal insufficiency, hypertension and generalized atherosclerosis may contribute to the problem. Kennedy[44] and his co-workers in Belfast have pointed out that there is an association between ischaemic necrosis of the lesser curvature and the addition of a Nissen fundoplication to highly selective vagotomy. In view of this link and the incidence of gas bloat which follows Nissen fundoplication, it is possible that marked gastric dilatation predisposes to the problem. In view of this important finding the two operations should not be combined. If the complication does occur it is heralded clinically by severe epigastric, shoulder tip or back pain, together with shock and generalized peritonitis. Free gas is usually present under the diaphragm, but may still be present following the laparotomy. Expeditious surgical treatment is required when the defect is closed. Extensive and delayed perforation may require treatment by gastric resection. Of 19 patients reported in the literature, nine died, underlining the serious nature of this problem.

Anterior Lesser Curve Seromyotomy with Posterior Truncal Vagotomy

This operation was first developed in 1979 predominantly for technical reasons.[57,58] By this time, proximal gastric vagotomy had been extensively investigated in animals and humans and had been shown to be associated with a low mortality.[59] The operation was, however, tedious and time consuming to perform, damage to the nerve of Latarjet could result in gastric stasis and there was a small risk of ischaemic necrosis of the lesser curvature of the stomach which, as has been said, was unpredictable and not uncommonly fatal.

Over the last decade it has become increasingly apparent that in the hands of many surgeons, recurrence rates have been unacceptably high. Even in expert hands such as those surgeons who were co-founders of the procedures in Copenhagen, recurrence rates of 30% have been quoted over a period of up to 18 years.[60,61] It seemed even before increasing rates of recurrent peptic ulceration were being described with highly selective vagotomy that there would be an advantage in the development of an operation which, while denervating the parietal cell mass could be more easily and expeditiously performed with neither risk of damage to the nerve of Latarjet nor ischaemic necrosis of the lesser curvature. Furthermore, anterior lesser curve seromyotomy with posterior truncal vagotomy would appear to offer a greater degree of gastric denervation while still preserving the pylorus and its anterior innervation.

It has been shown experimentally by Daniel and Sarner[62] that preservation of the antral branches of the anterior nerve of Latarjet permitted the delivery of nerve impulses not only to the anterior antral and pyloric walls but also to the posterior antrum and pylorus through intramural vagovagal arcs. Thus, gastric emptying should be similar to that after highly selective vagotomy with pylorus preservation and this indeed turned out to be the case. The incurables of dumping and diarrhoea were still largely overcome and gastric stasis, to any appreciable degree, did not occur.

In this procedure, the lower 6–8 cm of oesophagus are mobilized, the anterior vagus nerve is carefully preserved and dissected clear of the exposed length of oesophagus. The posterior vagus trunk is next divided and the oesophagus cleared of any residual nerve fibres which may go on to innervate the proximal fundix insitian intramurally. In performing these manoevres around the oesophagus the "criminal nerve of Grassi" must be sought and, if present, divided. At the oesophagogastric junction anteriorly is a constantly placed fibrofatty bundle which extends from the spatulate expansion of the distal anterior nerve trunk horizontally and to the left of the gastric fundus. This bundle contains numerous nerve strands from the anterior vagus and requires to be divided.

At a point 6 cm proximal to the pylorus and 1 cm lateral to the extreme of the lesser curvature the seromyotomy is commenced by making a transverse incision through the seromuscular layers. This allows the operator to insinuate scissors beneath the circular muscle fibres and to develop a plane along which to do the seromyotomy close to the lesser curvature. In the beginning of this dissection the lower branches of the crow's foot are divided and ligated with fine ligatures. The nerve fibres separate widely as the circular muscle is dissected off the underlying submucosa. Once the correct plane of dissection is achieved immediately adjacent to the submucosa, the scissors may be gently and easily spread to facilitate the more proximal dissection up to a point just below the oesophagogastric junction staying on the serosa-coloured stomach. The myotomy is finally extended laterally across the front of the stomach distal to the lower oesophageal sphincter which must remain intact.[63]

On completion of the lesser curve seromyotomy the submucosa can be seen pouting through the muscular defect along the length of the incised area. The vagus nerves which run with the serosa are widely separated by the gap which develops. The defect created by the seromyotomy is closed, employing a method of "overlap repair". This is achieved by tacking the serosa on the lesser curve aspect over the serosa on the gastric side of the myotomy using a continuous absorbable suture. This overlap repair is done so as to overcome the theoretical possibility of nerve sprouting occurring from divided nerve endings and thus permitting reinnervation of the mucosa. There is no evidence that sprouting nerve fibres can penetrate an intact seromuscular layer which they would be required to do following the overlap repair in order to reinnervate the gastric mucosa.[64] This overlap completes the procedure and overcomes any possibility of a hole in the mucosa having been overlooked or of ischaemic change occurring. It must be emphasized that there has been no report of ischaemic necrosis of the lesser curvature having occurred following this procedure.

The operation of anterior lesser curve seromyotomy with posterior truncal vagotomy would seem to satisfy many of the criteria which might at the present time be applied in devising an operation for peptic ulcer:

1. As much of the stomach as possible should be denervated without impairing gastric emptying.
2. The pylorus should be preserved.
3. Gastric emptying should be near normal.
4. The loss of adaptive relaxation after all forms of vagotomy giving rise to distension should be compensated for.
5. Dumping, diarrhoea and duodenogastric reflux must be minimized.

6. The operation must be safe and simple to perform. It must also be reproducible and feasible for performance by the general surgeon as well as the gastroenterological enthusiast.
7. The risks of damage to the nerve of Latarjet and of ischaemic necrosis of the lesser curvature must be overcome.
8. The incidence of recurrent ulceration must be acceptably and competitively low compared with other forms of vagotomy.

In anterior lesser curve seromyotomy with posterior truncal vagotomy the whole of the posterior wall of the stomach is denervated and our initial experience with the procedure has suggested that the anterior seromyotomy adequately denervates the anterior parietal cell area of the stomach. Stimulation of the antral musculature through the anterior nerve of Latarjet produces contractile activity throughout the whole antrum. It was felt that performing a myotomy to the lesser curvature of the stomach might in part compensate for the lack of adaptive relaxation of the stomach inherent in all other forms of gastric vagotomy which gave rise to the sensation of early fullness and bloating. Liquid and solid phase gastric emptying studies were performed in 17 controlled subjects, 14 patients before and at least six months after anterior lesser curve seromyotomy and posterior truncal vagotomy, 14 after vagotomy and pyloroplasty, 11 after vagotomy and gastroenterostomy and seven after polyagastrectomy.[65] Of the 14 patients in the vagotomy and pyloroplasty group, eight had no postvagotomy sequelae and six had postvagotomy diarrhoea. This study showed that there was no delay in emptying time for liquids or solids between anterior lesser curve seromyotomy with posterior truncal vagotomy and controls. There was, however, a little increase in the early emptying of liquids which has been observed after all other forms of vagotomy and is probably less marked after this procedure than any other.

Some concern has been expressed about complete division of the posterior vagus nerve trunk in terms of inducing postvagotomy sequelae. We have found a very low incidence of diarrhoea and virtually no dumping following this procedure. Three factors may contribute to dumping and diarrhoea produced after truncal vagotomy and drainage. These are:

1. division of the hepatic branches of the anterior vagus;
2. division of the coeliac branches of the posterior vagus;
3. destruction of the pylorus by pyloroplasty.

Of these, the last would appear to be the most significant contributory factor to emptying problems following vagotomy. Clearly division of the coeliac branches of the posterior vagus nerve may contribute in part to postvagotomy sequelae but when the integrity of the pylorus and of the hepatic branches of the anterior vagus are maintained then it is unlikely that division of the coeliac branches of the vagus will in itself produce any significant clinical problems.

In 1985 a survey was performed to assess the mortality and morbidity of this procedure in the elective treatment of chronic duodenal ulcers. From six participating centres a total of 600 cases were studied. There was one death in the postoperative period due to a myocardial infarction which occurred three weeks postoperation, and an overall mortality of 0.16%. There were no cases of ischaemic necrosis of the lesser curvature nor was there any postoperative bleeding necessitating reoperation.[66]

By the late 1980s several groups had reported their experience with this procedure. In Scotland Gunn and his colleagues described their experience of treating 241 patients, all of whom had chronic duodenal ulcer.[67] The postoperative mortality was 0.4% and 1.6% required a drainage procedure for gastric stasis. The five year recurrent ulcer rate in a consecutive group of 175 of these patients was 3%. This was after an initial learning curve on 66 patients in whom the recurrent ulcer rate was 14%. The authors concluded that the immediate and five year results following this procedure were at least comparable with those following conventional highly selective vagotomy and that the procedure of lesser curve seromyotomy with posterior truncal vagotomy presented an easy and rapid alternative to conventional highly selective vagotomy. In 1985 and again in 1988, Oostvogel and van Vroonhoven described their experience in a trial comparing anterior lesser curve seromyotomy with posterior truncal vagotomy (ASPTV) with conventional proximal gastric vagotomy in 91 patients.[68] Two years after surgery satisfactory results (Visick grades 1 and 2) were found in 84.2% of patients after PGV and in 88.9% after ASPTV. There was a significant difference in the duration of surgery, the latter procedure being more rapidly performed. The incidence of recurrent ulceration in both groups of patients was 9% at four years. The authors anticipated that as ASPTV was technically simpler and less time consuming than conventional PGV, it would replace the latter procedure as the operation of choice in the surgical treatment of chronic duodenal ulcer.[69]

ASPTV was compared with truncal vagotomy and pyloroplasty by our own group in a series of 146 patients with chronic duodenal ulcer. They had a mean duration of symptoms of seven years.[70] The mean follow-up time was 4.5 years with a range of 2–7 years. One elderly patient died from a myocardial infarction in the truncal vagotomy group. Acid secretory inhibition in response to insulin and pentagastric stimuli was equal in both groups, indicating a similar degree of vagal denervation. Recurrent ulcers occurred in five patients after ASPTV and two after truncal vagotomy and pyloroplasty. Dumping and diarrhoea were significantly more common after the truncal vagotomy and drainage with 31 incidences compared with eight following ASPTV. The mean operating time was increased by only six minutes when ASPTV was performed rather than TVP. The results of this study show that ASPTV was associated with a lower incidence of dumping and diarrhoea and achieved better overall Visick gradings than truncal vagotomy and pyloroplasty.

Thus overall the international series describing the procedure of ASPTV have shown it to be a simple, safe and rapidly performed procedure with a low incidence of postoperative sequelae in the early period. There has been no reported incidence of ischaemic necrosis of lesser curvature and the overall mortality is of the order of 0.16%. Dumping virtually never complicates this procedure and the incidence of diarrhoea is less than 3%. Delayed gastric emptying occurs in approximately 2% of patients who may need either pyloric dilatation or pyloroplasty. The evidence consistently portrayed throughout the medical literature in the last five years shows that the operation of ASPTV is as effective as conventional highly selective vagotomy and may have the additional advantage of simplicity, speed and safety over HSV.

MEDICAL VERSUS SURGICAL TREATMENT

In view of the high recurrence rates when H_2 receptor antagonist therapy is ceased, it is clear that there comes a time in the management of a chronic duodenal ulcer when the decision is made between long term or permanent drug treatment, often using full therapeutic doses, and operation. Prospective clinical trials of elective surgery against medical therapy are important but few exist. Harling *et al.* reported a controlled trial of 86 duodenal ulcer patients with severe symptoms who were randomized to full dose cimetidine plus maintenance therapy for one year or highly selective vagotomy without pyloroplasty.[71] These patients were followed up for 57 months. In the cimetidine treated group only 12% remained symptom-free and 35% had operations for recurrent symptoms while 53% had regular medical treatment. The overall recurrence rate after highly selective vagotomy was 17% and the final Visick grading was 75%, excellent or good. The authors concluded that the operation was the treatment of choice in patients with a history of severe symptoms from peptic ulceration and rapid recurrence after medical treatment. Graffner and his colleagues analysed the results of 405 consecutive parietal cell vagotomies over ten years[72] and confirmed that:

1. recurrences occur earlier in patients with pyloric and prepyloric ulcers;
2. the postoperative peak acid output to pentagastrin is higher in those who develop recurrent duodenal ulcer than in those who do not;
3. the recurrence rate depended upon surgical expertise;
4. over half the recurrent ulcers were successfully treated medically.

Anderson reported that long term medical treatment and surgery were equally acceptable options for most patients, but he pointed out that, in Denmark, in the long term, operation was cheaper for the patient.[73] He also made the point that in these days of powerful ulcer healing drugs, recurrent ulceration may no longer be the main criterion for success of surgery. Lack of side effects, in particular the incurables of dumping and diarrhoea, is now more important because recurrence of ulceration often responds to a further course of H_2 receptor antagonists or more certainly to omeprazole.

The debate about the most appropriate treatment for uncomplicated duodenal ulcer has continued over recent years. One message that has certainly come across strongly is that if surgery is indicated then highly selective vagotomy or pylorus preserving vagotomy is the operation of choice because it is associated with minimal morbidity and virtually no mortality. The somewhat high ulcer recurrence rate after highly selective vagotomy is, however, of some concern. It is still only 20 years since these operations were first described. By the mid-1980s recurrence rates in those long term studies following highly selective vagotomy were creeping up, and in the studies of Herrington *et al.*,[74] von Holstein,[75] Enskog,[76] Marceau[77] and Paimela[78] they average 9.2%, 18%, 13.8%, 12% and 16% respectively. The variable incidence of recurrence is due in part to differing surgical technique and experience and seniority does not necessarily guarantee success. Undoubtedly, however, highly selective vagotomy is an operation which must be learnt from the experienced vagotomist and at the present time very many fewer vagotomies are being performed so that it may become a procedure to be carried out by the surgical superspecialist.

In selecting patients for peptic ulcer surgery some emphasis should clearly be placed on the identification of the group or groups of patients who will do badly. Primrose and his colleagues[79] were able to link poor results to both medical and surgical treatment with smoking habits. Several papers have reported poor results following highly selective vagotomy when the ulcer was pyloric or prepyloric; Jordan and Thornby[80] noted recurrence rates after highly selective vagotomy of 6% and 21% for duodenal and pyloric or prepyloric ulcers respectively while Muller[81] noticed recurrence rates of 14% and 35% for the same conditions. Muller suggested the addition of a drainage procedure to a highly selective vagotomy would be beneficial when treating pyloric canal and prepyloric ulcers. Jordan and Thornby stated that when selective vagotomy and antrectomy and highly selective vagotomy were compared prospectively the recurrence rate was significantly reduced after selective vagotomy and antrectomy (2.2% vs. 10.0%).[80] However, if the pyloric ulcers were excluded no significant difference in ulcer recurrence could be demonstrated between the two groups.

One is left with the question as to whether there is any role for elective peptic ulcer surgery in the 1990s? Contemporary surgical gastroenterologists must have posed this question and many medical peers must have dismissed elective surgical treatment to the history books. The latter view has had a most profound effect for how many of today's gastroenterologists refer cases for surgery? Their argument is at first sight a good one. Virtually all chronic peptic ulcers will succumb to the powerful H_2 receptor antagonists cimetidine, ranitidine or femotidine.[82] The occasional resistant ulcer will thereafter almost inevitably heal with omeprazole. Using acid secretory inhibition to heal ulcers, great strides have been made in the past 15 years. A problem arises, however, in maintaining ulcer healing. Stopping a two month course of any of the above drugs results in recurrence rates of up to 90% at one year. Even long term low dose maintenance therapy has a recurrence rate of 2.5% per month, 30% per year.[83]

Over the past 15 years there has been no reduction in ulcer associated mortality in England and Wales despite the vast investment in H_2 receptor antagonists. The number of deaths from peptic ulcers, nearly 4500 per year, is as high as that from oesophageal or rectosigmoid cancers in these countries.[84] Indeed, ulcer mortality is rising, year by year, particularly in the elderly female.[85] Moreover, this increase is occurring at a time when the overall prevalence of the disorder is estimated to be declining. What is the reason for this? The rise cannot be attributed to increased rates of colonization or virulence by *Helicobacter pylori* although detailed studies of the natural history of different strains of this organism bear further investigation. It has been suggested that some strains of organism are more pathogenic or ulcerogenic than others.[86] It is possible, though unlikely, that a particular strain is more virulent in terms of producing ulcer perforation or bleeding, particularly in the elderly female. A more likely explanation relates to the increasing use of non-steroidal anti-inflammatory drugs, particularly in the elderly. Over 22 million prescriptions for these drugs are dispensed annually in the UK and 44 million in the USA.[87] These figures do not allow for the even greater volume sold over the counter. Even the use of ultra low dose aspirin (75 mg per day) in the prophylaxis of coronary artery disease is a significant risk factor for ulcer bleeding.[88] In a study within three months of taking non-steroidal anti-inflammatory drugs (NSAIDs), 17% of the patients developed ulcers, 14% developed gastric erosions and over 70% developed gastric erythema.[89] These drugs are, however, potent in the relief of rheumatic pain and may alleviate unexplained abdominal pain in the elderly. If further proof of their irritant effect was needed, merely stopping the drug frequently results in alleviation of dyspepsia and ulcer healing. These drugs are probably the major cause of the rise in ulcer associated mortality which we are witnessing.

Another factor, equally difficult to assess in absolute terms, may be the dramatic reduction in the use of elective peptic ulcer surgery in the last 15 years. This may have played a role in the increased mortality because definitive acid reducing surgery results in long term, if not permanent, ulcer healing. The ulcers which do recur after surgery rarely perforate or bleed because acid secretion has been reduced and the ulcer diathesis blunted. MacLaine Ross *et al.*, in a 15 year follow-up of 779 patients from south east Scotland who had undergone acid reducing surgery, showed that though mortality was high from smoking related diseases, no patient died from perforation or bleeding of a recurrent peptic ulcer.[90] Many of these patients must have been taking NSAIDs. It would seem, therefore, that a potential exists for reducing the ulcer associated mortality by permanent reduction in acid secretion. This argument would seem to proffer a policy in favour of the more widespread use of vagotomy but year by year decreasing numbers of these procedures are being performed.

The open operative procedures carry short term morbidity and an economic burden, due entirely to a long abdominal incision, in contrast to the rapid recovery made when, for example, a cholecystectomy is performed laparoscopically. Few would now question that laparoscopic cholecystectomy is here to stay. Both conventional highly selective vagotomy and lesser curve seromyotomy with posterior truncal vagotomy can now be performed through the laparoscope. Feasibility, however, is not the hallmark of justification for the widespread adoption of these techniques. So far, only a handful of studies exist in the literature which are largely animal based.[91–93] Not only do they confirm the feasibility of the laparoscopic technique but it has also been shown that acid inhibition of the order of "open vagotomy" can be achieved. One study compared truncal vagotomy, highly selective vagotomy and anterior lesser curve seromyotomy with posterior truncal vagotomy in 20 pigs. The anterior lesser curve seromyotomy with posterior truncal vagotomy was found to be technically the most feasible and may well lend itself to the use of a laser. If laparoscopic vagotomy is to be encouraged then only highly selective or anterior lesser curve seromyotomy with posterior truncal vagotomy can be considered in view of the necessity to eliminate the incurables of dumping and diarrhoea. Katkhouda in Nice has now performed anterior seromyotomy with posterior truncal vagotomy in 80 patients with excellent short term results (personal communication, 1993). Few long term studies have yet been published and it will take several years to assess their safety and long term rates of recurrent ulceration.

Laparoscopic vagotomy may also have cost advantages on its side by producing permanent acid inhibition to safe levels for the cost of some two hours of operating time and two days in hospital, with a rapid return to work thereafter. The cost of low dose maintenance therapy with H_2 receptor antagonists is at least £1000–2000 per decade.[94] A problem of great importance in employing laparoscopic vagotomy more widely will undoubtedly be that of surgical training and surgical skill. Untrained and unskilled laparoscopists could undoubtedly gain these procedures a bad reputation and, more importantly, make them dangerous. This is now coming to light with laparoscopic cholecystectomy, where the incidence of common bile duct injury has been much higher than in the days of open gall bladder removal. If these procedures can be performed with skill, safety and precision, then they may have an important role in reducing the considerable mortality of peptic ulceration which still exists.

REFERENCES

1. *Mortality Statistics (General): Review of the Registrar General on Deaths in England and Wales 1990.* Series DH1 number 24, p. 32. London, HMSO.
2. Taylor TV. Deaths from peptic ulceration. *Br Med J* 1985; **291**: 653–5.
3. Taylor TV. Current indications for elective peptic ulcer surgery. *Br J Surg* 1989; **76**: 427 8.
4. Bauerfeind P, Koelz HR, Blum AL. Ulcer treatment: regimens and duration of inhibition of acid secretion: how long to dose. *Scand J Gastroenterol* 1988; **23** (suppl): 153 (23–32).
5. Rubin R. Medical treatment of peptic ulcer disease. *Med Clin N Am* 1991; **75**: 981–98.
6. Bardhan KD. Omeprazole in the management of refractory duodenal ulcer. *Scand J Gastroenterol* 1989; **24** (suppl): 168 (63–73).

7. Naschitz JE, Yeshurun D, Odehm A. *et al.* Overt gastrointestinal bleeding in the course of chronic aspirin administration for secondary prevention of arterial occlusive disease. *Am J Gastroenterol* 1990; **85**: 408–10.
8. Walt R, Logan R, Katschinski BD, Ashley J, Langman M. Rising frequency of ulcer perforations in elderly people in the United Kingdom. *Lancet* 1986; **1**: 489–92.
9. Crabtree JE, Taylor JD, Wyatt JI, Heatley RV, Shallcross TM, Tomkinson DS. Mucosal IgA recognition of *Helicobacter pylori* 120 kDa protein, peptic ulceration and gastric pathology. *Lancet* 1991; **338**: 332–5.
10. Shapiro S, Gordon L, Dayhkovsky L, Grundfest W, Chandra M. Development of laparoscopic anterior seromyotomy and right posterior truncal vagotomy for ulcer prophylaxis. *J Laparosc Endosc Surg* 1991; **1**: 277–86.
11. Voeller GR, Pridgen WL, Mangiante EC. Laparoscopic posterior truncal vagotomy and anterior seromyotomy: a pig model. *J Laparosc Endosc Surg* 1991; **1**: 375–9.
12. Hunter JG, Becker JM, Lee RG, Christian PE, Dixon JA. Anterior lesser curve laser seromyotomy with posterior truncal vagotomy: a potential treatment for peptic ulcer disease. *Br J Surg* 1989; **76**: 949–52.
13. Graham DY, Lew GM, Klein PD *et al.* Effect of treatment of *Helicobacter pylori* infection on the long term recurrence of gastric or duodenal ulcer. A randomised controlled study. *Ann Intern Med* 1992; **116**: 705–8.
14. Silvoso GR, Ivey KJ, Butt JH, Lockard OO, Holt SD, Sisk C. Incidence of gastric lesions in patients with rheumatic disease on chronic aspirin therapy. *Ann Intern Med* 1979; **91**: 517–20.
15. Graham DY. *Helicobacter pylori*: future directions in research. In: *Helicobacter pylori, Gastritis and Peptic Ulcer* (eds Malfertheiner P, Ditschuneit H), pp. 463–70. Berlin, Springer Verlag, 1990.
16. Graham DY, Lew GM, Kuwayama H. *Helicobacter pylori*: its clinical significance in gastroduodenal disease. *Endoscopia Digestiva*, 1992; **4**: 429–47.
17. Graham DY. *Campylobacter pylori* and peptic ulcer disease. *Gastroenterology* 1989; **96** (suppl): 615–25.
18. Hentschel E, Brandstatter G, Dragosics B. Effect of ranitidine and amoxicillin plus metronidazole on the eradication of Helicobacter pylori and the recurrence of duodenal ulcer. *N Eng J Med* 1993; **328**: 308–12.
19. Graham DY, Lew GM, Malarty HM *et al.* Factors influencing the eradication of *Helicobacter pylori* with triple therapy. *Gastroenterology* 1992; **102**: 493–6.
20. Graham DY. Gastroenterology today and tomorrow. *Am J Gastroenterol*, 1992; **87**: 559–61.
21. Tytgat GTN. Colloid bismuth subcitrate in peptic ulcer disease – a review. *Digestion* 1987; **37** (suppl 2): 31–41.
22. Marshall BJ, Warren JR, Blincow ED, Philips M, Goodwin CS. Prospective double blind trial of duodenal ulcer relapse after eradication of *campylobacter pylori. Lancet* 1988; **2**: 1427–1431.
23. Rauws EAJ, Tytgat GNJ. Cure of duodenal ulcer associated with eradication of *Helicobacter pylori. Lancet* 1990; **335**: 1233–5.
24. Wolfler A. Gastroenterostomie. *Zentrable Chir*, 1883; **8**: 705–7.
25. Moynihan BGA. Observations upon the treatment of chronic diseases of the stomach. *Surg Gynecol Obstet* 1908; **6**: 4.
26. Mayo WJ. A study of gastric and duodenal ulcers with special reference to their surgical cure. *Surg Gynecol Obstet* 1908; **6**: 600.
27. Lewisohn R. The frequency of gastro-jejunal ulcers. *Surg Gynecol Obstet* 1925; **40**: 70–4.
28. Ordahl NV, Ross RP, Baker DV. The failure of partial gastrectomy with gastroduodenostomy in the treatment of duodenal ulcer. *Surgery*, 1955; **38**: 158–61.
29. Golligher JC, Moir PJ, Rigley JH. Billroth 1 and polyagastrectomy operations for duodenal ulcer: a comparison. *Lancet* 1956; **2**: 220–2.

30. Farmer DA, Smithwick RH. Hemigastrectomy combined with resection of the vagus nerves. *New Eng J Med* 1952; **247**: 1017–22.
31. Farmer DA, Harrower HW, Smithwick RH. The choice of surgery in peptic ulcer disease. *Am J Surg* 1970; **120**: 295–9.
32. Herrington JL Jr, Sawyers JL, Scott HW Jr. A 25 year experience with vagotomy/antrectomy. *Arch Surg* 1983; **106**: 469–75.
33. Herrington JL Jr. Truncal vagotomy and antrectomy. Symposium on peptic ulcer disease 1976. *Surg Clin Am* 1976; **56**: 1335–49.
34. Dragstedt LR. Acid ulcer. *Ann Surg* 1936; **62**: 118–22.
35. Dragstedt LR, Overhelman HA, Smiktt CA. Experimental hyperfunction of the gastric antrum with ulcer formation. *Ann Surg* 1951; **134**: 332–6.
36. Weinberg JA, Stempien SJ, Movius HJ. Vagotomy and pyloroplasty in the treatment of duodenal ulcer. *Am J Surg* 1956; **92**: 202–6.
37. Dragstedt LR, Owens FM Jr. Supradiaphgramatic section of the vagus nerves in the treatment of duodenal ulcer. *Proc Soc Exp Biol Med* 1943; **53**: 152–4.
38. Ferguson GH, Rose M, MacLennan I, Taylor TV, Torrance HB. Vomiting following Roux en Y biliary diversion: relation to surgical technique. *Br J Surg* 1990; **77**: 584–91.
39. Ferguson GH, MacLennan I, Taylor TV, Torrance HB. Outcome of revisional gastric surgery using a Roux en Y biliary diversion. *Br J Surg* 1990; **77**: 551–5.
40. Taylor TV. The post vagotomy and cholecystectomy syndrome. *Ann Surg* 1981, **194**: 625–9.
41. Taylor TV, Lumbert ME, Qureshi A, Torrance HB. Should cholecystectomy be combined with vagotomy and pyloroplasty? *Lancet* 1978; **1**: 635–6.
42. Franksson C. Selective abdominal vagotomy. *Acta Chir Scand* 1948; **96**: 409–12.
43. Jackson RG. Anatomic study of the vagus nerves with a technique of transabdominal selective gastric vagus resection. *Arch Surg* 1948; **57**: 333–5.
44. Kennedy T, Magill P, Johnston GW. Proximal gastric vagotomy, fundoplication and lesser curve necrosis. *Br Med J* 1979; **1**: 1455–6.
45. Griffith CA, Stavney LS, Kato T, Harkins HN. Selective gastric vagotomy. *Am J Surg* 1963; **105**: 13–23.
46. Harkins HN, Stavney LS, Griffith CA, Savage LE, Kato T, Nyhus LM. Selective gastric vagotomy. *Ann Surg* 1963; **158**: 458–60.
47. Sawyers JL, Scott HW, Edwards WH, Shull HJ, Law DH. Comparative studies of the clinical effects of truncal and selective vagotomy. *Am J Surg* 1968; **115**: 165–72.
48. Andrup E, Jennsen HE. Selective vagotomy of the parietal cell mass preserving innervation of the undrained antrum. *Gastroenterology* 1970; **59**: 522–5.
49. Johnson D, Wilkinson AR. Highly selective vagotomy without a drainage procedure for duodenal ulcer. *Br J Surg* 1970; **57**: 289–93.
50. Griffith CA, Harkins HN. Partial gastric vagotomy: an experimental study. *Gastroenterology* 1957; **32**: 96–102.
51. Holle F, Hart W. Neue wede der chirurgie des gastroduodenulkus. *Med Klin* 1967, **62**: 441–5.
52. Joffe SM, Crockett A, Chang M, Bracket K. *In vitro* and *in vivo* technique for assessing vagus nerve regeneration after parietal cell vagotomy in the rat. In: *Vagal Nerve Function. Behaviour and Methodological Considerations* (eds Kral JG, Plowle PL, Brooks CM). Amsterdam, Elsevier, 1983.
53. Joffe SM, Crockett A, Doyle D. Morphological and functional evidence of reinnervation of a gastric parietal cell mass following a parietal cell vagotomy. *Am J Surg* 1982; **143**: 80–4.
54. Holle GE, Reiser SB. Effect of selective proximal gastric vagotomy without and with pyloroplasty on gastro-duodenal motility. *Am J Dig Sci* 1985; **36**: 773–7.
55. Holle F. Randomised study: SPV with versus without pyloroplasty. In: *Vagotomy – Latest Advances* (ed. Holle, F), pp. 182–3. Berlin, Springer-Verlag, 1974.

56. Johnston D. Operative mortality and postoperative morbidity of highly selective vagotomy. *Br Med J* 1975; **4**: 545–7.
57. Taylor TV. Lesser curve superficial seromyotomy – an operation for duodenal ulcer. *Br J Surg* 1979; **66**: 733–5.
58. Taylor TV. Lesser curve myotomy in the dog: an experimental study. *Ann Surg* 1980; **191**: 414–18.
59. Golligher JC, Hill GL, Kenny JE, Nutter E. Proximal gastric vagotomy without drainage for duodenal ulcer: results after 5–8 years. *Br J Surg* 1978; **65**: 145–8.
60. Andrup E, Anderson D, Jensen HE. Parietal cell vagotomy for peptic ulcer disease. *World J Surg* 1977; 119–23.
61. Hoffman J, Jensen HE, Ponsen PE *et al.* Prospective controlled vagotomy trial for duodenal ulcer. *Br J Surg* 1984; **73**: 583–7.
62. Daniel EE, Sarner SK. Distribution of excitatory vagal fibres in canine gastric wall to control motility. *Gastroenterology* 1976; **71**: 608–12.
63. Taylor TV, Gunn AA, MacLeod DA, MacLennan I. Anterior lesser curve seromyotomy with posterior truncal vagotomy in the treatment of chronic duodenal ulcer. *Lancet* 1982; **2**: 846–9.
64. Walker WS, Taylor TV. A modification to the technique of lesser curve seromyotomy. *Ann Roy Coll Surg Eng* 1982; **64**: 123–4.
65. Taylor TV, Holt S, Heading R. Gastric emptying after anterior lesser curve seromyotomy with posterior truncal vagotomy. *Br J Surg* 1985; **72**: 620–3.
66. Taylor TV, Gunn AA, MacLeod DAD *et al.* Morbidity and mortality following anterior lesser curve seromyotomy and posterior truncal vagotomy for duodenal ulcer. *Br J Surg* 1985; **72**: 950–1.
67. Moss JG, Gunn AA, MacLeod DAD. Anterior lesser curve seromyotomy and posterior truncal vagotomy for duodenal ulcer. *J Roy Coll Surg Edinb* 1985; **30**: 239–41.
68. Oostvogel HG, van Vroonhoven TMJ. Anterior lesser curve seromyotomy with posterior truncal vagotomy versus proximal gastric vagotomy. *Br J Surg* 1988; **75**: 121–4.
69. Oostvogel HJ, van Vroonhoven TMJ. Anterior lesser curve seromyotomy and posterior truncal vagotomy – technique and early results of a randomised trial. *Neth J Surg* 1985; **37**: 69–74.
70. Taylor TV, Thomas PE, Lythgoe PJ, MacFarland JB. Anterior lesser curve seromyotomy and posterior truncal vagotomy and pyloroplasty in the treatment of chronic duodenal ulcer – results of a prospective controlled trial. *Br J Surg* 1990; **77**: 1007–9.
71. Harling H, Balsley I, Bentzen E. Parietal cell vagotomy or cimetidine maintenance therapy for duodenal ulcer? *Scand J Gastroenterol* 1985; **20**: 747–50.
72. Graffner HO, Liedberg GF, Oscarson JEA. Parietal cell vagotomy in the surgical treatment of chronic duodenal, pyloric and prepyloric ulcer disease. *Int Surg* 1985; **70**: 139–42.
73. Anderson D. Prevention of ulcer recurrence – medical versus surgical treatment. A surgeon's view. *Scand J Gastroenterol* 1985; **20** (suppl. 110): 89–92.
74. Herrington JL Jr, Davidson J, Shumway SJ. Proximal gastric vagotomy: follow-up of 109 patients for 6–13 years. *Ann Surg* 1986; **204**: 108–13.
75. Von Holstein C, Graffner H, Oscarson J. One hundred patients ten years after parietal cell vagotomy. *Br J Surg* 1987; **74**: 101–3.
76. Enskog L, Rydberg B, Adamai HO, Enander LK, Invar C. Clinical results one to ten years after highly selective vagotomy in 306 patients with prepyloric and duodenal ulcer disease. *Br J Surg* 1986; **73**: 357–60.
77. Marceau P, Bourque RA, Piesch EP, Biron S, Potvin M. Long term results of hyperselective vagotomy for duodenal ulcer. *Canad J Surg* 1986; **29**: 421–3.

78. Paimela H, Hallikainen D, Ahonen J, Hockersted K, Palmu A, Scheinin TM. The prognostic significance of radiological determined gastric emptying time before proximal gastric vagotomy. *Acta Chir Scand* 1986; **152**: 611–15.
79. Primrose JN, Axon ATR, Johnston D. Highly selective vagotomy and duodenal ulcers that fail to respond to H_2 receptor antagonists. *Br Med J* 1988; **206**: 1031–5.
80. Jordan PH Jr, Thornby J. Should it be parietal cell vagotomy or selective vagotomy/ antrectomy for the treatment of duodenal ulcer? A progress report. *Ann Surg* 1987; **205**: 572–87.
81. Muller C, Liebermann-Meffert D, Allgower M. Pyloric and prepyloric ulcers. *World J Surg* 1987; **11**: 339–44.
82. Bauerfeind P, Koelz HR, Blum AL. Ulcer treatment: regimens and duration of inhibition of acid secretion: how long to dose. *Scand J Gastroenterol* 1988; **23** suppl 153: 23–32.
83. Ruben R. Medical treatment of peptic ulcer disease. *Med Clin N Am* 1991; **75**: 981–98.
84. Her Majesty's Stationery Office. Mortality statistics (general): review of the Registrar General on Deaths in England and Wales. 1990: Series DHI 24/32.
85. Katschinski BD, Logan R. Changes in the birth cohort pattern of peptic ulcer mortality in England and Wales. *Post Grad Med J* 1991; **67**: 825–8.
86. Crabtree JE, Taylor JD, Wyatt JI, Heatley RV, Shallcross TM, Tomkinson S. Mucosal IgA recognition in Helicobacter pylori 120 kDa protein, peptic ulceration and gastric pathology. *Lancet* 1991; **338**: 332–5.
87. Walt R, Logan R, Katschinski BD, Ashley J, Langman M. Frequency of ulcer perforations in elderly people in the United Kingdom. *Lancet* 1986; **1**: 489–92.
88. Naschitz JE, Zeshurun D, Odeh M, Basan H, Rosner I, Stermer E. Overt gastrointestinal bleeding in the course of chronic aspirin administration for secondary prevention of arterial occlusion disease. *Amer J Gastroenterol* 1990; **85**: 408–10.
89. Silvoso GR, Ivey KJ, Butt JH, Lockard OO, Holt SD, Sisk C. Incidence of gastric lesions in patients with rheumatic disease on chronic aspirin therapy. *Ann Intern Med* 1979; **91**: 517–20.
90. MacLaine Ross AH, Smith AA, Anderson JR, Small WP. Late mortality after surgery for peptic ulcer. *New Eng J Med* 1982; **307**: 519–22.
91. Shapiro S, Gordon L, Dayhkovsky L, Grundfest W, Chandra M. Development of laparoscopic anterior seromyotomy and right posterior truncal vagotomy for ulcer prophylaxis. *J Laparo Endosc Surg* 1991; **1**: 277–86.
92. Voeller GR, Pridgen WL, Mangaint EC. Laparoscopic posterior truncal vagotomy and anterior seromyotomy. A pig model. *J Laparo Endosc Surg* 1991; **1**: 375–9.
93. Hunter JG, Becker JM, Lee RG, Christian PE, Dixon JA. Anterior lesser curve seromyotomy with posterior truncal vagotomy: a potential treatment for peptic ulcer disease. *Brit J Surg* 1989, **76**: 949–52.
94. British Medical Association and the Pharmaceutical Press. *British National Formulary*, pp. 31–4. London British Medical Association and the Pharmaceutical Press, 1992.

10.2

Laparoscopic Posterior Truncal Vagotomy and Anterior Seromyotomy

J. MOUIEL and N. KATKHOUDA

INTRODUCTION

Posterior truncal vagotomy and anterior seromyotomy is the operation of choice when the laparoscopic approach is used for the treatment of chronic duodenal ulcer disease. In comparison to other operative techniques of vagotomy, the operation described by Taylor is the most simple and rapid and is extremely effective, as has been confirmed by our own results from 1989, at which time the procedure was undertaken at open surgery.[1,2]

PRINCIPLES

The principle of the operation is based on the anatomical works of Latarjet which showed that the nerves responsible for stimulating acid secretion arose from the anterior and posterior gastric nerves. These nerves pass in the superficial seromuscular layer before penetrating the gastric wall, along with the vascular pedicles. The division of the seromuscular layer down to the mucosa therefore leads to the division of the secretory pneumogastric branches (Fig. 10.2.1) and it has been established experimentally that, to be effective, the seromyotomy must be undertaken exactly 1.5 cm parallel to the lesser curve.

The technique originally described by Taylor in 1979[3] consisted of a division of the seromuscular layer along the lesser curve on both the anterior and posterior layers of the stomach from the oesophagogastric junction down to the incisura, thereby producing a selective denervation of the fundus. In 1982, the same author[4] proposed that the posterior seromyotomy be replaced with a posterior truncal vagotomy, a procedure which had already been undertaken in 1979 by Hill and Barker[5] as part of the selective vagotomy. This division of the

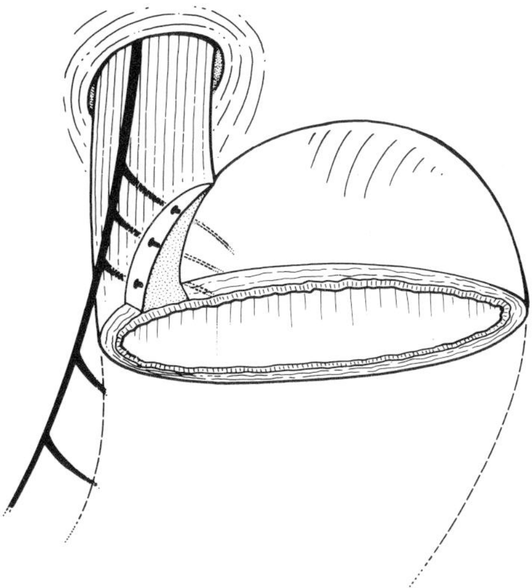

Figure 10.2.1. The principles of Taylor's operation. Posterior truncal vagotomy assures the denervation of the posterior cellular mass. The anterior seromyotomy assures the highly selective denervation of the anterior cellular mass.

posterior vagus nerve guarantees a complete denervation of the posterior territory and, as Smith[6] and Burge[7] have shown, produces no secondary effects associated with the denervation of the pancreas and the intestine. In particular, postoperative diarrhoea is avoided and the motility in the pyloric and antral region is maintained. Similarly, the anterior seromyotomy preserves the pyloric branches of the nerve of Latarjet (Fig. 10.2.2), thereby preserving the antral pump and avoiding pylorospasm. This, in turn, ensures the physiological emptying of the stomach by dispensing with the need for an associated drainage procedure. The experimental validity of this has been established by Daniel[8] who has shown that the pyloric branches of the anterior nerve of Latarjet in the dog are sufficient to ensure maintenance of gastric emptying.

SELECTION OF PATIENTS AND OPERATIVE INDICATIONS

The preoperative evaluation of patients with duodenal ulceration is the same for those patients to be operated on laparoscopically as those submitted to open surgery. The investigation comprises a general assessment of risk factors and an evaluation of the ulcer disease by endoscopy, in addition to radiological and secretory studies. The endoscopy provides an accurate localization of the ulcer, detects the presence of superinfection with *Helicobacter pylori*[9] and excludes disease elsewhere. The barium swallow and meal, to which we have remained

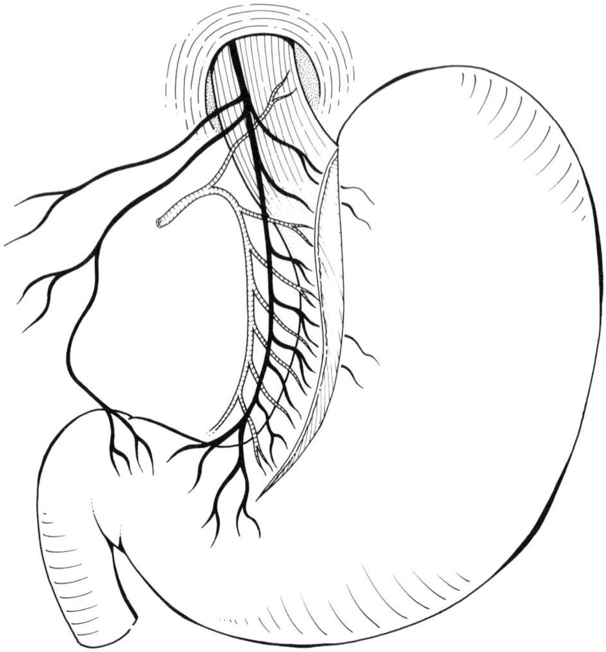

Figure 10.2.2 The anterior seromyotomy begins at the oesophagogastric junction extending parallel with the lesser curve at 1.5 cm exactly from its border and ending at the crow's foot, preserving the last few pyloric and antral branches.

faithful, provides the morphological evaluation, notably of the dynamic state of the fundus, in addition to the function of the antral pump and duodenal emptying, which can also be studied using isotope scans. These examinations allow the presence of a prepyloric ulcer to be excluded, which at the present time we believe is a poor indication for laparoscopic treatment[10,11] and establish the presence of oesophagitis associated with gastro-oesophageal reflux with or without an associated hiatus hernia. The presence of significant pyloric stenosis must also be excluded. The secretory study comprises an assessment of basal acid output and a pentagastrin stimulation test. These investigations are necessary to assess the degree of hyperacidity in those patients who have been resistant to medical treatment. This preoperative evaluation will also provide useful information on the effectiveness of operative treatment by measuring the drop in postoperative acid secretion. In addition to these assessments, the blood gastrin level is established to eliminate the presence of a gastrinoma.[10,12]

The operative indications in the elective situation are for ulcers resistant to medical treatment in patients who have been well followed-up during treatment for at least two years with the relevant endoscopic assessment and without the development of complications. Surgery can be proposed, however, in those patients who are unwilling to consider long term medical treatment or who cannot be followed up for geographical or socioeconomical reasons.

New perspectives have opened up with minimally invasive therapy and allowed the opportunity for an informed choice by the patient, who may opt for long term medical treatment on the one hand or a laparoscopic cure on the other.

OPERATIVE PROCEDURE

The preoperative evaluation of the patient, the general anaesthetic and the peroperative monitoring are the same as for those employed at open surgery. In the same way, the creation and maintenance of the pneumoperitoneum, the use of video endoscopy, the techniques of suction, irrigation, diathermy and coagulation are the same as for those of other laparoscopic procedures and are described in the preceding chapters in this book. The specific problems related to laparoscopic vagotomy, including the positioning of the patient, the instruments, the access and the techniques of haemostasis are described.

Positioning

The positioning of the patient for vagotomy is similar to that for cholecystectomy. It is preferable to have a tilting operating table, allowing a 15° tilt (reverse Trendelenburg) and a left lateral rotation of 15°. It is our practice to place a small support between the shoulder blades which are raised by about 10 cm. With the patient under general anaesthesia and tracheal intubation, a nasogastric tube is passed. The surgeon stands between the legs of the patient with the nurse assistant to the patient's left, with the video endoscopy and suction equipment, and a second monitor is placed on the right, with the laser and electrocoagulation. Two assistants are helpful; one on the left and other on the right of the patient.

Instrumentation

In addition to the normal instruments for laparoscopic surgery, we recommend the use of a 30° laparoscope or a retractor. We employ an endoretractor to raise the anterior abdominal wall. It is useful to have a coagulating hook with a channel which allows any smoke to escape. We also routinely use a dissector which can hold small dissecting swabs, curved coagulating scissors, a dissector or a curved memory instrument or an articulated curved instrument. For haemostasis we either use single or multiple clip applicators. For any suturing that is required, two needle holders are required with curved needles (32 mm and 26 mm), in addition to ski needles mounted with non-absorbable suture material (2/0 and 4/0).

Access (Fig. 10.2.3)

We routinely employ five ports (Fig. 10.2.3) which are inserted under CO_2 pneumoperitoneum which is controlled electronically at a pressure of 14 mmHg. The first port for the laparoscope is positioned two finger breadths to the right and above the umbilicus which allows the insertion of the other cannulae under vision. The second port is placed in the epigastric region, for the retractor; the third is positioned in the right subcostal region; and the fourth in the left subcostal region, for the dissectors. The fifth is positioned two finger breadths above and to the left of the umbilicus, for the main operating channel. It is useful to use 10 mm cannulae for the laparoscope, the operating channel and the left subcostal port, which allows the movement of the laparoscope and the instruments from one port to the other, thereby improving access, in particular in the region of the oesophagogastric angle. We recommend, however, that a device is used to retract the complete anterior abdominal wall with a pneumoperitoneum of around 8 mmHg to avoid the risk of pneumomediastinum and pneumothorax. These risks are not insignificant in the obese patient, where there is a large left

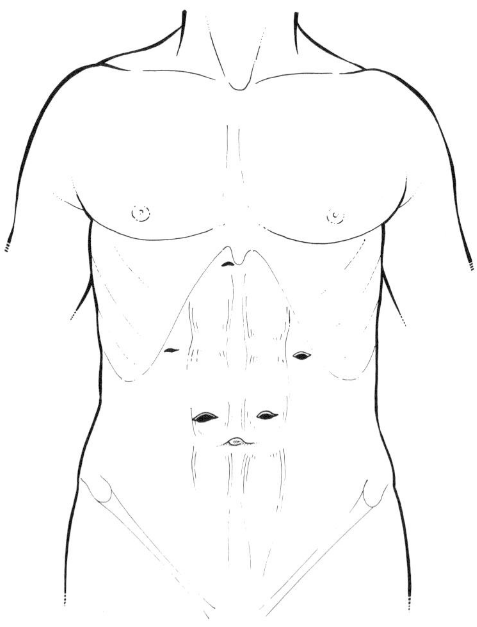

Figure 10.2.3 Access using five trocars for the endoscope, the liver retractor, the grasping forceps and other instruments.

lobe of liver, in patients previously operated on and where the dissection time is prolonged because of the need for adhesiolysis.

Exploration

The operation starts following the insertion of the laparoscopic port, allowing the diagnosis to be confirmed and, following mobilization of the intra-abdominal structures and in particular the left lobe of the liver, verifying that the operation can be undertaken safely by the laparoscopic approach. In cases of difficulty, open surgery is to be preferred, the patient having already agreed preoperatively that this may be required.

The surgeon must firstly confirm the diagnosis of duodenal ulceration, confirming its precise localization and appreciating the anatomical relationships. The lesser omentum must be carefully examined, in particular to exclude the presence of an aberrant left hepatic artery. An assessment of the oesophago-gastric angle, the distribution of the short gastric vessels and the recognition of the anterior branches of the nerve of Latarjet must be undertaken. This evaluation is made easier with the use of a 30° laparoscope and by an indirect form of bimanual palpation using an atraumatic dissector and a probe or dissecting swab. It is important to complete this examination by establishing the presence of associated gastric pathology (such as hiatus hernia) with the stomach above and below the transverse mesocolon (adhesions, cholecystitis, biliary cysts, diverticulitis and pelvic pathology in the female).

Laparoscopic Dissection

Sharp dissection is undertaken with the coagulating scissors and the coagulating hook, with the access to the hiatus and the seromyotomy. Blunt dissection is undertaken with a small dissecting swab to facilitate the mobilization of the oesophagus and in particular to locate the posterior vagal trunk. Haemostasis is achieved with electrocautery for small vessels and with clip or ligation for larger vessels. The approximation of tissues is achieved with interrupted or continuous sutures, which are tied using either intra- or extracorporeal techniques. It is useful to secure the approximation of the anterior wall of the stomach with the application of some fibrin glue.

The procedure is undertaken in three stages: access to the hiatus, posterior vagotomy and the anterior seromyotomy.

1. Access to the Hiatus

The left lobe of the liver is raised with the help of the retractor placed in the epigastric port. The surgeon gains access to the hiatal region by opening the lesser omentum which is stretched by two retracting dissectors at the level of the

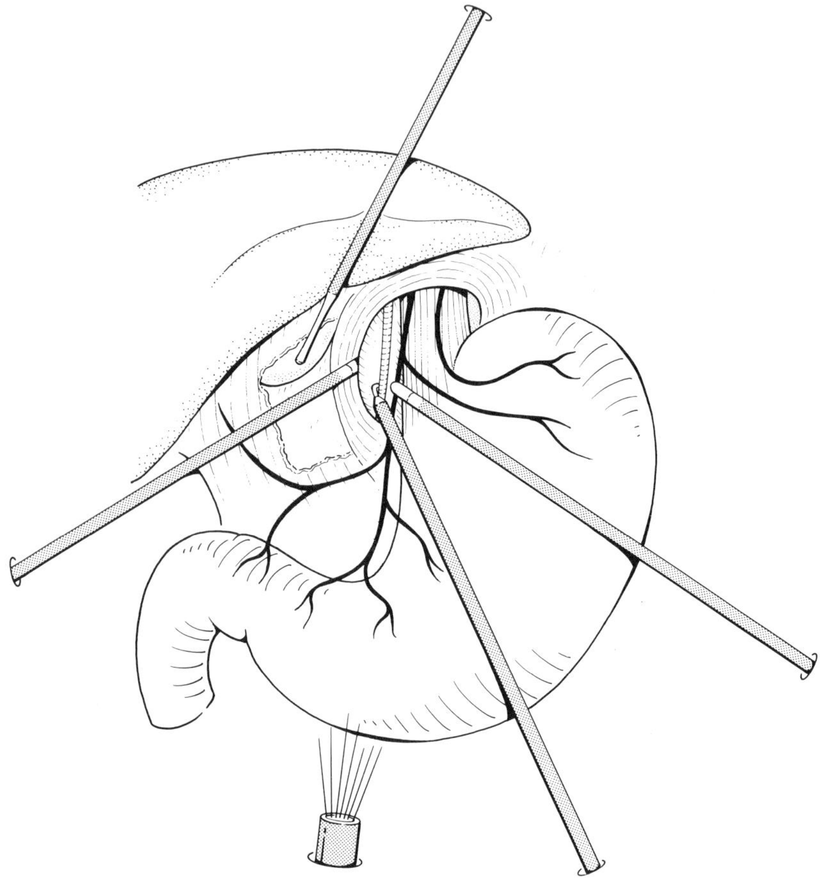

Figure 10.2.4 Approach to the oesophageal hiatus and the posterior vagus curve.

right crus of the diaphragm (Fig. 10.2.4). This division gives access to the upper part of the lesser sac, whilst respecting the gastrohepatic nerves of the anterior nerve of Latarjet. The incision is carried down to the region of the right crus and is mobilized along its length.

2. The Posterior Truncal Vagotomy

The two landmarks for laparoscopic posterior truncal vagotomy are the caudate lobe (segment I) on one side and the right crus of the diaphragm on the other (Fig. 10.2.5). The right crus is grasped by a dissector and is drawn towards the right, thereby providing access to the paraoesophageal peritoneum. The peritoneal incision along the border of the right crus allows access to the posterior aspect of the oesophagus into the meso-oesophagus by retracting outside and to the left of the abdominal oesophagus. It is in this area that the white cores of the

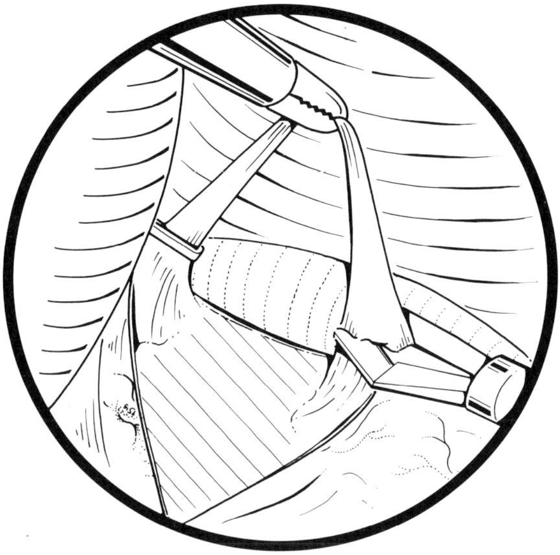

Figure 10.2.5 Posterior truncal vagotomy: the posterior trunk of the vagus nerve is clipped before being divided.

posterior vagus can be easily identified within this angle. It is grasped by a dissector and held taut, cleared of any associated small vessels with the coagulating hook and a segment is resected between two clips for histological confirmation of the completeness of vagotomy.

3. The Anterior Seromyotomy

The anterior wall of the stomach is displayed with the help of grasping forceps inserted into the right and left subcostal ports and the position of the seromyotomy marked out with the coagulating hook from the oesophagogastric junction to the crow's foot following the lesser curve at a distance of about 1.5 cm. This seromyotomy is undertaken with the coagulating hook using monopolar coagulation. The hook is used to successfully incise the serosa and the oblique and circular muscle layers. The two grasping forceps can be used to hold the two edges of the incision in this way, allowing the deep circular muscle fibres to be better displayed (Fig. 10.2.6). These muscles are therefore torn by the mechanical effect of traction and eventually completed by the coagulating hook. After having divided the last muscular fibres, it is easy to verify the integrity of the protruding mucosa, since the field division is magnified by the endoscopy. The hook is manipulated from above to below to divide the superficial muscular layer and from below to above to isolate the submucosal layer, as if one were undertaking a Heller cardiomyotomy. The seromyotomy is undertaken progressively using almost the same technique.

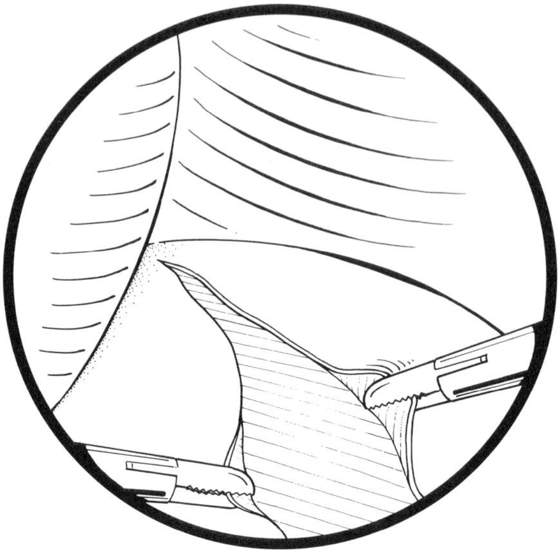

Figure 10.2.6 Elevation of each side of the incision during the seromyotomy with gastric mucosa visible between them.

During this dissection, as in open surgery, three to five short vessels can be encountered in the line of dissection and need to be divided following haemostasis. For this, one can employ the technique used by Taylor himself in his first few cases, isolating the seromuscular vessels with the hook passing under the vessels and then dividing these between clips or, alternatively, these vessels can be secured with interrupted sutures. It is necessary to be extremely careful in achieving adequate haemostasis during the course of the seromyotomy. The completed seromyotomy leaves an incision 7–8 mm wide following the division of the circular muscle layers. Having verified the integrity of the mucosa, the seromyotomy is closed with two or three running sutures with the knots being tied either intra- or extracorporeally (Fig. 10.2.7). It is useful to further secure this incision with fibrin glue. Having confirmed haemostasis with suction irrigation, the pneumoperitoneum is discontinued under hyperventilation and the cutaneous access ports are closed with subcutaneous sutures following infiltration with bupivacaine.

Two variations of the technique have been described. The seromyotomy can be undertaken using a contact Nd.Yag laser.[13] Alternatively, a linear anterior gastrectomy[14] can be undertaken using a 3 and 6 cm Endo GIA. The "tissue thickness measuring device" confirms that the Endo GIA can be used for the staple resection of the anterior gastric wall. The inferior landmark in the region of the crow's foot is grasped and this serves as a guide for the stapling device which is fired parallel to the lesser curve up to the oesophagogastric angle. A 60 F gauge oesophageal bougie prevents any stricturing in this area. The anterior gastrectomy specimen is removed and the presence of all the layers of the gastric

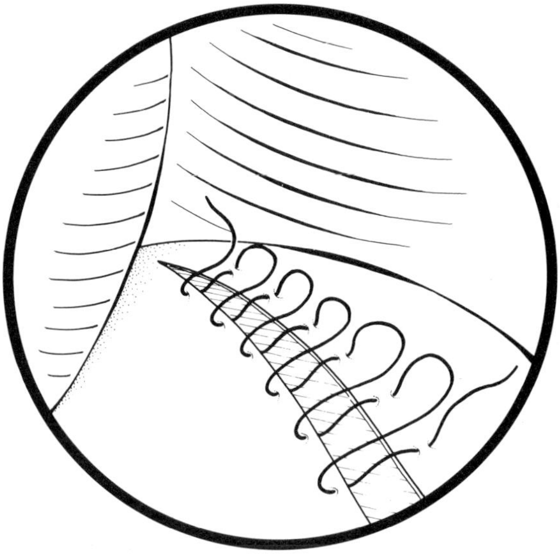

Figure 10.2.7 Overlapping suture closure of the seromyotomy.

wall are verified. The experimental and clinical results of this approach appear to have confirmed that this is effective.[14,15]

Peroperative Assessment

Assessment of the mucosal integrity is essential and it is useful to distend the stomach with 150–250 ml of methylene blue stained saline passed through the nasogastric tube. The completeness of vagotomy can be undertaken with a Congo red test[16] since it is easy to confirm the colour change to black in the acid zone under peroperative endoscopic control. The presence of an island of mucosa stained black in the region of the fundus suggests that the denervation has been incomplete and a search will be made to verify the completeness of the seromyotomy. Finally, the patency of the duodenum and the absence of pyloro-spasm can be confirmed peroperatively by endoscopic means.

Treatment of Associated Lesions

Any associated lesions in the supracolic compartment should be dealt with at the same time, as is the case in open surgery; cholecystectomy for cholelithiasis, fundoplication for reflux oesophagitis associated with a hiatus hernia and resistant to medical treatment, deroofing of hepatic cysts and adhesiolysis for any associated adhesions. In these situations, the use of an abdominal wall retractor under low pressure pneumoperitoneum avoids the secondary effects of prolonged insufflation with CO_2.

POSTOPERATIVE COURSE

The postoperative course, as for all laparoscopic surgery, is usually uneventful. Postoperative pain is significantly reduced because of the minimal access procedure and the use of local anaesthetic infiltration for the wounds. It is therefore unusual for analgesics to be prescribed by injection in the postoperative period. The postoperative recovery period is very short in the absence of any invasive perioperating monitoring. The nasogastric tube is maintained for the first 24 hours, but thereafter oral nutrition is gradually introduced and the patients are normally discharged on the third or fourth postoperative day.

PRESENT EXPERIENCE

At the present time, we have undertaken 62 such operations in the elective situation in 12 females and 50 males (19–61 years) who have had a duodenal ulcer resistant to medical treatment and followed for at least two years. In the majority of these patients, this treatment has included antacids, H_2 receptor antagonists with or without omeprazole and with or without a course of amoxycillin where *Helicobacter pylori* has been implicated in the ulcer diathesis. These patients have presented with an average of 2.8 ulcer recurrences each year under treatment and six of them have presented with significant gastrointestinal bleeding which has responded well to medical treatment.

The procedure has lasted on average 140 minutes (range 120–220 minutes). In a few patients there was a significant episode of hypercapnia which responded well to appropriate measures, but which led us to consider more often the use of an abdominal wall retractor to minimize the pneumoperitoneal pressure. There has been no breach of the gastric mucosa and we have not needed to convert any patient to an open procedure. The postoperative course has been uneventful without any death and postoperative morbidity limited to a pneumothorax in one patient which was treated by a chest drain for 24 hours.

In the longer term, one patient has developed significant reflux oesophagitis. Two patients developed intragastric food boluses which settled on medical treatment and two patients developed transitory diarrhoea. Follow-up at two months following surgery has shown healing of the ulcer in 59 cases and the presence of a scar in three further patients. The secretory tests have shown a diminution in the basal acid output of 78% and 80% reduction in pentagastrin stimulated acid secretion. Follow-up at two years has shown two recurrences which have responded to medical treatment and in both patients the ulcers were prepyloric. At two years the reduction in acid output has been maintained with basal acid output and pentagastrin stimulated acid secretion being reduced by 65%. Other authors have confirmed this laparoscopic experience using Taylor's technique such as Lirici,[17] Cuschieri,[18] Pietrafitta[19] and Shapiro.[20] Others have followed variations of this operation using a linear gastrectomy.[14,15]

DISCUSSION

Posterior truncal vagotomy with anterior seromyotomy has been validated in open surgery in a multicentre study comprising 605 patients operated on by 11 different teams using the same technique.[21] Postoperative mortality was very low, with only one postoperative death (0.5%) from a myocardial infarct. Morbidity has been extremely low; in particular, necrosis of the lesser curve and gastric fistulation have not been observed. The duration of hospitalization has been short, as in the case of highly selective vagotomy, and has generally been less than a week. The assessment of outcome has been satisfactory with 94% of patients having been graded Visick 1 or 2. It was noted, however, that 12% of patients had problems with gastric emptying which required a drainage procedure. More recently, an endoscopic dilatation of the pylorus has replaced this.[22] No cases of dumping syndrome have been identified, although two patients have complained of persistent diarrhoea. The recurrent ulcer rate was 1.5% in the 181 patients who had been followed for a period of at least five years. In contrast, the variation described by Hill and Barker[5] combining a posterior truncal vagotomy and highly selective anterior vagotomy has never been submitted to formal validation at open surgery. The initial study comprised only 25 patients without a controlled population.

Controlled studies have compared Taylor's procedures to other operative approaches such as truncal vagotomy and highly selective vagotomy. In one study[23] seromyotomy was thought to be as straightforward and effective as truncal vagotomy, with a similar reduction in acid production with the recurrent ulcer rate of 3% compared with 6% for truncal vagotomy. The advantage, however, was the absence of secondary effects such as dumping syndrome and diarrhoea and no evidence of delayed gastric emptying. In the same way, seromyotomy was judged to be as effective in terms of reducing acid production and maintaining gastric motility as highly selective vagotomy.[24] Equally, the technique has provided other undeniable technical advantages which have been confirmed by authors using the technique. It is an easier procedure to undertake and more rapid, providing constant results, even in the obese patient, since the success of the operation is independent of the anatomic variation of the nerves of Latarjet.

The experience of colleagues[25,26] and of our own team convinced us to transpose this procedure to one which could be undertaken by laparoscopic means.[1,2,27–31] This minimally invasive approach has posed the question regarding the therapeutic indications over the last few years where the role of surgery has been considerably limited.[3] The reduction in the surgical indications can be explained in some part by a better understanding of the ulcer diathesis and the factors associated with recurrence.[32] The recognition of factors such as stress, tobacco and alcohol, along with the recognition of superinfection with *Helicobacter pylori*,[9] have paralleled the introduction of effective medical treatment such as H_2 receptor antagonists, omeprazole and gastric mucosal protectors to the point where one could have said that the ulcer resistant to medical treatment no longer existed.[33,34] This reduction in surgical indications can also be explained on the evidence of the long term secondary effects of classical surgical treatments, with a high risk of ulcer recurrence following highly selective vagotomy[35–37] or with complications of dumping or diarrhoea often associated with truncal vagotomy.[10,34,38,39]

However, there are a number of drawbacks to medical treatment. The natural history of the disease[32] is not free from complications which are not often taken into account in reports in the medical literature. Whereas it is true that the medical treatments are generally accepted as being very effective,[33] recurrence develops on cessation of treatment no matter which drug is used in 70–90% of cases. It has been suggested that maintenance treatment be continued for five years[40] with, despite all this, the recognition of recurrences following cessation of prolonged treatment of the order of 16%. [Eradication of *Helicobacter pylori* and taking into account risk factors predicting recurrence such as alcohol and tobacco are likely to reduce the incidence of ulcer recurrence,[33] but in all of these cases, compliance with prolonged preventive medical treatment is difficult to obtain in a condition which can continue to cause problems over a number of years.[32]] Laparoscopic surgery is likely to be used to treat this type of severe ulcer in patients who are non-compliant to medical treatment. Furthermore, doubt still exists over the long term secondary effects of antisecretory drugs such as omeprazole.[41,42]

The choice is clear and must lie between a prolonged medical treatment and an effective minimally invasive surgical treatment, with the patient being well informed of the therapeutic options. In this way, all the various types of vagotomy have been proposed: truncal vagotomy by laparoscopic or thoracoscopic means with endoscopic dilatation of the pylorus to avoid problems with gastric emptying,[27,43] or a posterior truncal vagotomy and anterior highly selective vagotomy as described by Bailey and Zucker,[44,45] or the highly selective vagotomy as described by Weerts and Dallemagne.[46] It is argued that this is the operation of choice in open surgery.[47] The long term results appear to depend essentially on the experience of the surgeon,[48] with the recurrence rate at ten years ranging from 2% for Johnston[47] to 30% for Hoffmann.[38] It is for this reason that we proposed this form of ultraselective vagotomy which comprises a posterior truncal vagotomy with anterior seromyotomy, an operation which is rapid and constantly reproducible.[1,21,30]

CONCLUSIONS

Posterior truncal vagotomy and anterior seromyotomy is a procedure that has been validated by multicentre studies and by controlled study at open surgery. It combines the rapidity and effectiveness of a truncal vagotomy with the advantage of maintaining the gastric antral pump with an ultraselective vagotomy. Convinced by this conventional surgical experience, we have undertaken laparoscopically the approach first described by Taylor with the same initial results. It is for this reason that we believe that this minimally invasive surgery has opened a new era in the effective treatment of ulcer disease which will have to be balanced in the future with the long term medical treatments. Nonetheless, like all new techniques, this laparoscopic procedure must be the subject of multicentre controlled studies to evaluate the long term results.

REFERENCES

1. Mouiel J, Katkhouda N, Gugenheim J, Fabiani P, Goubaux B. Traitement de l'ulcere duodenal par vagotomie tronculaire posterieure et seromyotomie anterieure sous video-laparoscopie. Note preliminaire avec presentation de film. Academie de Chirurgie, Paris, Seance du 6 juin 1990. *Chirurgie* 1990; **116**: 546–51.
2. Katkhouda N, Mouiel J. A new surgical technique of treatment of chronic duodenal ulcer without laparotomy by videocoelioscopy. *Am J Surg* 1991; **161**: 361–4.
3. Taylor TV. Lesser curve superficial seromyotomy. An operation for chronic duodenal ulcer. *Br J Surg* 1979; **66**: 733–7.
4. Taylor TV, MacLeod DAD, Gunn AA, MacLennan I. Anterior lesser curve seromyotomy and posterior truncal vagotomy in the treatment of chronic duodenal ulcer. *Lancet* 1982; **ii**: 846–8.
5. Hill GL, Barker MCJ. Anterior highly selective vagotomy with posterior truncal vagotomy: a simple technique for denervating the parietal cell mass. *Br J Surg* 1978; **65**: 702–5.
6. Smith GK, Farris JM. Some observations upon selective gastric vagotomy. *Arch Surg* 1963; **86**: 716.
7. Burge HW, Hutchinson JSF, Longland CJ *et al.* Selective nerve section in the prevention of post-vagotomy diarrhoea. *Lancet* 1964; **1**: 577.
8. Daniel EE, Sarna SK. Distribution of excitatory vagal fibres in canine gastric wall to central motility. *Gastroenterol* 1986; 295–420.
9. Hentschel E, Brandstatter G, Dragosics B *et al.* Effect of ranitidine and amoxicillin plus metronidazole on the eradication of *Helicobacter pylori* and the recurrence of duodenal ulcer. *New Eng J Med* 1993; **328**: 308–12.

10. Hautefeuille P, Picaud R. *Les Recidives apres Vagotomies pour Ulcere Duodenal.* Rapport presente au 85e Congres de Chirurgie, Monographies de l'Association Francaise de Chirurgie. Paris, Masson, 1983.
11. Johnston D, Blackett RL. Recurrent peptic ulcers. *World J Surg* 1987; **11**: 274–82.
12. Mignon M, Ruszniewski PH, Haffar S, Rigaud D, Rene E, Bonfils S. Current approach to the management of tumoral process in patients with gastrinoma. *World J Surg* 1986; **10**: 703–10.
13. Pietraffita JJ, Schultz LS, Graber JN *et al.* Laser laparoscopic vagotomy and pyloromyotomy. *Gastrointest Endosc* 1991; **37**: 338–43.
14. Gomez-Ferrer F, Arenas J, Marin M, Pardo J. Gastrectomie lineaire fundique et vagotomie tronculaire posterieure. *J Coeliochis* 1993; **4**: 34–7.
15. Hannon JK, Snow LL, Weinstein SL. Endoscopic staple assisted anterior highly selective vagotomy combined with posterior truncal vagotomy for treatment of peptic ulcer disease. *Surg Laparosc Endosc* 1992; **2**: 254–257.
16. Donahue PE, Bombeck CT, Yoshida J, Nyhus LM. The simplified endoscopic Congo Red test for completeness of vagotomy. *Surg Gynecol Obstet* 1986; **163**: 287–9.
17. Lirici MM, Buess G, Becker HD. The laparoscopic approach to modified Taylor's procedure in the treatment of chronic duodenal ulcer: an improved technique. *Surg Laparosc Endosc* 1992; **2**: 199–204.
18. Cuschieri A. Personal communication.
19. Pietrafitta JJ. Laparoscopic peptic ulcer surgery. In: *Laparoscopic Abdominal Surgery* (eds Graber JN, Schultz LS, Pietrafitta JJ, Hickok DF), pp. 233–44. New York, McGraw-Hill, 1993.
20. Shapiro S, Gordon L, Dayhkovsky L, Grundfest W, Chandra M. Development of laparoscopic anterior seromyotomy and right posterior truncal vagotomy for ulcer prophylaxis. *J Laparoendosc Surg* 1991; **1**: 279–86.
21. Taylor TV, Gunn AA, MacLeod DAD *et al.* Morbidity and mortality after anterior lesser curve seromyotomy and posterior truncal vagotomy for duodenal ulcer. *Br J Surg* 1985; **722**: 950–1.
22. Taylor TV. Experience with the Lunderquist Ownman dilator in the upper gastro-intestinal tract. *Br J Surg* 1983; **70**: 445.
23. Taylor TV, Lythgoe JP, McFarland JB, Gilmore IT, Thomas PE, Ferguson GH. Anterior lesser curve seromyotomy and posterior truncal vagotomy versus truncal vagotomy and pyloroplasty in the treatment of chronic duodenal ulcer. *Br J Surg* 1990; **77**: 1007–9.
24. Oostvogel HJM, van Vroonhoven TJMV. Anterior seromyotomy and posterior truncal vagotomy. Technique and early results of a randomized trial. *Neth J Surg* 1985; **37**: 69–74.
25. Kahwaji F, Grange D. Ulcere duodenal chronique. Traitement par seromyotomie fundique anterieure avec vagotomie tronculaire posterieure. *Presse Med* 1987; **16**: 28–30.
26. Mouiel J. *Actualites Digestives Medico-Chirurgicales*, 10e edition, pp. 20–2. Paris, Masson, 1989.
27. Triboulet JP. Progres dans le traitement de l'ulcere duodenal. La seromyotomie avec vagotomie. In: *Actualites Digestives Medico-Chirurgicales*, 10e edition (ed. Mouiel, J), pp. 15–22. Paris, Masson, 1989.
28. Mouiel J, Katkhouda N. Laparoscopic truncal and selective vagotomy. In: *Surgical Laparoscopy*, (eds Zucker K, Bailey RW), pp. 263–79. St Louis, Missouri, QMP, 1991.
29. Mouiel J, Katkhouda N. Traitement de l'ulcere duodenal non complique. In: *La Chirurgie Digestive par Voie Coelioscopique* (eds Testas P, Delaitre B), pp. 137–45. Paris, Vigot Ed, 1991.
30. Mouiel J, Katkhouda N. Laparoscopic vagotomy in the treatment of chronic duodenal ulcer disease. In: *Problems in General Surgery* (eds Nyhus LM, Berci G), pp. 358–65. Philadelphia, Lippincott, 1991.

31. Mouiel J, Katkhouda N. Laparoscopic anterior seromyotomy and posterior truncal vagotomy. In: *Operative Manual of Endoscopic Surgery* (eds Cuschieri A, Buess G, Perissat J), pp. 263–72). Berlin, Springer-Verlag, 1992.
32. Waisbren SJ, Modlin JM. The evolution of therapeutic vagotomy. *Surg Gynecol Obstet* 1990; **170**: 261–72.
33. Wormsley KG. Histoire naturelle et facteurs predictifs de la recidive des ulceres duodenaux pendant le traitement d'entretien. In: *Controle de la Secretion Acide* (eds Mignon M, Galmiche JP, Ruszniewski Ph, Pappo M), pp. 171–80. Paris, John Libbey Eurotext, 1988.
34. Tytgat GNJ, Lamers CBHW, Hameeteman W *et al.* Omeprazole in peptic ulcers resistant to histamine H_2 receptor antagonists. *Aliment Pharmacol Therapeut* 1987; **1**: 31–8.
35. Hollender LF, Marrie A. *La Vagotomie Supra-selective.* Paris, Masson, 1977.
36. Jordan PH. An interim report on parietal cell vagotomy versus selective vagotomy and antrectomy for treatment of duodenal ulcer. *Ann Surg* 1979; **5**: 643–53.
37. Andersen D, Andrup E, Hostrup H, Sorensen FH. The Aarhus County vagotomy trial: trends in the problem of recurrent ulcer after parietal cell vagotomy and selective gastric vagotomy with drainage. *World J Surg* 1982; **6**: 86–92.
38. Hoffmann J, Olesen A, Jensen HE. Prospective 14 to 18-year follow-up after parietal cell vagotomy. *Br J Surg* 1987; **74**: 1056–9.
39. Dragstedt LR, Lulu DJ. Truncal vagotomy and pyloroplasty: critical evaluation of one hundred cases. *Am J Surg* 1974; **128**: 344–6.
40. Penston JG, Wormsley KG. Efficacy and safety of long-term maintenance therapy of duodenal ulcers. *Scand J Gastroenterol* 1989; **24**: 1145–52.
41. Ekman L, Hansson E, Havu N, Carlsson E, Lundborg P. Toxicological studies on omeprazole. *Scand J Gastroenterol* 1985; **20** (suppl. 108); 53–69.
42. Lambert R, Creutzfeldt W, Stockmann F, Jacubaschke U, Maas S, Brunner G. Long-term omeprazole treatment in man: effects on gastric endocrine cell population. *Digest* 1988; **39**: 126–35.
43. Dubois F. Laparoscopic vagotomy. In: *Operative Manual of Endoscopic Surgery* (eds Cuschieri A, Buess G, Perissat J), pp. 254–62. Berlin, Springer-Verlag, 1992.
44. Bailey RW, Flower JL, Graham SM. Combined laparoscopic cholecystectomy and selective vagotomy. *Surg Laparosc Endosc* 1991; **1**: 45–9.
45. Bailey RW, Zucker KA. Laparoscopic management of peptic ulcer disease. In: *Surgical Laparoscopy Update* (ed. Zucker KA), pp. 241–86. St Louis, Missouri, QMP, 1993.
46. Weerts JM, Dallemagne B, Jehaes C, Markiewicz S, Lombard R. La chirurgie gastrique per-laparoscopique: une proche realite. *Med Chir Dig* 1992; **21**: 205–6.
47. Johnston D, Axon ATR. Highly selective vagotomy for duodenal ulcer: the clinical results after 10 years. *Br J Surg* 1979; **66**: 874.
48. Johnston D, Goligher JC. The influence of the individual surgeon and of the type of vagotomy upon the insulin test after vagotomy. *Gut* 1971; **12**: 963–7.

10.3

Laparoscopic Highly Selective Vagotomy

J. M. WEERTS, B. DALLEMAGNE, C. JEHAES, S. MARKIEWICZ and R. LOMBARD

Since the first publication of Dragstedt, the role of the vagus nerves in the pathogenicity of recurrent duodenal ulcer disease has been well demonstrated and for many years, surgery was the only treatment for intractable ulcers.

However, in the late 1970s, the appearance of H_2 receptor antagonists made a dramatic change in the treatment of such disease. Patients could rely on a long term effective treatment without major side effects. More recently, the introduction of omeprazole has pushed this balance further towards medical treatment.

The use of these drugs implies the necessity of permanent treatment, as all the symptoms recur as soon as the patient stops the therapy. A more definitive treatment might therefore be required at some stage.

In 1967, Holle and Hart described the first clinical application of highly selective vagotomy (HSV) or proximal cell vagotomy.[1] The principles of the procedure are well known: the denervation is obtained by dividing all the secreting branches, located on the left of the Latarjet nerve. This dissection starts on the left side of the crow's foot and is performed by division of the neurovascular bundles of the lesser curvature. It is also carried on the gastric pouch and on the oesophageal wall (6–7 cm).

Long term studies have shown almost a 5% recurrence rate per five years.[2–4] This compares favourably with medical treatment, especially when this is discontinued.

The onset of laparoscopy and the advantages of minimal invasive surgery have led teams to adapt the HSV to this approach. This operation can be demanding and time consuming and other procedures have also been adapted such as Taylor's seromyotomy associated with a posterior truncal vagotomy or the association of the posterior truncal vagotomy with an anterior HSV.

In this chapter we shall present the technique of the HSV and the results of our team in this field.

PATIENT SELECTION

The selection of the patients is based on a long story of recurrent duodenal ulcer. Prepyloric ulcers can be induced due to the same aetiopathogenicity. Strong reserve should be made for other types of ulcers.

The recurrences should be well documented by endoscopies and a screening for *Helicobacter pylori* should be negative. A recent barium meal should exclude any pyloric or bulbar stenosis.

An acid study with stimulation by pentagastrin will exclude any contraindication for HSV, as will assessment of gastrin and parathormone blood levels.

In case of suspicion of gastro-oesophageal disease, oesophageal manometry and a 24-hour pH study should be carried out as well.

PROCEDURE

As for any other upper GI laparoscopic procedure, the patient will be under general anaesthesia, in a lithotomy position. The surgeon will be standing between the legs of the patient, facing the monitor(s) on the right and/or the left side of the patient's head. One assistant will be standing on each side, for retracting the liver, holding the camera and grasping the stomach.

For a HSV, six ports are usually used. The positioning is similar to the Nissen fundoplication, i.e. one 10 mm port above the umbilicus for the camera, one 10 mm under the xiphoid process, one in the right hypochondrium and two in the left hypochondrium. One extra 10 mm port (D) is placed high in the left hypochondrium, under the subcostal margin. It will be used for the introduction of a clip applicator, in order to save as much time as possible (Fig. 10.3.1).

The operator will use ports A and B, while the camera will be introduced in port C. Port H will be used for retracting the liver while the far left port (G) will help in presenting the stomach.

The first step of the procedure will be the recognition of the various landmarks for the dissection. The major structure is the crow's foot with the nerve of Latarjet. It is usually recognized 4–5 cm to the left of the pylorus. All the dissection will then be performed on the left side of this nerve. It is very important to dissect smoothly, to prevent any haematoma formation that will render any further dissection more difficult. All the neurovascular bundles along the lesser curvature must be divided.

The first layer usually includes large vessels: the peritoneum will be opened with electrocautery to allow the dissection of the bundles. A hook is very useful to separate the different vessels without harming them. Once they are freed from adjacent tissues, clips can be applied on several vessels in one go. Then the vessels are divided. This way of proceeding will save time.

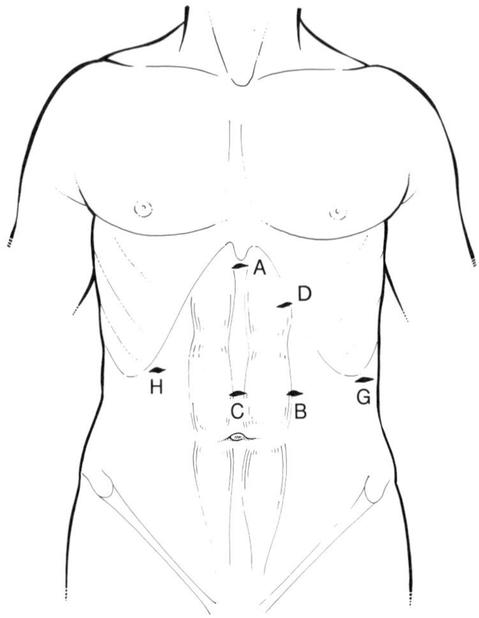

Figure 10.3.1 Positioning of ports.

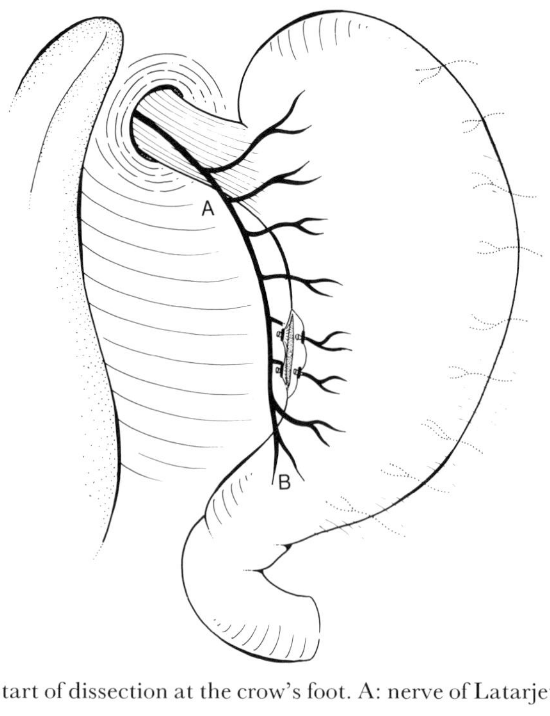

Figure 10.3.2 Start of dissection at the crow's foot. A: nerve of Latarjet; B: crow's foot.

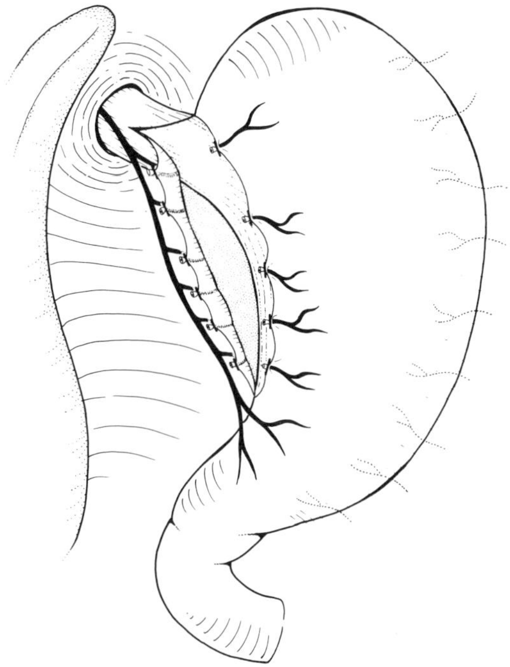

Figure 10.3.3 Dissection of the lesser curvature.

Once the first layer has been separated from the crow's foot to the cardia, the dissection will be carried on the second layer. The vessels are much smaller and most of time, cautery is quite sufficient; one must be careful, though, as bleeding will create a haematoma or will retract in the muscular layer of the gastric wall. The different layers will be dissected in the same way. Once the posterior layer is reached, the vessels are once again much larger and must be divided between clips. The lesser curvature must gradually be everted by the first assistant, to obtain the best exposure.

The lesser sac will be more easily opened on the medial part of the lesser curvature. The dissection is then carried out towards the crow's foot and towards the cardia. It is important to divide any posterior adhesions between the stomach and the pancreas. Clips are used to divide the vessels on the posterior layer of the lesser curvature.

The dissection of the lesser sac is of course the first part of the procedure. It is important to free the oesophagus from all the bundles that emerge from the main trunks. Therefore, the serosa on the anterior wall of the cardia will be opened and dissection will aim to the left side of the oesophagus. The gastric fundus will be fully mobilized right to the first short gastric vessel. This part of the dissection can also be done through the lesser sac on the posterior side of the gastric fundus.

The dissection will be carried on the posterior wall of the oesophagus, keeping the posterior trunk [of the vagus nerve] to the right of the patient. At least 6 or 7 cm of oesophagus should be skeletonized.

The anterior and posterior trunks are preserved by keeping them on the right side of the dissection. Usually, the criminal nerve of Grassi can easily be identified and divided.

Once the whole oesophagus has been skeletonized on all sides, one must check that the dissection has been fully completed on the lower edge of the lesser omentum, particularly on the posterior side of the crow's foot. This part is sometimes very difficult to expose and one must not hesitate to change the site of the optic (i.e. use one of the other 10 mm ports) to make sure that the dissection is adequate.

As in gastro-oesophageal repair, a rubber sling can be brought in to be placed around the cardia to help its manipulation.

In case of an associated gastro-oesophageal disease, a fundoplication is done, providing there is no contraindication on preoperative manometry. The 360° wrap is usually done without dividing the short gastric vessels, because of the fear of jeopardizing the blood supply of the lesser curvature. The wrap is created in the same way as previously described, bringing the posterior gastric pouch around the oesophagus without any traction. The first stitch will be passed through the oesophageal wall. The wrap will be done loose and short.

In all the other cases, the oesophagogastric junction is left without any reconstruction or an angle will be reconstructed by suturing the gastric pouch to the left side of the oesophagus, or a posterior hemifundoplication will be created (so-called Toupet fundoplication). This is done to prevent gastro-oesophageal reflux in the future as the angle has been totally disrupted by the nerve dissection. The gastric pouch is brought behind the oesophagus and sutured by a continuous stitch to the right side of the oesophagus. The length of the suture will be 3 cm. On the left side of the oesophagus the gastric pouch will also be sutured in order to have a posterior 210° hemifundoplication. This will probably avoid any further non-acid reflux although this is not proven.

The lesser curvature can also be sutured by a running suture of absorbable material to avoid any perforation due to necrosis of the gastric wall. We do not do this routinely in our unit.

The pneumoperitoneum is then released after washing the peritoneal cavity with warm saline to remove all the clots. Before withdrawing the camera, inspection of the different port sites will be done to check for any bleeding.

A nasogastric tube is usually left for the recovery period and then removed; the patients are allowed to drink the next day and are discharged on the third or fourth day, after a barium meal to determine the presence of delayed emptying of the stomach and the positioning of the valve, if present, for further follow-up.

RESULTS

From January 1991 to December 1992, 44 patients were operated on for chronic duodenal ulcer disease, with or without gastro-oesophageal disease. All the patients were suffering from intractable disease, with a relapse of the symptoms each time they stopped their medical treatment. The mean duration of medical treatment was 64 months, ranging from 19 to 200 months.

All the patients underwent a barium meal, which showed an active duodenal ulcer in 37 patients, mild stenosis of the pylorus in one and one more severe stenosis of the 1° duodenum with no dilatation or gastric emptying delay.

Endoscopy was performed in all patients, but *Helicobacter pylori* was not searched for in every patient. It was negative in 21 patients. Seventeen patients presented with at least a stage 2 oesophagitis which justified the antireflux repair.

Acid studies were also performed with pentagastrin; the mean basal acid output was 4 meq HCL $hour^{-1}$ (range 0–9) and the mean maximal acid output was 34.8 meq HCL $hour^{-1}$ (range 10–56).

One patient had a perforated duodenal ulcer that was first repaired by laparoscopy and the HSV was performed three months later as the patient had a long story of duodenal ulcer disease.

All the patients were classified ASA I according to the American Society of Anesthesiology.

All the patients underwent a classical HSV but an additional antireflux procedure was performed in 32 patients, i.e. 17 Nissen–Rossetti fundoplications and 15 posterior hemifundoplications as described by Toupet. The average operating time was 145 minutes but was obviously shorter for patients undergoing a formal HSV with no antireflux procedure (119 minutes).

The patients were all back on oral feeding on the first postoperative day and the mean hospital stay was 3.1 days. There was no death and no severe complications occurred. One mild chest infection was noted; on control barium meal, performed on the second postoperative day, there was no delayed emptying of the stomach, but severe oedema of the lesser curvature was noted in several patients.

On follow-up, one patient returned with a recurrence of his ulcer (melaena); one patient presented within the first month with a 1 cm ulcer on the angle of the lesser curvature; the nature of this ulcer was probably ischaemic and the patient is currently under investigation. All the other patients are asymptomatic.

Some of the patients (17) accepted to undergo postoperative endoscopy and acid studies. On endoscopy, all the previous ulcers were healed. No oesophagitis was noted. Acid studies performed at least three months after the operation demonstrated a marked reduction in acid secretion with the pentagastrin test: 65% reduction on basal acid output and 60% reduction on maximal acid output.

Two patients presented three and six months after operation with a small incisional hernia at one of the port sites.

CONCLUSION

Laparoscopic highly selective vagotomy is certainly feasible. The first results are in favour of such an approach. However the procedure is demanding and requires a certain expertise in laparoscopic surgery in order to achieve at least the same results as for open surgery.

In certain obese patients, other procedures should be recommended, such as seromyotomy or gastric linear resection. But long term follow-up is certainly mandatory for all these procedures.

REFERENCES

1. Holle F, Hart W. News in the surgery of the gastro-duodenal ulcer. *Med Klin* 1967; **62**: 441.
2. Johnston D, Wilkinson M. Highly selective vagotomy without a drainage procedure in the treatment of duodenal ulcer. *Br J Surg* 1970; **57**: 289–96.
3. Jordan PH. An interim report on parietal cell vagotomy versus selective vagotomy and antrectomy for treatment of duodenal ulcer. *Ann Surg* 1979; **189**: 645–52.
4. Andersen D, Andrup E, Hostrup H, Sorensen F. The Aarhus County vagotomy trial: trends in the problem of recurrent ulcer after parietal cell vagotomy and selective vagotomy with drainage. *World J Surg* 1982; **6**: 82–5.

10.4

Thoracoscopic Truncal Vagotomy

J. MOUIEL and N. KATKHOUDA

As long ago as 1943, Dragstedt[1] proposed a thoracoscopic approach for truncal vagotomy in the treatment of ulcer disease, but this approach was subsequently abandoned for an abdominal approach, given the requirement for a drainage procedure which was usually achieved by means of a gastroenterostomy or pyloroplasty.[2] Since then, truncal vagotomy via the thoracic route has been reserved for the rare occasion when there was concern regarding the use of the abdominal route in a patient with recurrent ulceration and multiple previous abdominal operations.[3–6] In 1956, thoracoscopic truncal vagotomy had been proposed in the elective treatment of ulcer disease by Wittmoser[7] and it was suggested that after an interval of three weeks this be associated with a splanchnicectomy as a means of avoiding pylorospasm. This important and original experience has, however, remained isolated and anecdotal, there having been no controlled studies undertaken and no long term results reported.

The attraction of this approach has been recognized by Dubois,[8,9] who has demonstrated that thoracoscopy is a rapid, efficacious and simple intervention and embraces the overall concept of minimally invasive surgery. Furthermore, the early results have once again questioned the secondary physiological effects of a truncal vagotomy by raising the need for an associated drainage procedure.[10]

PRINCIPLES

The fact that vagotomy heals duodenal ulceration by a reduction in the secretion of acid has been well recognized since the early works of Dragstedt.[1] He demonstrated that truncal vagotomy produced an almost complete abolition of acid production, but that this was accompanied by pyloric hold-up which therefore required a drainage procedure, such as pyloroplasty or gastrojejunostomy, to avoid gastric stasis.[2] It has been evident over the years from the large reported series of oesophagectomy that the pyloric hold-up which accompanies the associated truncal vagotomy is not always invariable and that it is possible to replace surgical drainage with simple balloon dilatation of the pylorus.[11] From an anatomical point of view,[12] the vagal nerves are distributed in a plexus in the inferior part of the posterior mediastinum and in 90% of cases form well-defined anterior and posterior trunks in the region of the oesophageal hiatus. For

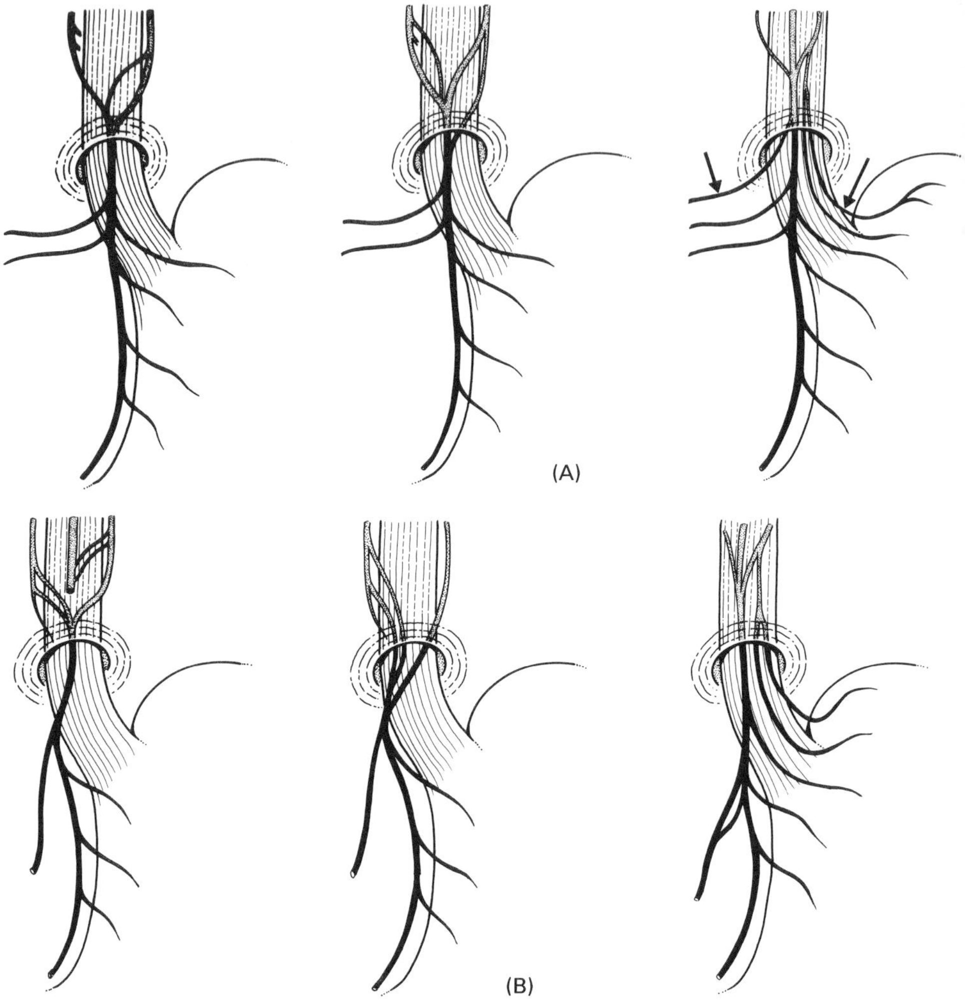

Figure 10.4.1 Anatomy of the vagal system, above the level of the hiatus the "multiple nerves" of the oesophageal plexus, below the two vagal trunks. A: anterior vagal nerve; B: posterior vagal nerve.

thoracic vagotomy to be complete, therefore, all of these nerve fibres surrounding the oesophagus at this level require to be divided, taking care not to miss any aberrant nerves or fibres which have branched at a higher level (Fig. 10.4.1).

PATIENT SELECTION AND OPERATIVE INDICATIONS

The preoperative evaluation for patients being considered for thoracoscopic vagotomy comprises, firstly, a general assessment to evaluate risk factors such as those involving the respiratory tract. Severe respiratory insufficiency or preceding pleural or pulmonary disease may prevent a thoracic approach. Secondly, the ulcer disease itself requires to be properly assessed by means of endoscopy, radiology and secretory studies. Endoscopic examination is required to establish the presence of a duodenal ulcer which has persisted despite carefully monitored medical treatment. It may also demonstrate recurrent ulceration, despite a previous abdominal vagotomy or an anastomotic ulcer which has occurred following gastric bypass or gastrectomy. Endoscopic biopsy should be used to exclude the presence of Barrett's ulceration, metaplastic change or a superinfection of the duodenal ulcer by *Helicobacter pylori*. It is important to exclude the presence of oesophageal reflux, impaired oesophageal clearance, an associated oesophageal stenosis or impaired gastric emptying. All of these features are best demonstrated by barium swallow and meal, which we have found indispensable in this regard. An alternative approach would be to employ an isotope scan using technetium^{99} to assess the solid phase emptying and indium^{111} to assess the liquid phase.[13]

Secretory studies include those assessing basal acid output and pentagastrin stimulated acid secretion. In those instances where vagotomy has previously been undertaken, it has been our practice to assess acid production in response to insulin induced hypoglycaemia. This final assessment correlates well with basal acid output and provides a reasonable assessment of the completeness of the previously undertaken vagotomy. At the same time, the presence of the normal gastrin level will eliminate the diagnosis of Zollinger–Ellison syndrome as being a cause for ulcer recurrence.[14] This protocol of investigation undertaken before surgery and 1–3 months following thoracoscopic vagotomy is essential in this evaluation phase, providing confirmation that there is a drop in acid production and a lack of significant problems with gastric emptying.

At the present time, the proposed operative indications are restricted to those patients previously operated on using an abdominal approach and followed up on a number of occasions. These patients comprise those with recurrent peptic ulcer disease after an attempt at reducing acid production by means of abdominal vagotomy or resection. Patients considered for thoracoscopic vagotomy also include those being considered for a gastric bypass procedure for incapacitating reflux after a failure of a previous surgical attempt dealing with gastro-oesophageal reflux, with or without an associated hiatus hernia. It is apparent that thoracoscopic vagotomy provides an elegant and rapid solution for patients with severe symptoms and those in whom an approach to the subphrenic space is not an option.[10,15,16,17]

The indications have widened under the influence of Dubois[8,9] to include the elective treatment of ulcer disease for the non-compliant patient and to those individuals who have not complied with medical therapy. In this group of patients is also included those individuals who, for geographical or socioeconomical reasons, could not be adequately followed but these indications remain under evaluation.

SURGICAL PROCEDURE

Anaesthesia and Monitoring of Patient

The operation is performed under general anaesthesia with selective intubation to allow collapse of the left lung during the thoracoscopic dissection. Careful peroperative monitoring is undertaken and comprises electrocardiography, assessment of blood pressure and central venous pressure, along with CO_2 monitoring to assess the effects of CO_2 insufflation which is maintained in low pressure. Insufflation for thoracoscopic work is not always essential.

Operative Position

The patient is placed in a right lateral decubitus position as if for a left thoracotomy, with the surgeon behind the patient's back and the assistant to the left. This provides both operators with the same operative field, looking at the monitor placed opposite.

Equipment and Instrumentation

For this procedure, a 0° or 30° thoracolaparoscope can be employed and is connected to a video system and camera. An insufflator, a suction irrigation system and mono or bipolar electrocoagulation are required. We employ 5 mm and 10 mm ports for access and use reducing sleeves as required. Standard laparoscopic instruments are used and include atraumatic grasping forceps, Babcock forceps and a clip applicator. In principle, ligatures are not particularly useful with this approach.

A number of instruments have now been designed specifically for thoracoscopic surgery and these include malleable ports, allowing the introduction of curved instruments. It is possible, however, to use standard instruments through short incisions in the chest wall without the need for ports. A set amount of instrumentation is required to facilitate pyloric dilatation and this includes a gastroduodenoscope with an operating channel of 2.8 mm, dilating balloons measuring between 15 mm and 25 mm in diameter (Rigiflex, Microvasive, Boston Scientific Company) and a graduated syringe with manometric pressure control which allows insufflation of the balloon to 45 psi (Rigiflator, Microvasive, Boston Scientific Company).

Creation of Pneumothorax

The pneumothorax can be created either with the aid of a retractable needle or with an open thoracoscopic technique. A dissector is passed through a 1 cm incision in the eighth intercostal space in the posterior axillary line. The jaws of the instruments can be used to separate the intercostal muscles and to reach the pleura, allowing the characteristic indrawing of air into the pleural cavity. The pneumothorax should be maintained with a controlled pressure of CO_2 to a maximum of 8 mmHg so as to avoid mediastinal displacement which may result in arrhythmias and hypotension. The utilization of CO_2 in this form of thoracoscopic surgery is not essential but does have the advantage of contributing to the collapse of the left lung, avoiding the theoretical risk of gas embolus in the small pulmonary veins when opened and the risk of accidental injury from the use of monopolar coagulation in a humid environment.

Access (Fig. 10.4.2)

We would advise the use of four ports for this procedure. The first port is inserted in the eighth interspace in the posterior axillary line to allow introduction of the laparoscope. It is important to place the posterior port 2 cm in front of the costal angle to avoid damage to the intercostal nerves and the transverse processes of the vertical column. The remaining trocars are placed under direct vision. The second and third ports (5 mm) are placed in the midaxillary line as far apart as possible from each other. The lowest of these is used for the suction irrigation cannula, which is held in the left hand and serves as a retractor. The higher of the two is used for the scissors and for the dissecting hook in the right hand. Finally, a 5 mm trocar is placed anteriorly to produce a diamond-shaped operative field and this allows the use of a further retractor or dissector.

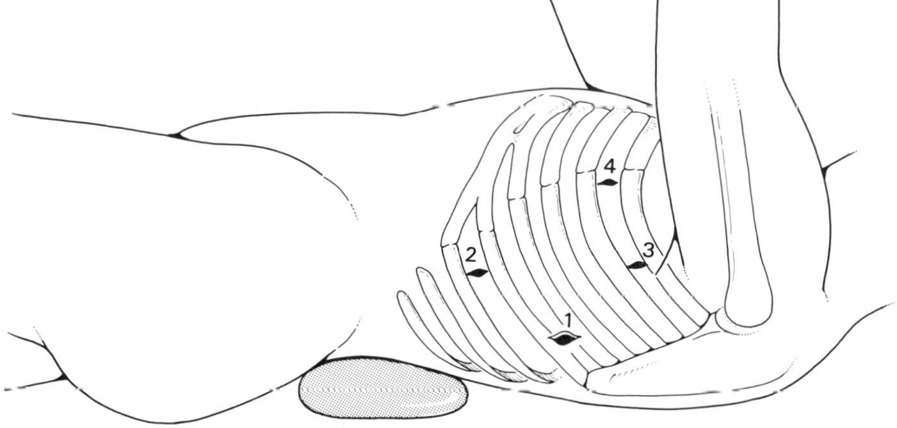

Figure 10.4.2 Surgical access and placement of trocars.

OPERATIVE TECHNIQUE

Examination

After freeing the pleuropulmonary adhesions with the help of a 30° laparoscope, the boundaries of the operating field are defined, with the left hemidiaphragm below, the longitudinal projection of the aorta behind, the pericardium in front and the retracted lung above (Fig. 10.4.3). It is perhaps useful, particularly at the beginning of the surgeon's experience (as recommended by Cuschieri[18]), to use at the same time a flexible endoscope which, when introduced through the flank, will enable rapid identification of the transilluminated oesophagus and will assist in the mobilization of the oesophagus which can be displaced by a combination of flexion and rotation with the tip of the endoscope.

Thoracoscopic Dissection

The oesophagus is dissected out as low as possible in front of the triangular ligament which can be divided with coagulation only if it interferes with access. The pleura is incised longitudinally in front of the aorta and the oesophagus, which is dissected out with the aid of the dissecting hook and the retractor on its anterior and then its posterior aspect. The entire oesophagus can be mobilized in this way, carefully displacing the right pleura in such a way as to free its right posterior aspect. It is useful to pass a tape or sling once this dissection has been completed and before proceeding to the vagotomy. In principle, all longitudinal fibres corresponding to the pneumogastric nerves should be divided but it is useful to proceed in a stage manner from the left anterior surface to the right

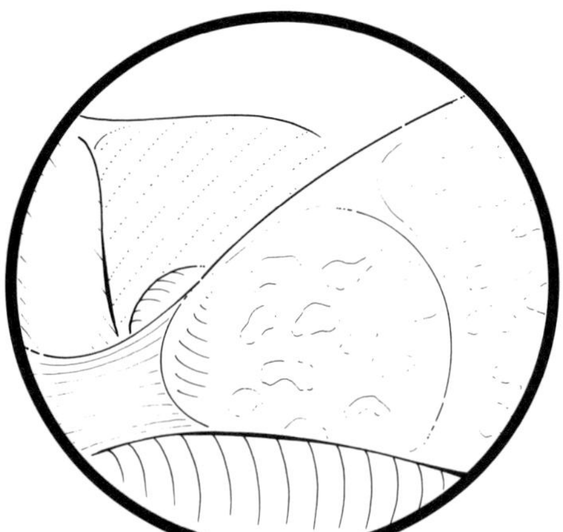

Figure 10.4.3 Thoracoscopic view into left side of pleural cavity with dome of left diaphragm on the left and the lung on the right.

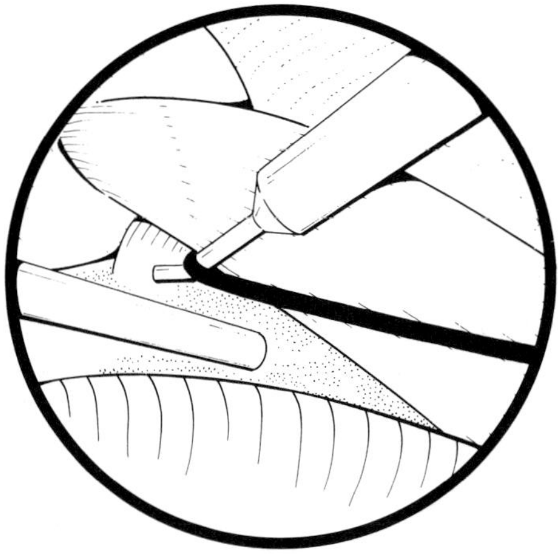

Figure 10.4.4 Coagulation hook used to dissect out the posterior vagal trunk. Access to the left aspect of the oesophagus and anterior truncal vagotomy.

anterior surface and from there exposing the oesophagus with the help of the tapes and by lifting the inferior part with the help of the irrigation suction device.

Where exposure is difficult, an atraumatic Babcock dissector can be used to grasp the oesophagus. Normally, the left anterior and right posterior vagal trunks separate in the lowermost part of the mediastinum and are seen as a plexus of nerve bundles immediately above this. In this way it is usually necessary to divide three or four nerve bundles on each side of the oesophagus, with one of the nerve bundles being more prominent than the others. This dissection is generally achieved without much in the way of blood loss, since there are few paraoesophageal vessels at this level and it usually suffices merely to identify the nerve trunks with the coagulating hook (Fig. 10.4.4) or the scissors (Fig. 10.4.5). These can be divided with electrocautery or with sharp dissection after having obtained a fragment of the vagal trunk for histological analysis.

Reinflation of the Lung and Drainage

The procedure finishes by verifying that there is no continued bleeding and that the left lung has fully re-expanded. In those cases where an accidental pleural injury is suspected, it will only be necessary to hyperinflate the lungs to clear the CO_2. In this way, the released oesophagus seals the breach by returning to its previous position in the mediastinum. The ports are removed and the airtightness of the wounds are assured whilst the hyperinflation of the lungs is continued. In the absence of any bleeding or obvious air leak from a damaged lung, no drainage is necessary and this is psychologically preferable for the patient.

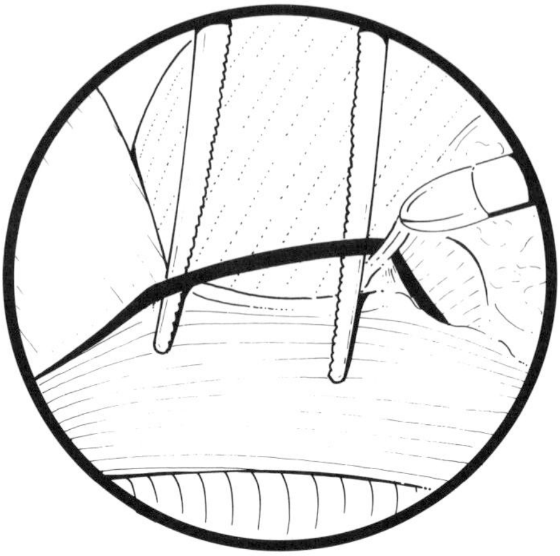

Figure 10.4.5 Identification of anterior vagal trunk before division. Access to the right aspect of the oesophagus and truncal vagotomy.

Otherwise, an underwater drainage is instituted through one of the cannula wounds for 24 hours. The intercostal spaces are infiltrated with a long-acting local anaesthetic such as bupivacaine.

Endoscopic Dilatation of Pylorus

The endoscopic dilatation of the pylorus was undertaken in our early experience during the same operative intervention, but as our experience has progressed this is normally undertaken on the third week following the truncal vagotomy and where there remains persistent pylorospasm. This latter complication is normally observed in about 10% of cases.[19,20] The pyloric dilatation is undertaken using controlled pressure, passing the dilating balloon through the operating channel of the endoscope. This dilatation is usually completed within ten minutes and its effectiveness is comparable to that of a pyloroplasty. Where pyloric dilatation fails to control symptoms, this procedure can easily be repeated.[21,22]

RESULTS

The immediate results are those normally observed with any form of coelioscopic surgery. The recent experience has limited follow-up and is limited to 50 cases without peroperative complication and excellent short term results.[8,9,10,15] Complications of delayed gastric emptying have been noted in only 10% of cases, requiring a pyloric dilatation after failure to control symptoms with simple dietetic measures and treatment with prokinetic agents, such as cicapride. Postoperative endoscopy has in all cases confirmed healing of the ulcer with, in the cases where gastric emptying has been delayed, the persistent presence of a food bolus. Radiology of the upper gastrointestinal tract has shown moderate stasis with slight distension of the stomach in all patients undergoing total vagotomy but delayed gastric emptying has been observed in only 10% of cases. Other authors have had very similar results.[23]

DISCUSSION

The place of conventional surgery in the treatment of ulcer disease has reduced considerably with the advent of effective medical therapy, such as H_2 receptor antagonists and the newer proton pump blockers such as omeprazole. Truncal vagotomy itself has been superseded by highly selective vagotomy and the variant of posterior truncal vagotomy with anterior seromyotomy. These procedures have a mortality less than 0.1% and a comparable efficacy, but having the advantage of a reduction in morbidity.[15]

There is no doubt that laparoscopic or thoracoscopic vagotomy will once again raise the question of the optimal therapy for ulcer disease.[1,24,25] Truncal vagotomy undertaken by the thoracoscopic route is the least invasive of the surgical procedures and can be undertaken in a straightforward, rapid and effective manner. The foreseeable physiological consequences, however, have largely occurred in patients with recurrent ulcer disease and those who have already undergone a surgical procedure which has included a gastric drainage procedure. After thoracoscopic surgery, however, in previously non-operated patients, the delay in gastric emptying is much less noticeable than might have been expected, so challenging the previously well-established physiological concepts. A number of explanations have been proposed.[10,13] The effectiveness of medical treatment may have considerably reduced the degree of inflammatory scarring around the ulcer and have therefore reduced the incidence of pyloroduodenal stenosis. The dangers of postoperative adhesions are avoided by employing a thoracoscopic approach in the same way that a postoperative ileus can be avoided. Furthermore, the delays in gastric emptying can be avoided by prescribing appropriate diet and by utilizing prokinetic gastric agents.[5] The fact that these agents may be useful in such patients is supported by the finding of food boluses thought to be due to poor antral contractions and as a finding of postoperative distension which is thought to be due to the loss of gastric relaxation. In cases where delays in gastric emptying persist, endoscopic dilatation appears to be an appropriate solution whilst respecting the concept of minimally invasive surgical techniques.

The simplicity and efficacy of this surgical intervention, the minimal scarring, the uneventful postoperative course and early return to normal activity support the wider use of thoracoscopic truncal vagotomy, associated if necessary with endoscopic pyloric dilatation, but it will be necessary to validate this initial experience with prospective studies and adequate long term follow-up.

REFERENCES

1. Dragstedt LR, Owen FM. Supra-diaphragmatic section of vagus nerve in the treatment of duodenal ulcer. *Proc Soc Exp Biol Med* 1943; **53**: 152–4.
2. Dragstedt LR, Lulu DJ. Truncal vagotomy and pyloroplasty: critical evaluation of one hundred cases. *Am J Surg* 1974; **128**: 344–6.
3. Fawcett AN, Johnston D, Duthie HC. Revagotomy for recurrent ulcer after vagotomy and drainage for duodenal ulcer. *Br J Surg* 1969; **56**: 111–16.
4. Taylor TV, Pearson KW, Torrance B. Revagotomy for recurrent peptic ulcer. *Br J Surg* 1977; **64**: 477–81.
5. Hede TE, Temple JG, MacFarland J. The place of transthoracic vagotomy in the management of recurrent peptic ulceration. *Br J Surg* 1977; **64**: 332–5.
6. Lehr L, Pichlmayr R. Low-risk thoracic vagotomy for anastomotic ulceration. *World J Surg* 1982; **6**: 93–7.
7. Wittmoser R. Thoracoscopic sympathetic and vagotomy. In: *Endoscopic Surgery* (eds Cuschieri A, Buess G, Perissat J), pp. 110–33. Berlin, Springer-Verlag, 1992.
8. Dubois F. La chirurgie de l'ulcere duodenal non-complique. In: *La Chirurgie Digestive par Voie Coelioscopique* (eds Testas P, Delaitre B), pp. 133–6. Paris, Vigot, 1991.
9. Dubois F. Laparoscopic vagotomy. In: *Operative Manual of Endoscopic Surgery* (eds Cuschieri A, Buess G, Perissat J), pp. 254–62. Berlin, Springer-Verlag, 1992.
10. Mouiel J, Dubois F, Champault G. La vagotomie tronculaire par thorascopie. In: *Encycl Medi Chir, Technikques Chirurgicales, Chirurgie Digestive* 40; 292, Paris, France, 1993.
11. Bemelman WA, Brummelkam WH, Bartelsman JFWM. Endoscopic balloon dilation of the pylorus after esophagogastrostomy without a drainage procedure. *Surg Gynecol Obst* 1990; **170**: 424–6.
12. Hollender LF, Marrie A. *La Vagotomie Supra-selective*. Paris, Masson, 1977.
13. Jian R. Clinical relevance of gastrointestinal manometry. *Front Gastrointest Res* 1990; **17**: 274–87.
14. Hautefeuille P, Picaud R. *Les Recidives apres Vagotomies pour Ulcere Duodenal*. Paris, Masson, 1983.
15. Champault G, Belhassen A, Rizk N, Vazzana G, Boutelier P. Ulcere duodenal le retour de la vagotomie tronculaire. *Presse Med* 1993; **22**: 225.
16. Festen HPM, Lamers CBH, Driessen WMM, Van Tongern JHM. Cimetidine in anastomotic ulceration after partial gastrectomy. *Gastroenterology* 1979; **76**: 83.
17. Heppell J, Bess MA, McIlrath DC, Dozois RR. Surgical treatment of recurrent peptic ulcer disease. *Ann Surg* 1983; **198**: 1–4.
18. Cuschieri A, Shimi S, Banting S. Endoscopic oesophagectomy through a right thoracoscopic approach. *J R Coll Surg Edinb* 1992; **37**: 7–11.
19. Chisholm EM, Chung SCS, Sunderland GT, Leong HT, Li AKC. Thoracoscopic vagotomy: a new use for the laparoscope. *Br J Surg* 1992; **79**: 254.
20. Craig PI, Gillespie SK. Through the endoscope balloon dilation of benign gastric outlet obstruction. *Br Med J* 1988; **297**: 396.
21. Mouiel J, Katkhouda N. Laparoscopic truncal and selective vagotomy. In: *Surgical Laparoscopy* (ed. Zucker KA), pp. 263–79. Saint Louis, Missouri, QMP. 1991.

22. Taylor TV. Experience with the Lunderquist Ownman dilatator in the upper gastro-intestinal tract. *Br J Surg* 1983; **710**: 445.
23. Laws HL, Naughton MJ, McKernan JB. Thoracoscopic vagotomy for recurrent peptic ulcer disease. *Surg Laparosc Endosc* 1992; **2**: 24–8.
24. Mouiel J, Katkhouda N. Traitement de l'ulcere duodenal non complique par vagotomie sous coelioscopie. In: *La Chirurgie Digestive par Voie Coelioscopique* (eds Testas P, Delaitre B), pp. 137–45. Paris, Vigot, 1991.
25. Mouiel J, Katkhouda N. Laparoscopic vagotomy in the treatment of chronic duodenal ulcer disease. In: *Problems in General Surgery: Vol. 8 Laparoscopic Surgery* (ed. Berci G), pp. 358–65. Philadelphia, JB Lippincott, 1991.

Overview

Antiulcer surgery

There has been a steady and progressive decline in the number of surgical procedures undertaken for ulcer disease over the last 20 years. This can be accounted for largely by the successful introduction of antiulcer therapy. In the same way, there has been a resurgence in interest in surgical treatment of reflux oesophagitis, so the introduction of laparoscopic surgical techniques has redirected the surgeon's attention to the treatment of peptic ulcer disease. Taylor's excellent contribution (Chapter 10.1) charts the development of modern ulcer surgery and highlights the potential pitfalls awaiting the laparoscopic surgeon. The lessons of open surgical treatment for ulcer disease seem clear, namely, the careful selection of the patient and the surgical procedure, while at the same time ensuring that the experience in the treatment of this condition is concentrated in the hands of a few surgeons.

There are many attractions to considering laparoscopic treatment of ulcer disease and, at present, highly selective vagotomy or anterior seromyotomy combined with posterior truncal vagotomy would appear to be the operations against which all others will be judged. It remains to be seen whether the economic drive to laparoscopic treatment of ulcer disease in some countries will be matched elsewhere.

11.1

Expectations of Oesophageal Resection

T. HENNESSY

INTRODUCTION

The low resectability rate, high perioperative mortality and poor long term survival reported by Earlam and Cunha-Melo[1] in an extensive review of the literature on the surgical treatment of oesophageal cancer published in 1980, reflected the unsatisfactory nature of surgical techniques and pre- and postoperative care during the period 1953–78. A subsequent meta-analysis[2] covering the period January 1980 to December 1988 and examining the outcome of surgical treatment in 76 911 patients demonstrated that while resectability rates had improved and mortality rates had fallen there had been no improvement in long term results.

However, although this latter report establishes a baseline for assessing the outcome of present day treatment it should be understood that it reflects an approach to treatment which is a decade out of date. While some series in the report include the three phase operation described by McKeown[3] for intrathoracic tumours, others carried out conventional procedures using a right thoracotomy for midthoracic tumours and a leftsided approach for adenocarcinomas. Transhiatal resection was also employed. The extent of lymphadenectomy varied considerably. Most surgeons carried out some form of lymph node dissection. Approximately one third of the authors carried out a detailed abdominal lymphadenectomy including the coeliac axis nodes, those along the splenic, left gastric and hepatic arteries and the paracardial nodes. Fifty percent of surgeons dissected the intrathoracic lymph nodes but only a few surgeons performed a cervical lymph node dissection. Less than 25% of authors carried out any kind of adjuvant therapy. Chemotherapy alone was used preoperatively in 11 prospective trials. A combination of chemotherapy and irradiation was used preoperatively in a further 11 trials. All had small numbers and only two compared the results with surgical resection alone.

While we do not yet have irrefutable evidence that combined therapy improves the chances of long term survival, many of the trials now ongoing have indicated that such treatment downgrades the tumour and improves resectability rates. Trends towards better long term survival have also been demonstrated. In many instances, however, these advantages are offset by an increased morbidity and mortality due to toxicity.

The failure of conventional treatment to ensure long term survival can be attributed to a number of factors, of which late presentation is one of the most important. Symptoms of dysphagia are often present for up to six months before patients seek medical advice. Since very significant narrowing of the lumen is necessary to produce dysphagia this means that the lesion is locally quite advanced at the time of presentation. In our own experience, 90% of patients have full wall penetration and 65% have lymph node involvement at the time of surgery.[4]

Failure to control locoregional disease is another reason why long term survival has not been achieved and of course this situation is strongly linked to late presentation. Many patients die from local recurrence rather than distant metastases and Guili *et al.* have shown, in a review of 2400 patients with oesophageal cancer, that 50% developed a recurrence at the anastomosis or in the mediastinum.[5]

The two most important prognostic factors are wall penetration and lymph node involvement. Skinner[6] states that when both these factors are absent, five year survival is 55% but is less than 12% if more than five local lymph nodes are involved and the tumour has gone completely through the wall. Our own experience has demonstrated similar results.

Failure to eliminate locoregional disease is not entirely related to late diagnosis and the presence or absence of involved lymph nodes and penetration through the wall of the oesophagus. In oesophageal cancer the propensity for extensive submucosal infiltration to a length of several centimetres beyond the visible extent of the tumour is well known and contributes to the high incidence of anastomotic recurrence due to microscopic involvement, particularly of the proximal margin. Wide resection margins are needed to achieve satisfactory clearance and it is considered that a vertical clearance of 10 cm is needed to avoid the risk of anastomotic recurrence. It is equally important when resecting adenocarcinomas involving the cardia that adequate clearance is achieved, particularly along the lesser curvature of the stomach. In cases where the tumour appears to arise primarily in the stomach rather than the cardia, we agree with McKeown[7] that total gastrectomy is indicated in addition to resection of the lower half of the oesophagus. When the cervical oesophagus is involved it is difficult to obtain adequate proximal clearance without resection of the larynx and pharynx.

The gratifying fall in perioperative mortality during the past decade or so is due to a number of different factors. Improved preoperative preparation, particularly in regard to nutrition, has been of benefit and where there has been weight loss in excess of 10% of the patient's ideal weight, it is considered beneficial to spend a week or two improving the patient's nutritional status.

Prophylaxis against postoperative problems such as atelectasis and pulmonary infection, cardiac arrhythmias and pulmonary embolus can be implemented. Preoperative chest physiotherapy and early extubation postoperatively minimize the risk of pulmonary problems and continuous monitoring allows early intervention and treatment of cardiac arrhythmias. Graduated pressure stockings and prophylactic heparin reduce the likelihood of deep vein thrombosis and pulmonary embolus.

Since stapling instruments[8] are useful in high anastomoses and may be less likely to leak than those sutured by hand, there has been a great increase in their use. On the other hand, cervical anastomoses, which have become more frequent, are more prone to leakage than intrathoracic anastomoses.[9] More precise methods of estimating fluid requirements and better control of infection also contribute to the reduction in perioperative mortality.

There was a significant improvement recorded in resectability rates between 1980 and 1990, rising from 39% to 56%. These figures bear little relationship to the situation as a whole in a particular area or country and reflect a specific referral pattern for a hospital or a unit in combination with the conservative or aggressive approach of the surgeon to treatment. The improvement in resection figures between 1980 and 1990 suggests more confidence in the general condition of the patient and probably a greater recognition of the inadequacies of alternative palliative treatments. Surgical techniques other than the three stage methods have not changed appreciatively but have been greatly facilitated by improved anaesthetic techniques such as selective pulmonary ventilation with double lumen endotracheal tubes.

Combined therapy has been employed in a number of different formats over the last decade. The best results of chemotherapy are obtained by the use of two or more agents and some of the best response rates have been reported with a combination of 5-fluorouracil and cis-platin.[10,11] Further improvement in results has been gained by the combined use of chemotherapy and irradiation in the preoperative period with the cytotoxic agents acting simultaneously as radio sensitizers and cellular toxins. Although complete response with no histological evidence of tumour is achieved in a small number of cases there is not sufficient evidence of permanent ablation of the tumour to omit the subsequent surgery.

Combined therapy is most effective when administered preoperatively and the response rate in squamous cell carcinoma is greater than that obtained with adenocarcinomas. Even when responses are incomplete, the downgrading of tumours achieved with combined therapy significantly increases the resectability rates even with advanced tumours.

The toxicity of these regimens is variable but considerable and most series report a significant morbidity and mortality. Myelosuppression, nephrotoxicity and pulmonary fibrosis are among the principal problems encountered.[12]

Currently, the options available in the treatment of oesophageal cancer (excluding palliative procedures) are oesophagogastrectomy using a thoraco-abdominal incision or a midline epigastric incision and left thoracotomy; the Lewis–Tanner oesophagectomy usually employed for middle third tumours; transhiatal oesophagectomy using Orringer's technique[13] or the inversion–

extraction techniques[14]; three phase oesophagectomy using the McKeown technique or the en bloc oesophagectomy of Skinner[15]; or three phase oesophagectomy with three field lymph node dissection which resects the regional lymph nodes in the abdomen, the mediastinum and bilaterally in the neck.[16]

Preoperative treatment with a combination of irradiation and chemotherapy may be added to any of the above procedures. The combination of irradiation and chemotherapy may also be used on its own.[17] Hyperthermia using an intracavitary device to raise the local temperature to 40° has been used to enhance the effect of irradiation on hypoxic cells and tumour cells in the S-phase.[18,19] It also enables the same effect to be achieved with a lower dose of radiation. Radiation alone is still used as definitive treatment in some centres.[20]

The following is an account of the results of these individual approaches to oesophageal cancer including perioperative mortality, early and late complications, recurrence rate and long term survival.

RADICAL RADIOTHERAPY

There have been no prospective randomized trials comparing radiotherapy and surgery. Pearson's[21] study, which is frequently cited, compared his radiotherapy results with the results of a group of patients undergoing surgery at a different time. Nevertheless Pearson's results are impressive, showing a 25% survival in patients with cervical lesions, 16% survival for tumours of the mid-oesophagus and 12% for lower third tumours. Huang and Wu[22] also report a remarkably high five year survival rate of 32.3% in patients with cervical tumours. The superior results obtained with radiotherapy for cervical lesions probably reflect a different referral pattern for lesions of the upper and lower oesophagus with a higher radiation referral rate of early lesions of the cervical oesophagus because of perceived surgical difficulties. In contrast, more advanced and inoperable lesions of the middle and lower oesophagus are referred for radiotherapy, with earlier lesions accepted for surgery.

Small squamous cell tumours with a good blood supply respond best to irradiation. Anaemia should be corrected prior to treatment and nutritional support given either parenterally or via an enteral tube. Radical radiotherapy is generally regarded as a dosage of 50 Gy given over a period of four weeks. Doses of up to 60 or 70 Gy may also be used. A variety of techniques may be employed using rotational fields, opposing fields or three fields.

Complications include radiation pneumonitis, oesophagitis or myelitis.[23,24] Massive haemorrhage may occur in the course of treatment. Perforation of the oesophagus can occur with mediastinitis or fistula formation. Benign stricture of the oesophagus due to fibrosis occurs in about 50% of treated patients and may require repeated dilatation. Dilatation in the early post-treatment period is dangerous and there is a real risk of instrumental perforation.

Radiation is seldom used alone nowadays and is usually combined with chemotherapy, either as sole treatment or as a preliminary to surgical resection. Hyperthermia may be added to the combination to enhance the effect. A recent study comparing radiation therapy alone and in combination with 5-fluorouracil and cis-platin showed distinct advantages with the combined treatment.[12] The median survival with combined therapy was 12.5 months as against 8.9 months for radiation alone. Survival at 12 and 24 months was 50% and 38% respectively for the combined therapy group and 38% and 10% for the radiotherapy group. The combined therapy group also demonstrated fewer instances of local and distant recurrence. There was, however, a significantly greater incidence of severe and life-threatening side effects in the combined therapy group.

COMBINED RADIOTHERAPY AND CHEMOTHERAPY

Franklin *et al.*,[25] having reported a local recurrence rate of only 13% following a preoperative regimen of 5-fluorouracil and mitomycin C plus radiation to 30 Gy for squamous cell tumours and having identified a subgroup with no tumour in the resected specimen as long term survivors, went on to suggest that an increased dosage of radiotherapy and two courses of chemotherapy might obviate the need for surgery. A pilot study by Coia *et al.*[26] also reported encouraging results using chemotherapy and irradiation alone. A more extensive study by the same group[27] demonstrated that of 30 patients with stage 2 and 3 disease the overall response rate was 87%, the local relapse-free rate at one year was 73% and the two year survival rate was 47%. Similar relapse-free rates and two year survival rates were obtained by Keane *et al.*[28] using a similar regimen. A number of trends appear in these and other trials which have yet to be fully validated. The relapse-free rate of squamous cell tumours is greater than for adenocarcinomas. Similarly there seems to be a trend towards improved survival in tumours of the upper two thirds of the thoracic oesophagus when compared with tumours of the lower third of the oesophagus.

HYPERTHERMIA, CHEMOTHERAPY AND RADIOTHERAPY

The combination of hyperthermia with radiotherapy and chemotherapy (HCR) has been shown to be more effective than chemotherapy and radiotherapy (CR) alone. The histopathological effectiveness of both regimens were compared by

Matsuda *et al.*[29] In the HCR group 69% of tumour cells were rendered non-viable or were severely damaged. In the CR group the percentage of tumour cells similarly affected was 48%. The difference was found to be statistically significant. Following resection this difference in preoperative tumour cell damage was reflected in the survival rates. The three year survival rate for the HCR group was 31.3% and for the CR group 19.3%. The combination of hyperthermia, radiotherapy and chemotherapy was also shown to improve survival in advanced and inoperable tumours of the oesophagus.

SURGICAL RESECTION FOR ADENOCARCINOMA OF THE OESOPHAGUS AND CARDIA

According to Muller and colleagues,[2] most authors reporting their experience with oesophageal resection for carcinoma during the period 1980–88 felt that adenocarcinomas of the gastro-oesophageal junction required only partial resection of the thoracic oesophagus to the level of the aortic arch or the azygos vein, depending on which approach was used. The most favoured approach was the thoracoabdominal followed by the left thoracic. Transhiatal resection, however, was also popular allowing the area of the tumour to be dissected under vision and the "blind" mobilization to be carried out on the normal oesophagus.

In general, adenocarcinomas in the region of the cardia, including those arising in Barrett's ectopic epithelium, have a poor prognosis.[30,31] McKeown's division of tumour sites in the oesophagus into seven different areas is a helpful convention. Sites 5, 6 and 7 in his nomenclature include the lower oesophagus and gastro-oesophageal junction. Site 5 is located in that portion of the oesophagus immediately above the diaphragm and sites 6 and 7 identify the abdominal oesophagus and the gastro-oesophageal junction respectively. In McKeown's view, with which we concur, tumours at site 5 require resection of the lower oesophagus to the arch of the aorta, the spleen, distal pancreas and proximal stomach to the antrum and all associated lymph node groups. Tumours at sites 6 and 7 require a similar resection which includes total gastrectomy.

In Muller's analysis[2] no significant difference in mortality rates was found between patients with tumours at different sites, including those located at the gastro-oesophageal junction with a mean of around 18%. The mortality was also unaffected by whether the approach was through the right or left chest. However, three stage resection with cervical anastomosis reduced mortality to around 12% and for transhiatal blunt dissection, the figure was 11%. Adenocarcinoma of the cardia had a lower five year survival rate than squamous cell carcinoma and a recent report gave a mean survival time of 11 months.[32] Our own experience of 18% five year survival is somewhat higher than the overall figure of 15%.[33] Muller and colleagues found a 24% five year survival for squamous cell carcinoma.

TRANSHIATAL RESECTION OF THE OESOPHAGUS

Orringer's two main reasons for advocating transhiatal resection of the oesophagus without thoracotomy are the avoidance of the mortality associated with thoracotomy and the disastrous consequences of an intrathoracic anastomotic leak.[34] There is certainly evidence to show that pulmonary complications such as atelectasis, pneumonia and pulmonary insufficiency are more frequent after transthoracic oesophagectomy. Anastomotic leakage into the neck is undoubtedly less likely to be fatal than an intrathoracic leak but it is also true that anastomotic leakage is more frequent after cervical anastomosis and leakage into the mediastinum can also occur with a cervical anastomosis. However, the low mortality of 5% with transhiatal resection reported by Orringer is reflected in most reports of this technique. The technique was originally designed as a palliative procedure and although the two year survival of 32% and the four year survival of 17% is not greatly different from the results of more extensive procedures, clearly any improvement is only likely to be achieved by combining the technique with some form of adjuvant therapy.

Although generally regarded as a "blind" dissection, Orringer has pointed out that most tumours of the lower 10 cm of the thoracic oesophagus and the upper 5 cm can be dissected under vision. Nevertheless, there is a genuine risk of significant bleeding or injury to the membranous posterior wall of the trachea. Conversion to thoracotomy should be undertaken if there is any difficulty in mobilizing the tumour.

The incidence of thoracic duct injury is also high with transhiatal oesophagectomy and Orringer has reported a rate of 2.5%.[35] Our experience has been similar with only two patients developing chylothorax out of more than 500 patients operated on by the transthoracic route while 5% of a small series of transhiatal oesophagectomies sustained an injury to the thoracic duct.[36] There is also an increased risk of laryngeal nerve injury.

Our experience with transhiatal techniques has not been very satisfactory. The perioperative mortality was no better than with transthoracic operations and although there were no instances of serious haemorrhage or tracheal injury, the increased incidence of chylothorax with its attendant morbidity and mortality is a significant deterrent.

INVERSION–EXTRACTION OESOPHAGECTOMY

This is a variation in the transhiatal technique in which an instrument similar to a varicose vein stripper is passed through the oesophageal lumen from an oesophagotomy below.[14] After transection of the cervical oesophagus and after securing the distal divided end of the oesophagus around the stripper with a strong ligature, the oesophagus is stripped out of the mediastinum by inversion into the lumen. The technique is suitable only in situations where the intrathoracic oesophagus is normal.

Our experience with this technique is limited but we found difficulty in delivering the gastric tube into the cervical region through the narrow "tunnel" provided by this technique.

THE LEWIS–TANNER RESECTION

The Lewis–Tanner resection[37,38] mobilizing the stomach through a midline abdominal incision and approaching the oesophagus through a rightsided thoracotomy is probably still the most frequently used technique for resection of squamous carcinoma of the oesophagus. The advantages include dissection of the intrathoracic oesophagus and regional lymph nodes under vision. For the majority of midthoracic tumours whose upper margins are usually around the level of the arch of the azygos vein, the proximal clearance is adequate. High intrathoracic anastomosis is not technically a problem provided that the approach has been made sufficiently high, resecting the fifth rib.

Wong[39] has pointed out that the difference between a high intrathoracic anastomosis carried out at the apex of the right chest and a cervical anastomosis is no more than 2 cm. The aim should be to achieve proximal clearance of around 10 cm.

The advantages of the technique must be balanced against the increased risk of pulmonary complications and the risk of an intrathoracic anastomotic leak with its high mortality. Mortality rates are no different from those found with left thoracotomy and overall five year survival is similar at 20%. It is disappointing that the Lewis–Tanner technique, despite the fact that it affords the opportunity for adequate proximal and distal clearance and the dissection of coeliac and mediastinal lymph nodes, provides no additional benefit in terms of duration of survival.

THREE PHASE RESECTION

McKeown's three phase oesophageal resection[40] provides good proximal and distal margins and offers the added safety of a cervical anastomosis. The disadvantages include the sequential dissections in the abdomen, thorax and neck which make the operation a lengthy one and the difficulty of delivering a bulky tumour through the narrow thoracic inlet. We have modified the operation to obviate these problems.[41]

In the modified technique the operation is commenced in the chest and the thoracic oesophagus and mediastinal lymph nodes are dissected via a right thoracotomy. The cervical and abdominal dissections are carried out simultaneously by two surgeons using left cervical and midline epigastric incisions respectively. After division of the cervical oesophagus a length of Penrose drain is attached to the distal cut end and the thoracic oesophagus withdrawn through the posterior mediastinum into the abdomen where it is removed with the cardia and part of the lesser curvature of the stomach. The stomach is then reconstructed in a tubular fashion and, after suture to the Penrose drain still in situ in the posterior mediastinum, is drawn through the mediastinum into the neck. Anastomosis is then carried out between the cervical oesophagus and the gastric fundus. Usually the most suitable site is the posterior wall.

Pulmonary complications occur with a similar frequency to other transthoracic techniques and cardiac arrhythmias are also common. There is an increased risk of injury to the recurrent laryngeal nerve which can be minimized by avoiding the use of metal retractors in the neck dissection. Anastomotic leaks are uncommon but can undoubtedly leak into the mediastinum as well as externally in the neck. Gastric stasis is more common after three phase resection and there is a risk of regurgitation and pulmonary aspiration in the early postoperative weeks in debilitated patients. The question of whether or not pyloromyotomy or pyloroplasty should be employed remains unresolved although we have had occasional dramatic evidence of its effectiveness when carried out as a secondary procedure for persistent gastric stasis.

Three stage oesophagectomy has reduced the incidence of microscopic tumour at resection margins from 19% to 7% in our experience and this should have a positive effect on locoregional control of the tumour. However, there are not yet sufficient numbers in our series who have undergone surgery more than five years ago to observe any trend towards long term survival. In Muller's review long term survival was not improved with the three phase technique, nor did the addition of extensive mediastinal lymph node dissection confer any additional survival benefit.

EN BLOC RESECTION OF THE OESOPHAGUS

The rationale underlying the en bloc resection advocated by Skinner[42] is based on the conviction that if wall penetration is absent or minimal, with no more than four local lymph nodes involved, and if there is no evidence of distant metastases, it is possible to eradicate the tumour locally and improve the prospects of long term survival. The resection includes 10 cm margins proximally and distally and includes a block of tissue which, in addition to the thoracic oesophagus, encompasses both pleural surfaces, the azygos vein, thoracic duct, posterior pericardium and all adjacent lymphatic and fibrofatty tissue. Either stomach or colon can be used for the reconstruction. The latter is preferred by Skinner because of fewer problems with reflux oesophagitis and stricture formation. Very accurate preoperative staging is required as the oesophageal tumour is not evaluated until quite late in the dissection and such an extensive dissection is unjustified unless the criteria listed above with regard to staging are met.

Skinner's overall five year survival rate for en bloc resection was 21%. He also reported a three year survival rate of 44% and 50% respectively for patients with wall penetration or lymph node involvement. Mortality rate is not increased by the extensive dissection involved in this technique and the incidence of vocal cord paralysis is low at 2%.[43] The author conceded that the technique is likely to benefit only those patients with early wall penetration or early lymph node involvement of one to four glands. Nevertheless an analysis of the site of recurrence in 20 patients with adenocarcinoma arising in Barrett's epithelium who died of metastatic disease demonstrates the excellent local control afforded by en bloc resection. Only one patient had a mediastinal recurrence while four patients developed metastatic disease in cervical lymph nodes.[31] These results, of course, also raise the important question of whether formal cervical lymph node dissection should be carried out.

CERVICAL LYMPH NODE DISSECTION

The inclusion of cervical lymph node dissection in radical operations for carcinoma of the oesophagus is both novel and controversial at the present time. In the past, involvement of cervical nodes was classified as distant metastases and was seen as evidence of systemic disease if it was associated with lower third or even middle third tumours. There is now increasing evidence to suggest that despite spread to cervical nodes, the tumour may be regarded as regionally confined.

The variability of lymph node dissection is very considerable. Most surgeons carry out a fairly complete abdominal lymph node dissection and the majority are equally thorough in dissecting nodes in the lower and middle mediastinum.

Few, however, embark on lymph node dissection in the neck. Kato *et al.*[44] recorded a five year survival of 20% for operations of this magnitude. Whether extension of the thoracic dissection to include the upper mediastinal but not the cervical lymph nodes would improve long term survival has not been established although one Japanese study demonstrated a 60% actuarial five year survival for mediastinal dissection only, when more extensive node dissection was excluded on the basis of preoperative staging using ultrasound computerized tomography and endoscopic ultrasonography.[45] The need for dissection of the superior mediastinum is emphasized by Akiyama's[46] report that metastatic lymph nodes in the superior mediastinum are found in 36% of tumours of the upper thoracic oesophagus, in 12% of midthoracic oesophageal tumours and 11% of lower thoracic oesophageal tumours. Since lymphatic drainage of the oesophagus is bidirectional, this distribution pattern of lymph node involvement is to be anticipated.

Even among those who favour extended lymph node dissection in three fields, controversy exists on whether this should be done on a selective basis. It has been reported that while patients without lymph node metastases benefit from three field dissection the benefits are less certain when lymph node involvement is present.[47] But evidence has also been presented that survival is improved in patients with nodal metastases and that survival is uninfluenced by extended dissection if the lymph nodes are clear.[48] To complete the picture Isono *et al.*[49] claim that both categories of patients benefit from the three field technique.

The importance of lymphadenectomy is not only related to its effect on prognosis but also to its prophylactic function against local recurrence and not least to its value in diagnostic staging. There is no other reliable method of staging available at present. A minimum number of dissected lymph nodes is required for reliable staging and Siewert[50] has suggested that the minimum requirement should be 15–20 nodes for each oesophagectomy specimen.

The impact of lymphadenectomy on local recurrence is illustrated by the reduced local recurrence rate of 5.3% found by Siewert after en bloc resection. By contrast, Barbier *et al.*[51] found a local recurrence rate of more than 50% after incomplete lymphadenectomy.

Evaluation of extended lymph node dissection is hampered at present by the absence of prospective randomized trials. Most analyses are retrospective and compare groups of patients operated on during different time spans. The only randomized study available at present was carried out by Kato *et al.*[44] and this study has been criticized on the grounds that one group had older patients and a higher mortality in the two field group who were also operated on by a different surgical team. The two field group also had more tumours located in the upper mid oesophagus which might have adversely affected the results. Allowing for these disparities, the results in the three field group are impressive. The hospital mortality for this group was 2.6%. The five year survival rate was 49% versus 34% for the two field group. The percentage of patients with positive nodes was comparable in both groups, 64% versus 66%, and no difference was seen in the incidence of complications, including anastomotic leakage. However, the limited dissection in the two field group and the greater number of upper mid thoracic tumours makes it at least possible that the two field group was understaged in relation to lymph node involvement with consequent effect on the prognosis.

Peracchia *et al.*[52] studied a group of 240 patients with carcinoma of the thoracic oesophagus operated on between 1980 and 1986 by transthoracic oesophagectomy and standard lymphadenectomy and also a group of 40 patients undergoing oesophagectomy with three field lymphadenectomy between 1987 and 1990. Although the groups were comparable in terms of age, sex and tumour location the authors felt that a valid comparison could not be made because patient selection had been employed in the extended dissection group. Nevertheless some of the results are worth noting. The mortality rate was

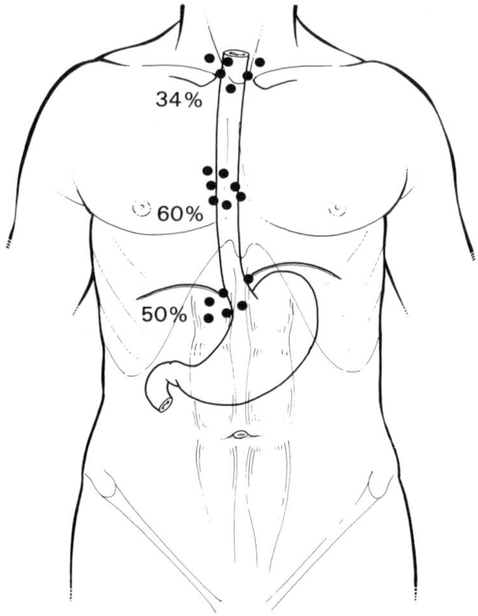

Figure 11.1.1 Distribution of involved lymph nodes.

roughly similar, being 7.5% and 5% respectively for standard and extended resection. The incidence of recurrent laryngeal nerve lesions was also similar at 6.2% for standard resection and 7.5% for extended resection, lending further support to the belief that most of these injuries arise during dissection of the superior mediastinum. The frequency of locoregional recurrence was 43% and the five year survival was a predictable 20.8% in the patients who underwent a standard dissection. The lymph node status proved the most important prognostic factor and five year survival rose to 35% for patients with negative lymph nodes. Another significant observation was that although the location of the tumour had no influence on survival if lymph nodes were involved, upper thoracic tumours had a worse prognosis in node negative patients. The implication of this finding is that the limitations of standard resection in upper thoracic tumours lead to understaging and the allocation of a false negative lymph node status. According to the same author, similar understaging appears to occur in transhiatal oesophagectomy with 29% five year survival after the transhiatal technique and 41% after transthoracic oesophagectomy in the absence of lymph node involvement.[53]

The distribution of lymph node metastases has been studied by Tsurumuru *et al.*[54] who reported that in 34.1% of patients, cervical lymph nodes were involved, 59.9% of patients had positive mediastinal nodes and 50% of patients had abdominal lymph node metastases (Fig. 11.1.1). They also found that 21.4% of patients had positive lymph nodes in all three regions simultaneously.

Looking separately at cervical lymph node metastases they found that 90% of positive nodes were confined to the triangle bounded by the omohyoid muscle, the clavicle and the oesophagus. Positive nodes were slightly more common on the right side compared with the left (24.2% vs. 18.1% respectively) and bilateral involved cervical nodes occurred in 8.2% of patients. Positive cervical nodes alone or positive cervical and abdominal nodes without mediastinal involvement occurred but rarely.

Ide *et al.*[45] carried out a study in which extent of dissection was matched to preoperative staging determined by conventional and endoscopic ultrasound. The study was stimulated by failure of standard dissection plus postoperative T-shaped irradiation to improve five year survival beyond 22–23%. Depending on ultrasound findings, patients received either a standard dissection, a standard plus leftsided neck dissection or an extended dissection including bilateral cervical lymph nodes. Despite the greater incidence of advanced disease and upper thoracic tumours in patients undergoing three field dissection, three and four year survival was similar in all three groups. It is of interest to note that apart from anastomotic leak, the incidence of which was similar in all three groups, postoperative complications such as pneumonia and recurrent nerve paralysis were considerably less in patients receiving leftsided neck dissection only. The mortality rate was also greater in patients undergoing the full three field dissection.

A number of reports on three field dissection give an operating time of around eight hours and emphasize the need for several days' postoperative ventilatory support. This may have an adverse effect on postoperative morbidity and mortality. It has been our experience that when routine overnight mechanical ventilation was abandoned there was a significant reduction in postoperative morbidity.

The recently reported Japanese nationwide study[49] compared almost 1800 cases of three field oesophagectomy with almost 2800 patients undergoing two field oesophagectomy. Ninety-six institutions participated in the study. The 30 day mortality for the extended operation was 2.8% compared with 4.6% for the standard operation. Lymph node metastases were present in 73% of patients in the extended operation group and 59% of patients in the standard group. The overall rate of metastatic cervical nodes was 27% but rose to 42% for upper oesophageal tumours and fell to 19% for lower oesophageal tumours. Abdominal nodes exhibited a trend in the opposite direction with a rate of 64% for lower oesophageal tumours and 41% and 19% respectively for middle and upper oesophageal tumours. Laryngeal nerve paralysis was more frequent after three field oesophagectomy than after two field oesophagectomy but the incidence was high in both operations at 20% and 14% respectively. The five year survival was better overall for the extended operation; 34% vs. 27%, and the difference was statistically significant. Extended oesophagectomy provided better long term survival in patients without nodal metastases (57% vs. 45%) and also in patients with involved lymph nodes (33% vs. 29%). Patients with tumours staged as T1, T2 or T3 all survived longer with the three field operation but the prognosis of T4 tumours was unaffected. It is worth noting that even with the standard two field oesophagectomy the five year survival figures are better than average.

Perhaps the most interesting survival figures recently reported are those of Udagawa and Akiyama[55] who obtained a five year survival rate of 100% for stage 1 tumours after three field oesophagectomy compared with 59% survival for those undergoing two field oesophagectomy. The figures for stage 2 patients were 84% and 58% respectively. While such differences could be attributed to more accurate staging in three field oesophagectomy, there was also a better prognosis after the extended operation in patients with stage 4 disease with distant nodal metastases (25% vs. 14%) and this difference cannot be due to inaccurate staging.

A difference in the recurrence patterns was noted by Desai *et al.*[56] between patients undergoing three field oesophagectomy and standard oesophagectomy. In the latter group recurrence was predominantly in lymph nodes whereas recurrence after the extended operation tended to be in distant sites such as lungs and liver and nodal recurrence tended to be in the cervical region following resection of more proximally placed lesions.

A definitive statement on the value of oesophagectomy with three field lymphadenectomy must await the outcome of prospective controlled randomized trials. However, the evidence to date suggests that the more radical operation makes a number of valuable contributions. The accuracy of staging is improved and it reduces the incidence of locoregional recurrence. It improves overall survival and the prognosis in upper thoracic oesophageal tumours. The extended operation does not seem to have an adverse effect on perioperative mortality but there is a significant increase in the incidence of laryngeal nerve injury and vocal cord paralysis. Clearly all the beneficial effects of oesophagectomy with three field lymphadenectomy derive from better clearance of locoregional disease. No benefit is likely to accrue from the procedure if micrometastases are present elsewhere. The presence of five or more positive lymph nodes according to Skinner is a strong indicator that distant metastases are present. Combination therapy with preoperative irradiation and chemotherapy using more than one agent is designed to deal with this situation and is under extensive investigation at present (see Table 11.1.1).

Table 11.1.1 Complications scale with different techniques

	Standard resection	THR	Three stage	Three field
Anastomotic leak	+	++	++	++
Thoracic duct leak	+	++	+	+
Laryngeal n. paralysis	−	+	+	++
Tracheal bronchial injury	−	++	−	−

THR: transhiatal resection

COMBINED THERAPY

Multimodality or combined therapy is based on the conviction that the radio-sensitizing properties of the chemotherapeutic agents used will enhance the effects of the radiotherapy and that the cytotoxic properties of the drugs used will have a systemic effect also. The suggestion that resection is unnecessary is unwarranted even if endoscopy and biopsy suggest that the tumour has been eliminated. Resection offers the best available means of detecting and at the same time eliminating residual tumour and is an essential part of the combined treatment. The best results appear to accrue from a combination of 5-fluorouracil and cis-platin, and mitomycin, adriamycin, vincristine and bleomycin are also used. Experimental evidence suggests that the best results are achieved by preoperative administration. Radiation dosage is generally in the region of 30 Gy. Complete eradication of the tumour is the best prognostic indicator but complete remission of this sort is infrequent and was recorded in only 18% of Poplin's[57] series, although Orringer *et al.*[58] found that one quarter of their patients had no tumour in the resected specimen. Toxicity with some multimodality regimens is high with significant morbidity and mortality and although Leichman *et al.*[59] obtained a 25% eradication of tumour with a regimen of 5-fluorouracil, cis-platin and radiotherapy, the hospital mortality following resection was a forbidding 27%.

Multimodality regimens have been used successfully for both squamous tumours and adenocarcinomas of the oesophagus. Pilot studies and comparisons with radiotherapy and historical controls have been reported but there is a need for controlled prospective randomized trials to determine the advantages of these multimodality treatments.

The trial conducted by Coia *et al.*[26] combined radiotherapy and chemotherapy which included 5-fluorouracil and mitomycin for patients with adenocarcinoma of the gastro-oesophageal junction. Although seven out of eight patients in the definitive treatment group had a complete response, there were two local recurrences in regional nodes and two patients in whom distant metastases appeared. All these recurrences appeared in the first year after treatment. The need for oesophagectomy after initial combined treatment is obvious and is further emphasized by the fact that a patient with local failure of treatment and persistent primary tumour underwent oesophagectomy ten months after treatment and was disease-free 46 months later. Failure to respond fully was followed by rapid development of local and disseminated disease. Urba *et al.*[60] found no improvement in survival with a regimen of 4900 cGy fractionated to 350 cGy five days per week and 5-fluorouracil followed by transhiatal oesophagectomy. They also found significant toxicity due to the radiotherapy. This unsatisfactory regimen differs from others in which better results were obtained by the high radiation dosage concentrated in 14 fractions and the use of only a single cytotoxic agent. The results obtained by MacFarlane *et al.*[61] with irradiation, 5-fluorouracil, cis-platin and mitomycin for adenocarcinomas of the gastro-oesophageal junction were much better, with downgrading of the tumour and a trend towards improved survival when compared with historical controls who had surgery only. The numbers, however, are very small and historical controls are unsatisfactory and the inclusion of squamous cell tumours of the lower end of the oesophagus, although separately analysed, causes a certain amount of confusion.

It is of interest to note that while, after resection alone, the extent of local disease as indicated by lymph node status was a reliable indicator of survival, this was not the case after preoperative chemoradiation. This paper also emphasizes the importance of resection in the combined therapy approach, noting the improvement in survival after resection of residual local disease. Hilgenberg *et al.*[62] studied the effect of 5-fluorouracil and cis-platin combined with resection on survival in patients with squamous cell tumours. Radiation was used postoperatively in patients at particular risk of local recurrence. Postoperative chemotherapy was given to diminish the incidence of systematic disease. Actuarial survival at 42 months was 54%. Multivariate analysis showed that the significant factors associated with three year survival were complete clinical response to the preoperative regimen, absence of tumour or, at most, only microscopic evidence of tumour in the resection specimen and absence of wall penetration. Permanent renal failure occurred in one patient after receiving cis-platin. Five patients required adjustment of the cis-platin dosage because of diminished renal function.

The report by Orringer *et al.*[58] further emphasizes the risk of serious, including fatal toxicity from multimodality regimens. Patients received 5-fluorouracil, cis-platin and vinblastine with radiation to a dosage of 45 Gy prior to transhiatal oesophagectomy. Two patients died of toxic complications but more significantly, only 26% of patients were able to tolerate the full planned dosages of all three drugs. As is usual, total responders did well and there was an overall survival rate of 60% at two years. Patients with adenocarcinoma appeared to have a survival advantage over those with squamous cell carcinoma but the difference was not statistically significant.

The studies reported above are from individual centres and because of the small numbers involved in each study, the results are difficult to evaluate.

The report of the Southwest Oncology Group[57] on combined therapy for squamous cell carcinoma of the oesophagus presents a study organized by eight separate institutions. There were 106 evaluable patients in the study. Complete response rate was 17%. If partial responses are included, the response rate was 37%. The overall resectability rate was relatively low at 49%. Total surgery associated mortality was 11%. The median survival rate was 12 months with a 28% survival at two years and a 16% survival rate at three years. When complete response was documented surgically median survival rose to 32 months with 67% survival after two years and 45% after three years. The protocol used in this study was 5-fluorouracil, cis-platin and 3000 cGy. While toxic reactions were reported as life-threatening in eight patients, no deaths were attributed to toxicity. The improvement in survival in complete responders

Table 11.1.2 Main complications of multimodality therapy

1.	Nausea and vomiting
2.	Myelosuppression
3.	Renal failure
4.	Pulmonary fibrosis
5.	Myelitis

identified at surgery was impressive but the overall median survival was no greater than could have been achieved with surgery or radiation alone, according to the authors. One of the difficulties in assessing the outcome of multimodality treatment is that restrictions in chemotherapy and radiation dosages imposed by toxic complications may result in considerable variations in total preoperative treatment. These anomalies may be further magnified when applicable to a number of different centres.

Kelsen *et al.*[63] had one of the highest median survival figures at 26 months using a protocol which consisted of cis-platin, vindesine and mitoguazone followed by surgery. The response rate was 42% and the resection rate was 86%. Median survival rates vary greatly in various studies and are a reflection of the small number of patients in individual groups with a consequently uneven distribution of early and late cases.

Our own experience with multimodality treatment has been encouraging although to date there are few hard data to report. Our study has been organized prospectively as a randomized controlled trial comparing surgery alone with a regimen of 5-fluorouracil, cis-platin and radiotherapy followed by surgery and the results with adenocarcinomas and squamous cell carcinoma will be analysed separately. To date, more than 100 patients have been included in the trial but because the trial contains four arms the numbers available for analysis are still small. However, complete response has been identified histologically in some patients. Complete response is more frequently seen in patients with squamous cell carcinoma than in those with adenocarcinoma. There is also a significant downgrading of the tumour after multimodality treatment. The principal toxic reactions observed have been myelosuppression, nausea and vomiting (Table 11.1.2). The gastrointestinal symptoms have been well controlled by the anti-emetic drug Zofran. There has been no significant effect on pulmonary or renal function. The preoperative regimen has not adversely affected perioperative morbidity or mortality. As yet, insufficient time has elapsed to make an assessment of the effect on survival. There is, however, a trend towards improved survival which is not yet statistically significant.

SUMMARY

Conventional surgery at the present time consists of partial oesophagectomy through a leftsided approach for lesions of the cardia or lower oesophagus and a

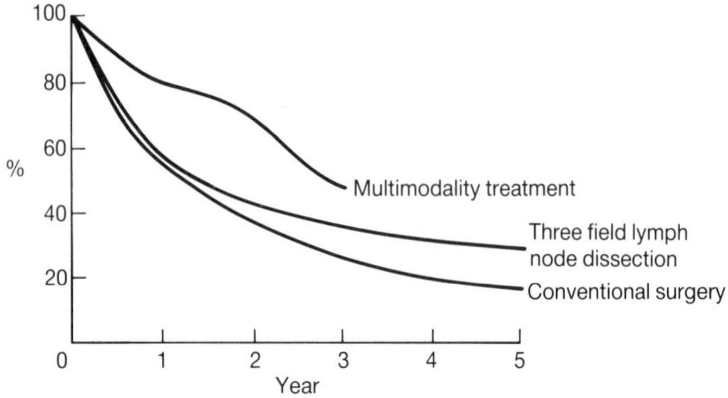

Figure 11.1.2 Survival rates with different regimens.

rightsided or Lewis–Tanner approach for lesions of the midthoracic oesophagus. Upper thoracic oesophageal tumours require a three phase oesophagectomy. The proximal resection margins with such conventional surgery should be at least 5–8 cm clear of the tumour. The associated lymphadenectomy should include left gastric, splenic, diaphragmatic and coeliac nodes in the abdominal dissection and lower and middle mediastinal nodes in the thoracic dissection. If resectability rates are limited to around 70%, thereby excluding very old or debilitated patients, those with severe concomitant disease or those with very advanced lesions, mortality should be in the region of 5–8%. Mean survival is unlikely to exceed 12 or 13 months and overall five year survival with a standard distribution of early and late cases will be between 15 and 20% (Fig. 11.1.2).

The most frequent complications will be pulmonary infection or cardiac irregularities but few of those should prove fatal. Anastomotic leaks should be not more than 1 or 2% but many of these are likely to have a fatal outcome. Recurrent laryngeal nerve paralysis after conventional surgery is rare and mostly associated with the three phase operation. Half or more of the patients will die of locoregional (mediastinal) recurrence between six months and five years after the operation, the majority in the first two years. Virtually all the five year survivors will have had no evidence of lymph node involvement in the resected specimens.

If transhiatal oesophagectomy is the operation of choice morbidity and mortality due to respiratory complications should be less but other complications such as tracheal injury, recurrent laryngeal nerve paralysis and injury to the thoracic duct will be greater. Five year survival should be similar to the figure for transthoracic oesophagectomy and reflects the percentage of patients without involvement of lymph nodes. Mean survival time is likely to be less than that for the transthoracic oesophagectomy because of the increased likelihood with this technique of leaving behind residual tumour outside the oesophageal wall and in the regional lymph nodes.

The inversion–extraction technique is probably best reserved for tumours around the cardia when the oesophagus in the area of the tumour can be dissected under vision. Results should be similar to those of conventional transhiatal oesophagectomy but the risk of tracheal or other mediastinal injury should be less.

If all Lewis–Tanner anastomoses were carried out at the apex of the chest cavity it is unlikely that there would be any difference between two stage resections via the right thoracic cavity and cervical anastomoses with regard to microscopic marginal involvement. However, since it is not always possible to carry out intrathoracic anastomoses at the desired high level there is a recordable advantage with cervical anastomosis in relation to microscopic marginal involvement which should be no more than 5% or even less than that.

Despite the possible defects in Kato's[44] controlled trial of oesophagectomy with three field lymph node dissection versus two field lymphadenectomy the results demonstrate what can be achieved with this technique, bearing in mind that many Japanese studies demonstrate superior results in terms of mortality and morbidity irrespective of the extent of lymph node dissection. Mortality for three field dissection was 2.6%. This can be compared with Peracchia's[52] 5% mortality rate for the same operation. The five year survival rate was an impressive 49%. However, even with standard dissection the five year survival was 34%. Perhaps the multicentric study of Isono *et al.*[49] is more representative with a five year survival of 34% for three field dissection. What is clear is that this extensive operation does not increase operative mortality. However, the incidence of laryngeal nerve paralysis rises sharply and an incidence of around 20% can be predicted.

The major benefit accruing from Skinner's en bloc dissection seems to be a reduction in mediastinal recurrence and a better two and three year survival without an increase in morbidity or mortality. However, five year survival is not significantly improved overall.

The effectiveness of multimodality therapy has still to be demonstrated from the outcome of prospective randomized trials but certain facts have already emerged from pilot studies. A combination of chemotherapeutic agents is more effective than a single agent and such a combination enhances the effect of radiotherapy. Squamous cell tumours respond more readily than adenocarcinomas. Downgrading of tumour is achieved in a substantial percentage of patients which improves resectability and reduces the risk of local recurrence. When complete histological response is achieved, i.e. no detectable tumour in the resected specimen, the two and three year survival rate is improved but non-responders derive no benefit from the regimen. There is a significant morbidity and mortality from most of the regimens in use, myelosuppression and renal failure being two of the principal problems. Since only around 20% of patients on average are complete responders likely to benefit from therapy, this has to be measured against 80% of patients who do not respond and do not benefit but may actually be harmed by the treatment. This problem can only be resolved by finding a reliable indicator of likely response. In the meantime the outcome of controlled trials currently in progress may give us a better knowledge of what we can expect of multimodality treatment in the future.

REFERENCES

1. Earlam R, Cunha-Melo JR. Oesophageal squamous cell carcinoma: a review of surgery. *Br J Surg* 1989; **67**: 381–91.
2. Muller JM, Erasmi H, Stelzner M, Zieren Y, Pichlmaier H. Surgical therapy of oesophageal carcinoma. *Br J Surg* 1990; **77**: 845–57.
3. McKeown KC. Resection of mid esophageal carcinoma with esophagogastric anastomosis. *World J Surg* 1981; **5**: 517–25.
4. Hennessy TPJ, O'Connell R. Carcinoma of the hypopharynx, esophagus and cardia. *Surg Gynecol Obstet* 1986; **162**: 243–7.
5. Giuli R, Gignoux M. Treatment of carcinoma of the esophagus. Retrospective study of 2400 patients. *Ann Surg* 1980; **192**: 44–52.
6. Skinner DB. Curative surgery for oesophageal carcinoma. In: *Surgery of the Oesophagus* (ed. Jamieson GG.), pp. 617–22. New York, Churchill Livingstone, 1988.
7. McKeown KC. Carcinoma of the oesophagus. *J Roy Coll Surg Edinb* 1979, **24**: 253–74.
8. Ravitch MM, Steichen FM. A stapling instrument for end-to-end inverting anastomoses in the gastrointestinal tract. *Ann Surg* 1979; **189**: 791–7.
9. Guo Jun Huang, Xian Zhi Gu, Liang Jun Wang *et al.* Combined preoperative irradiation and surgery versus surgery alone for squamous cell carcinoma of the midthoracic esophagus: A prospective randomized study in 360 patients. In: *Diseases of the Esophagus: Malignant Diseases* (eds Ferguson MK, Little AG, Skinner DB), pp. 275–81. New York, Futura Publishing Co, 1990.
10. Carey RW, Hilgenberg AD, Wilkins EW, Choi NC. Preoperative chemotherapy followed by surgery with possible postoperative radiotherapy in squamous cell carcinoma of the esophagus. *J Clin Oncol* 1986; **5**: 697–701.
11. Shields TW, Rosen ST, Hellerstein SM, Tsang T. Multimodality approach to treatment of carcinoma of the esophagus. *Arch Surg* 1984; **119**: 558–62.
12. Herskovic A, Martz K, Muhyi AS *et al.* Combined chemotherapy and radiotherapy compared with radiotherapy alone in patients with cancer of the esophagus. *New Eng J Med* 1992; **326**: 1593–8.
13. Orringer MB, Sloan H. Esophagectomy without thoracotomy. *J Thorac Cardiovasc Surg* 1978; **76**: 643.
14. Huang GJ, Wu YK. Operative technique for cancer of the oesophagus. In: *Carcinoma of the Oesophagus and Gastric Cardia* (eds Huang GJ, Wu YK), pp. 314, **366**: Berlin, Springer Verlag, 1984.
15. Skinner DB. En bloc resection for neoplasms of the esophagus and cardia. *J Thorac Cardiovasc Surg* 1983; **85**: 59–69.
16. Skinner DB. Cervical lymph node dissection for thoracic esophageal cancer. *Ann Thorac Surg* 1991; **51**: 884–5.
17. Lokich JJ, Shea M, Chaffey J. Sequential infusional 5-fluorouracil followed by concomitant radiation for tumors of the esophagus and the gastroesophageal junction. *Cancer* 1987; **60**: 275–9.
18. Li DJ, Wang CQ, Wiu ZL *et al. Intracavitary Microwave Hyperthermia in the Treatment of Esophageal Cancer.* Third International Symposium on Cancer Therapy by Hyperthermia, Drugs and Radiation, Colorado State University, Fort Collins, Colorado 1980.
19. Fujimaki M, Katol H, Tazawa K *et al.* Adjuvant hyperthermia in nonresectable esophageal carcinoma. In: *Diseases of the Esophagus: Malignant Diseases* (eds Ferguson MK, Little AG, Skinner DB), pp. 317–22. New York, Futura Publishing Co, 1990.
20. Earlam R, Cunha-Melo JR. Oesophageal squamous cell carcinoma II. A critical review of radiotherapy. *Br J Surg* 1990; **67**: 457–61.

21. Pearson JG. The present and future potential of radiotherapy in the management of esophageal cancer. *Cancer* 1977; **39**: 882–90.
22. Huang GJ, Wu YK. Radiotherapy for carcinoma of the esophagus. In: *Carcinoma of the Esophagus and Gastric Cardia* (eds Huang GJ, Wu YK), pp. 257–74. Berlin, Springer-Verlag, 1984.
23. Pearson JG. Radiotherapy for esophageal carcinoma. *World J Surg* 1981; **5**: 489–97.
24. Pearson JG. Present status and future potential of radiotherapy in the management of oesophageal cancer. In: *Carcinoma of the Oesophagus* (ed. Silber W), pp. 334–9. Rotterdam, Balkema, 1978.
25. Franklin R, Steiger Z, Vaishampayan G, Asfaw I. Combined modality therapy for esophageal squamous cell carcinoma. *Cancer* 1983; **51**: 1062–71.
26. Coia LR, Paul AR, Engstrom PF. Combined radiation and chemotherapy as primary management of adenocarcinoma of the esophagus and gastroesophageal junction. *Cancer* 1988; **61**: 643–9.
27. Coia LR, Engstrom PF, Paul A. Nonsurgical management of esophageal cancer: report of a study of combined radiotherapy and chemotherapy. *J Clin Oncol* 1987; **4**: 1783–90.
28. Keane J, Harwood A, Elhakim T. Radical radiation therapy with 5-fluorouracil infusion and mitomycin-C for oesophageal squamous carcinoma. *Radiother Oncol* 1985; **4**: 205–10.
29. Matsuda H, Tsutsui S, Nagamatsu M *et al.* Histopathologic and long term effects of hyperthermia combined with chemotherapy and irradiation for esophageal carcinoma. In: *Diseases of the Esophagus: Malignant Diseases* (eds Ferguson MK, Little AG, Skinner DB), pp. 311–15. New York, Futura Publishing Co, 1990.
30. Li H, Walsh TN, Hennessy TPJ. Carcinoma arising in Barrett's oesophagus. *Surg Gynecol Obstet* 1992; **175**: 167–72.
31. Altorki NK, Skinner DB, Ferguson MK, Little AG. Barrett's adenocarcinoma: long-term survival and recurrence patterns. In: *Diseases of the Esophagus: Malignant Diseases* (eds Ferguson MK, Little AG, Skinner DB), pp. 311–15. New York, Futura Publishing Co, 1990.
32. Fein R, Kelson D, Geller N *et al.* Adenocarcinoma of the upper esophagus and gastroesophageal junction: prognostic factors and results of therapy. *Cancer* 1985; **56**: 2512 18.
33. Hennessy TPJ, Keeling P. Adenocarcinoma of the esophagus and cardia. *J Thorac Cardiovasc Surg* 1987; **94**: 64–8.
34. Orringer MB. Technical aids in performing transhiatal esophagectomy without thoracotomy. *Ann Thorac Surg* 1984; **38**: 128–32.
35. Orringer MB. *Technical Aids in Performing Transhiatal Blunt Esophagectomy without Thoracotomy*. Abstracts of the International Society for Diseases of the Oesophagus, Rome, October 1983, E8-1.
36. Bolger C, Walsh TN, Tanner WA, Keeling P, Hennessy TPJ. Chylothorax following oesophagectomy. *Br J Surg* 1991; **78**: 587–8.
37. Lewis I. The surgical treatment of carcinoma of the oesophagus with special reference to a new operation for growths of the middle third. *Br J Surg* 1946; **34**: 18–31.
38. Tanner NC. The present position of carcinoma of the esophagus. *Postgrad Med J* 1947; **23**: 109–39.
39. Wong J. Esophageal resection for cancer: the rationale of current practice. *Am J Surg* 1987; **153**: 18–24.
40. McKeown KC. Total three-stage oesophagectomy for cancer of the oesophagus. *Br J Surg* 1976; **63**: 259–62.
41. Hennessy TPJ. Management of oesophageal cancer. In: *Progress in Surgery* (ed. Taylor I), pp. 32–46. Edinburgh, Churchill Livingstone, 1988.

42. Skinner DB. Surgical treatment for esophageal carcinoma. *Semin Oncol* 1984; **11**: 136–43.
43. Skinner DB, Belsey RHR. Resection for potentially curable esophageal cancer. In: *Management of Esophageal Disease* (eds Skinner DB, Belsey RHR). Philadelphia, WB Saunders, 1988.
44. Kato H, Hiroshi W, Tachimori Y, Iizuka T. Evaluation of neck lymph node dissection for thoracic esophageal carcinoma. *Ann Thor Surg* 1991; **51**: 931–5.
45. Ide H, Hanyu F, Murata Y, Kobayashi A, Yamada A, Kobayashi S. Extended dissection of thoracic esophageal cancer based on preoperative staging. In: *Diseases of the Esophagus: Malignant Diseases* (eds Ferguson MK, Little AG, Skinner DB), pp. 177–86. New York, Futura Publishing Co, 1990.
46. Akiyama H. Cardinals in the regional lymph node dissection in surgery of thoracic esophageal carcinoma. In: *Diseases of the Esophagus* (eds Siewert JR, Holscher AH), pp. 416–20. Berlin, Springer-Verlag, 1938.
47. Abe SI, Tachibana M, Shiraishi M, Nakamura T. Lymph node metastasis in resectable esophageal cancer. *J Thorac Cardiovasc Surg* 1990; **100**: 287–91.
48. Kakegawa TM, Fujita H. Arguments for extended three-field esophagectomy for thoracic esophageal cancer. Reported at the 13th Postgraduate Course of the Technical University of Munich, 1992 (unpublished report).
49. Isono K, Sato H, Nakayama K. Result of a nationwide study on the three-field lymph node dissection of esophageal cancer. *Oncology* 1991; **48**: 411–20.
50. Siewert JR, Roder JD. Lymphadenectomy in esophageal surgery. *Dis Esophagus* 1992; **5**: 91–7.
51. Barbier PA, Luder PJ, Schupper G, Becker CD, Wasner HE. Quality of life and patterns of recurrence following transhiatal esophagectomy for cancer: results of a prospective follow-up in 50 patients. *World J Surg* 1988; **12**: 270–6.
52. Peracchia A, Ruol A, Bardino A *et al*. Lymph node dissection for cancer of the thoracic esophagus: how extended should it be? *Dis Esophagus* 1992; **5**: 69–78.
53. Peracchia A, Ruol A. Lymphadenectomy for cancer of the cervical and thoracic esophagus. Reported at the 13th Postgraduate Course of the Technical University of Munich, 1992 (unpublished report).
54. Tsurumuru M, Akiyama H, Udagawa H, Ono Y, Suzuki M, Watanabe G. Cervical-thoracic-abdominal lymph node dissection for intrathoracic esophageal carcinoma. In: *Diseases of the Esophagus: Malignant Diseases* (eds Ferguson MK, Little AG, Skinner DB), pp. 187–96. New York, Futura Publishing Co, 1990.
55. Udagawa H, Tsurumuru M, Ono Y, Akiyama H. *Lymph Node Dissection and TNM Classification.* Proceedings of the 6th Congress of the Japanese section of the ISDE, Kurume, 1990.
56. Desai PB, Deshpande RK, Patil PK, Mistry RC. Radical lymphadenectomy in esophageal cancer: does it improve survival? *Dis Esophagus* 1992; **5**: 99–104.
57. Poplin E, Fleming T, Leichman L *et al*. Combined therapies for squamous-cell carcinoma of the esophagus; a Southwest Oncology Group Study (SWOG-8037). *J Clin Oncol* 1987; **5**: 622–8.
58. Orringer MB, Forastiere AA, Perex-Tamayo C, Urba S, Takasugi BJ, Bromberg J. Chemotherapy and radiation therapy before transhiatal esophagectomy for esophageal carcinoma. *Ann Thorac Surg* 1990; **49**: 348–55.
59. Leichman L, Steiger Z, Seydel HG, Vatikevicisu VK. Combined preoperative chemotherapy and radiation therapy for cancer of the esophagus: the Wayne Stage University, Southwest Oncology Group and Radiation Therapy Oncology Group experience. *Semin Oncol* 1984; **11**: 178–85.
60. Urba SG, Orringer MB, Perex-Tamayo C, Bromberg J, Forastiere A. Concurrent preoperative chemotherapy and radiation therapy in localized esophageal adenocarcinoma.

61. MacFarlane SD, Hill LD, Jolly PC, Kozarek RD, Anderson RP. Improved results of surgical treatment for esophageal and gastroesophageal junction carcinomas after preoperative combined chemotherapy and radiation. *J Thorac Cardiovasc Surg* 1988; **95**: 415–22.
62. Hilgenberg AD, Carey RW, Wilkins EQ, Choi NC, Mathiesen DJ, Grillo HC. Preoperative chemotherapy, surgical resection, and selective postoperative therapy for squamous cell carcinoma of the esophagus. *Ann Thorac Surg* 1988; **45**: 357–63.
63. Kelsen DP, Fein R, Coonley C, Heeland R. Cisplatin, vindesine and mitoguazone in the treatment of esophageal cancer. *Cancer Treatment Reports* 1986; **2**: 255–9.

11.2

Thoracoscopic Oesophagectomy – Minimally Invasive Direct Vision Oesophageal Mobilization for Cancer

A. DARZI, J. R. T. MONSON and A. HILL

INTRODUCTION

Total oesophagectomy is traditionally performed using either a full thoracotomy or a transhiatal approach in addition to a full gastric mobilization via laparotomy and finally a cervical anastomoisis. Open thoracotomy is highly invasive and is associated with considerable morbidity. Orringer first popularized blunt transhiatal oesophagectomy[1–4] for both benign and malignant disease, its main advantage over the two stage Lewis–Tanner procedure[5,6] or the three stage oesophagectomy[7] being the avoidance of a thoracotomy. The disadvantages of a blunt oesophagectomy include blood loss, trauma to the azygos vein, bronchus and recurrent laryngeal nerves. In addition nodal dissection is not possible with this technique. Mobilization of the oesophagus using a mediastinoscope has been described by Buess *et al.*[8] but once again this is associated with limited node dissection and in addition there may be difficulty in dissecting the lower end of the oesophagus.

We describe a technique which we have performed in ten patients in whom full thoracic mobilization of the oesophagus is undertaken thoracoscopically using a series of ports placed in the right chest. This is then followed by simultaneous gastric mobilization and oesophagogastric cervical anastomosis.

OPERATIVE TECHNIQUE

Thoracoscopic Phase

The operation is performed under general anaesthesia with a double lumen endotracheal tube to enable collapse of the right lung during the endoscopic

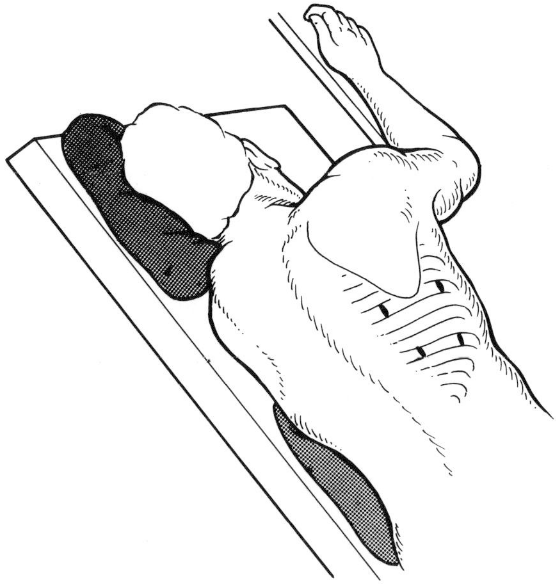

Figure 11.2.1 Position of ports for thoracoscopic oesophagectomy.

dissection. The first part of the operation consists of the endoscopic dissection of the thoracic oesophagus in the right thorax with the patient in the semiprone position. In the second stage of the operation the stomach is mobilized through an upper midline incision with the patient supine, while the cervical oesophagus is dissected through an incision anterior to the left sternocleidomastoid muscle in the neck. The cervical oesophagus is divided and the oesophagus and tumour are delivered through the abdominal wound. The stomach is then pulled through into the neck to be anastomosed to the cervical oesophagus.

In order to facilitate collapse of the right lung, an electronic pressure controlled CO_2 insufflator (Storz, Germany) is used, set at 1–3 mmHg. This pressure is used to avoid cardiac arrhythmias and mediastinal shift. Dissection of the oesophagus can be facilitated by the use of a flexible endoscope placed within the oesophagus. This aids identification of the oesophagus at the start of the procedure by visualizing the light within the lumen of the oesophagus. Movement of the endoscope within the oesophagus can be used to facilitate dissection.

Four thoracoscopic ports are used (Fig. 11.2.1). The upper two (one 5 mm and one 10 mm) are placed in front and behind the lower angle of the scapula. The lower two (both 12 mm) are placed several interspaces below these just above the diaphragm. The procedure is commenced with the camera in the lower anterior port.

For tumours located in the lower third of the oesophagus the thoracoscopic dissection begins at the level of the azygos vein. For those tumours elsewhere the dissection should commence in an area of normal oesophagus, either above or

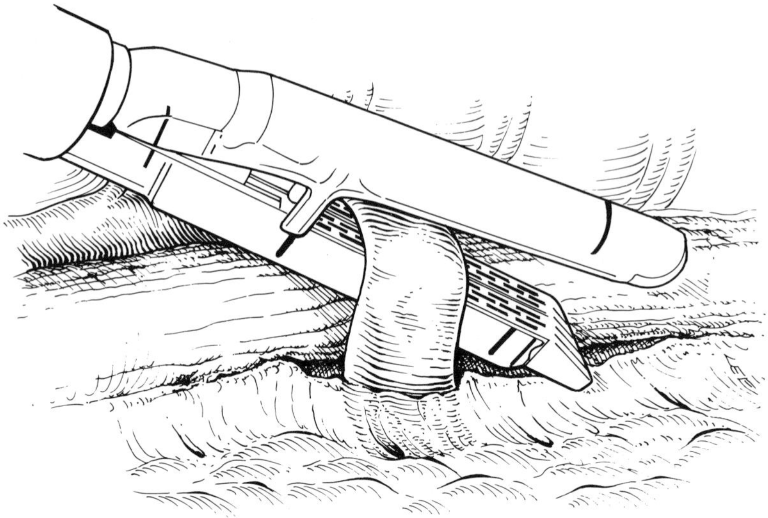

Figure 11.2.2 Division of the azygos vein. The stapler is inserted through the lower posterior port. In this view the laparoscope and camera have been inserted through the lower anterior port.

below, leaving dissection of the tumour until the remaining oesophagus has been fully mobilized. The pleura is divided above and below the azygos vein which is then dissected free from the underlying oesophagus. We routinely divide the azygos vein using an Endo GIA (Autosuture, Ascot, UK) linear stapler (Fig. 11.2.2). The mediastinal pleura over the entire oesophagus from the thoracic inlet to the inferior pulmonary vein is then divided. Above the azygos vein the dissection plane is between the oesophagus and the superior vena cava and trachea. An articulated dissector (Endodissect, Autosuture, Ascot, UK) can be used for the dissection and separation of these structures from the oesophagus. Any nodes encountered in this region can be dissected and removed en bloc with the oesophagus. Complete mobilization of the posterior aspect of the oesophagus is greatly facilitated by use of a variable curvature shape memory dissector.[8] Alternatively a soft rubber sling may now be passed around the mobilized upper oesophagus (Fig. 11.2.3).

The middle third of the oesophagus is mobilized by moving the rubber sling in a caudal direction. Any large arteries feeding the oesophagus from the aorta can be clipped and divided under direct vision. Separation of the oesophagus from the tracheal bifurcation, the pericardium, pericardiophrenic vessels and phrenic nerves is also completed under direct vision. Careful use of diathermy should be used to avoid thermal injury to the thoracic duct and the trachea. Again, enlarged lymph nodes can be dissected with the oesophagus or separately. On occasions it is useful to carry out this dissection using the harmonic scalpel (Ultracision Inc, USA) which produces less thermal damage to surrounding tissues than diathermy.

For dissection of the lower third of the oesophagus, the camera port should be moved to the upper posterior porthole. The inferior pulmonary ligament is divided with scissors (Autosuture, Ascot, UK), after electrocoagulation of the vessels within its fold. After mobilization of the thoracic oesophagus, two large bore chest tubes are inserted and the abdominal and cervical stages of the operation are performed simultaneously.

Abdominal Approach

The patient is placed in a supine position. To gain maximum access the upper left paramedian incision begins in the angle between the xiphisternum and the left costal margin and extends to the level of the umbilicus. In thin patients a midline abdominal incision is routinely employed. After insertion of a self-retaining retractor, the abdomen is explored to exclude hepatic or peritoneal secondaries. The disposition of the stomach and its vascular supply is reviewed.

Preparation of the Stomach

Adequate mobilization of the stomach for transfer through the chest is the key to the three stage procedure. The features concerned with gastric preparation are:

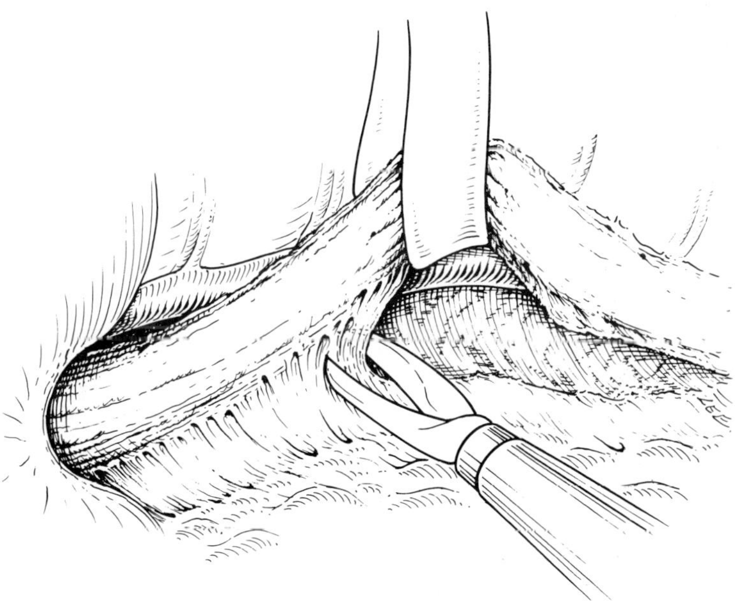

Figure 11.2.3 Oesophageal mobilization. The oesophagus has been encircled with a soft rubber sling. The laparoscope and camera have been inserted through the upper posterior port and the dissecting scissors through the lower posterior port.

selective ligation of the gastric vessels, duodenal mobilization, definition of the diaphragmatic hiatus and preparation of the pylorus.

Selective Ligation of the Gastric Vessels

The objective is to mobilize the stomach and yet preserve a blood supply from the right gastroepiploic and the right gastric vessels. This is best performed systematically in four stages.

1. The vasa brevia. The lowest of the vasa brevia is identified and, starting from below each individual vessel, is clamped and divided until the fundus of the stomach comes into view. Each vessel of the stomach wall must be tied individually to prevent the ligatures being pulled off when the stomach is drawn up through the thorax to reach the neck in subsequent stages of the operation. Great care and gentleness is needed when ligating the splenic origin of the vasa brevia so that injury to the spleen does not occur.

2. Left gastroepiploic vessels. The left gastroepiploic artery is tied as far laterally as possible so that the full extent of the gastroepiploic arcade is preserved.

3. Omental vessels. Omental vessels arising from the gastroepiploic arcade must be tied individually for two reasons; to prevent bunching and shortening of the gastroepiploic arcade and to prevent the ligatures being pulled off when the stomach and its vascular pedicle are put on the stretch.

4. Left gastric artery. After completion of the first three steps of vascular ligation, the stomach is pulled up by its greater curvature to expose its posterior surface. Upward traction on the stomach, combined with downward pressure on the pancreas, puts the left gastric vessels under tension. Since the point of the ligature is so close to the coeliac axis, it is important that pulsation in the splenic and hepatic arteries should be confirmed as the ligature is tied.

Duodenal Mobilization

Duodenal mobilization is more extensive than in Kocher's manoeuvre. The peritoneal reflection is incised lateral to the second part of the duodenum. The loose areolar tissue is divided so that the duodenum and the head of the pancreas can be brought forward as in the operation for pancreatectomy. Seven centimetres of the inferior vena cava and of the adjacent aorta should be exposed. This extensive mobilization allows the duodenum and the head of the pancreas to rotate to their embryological position in the midline. This procedure not only increases the reach of the stomach but also results in the pyloric outlet coming to lie between the crura of the diaphragm and being more in line with the direction of the oesophagus.

Definition of the Diaphragmatic Hiatus

The peritoneal reflections round the diaphragmatic hiatus should be divided to expose the fibres of the crura. The reflection on the right side of the abdominal oesophagus often contains an ancillary branch from the left hepatic artery. This should be divided between ligatures to prevent possible haemorrhage. It is easier to expose the crural fibres behind the oesophagus and this is further facilitated by forward traction on the abdominal oesophagus. The size of the hiatus is estimated by insertion of the fingers into the space between the two crura. If the aperture is too small to accommodate the pyloric antrum some of the muscle fibres of the crus should be divided with scissors. It is important that the crural hiatus should not be large enough to allow small gut to slide upwards and strangulate between the crura and the pyloric antrum.

Preparation of the Pylorus

Since total thoracic oesophagectomy inevitably results in total vagotomy, gastric stasis may result unless pyloric drainage is free and unobstructed. In many cases, if the pylorus is found to be wide and patulous, no measures to increase drainage are necessary. If, however, the pyloric muscle is thickened, pyloromyotomy without encroaching on the mucosa, as in Ramstedt's operation, is required. Alternatively, simple pyloroplasty may be performed.

Cervical Approach

The third stage of the operation can be carried out through a left or rightsided cervical incision. However, the right cervical approach has been found to have three distinct advantages: there is no danger to the thoracic duct, the right recurrent nerve is less liable to injury and the oesophagus, when mobilized during the right thoracotomy, moves to the right and is therefore more easily reached through a right cervical incision.

Position

The patient is positioned with slight neck extension as for thyroidectomy, but with the head turned slightly to the left side. Care is taken not to obstruct the thoracic drainage system during this stage of the operation as this may result in an accumulation of blood and serum in the oesophageal fossa and consequently in the right chest cavity.

Incision

An oblique incision is made on the right side of the neck, starting over the middle of the sternomastoid muscle and extending down to just above the jugular notch. After incision of the platysma and division of one or two branches of the anterior jugular vein, the anterior margin of the sternomastoid muscle is defined. The deep fascia medial to the sternomastoid is incised and the wound deepened to identify the infrahyoid muscles, the carotid sheath and the lateral aspect of the right lobe of the thyroid. If access is somewhat limited the lower fibrous portion of the sternomastoid muscle is divided and on occasions the omohyoid may require division. It should not be necessary to divide the entire sternomastoid muscle. By lateral traction on the carotid sheath and medial traction on the thyroid, the middle thyroid vein is put under tension. After division of this vein the correct plane has been reached and the right lateral aspect of the oesophagus can be exposed by dissection of the loose areolar tissue. This tissue is sometimes bloodstained as the result of the upper thoracic dissection and this acts as a guide. The right recurrent laryngeal nerve should be identified and preserved.

Delivery of the Cervical Oesophagus

A finger is passed behind the cervical oesophagus, entering the retropharyngeal space already defined in the thoracoscopic dissection. Keeping close to the oesophagus the finger is hooked forwards and the cervical oesophagus brought up into the wound. The presence of the indwelling nasogastric tube confirms the identify of the cervical oesophagus. Steady, slow and unhurried upward traction on the cervical oesophagus enables a non-crushing clamp to be placed around the oesophagus prior to division. A full length of nylon tape is then sutured to the distal cut end and the thoracic oesophagus including tumour is withdrawn into the abdomen, leaving the nylon tape as a guide in the posterior mediastinum. The lesser curve of the stomach is then divided using a linear stapling device (GIA 80, Autosuture, Ascot, UK) and the nylon tape is secured to the posterior aspect of the fundus. The tape and gastric tube are then gently drawn back up into the cervical incision. During this procedure the dome of the fundus appears first in the neck.

Oesophagofundic Anastomosis

The cervical oesophagus just below the cricopharyngeus muscle is approximated to the uppermost part of the dome of the fundus. Though it may be helpful to place a light clamp on the cervical oesophagus it is undesirable to clamp the dome of the fundus. A crescentic incision is made in the fundus and the gastric contents (often bloodstained) are aspirated. During this process it may be necessary to ligate some quite large gastric veins. The cervical oesophagus is divided obliquely so that the line of section will conform to the crescentic opening of the stomach wall. A posterior layer of simple sutures is inserted using 3/0 monofilament synthetic absorbable sutures on an atraumatic needle. The sutures are spaced at intervals of about 3 mm and after attaining perfect mucosal apposition, the knots are tied on the inside of the lumen. On completion of the posterior layer, the nasogastric tube is threaded from the cervical oesophagus down into the stomach for a distance of about 15 cm so that the tip of the tube is placed just proximal to the pylorus. The anterior layer of sutures is then completed in exactly the same way as the posterior layer. The clamp on the cervical oesophagus is removed and on completion of the anastomosis, the oesophagogastric stoma is allowed to fall back into the thoracic inlet. A stab drainage wound is inserted through the upper skin flap and the tube led down to the site of the anastomosis. The tube is attached to a separate underwater drainage system. The abdominal wound is then closed in a standard fashion.

RESULTS

Of the ten patients in the series thoracoscopic mobilization was abandoned or incomplete in three cases. In two patients the tumour proved to be unresectable due to tracheal invasion. Thoracoscopic mobilization of the oesophagus other than the tumour was completed leaving final tumour assessment to be completed at the time of laparotomy. Using a transhiatal approach tracheal invasion was confirmed and the procedure was abandoned. Both patients made an uneventful recovery and subsequently received chemoradiotherapy. In the third case thoracoscopic mobilization was abandoned due to equipment failure and the procedure was completed using a transhiatal approach. There has been no operative mortality and no patient suffered any unrecognized intrathoracic injuries.

DISCUSSION

This approach to oesophageal mobilization is safe and feasible. However, further experience will be needed before identifying its place in oesophageal surgery. The potential benefits of this procedure include better visualization, better nodal clearance and also the avoidance of the need for a thoracotomy. Nonetheless, there are some difficulties already apparent. Firstly, in advanced tumours the loss of tactile sense remains a problem. Specifically, assessment of tumour fixity to structures such as the trachea or aorta can be difficult. In such cases it has been our policy to complete the remaining oesophageal mobilization thoracoscopically – including division of the azygos vein – whilst avoiding final tumour dissection. This final step can then be easily completed by a transhiatal approach during the gastric phase of the procedure. In two such cases tracheal invasion rendered resection impossible and the operation was abandoned. We have been greatly impressed by the speed of recovery of these two patients in contrast to previous experience of unresectable cases in whom open thoracotomy had been performed.

As with other advanced laparoscopic procedures such as bowel resection, reduction in blood loss using this approach has been observed. In itself, the formal thoracotomy may be a bloody incision but in addition the requirement for meticulous haemostasis for video-directed surgery means that blood loss is kept to an absolute minimum. This is essential in order that image quality is not impaired due to light absorption by haemoglobin. Due to the high incidence of postoperative arrhythmias it is our current policy to administer digoxin prophylactically to all patients undergoing oesophageal resection. In addition, using a thorascopic approach we were concerned about the potential hazards of any mediastinal shift caused by the positive intrathoracic pressure. We have used a small positive pressure to aid in the pulmonary collapse so necessary for adequate visualization but in our more recent cases have abandoned insufflation once this has been achieved. Indeed, in those patients without significant chronic obstructive pulmonary disease such a technique is probably unnecessary. Despite these reservations no patients in the current series have experienced any cardiac problems either intraoperatively or postoperatively.

Whether the thoracoscopic approach can permit radical oesophageal dissection is unclear at this time. However, as with other endoscopic surgical procedures there seems little reason to suggest this will not be possible although instrumentation remains a problem for thoracoscopic procedures if only the dedicated ports are utilized. However, some surgeons have employed traditional long thoracic instruments inserted through small intercostal incisions. Obviously, the lack of necessity for high pressure insufflation in the chest cavity makes such an option possible and at least for pulmonary resections this approach appears to be successful.

Avoidance of a thoracotomy may lead to improved postoperative respiratory function with early discharge from the intensive care unit. Certainly, the level of postoperative thoracic discomfort is greatly reduced. Unfortunately, as the instruments are passed between the ribs, damage to intercostal nerves may occur due to vigorous "crowbarring" of the ribs and this should be avoided – even if further ports are required to aid surgical access. With this approach the risks of injury to intrathoracic structures and cardiac arrhythmias encountered with blunt transhiatal oesophagectomy are largely obviated. However, the procedure is time consuming in what is already a lengthy operation.

Technical difficulties may be encountered in patients with emphysema in whom air trapping may prevent collapse of the lung. Visualization of the oesophagus is therefore impaired in a situation where blunt retraction of the lung is very difficult. Some authorities have recently suggested the use of the full prone position for the thoracoscopic phase of the operation. In this way the lung will fall away from the operative field, as will any spilt blood. These options, along with further developments in instrumentation, may therefore make this operation technically easier and speedier.

Finally the role of preliminary thoracoscopy in staging of oesophageal cancer is an intriguing possibility. Endoluminal ultrasound is already proving to be a useful modality in the staging of oesophageal cancer and it may be that these two techniques may find a complementary role in the management of this disease.

REFERENCES

1. Godfaden D, Orringer MB, Appelman BD, Kalish R. Adenocarcinoma of the distal oesophagus and gastric cardia. Comparison of transhiatal oesophagectomy and throacoabdominal oesophagectomy. *J Thorac Cardiovasc Surg* 1986; **91**: 242–7.
2. Stewart JR, Sarr MG, Sharp KW. Transhiatal (blunt) oesophagectomy for malignant and benign oesophageal disease: clinical experience and technique. *Ann Thorac Surg* 1985; **40**: 343–8.
3. Orringer MB. Transhiatal oesophagectomy for benign disease. *J Thorac Cardiovasc Surg* 1985; **90**: 649–55.
4. Orringer MB. Transthoracic versus transhiatal oesophagectomy: what difference does it make? *Ann Thorac Surg* 1987; **44**: 116–18.
5. Tanner NC. The present position of carcinoma of the oesophagus. *Postgrad Med J* 1947; **23**: 109–39.
6. Lewis I. The surgical treatment of carcinoma of the oesophagus with special reference to a new operation for growths of the middle third. *Br J Surg* 1946; **34**: 18–31.
7. McKeown KC. Total three stage oesophagectomy for cancer of the oesophagus. *Br J Surg* 1986; **63**: 259–62.
8. Buess LF, Becker HD, Naruhn, Mentges B. Endoscopic esophagectomy without thoracotomy. *Prob Gen Surg* 1991; **8**: 478.

Overview

Oesophageal resection

In specialist centres, the morbidity and mortality rates associated with resection for oesophageal malignancy have shown continuing improvement, and oesophageal resection with radical clearance of regional lymph nodes has been associated with an improved duration of survival. Nonetheless, the poor prognosis and relatively high complication rate associated with oesophageal resection for malignancy makes the introduction of laparoscopic surgery an attractive alternative for some surgeons. However, the relative paucity of publications in the literature compared to other laparoscopic procedures reflects an underlying difficulty not previously suspected. As can be seen from Darzi and Monson's description of thoracoscopic mobilization (Chapter 11.2), the technique is straightforward but, as yet, there is not enough data on the possible benefit to the post-operative course. This will be influenced by the severity of the overall surgical insult, but more information is required on the pulmonary response to prolonged intrapleural dissection and insertion of several thoracic ports. The data available are still too few for direct comparison with open surgery. Instrumentation and techniques have improved and there has already been a move away from the blunt dissection techniques employed at mediastinoscopy. Continuing developments in thoracoscopic resection may yet prove that this major surgical procedure can be undertaken safely and without compromise to the patient.

12.1

Expectations of Hernia Surgery (inguinal and femoral)

R. BENDAVID

INTRODUCTION

The comparative analysis of traditional hernia techniques is an arduous task which must be handled with a great deal of perspicacity. Several factors account for the complexity of such an analysis and some of these must be dealt with in order to retain a relatively accurate meaning of the statistics gathered from the surgical literature.

Classification

No classification exists which can reliably differentiate the various types of groin hernias in terms of the extent of tissue damage and hence, which operation would best suit a particular situation. The classifications of Casten,[1] Gilbert[2] and Nyhus[3] do not, for example, differentiate between a simple indirect inguinal hernia and an inguinofemoral hernia, which represent the extremes of a spectrum. These two types of hernias will require entirely different approaches and yet, if the same surgical technique is used, results will not be comparable. No method exists of measuring and classifying tissue quality. As every surgeon knows, some inguinal ligaments shred easily when pierced by a suture needle to the extent that a herniorrhaphy seems tenuous. Tension is another crucial factor that cannot be measured and classified in order to determine the adequacy of a procedure or indicate the need for a prosthesis.

Corruption of Classical Techniques

Corruption of well-established operative procedures represents probably the single most important sin committed by surgeons. Very few perform a Bassini or a Shouldice repair; most do a "modified Bassini" or a "modified Shouldice".

This sin may be easily forgiven when the surgeon knows the exact, original description of the technique, but most often the modified version bears no resemblance to the original. Few surgeons realize that the Bassini operation dictates the resection of the cremaster and the division of the transversalis fascia from the deep inguinal ring to the pubic crest. These steps are of the utmost importance and rightly so. Imbrication of an inguinal floor is grossly inadequate. Can statistics on the Bassini operation then, be meaningful?

Statistics

A valid statistical analysis implies that the data being analysed are comparable. Unfortunately, this has not always been so. A glance at the surgical literature will often reveal the vagaries of statistics. Studies on the rate of recurrence of hernias, for example, may not distinguish between direct and indirect hernias. This is somewhat regrettable because the prognoses are entirely different for each. Whereas repair of a direct inguinal hernia may lead to a recurrence, through no fault of the surgeon, an indirect inguinal hernia should rarely fail and when it does, the surgeon may bear some of the responsibility.

Another drawback of statistics is noted when reports group primary and recurrent hernias without distinction. The outlook is entirely different for each, as demonstrated by Obney and Chan of the Shouldice Hospital.[4] Their report covered a series of 1057 recurrent inguinal hernia repairs on 964 patients between February 1970 and February 1972. The incidence of re-recurrence was from 2.3% to 20% (Table 12.1.1). The recurrence, however, when all patients are considered, is 1% or less. The introduction of mesh has largely corrected the problem to the extent that primary and recurrent hernias have the same expectation of success.[5]

Another study which illustrates the importance of differentiating between primary and recurrent hernias also came from the Shouldice Hospital. A series was reported by Bendavid dealing with 251 primary femoral hernias on 242 patients and 257 recurrent femoral hernias on 211 patients.[6] Whereas the recurrence rate in primary femoral repairs was 6.1%, with recurrent femoral repairs the failure rate ranged from 11.8% to 75% (Table 12.1.2).[6] Here again,

Table 12.1.1 Incidence of re-recurrence of inguinal hernias[4]

	Re-recurrence	Percentage
1× recurrent inguinal hernia	18/775	2.3
2× recurrent inguinal hernia	15/212	7.0
3× recurrent inguinal hernia	6/49	12.0
4× recurrent inguinal hernia	1/14	7.0
5× recurrent inguinal hernia	1/5	20.0
6× recurrent inguinal hernia	0/2	0.0

Table 12.1.2 Incidence of re-recurrence of femoral hernias[6]

	No. of cases	Recurrences	Percentage
1× recurrent femoral hernia	144	17	11.8
2× recurrent femoral hernia	72	25	34.7
3× recurrent femoral hernia	26	9	34.6
4× recurrent femoral hernia	10	3	30.0
5× recurrent femoral hernia	4	3	75.0
6× recurrent femoral hernia	1	0	—
	257	57	Average 22.0

the introduction of mesh has greatly improved the situation. Studies, therefore, should specify whether a technique was applied to a direct, indirect or inguinofemoral hernia and define these hernias as primaries or recurrences. Statistics must be viewed with circumspection in some instances. Time and accuracy of follow-up are significant factors in assessing a procedure. Some recurrences are still recorded after 30 years at the Shouldice Hospital and five year or ten year follow-up seems inadequate.

Multiple Hernias

All groin herniorrhaphies must include a diligent search for direct, indirect, femoral, interstitial, prevesical and prevascular hernias. Statistics of the Shouldice Hospital reveal that 13% of all patients have more than one significant hernia. This search must become routine if one is to avoid the "missed" hernia which can be a source of embarrassment and recurrence. In the series cited from Obney and Chan,[4] 37% of the 1057 recurrences operated revealed an indirect inguinal hernia! Such a recurrence is an extreme rarity with a Shouldice repair done in our institution.

Experience of the Surgeon

The experience of the surgeon is of paramount importance in every step of management: diagnosis, choice of incision, operative procedure, assessment of the quality of tissues, when to use prosthetic material and postoperative course. A study conducted by the Shouldice Hospital[7] revealed that a general surgeon in the Toronto area will perform an average of 50 hernia repairs a year. The surgeons in our institution will carry out from 600 to 900 procedures a year. This essentially means that a surgeon who dedicates all his or her time to hernia surgery may, in the space of one or two years, acquire the lifetime experience of the average general surgeon! This expertise is invariably reflected in their results. An old adage may be fitting to quote here: "The eyes of the master do more work than his hands".

Reconsideration of Some Concepts

The concept of high ligation of a hernial sac has been anchored for so long that it is seldom questioned. If an indirect sac is usually resected, why not a direct sac? In fact, neither need be resected. What is important is that the sacs be freed at the myoaponeurotic level deeply enough so that they may retract and disappear in the preperitoneal space, ensuring that there are no constricting bands. The important step lies in the reconstruction of the posterior inguinal wall. This seemingly heretic attitude is confirmed by the publications of Ryan[8] and subsequently Welsh,[9,10] both from the Shouldice Hospital. In their respective series of 313 and 3000 cases of sliding indirect inguinal hernias, the sacs were simply freed and returned to the preperitoneal space. The recurrence rate was 0.5%. Fifteen recurrences were identified, five as direct and ten as femoral hernias.

Another concept which must be re-examined is the nature and aetiology of the direct inguinal hernia. This type of herniation may well reflect a systemic disorder which Read[11] refers to as "metastatic emphysema". This concept should translate into the elimination of simple imbrication of the transversalis fascia for direct inguinal hernias and to more liberal guidelines in the use of mesh.

TRADITIONAL TECHNIQUES OF INGUINAL HERNIORRHAPHY

The Bassini Operation

Bassini presented his technique to the Italian Surgical Society in 1887 and his textbook appeared in 1889.[12,13] The details of his technique, however, were subsequently published by his student Attilio Catterina[14] in 15 plates which leave no doubt as to the method. The salient features must be pointed out, which are:

a) longitudinal incision of the cremaster, then its resection;
b) identification of an indirect sac which is ligated and resected at the level of the deep inguinal ring;
c) division of the transversalis fascia from the deep inguinal ring to the pubis;
d) reconstruction of the floor of the canal with interrupted silk sutures approximating the transversus arch to the inguinal ligament;

Table 12.1.3 Recurrence rate following the Bassini inguinal repair of primary inguinal hernias

Author	No. of cases	% follow-up	Years follow-up	Recurrence
Hagan[15]	–	–	–	2.9%
Bassini[12,13]	262	–	–	3.8%
Marsden[16]	367	–	–	4.0%
Houdard[17]	46	69.6	–	6.2%
Vayre[18]	305	–	–	7.2%
Callum[19]	186	–	5–12	7.5%
Chevrel[20]	119	50.0	–	8.4%
Magnusson[21]	305	–	6–7	9.6%
Berliner[22]	720	–	4–9	11.5%
Piper[23]	246	67.7	–	12.2%
Belanger[24]	1102	33.2	14	25.0%

e) replacement of the spermatic cord in its normal anatomical position with the external oblique aponeurosis closed anterior to the cord.

For primary hernias, the Bassini operation will yield good results if properly executed. Table 12.1.3 gives recurrence rates as gleaned from the surgical literature. I cannot help but feel that this method was applied to recurrences as well and possibly sometimes as a "modified Bassini"!

The Shouldice Operation

The Shouldice operation (Fig. 12.1.1) was introduced in 1945 and then modified in 1952 to its present form[25] It incorporates all the steps of the Bassini operation, particularly the resection of the cremaster and the division of the transversalis fascia from the internal ring to the pubic crest. In addition, using stainless steel wire, four lines of sutures are used in the repair. Starting near the pubis, the first line approximates the iliopubic tract; laterally, to the undersurface of the transversus arch (full thickness) medially, from pubic crest to the internal ring. When reaching the level of the internal ring, the suture will incorporate the lateral stump of the cremaster as a sling around the spermatic cord. The suture will then be reversed as the second line and will now approximate the free border of the transversus arch to the inguinal ligament. This will be done from internal ring to the level of the pubis. The third line begins near the internal ring and approximates the transversus arch again to the lower border of the inner aspect of the external oblique aponeurosis in such a manner as to create an artificial inguinal ligament superior to the existing one. At the level of the pubis, this third line of suture will reverse and become the fourth line of suture, incorporating again the external oblique aponeurosis more superiorly to the previous artificial inguinal ligament.

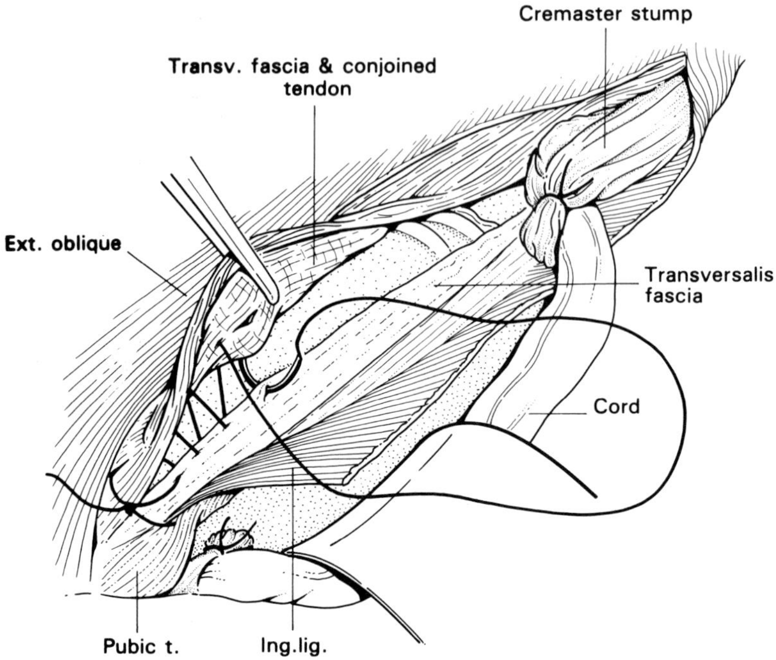

Figure 12.1.1 The Shouldice repair: first line of suture (courtesy of the *Encyclopedie Medico Chirurgicale*, Paris).

The division of the floor of the inguinal canal allows the search for femoral, prevascular and prevesical hernias, but above all, it allows the demonstration of all the structures that will be incorporated in the reconstruction of the floor. The lateral edge of the rectus becomes visible and is incorporated in the first line of suture as superiorly as feasible without tension.

As can be seen in Table 12.1.4, the results of various series show a marked improvement. It is fair to say that the Shouldice operation has benefited from the more recent means of diffusion and communication and direct contact by various surgeons with the Shouldice Hospital to observe the finer points of the technique.

The McVay Operation

This operation[35–37] (Fig. 12.1.2) is known by several names: the Cooper ligament repair, the Lotheissen repair, the Lotheissen–McVay repair. There is no doubt that the studies of Anson and McVay (1934–38) have popularized a procedure that had already been described by Lotheissen in 1897. It is a slightly more difficult operation to perform than the Bassini or Shouldice repairs but it is a procedure that every surgeon must perform well.

Table 12.1.4 Recurrence rate following the Shouldice operation of primary inguinal hernias

Author	No. of cases	% follow-up	Years follow-up	Recurrence
Shearburn[26]	550	100	13	0.2%
Volpe[27]	415	50	3	0.2%
Wantz[28,29]	2087	–	5	0.3%
Myers[30]	953	100	18	0.7%
Devlin[31]	350	–	6	0.8%
Flament[32,33]	134	–	6	0.9%
Wantz[28,29]	3454	–	1–20	1.0%
Shouldice Hospital[113]	2748	–	35	1.46%
Moran[34]	121	–	6	2.0%
Berliner[22]	591	–	2–5	2.7%

To do so, again, the transversalis fascia must be incised from the internal ring to the pubic crest. Omission of this step may lead to compression or laceration of the femoral vein, injury to the iliopubic vein(s) and the aberrant obturator artery. It is the only groin operation that is complicated by vascular injuries often enough to have been reported in series (Table 12.1.5). The retroinguinal space of Bogros can be markedly vascular and the site of preperitoneal haematomas[38]. The transition sutures which include the femoral sheath can be a delicate manoeuvre which requires direct vision and therefore demands the

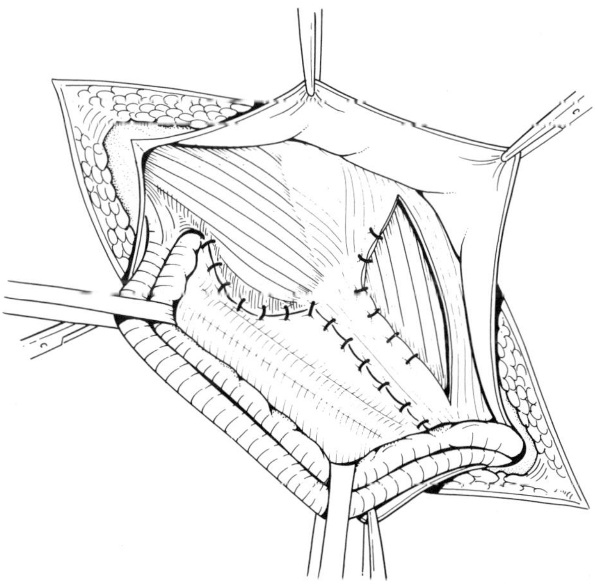

Figure 12.1.2 The McVay repair: final appearance prior to approximation of external oblique aponeurosis (courtesy of Editions Masson, Paris).

Table 12.1.5 Recurrence rate following the McVay operation of primary inguinal hernias

Author	No. of cases	% follow-up	Years follow-up	Recurrence
Flament[32,33]	135	–	6	1.5%
Rutledge[39]	1142	97.0	9	1.9%
Halverson[40]	1211	91.3	22	3.5%
Lubeth[41]	800	52.4	–	3.9%
Barbier[42,43]	1140	70.6	9–17	4.7%
Asmussen[44]	270	91.0	1–5	7.5%
Jones[45]	74	–	2	10.9%
Warlaumont[46]	373	85.1	1–10	15.5%

opening of the transversalis fascia. A relaxing incision is an integral part of the procedure and must be generous for the tension to be minimized. A common error is the fact that the sutures in the ligament of Cooper number one or two only and are inserted at the very medial portion of the ligament, leaving the lateral half to two thirds as a potential site of recurrence. When McVay repairs fail, those recurrences, in my experience, are among the most difficult to correct. Table 12.1.5 give a range of recurrence rates as gathered from the literature (1.5% to 15.5%).

The Nyhus Operation

The preperitoneal approach described by Annandale in 1876, used by Cheatle (1920), Henry (1936), McEvedy (1950), and several others was made popular by Nyhus of Chicago[3,47,48] (Fig. 12.1.3) The essential steps of the technique are as follows.

The skin incision is made horizontally two finger breadths superior to the pubis. The rectus sheath, once exposed, is incised transversely, allowing medial retraction of the rectus muscle. That same incision is extended laterally through the external oblique aponeurosis, the internal oblique and transversus muscles. The transversalis fascia then becomes evident and is in turn incised. Blunt dissection will reveal the posterior aspect of the inguinal floor. When the indirect, direct and femoral hernias have been dealt with, the repair consists of suturing the transversus arch and transversalis fascia superiorly to the iliopubic tract inferiorly. If necessary, sutures may also be inserted lateral to the internal ring.

My major criticism of this technique is that the iliopubic tract is a tenuous structure. Though always identified, it is strongest in its medial third where it can be quite thick. Rarely have I seen a solid iliopubic ligament extending from pubic crest to the level of the internal ring. McVay had already pointed out this fact in 1966.[36] No other operation has given such conflicting results and this can be seen in the following investigation by Gaspar and Casberg:[49] Dyson and

Pierce[50] – 2.7% recurrence in 88 indirect hernias and 35% in 51 direct hernias; Gregorie[51] – 1.2% recurrence for indirect hernias and 14.8% for direct hernias; Read[11] – no recurrences in 181 indirect inguinal hernias and four failures in 111 direct hernias (3.6%); Lindholm[52] – no recurrences in 172 indirect hernias and one recurrence in 41 direct hernias (2.4%).

The preperitoneal approach will acquire more converts with the introduction of prosthetic mesh in the "buttress" technique,[53] as will be seen below. Table 12.1.6 provides a glimpse of some of the results reported in the surgical literature.

RE-RECURRENCE FOLLOWING TRADITIONAL OPERATIONS ON RECURRENT HERNIAS

The failures of inguinal repairs may be ascribed to two causes: errors in judgement or technique on the part of the surgeon and endogenous causes.

Errors of Judgement and Technique

As stated earlier, 13% of patients present a second identifiable hernia which if overlooked becomes a "missed hernia". The large series presented by Obney

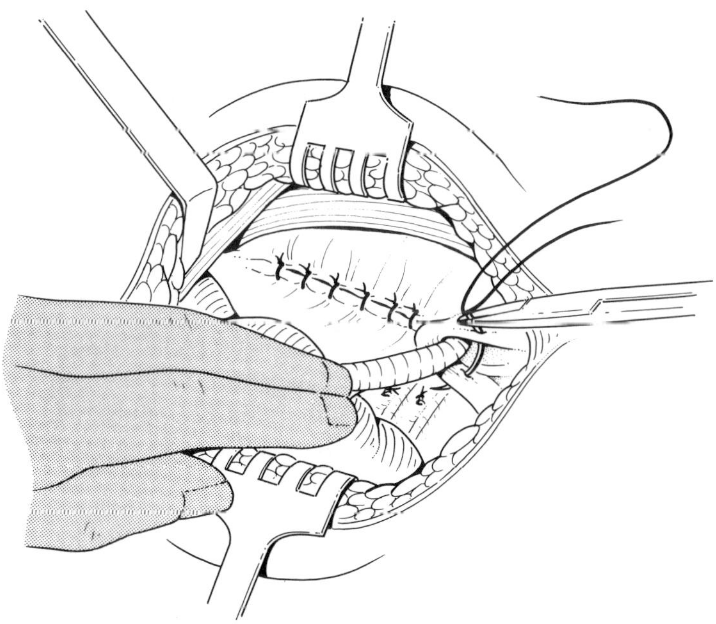

Figure 12.1.3 The Nyhus preperitoneal repair. Note the suture lateral to the spermatic cord (courtesy of JB Lippincott, Philadelphia).

Table 12.1.6 Recurrence rate following the Nyhus preperitoneal operation for primary inguinal hernias

Author	No. of cases	% follow-up	Years follow-up	Recurrence
Nyhus[3,47,48]	213	–	–	3.2%
Greenburg[54]	413	80.0	5	4.3%
Barbier[43]	806	77.5	9–17	4.7%
Nyhus[3,47,48]	1200	–	–	3.0–6.0%
Ljundahl[55]	402	90.3	1–5	6.4–16.7%
Read[11]	1420	79.0	3.5	6.8%
Callum[19]	186	–	5–12	7.5%
Brogeskov[56]	450	96.1	3	12.0%
Robertson[57]	63	98.4	3	17.0%
Gaspar[49]	233	90.0	10	21.0%

and Chan[4] proved 37% of the recurrences to be indirect inguinal hernias. These could be avoided when the cremaster is divided longitudinally from internal ring to the pubis. The incision of the transversalis fascia allows an excellent demonstration of the anatomy and hence the inclusion of the proper and substantial layers needed for repair. The inclusion of a relaxing incision must always be entertained when tension seems to be present. I have done over 1000 relaxing incisions without a single cause for regret. Still, recurrences will occur. The Shouldice experience proves that of our own 1% recurrence rate, two thirds will be femoral hernias and one third small direct inguinal hernias near the pubis. It may well be that an overzealous inguinal repair may place undue tension on the femoral ring, thereby promoting the subsequent recurrence. Why recurrences near the pubic crest? The best explanation, though not confirmed, was provided by Houdard[17] suggesting it may be due to a form of avascular necrosis due to the most medial suture which creates a triangular-shaped area with the apex at the pubis and the base formed by the suture.

Endogenous Causes

Though impossible to identify and quantitate, the quality of an individual's tissues varies considerably. Every surgeon has had the experience of redoing a repair at the same session – reinforcing it with mesh. The publications of Read[58] on protease–antiprotease imbalance provide us with an insight into this poorly understood mechanism of herniation through the transversalis fascia.

The more readily apparent causes of an increased failure rate when operating on recurrence are: the distorted anatomy, difficult access to the desired tissues and layers, predominance of scar tissue which does not hold sutures well, fear of injuries to adjacent vessel, viscus and cord components and above all, inability to approximate structures which may now be too far apart. Table 12.1.7 gives a summary of some of the re-recurrence rates in the surgical literature.

Table 12.1.7 Re-recurrence rate following traditional repairs of recurrent inguinal hernias

Author	Technique	No. of cases	% follow-up	Years follow-up	Recurrence
Tugnoli[59]	Bassini	60	–	–	6.5%
Cevese[60]	Bassini	142	74.0	11.3	13.4%
Kupcyk[61]	Shouldice	370	88.9	–	2.9%
Rotker[62]	Shouldice	73	83.5	2.3	5.9%
Wantz[28,29]	Shouldice	660	–	–	6.36%
Obney[63]	Shouldice	1057	–	11	3.9%
Rutledge[39]	McVay	127	–	17.4	2.4%
Halverson[40]	McVay	580	–	1–22	5.49%
Blaisdell[64]	Nyhus	101	–	–	12.0%
Lindholm[52]	Nyhus	15	–	–	27.0%
Barbier[42,43]	Nyhus	95	–	9–17	9.47%

TECHNIQUES OF INGUINAL HERNIORRHAPHIES UTILIZING MESH

The various studies of prosthetic materials since the beginning of this century (Milar, Steel, Teflon, Tantalum) tested the tolerance and quality of the implants. Since the mid 1950s, with the introduction of polypropylene (Marlex), Dacron (Mersilene) and more recently expanded polytetrafluoroethylene (ePTFE – Gore-Tex), prosthetics are now available which can be used safely. With safety came a surge of inventiveness as seen in the panoply of techniques introduced. Six techniques need be retained which have been tried and proven by well-known herniologists and these are the Rives technique,[65,66] the Nyhus buttress,[53] the Stoppa procedure[67,68] the unilateral Stoppa (Wantz),[69] the tension-free repairs[70,71] and the "plug" techniques.

The Rives Technique

Introduced in 1965 by Jean Rives (Rheims, France), the technique (Fig. 12.1.4) finds its use in recurrent inguinal and inguinofemoral hernias. Through an anterior approach, dissection is carried out with the aim of eliminating indirect, direct and femoral hernias. Careful dissection demonstrates the ligament of Cooper and the transversus arch. Dacron (Mersilene) is inserted into the preperitoneal space of Bogros and anchored to the ligament of Cooper inferiorly; more laterally, sutures anchor the mesh to the iliopubic tract and to the inguinal ligament. Laterally the mesh is cut to allow egress of the spermatic cord and the mesh closed snugly around the cord. Laterally and superiorly, the mesh is anchored through full thickness abdominal wall. I have personally eliminated the cut in the mesh and instead, I lateralize the cord, anchoring the mesh on

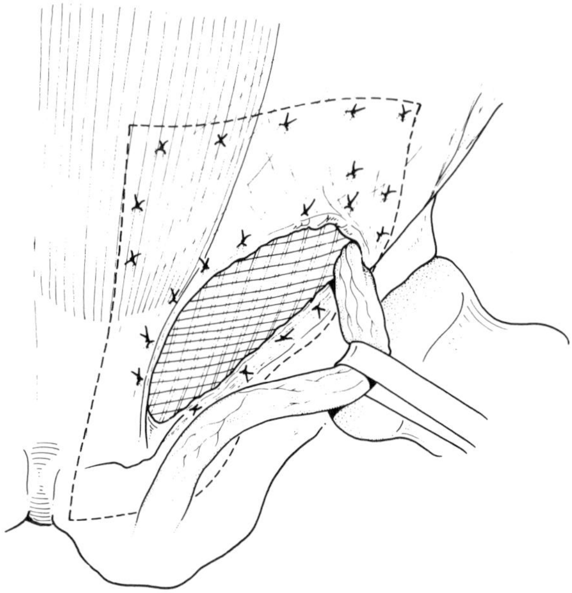

Figure 12.1.4 The Rives repair (as modified by Bendavid), eliminating the lateral incision in the mesh for the egress of the spermatic cord (courtesy of *World Journal of Surgery*).

Table 12.1.8 Recurrence rate following the use of mesh on primary repairs – the Rives technique

Author	No. of cases	% follow-up	Years follow-up	Recurrence
Rives[66]	65	–	–	0.0%
Rives[65]	183	66.1	1–9	1.6%
Flament[72]	586	80.0	5	1.7%
Galeone[73]	18	75.0	5	5.5%
Zagdoun[74]	185	80.0	1–7	7.0%
Barthes[75]	273	–	2	9.9%

either side of the cord, in a tunnel-like manner, providing a zig-zag course. This step has eliminated the oft-seen recurrence through the hole in the mesh (Table 12.1.8).

The Nyhus Buttress

Through a preperitoneal approach, where direct, indirect and femoral hernias are reduced (or resected), the Nyhus repair is carried out, namely transversalis

Table 12.1.9 Recurrence rate following the use of mesh on primary hernias – the Nyhus buttress technique

Author	No. of cases	% follow-up	Years follow-up	Recurrence
Nyhus[53]	115	–	0.5–10	1.7%
Rosenthal[76]	50	–	2.5	0.0%

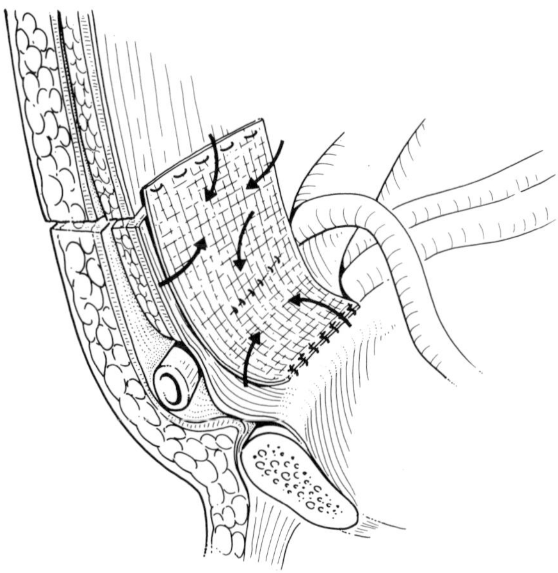

Figure 12.1.5 The Nyhus buttress technique (courtesy of JB Lippincott, Philadelphia)

fascia to the iliopubic tract or ligament of Cooper for direct hernias; anterior crus of the transversalis fascia and iliopubic tract about the internal ring for indirect hernias; iliopubic tract to Cooper's ligament for femoral hernias. These repairs are then reinforced by a covering of Marlex mesh (10 × 4 cm) anchored inferiorly to the ligament of Cooper and superiorly to the posterior inguinal floor. The buttress may be made as large as necessary (Fig. 12.1.5). The results are shown in Table 12.1.9.

The Stoppa Procedure

Introduced in 1968 by René Stoppa of Amiens, France, this procedure stands out as a daring and revolutionary method at first, but its simplicity can only be appreciated after several attempts. The technique must be well understood and seen first-hand before attempting it.

Table 12.1.10 Recurrence rate following the use of mesh on primary hernias – the Stoppa technique

Author	No. of cases	% follow-up	Years follow-up	Recurrence
VanDamme[77]	100	37.0	2	0.0%
Stoppa[68]	712	74.0	1–15	0.56%
Baeten[78]	150	–	1.5–5.5	0.66%
Montorsi[79a]	45	98.8	3	1.2%
Warlaumont[46]	285	91.3	1–10	1.2%
Stoppa[67]	255	91.3	2–10	2.5%
Pailler[79]	672	–	4	2.67%
Gross[80,81]	35	–	–	2.8%
Rignault[82]	568	–	–	4.0%
Wantz[69]	152	–	–	5.9%
Flament[83]	84	–	13	6.0%
Read[11]	83	–	4	7.0%

Essentially, it consists of exposing the posterior aspect of both groins from a preperitoneal approach through a subumbilical midline incision. Dissection is carried out through the prevesical space, then extended laterally. With the operating table in the Trendelenburg position, the peritoneum and contents are reflected cephalad. The spermatic cords are identified and lateralized as far as possible. When the hernias are dealt with (indirect, direct, femoral, prevascular), a chevron-shaped Mersilene mesh is inserted, the concave aspect of the chevron riding the neck of the bladder and each arm of the chevron extending laterally. The peritoneum is then allowed to fall back into place and, relying on the Pascal principle, the abdominal pressure keeps the mesh splayed against the abdominal wall (Fig. 12.1.6). Results have been impressive but they come from surgeons who are well experienced and from centres with a keen interest in hernia surgery (Table 12.1.10).

The Unilateral Stoppa (Wantz)

The unilateral Stoppa procedure represents a downsized version of the Stoppa operation as designed and performed by George Wantz of New York.

The operation begins with a suprapubic incision, lateral to the midline. The preperitoneal space is entered and after dealing accordingly with the hernia(s), a Mersilene mesh is anchored to the abdominal wall with the help of a Reverdin needle at the linea alba, along the arcuate line and laterally through the internal oblique, all sutures above the skin incision. The mesh is then allowed to fall and be splayed on the posterior aspect of the inguinal floor.

Wantz' series of 85 patients[69] (81 recurrences and four primaries) has not resulted in recurrences. The technique is simple, it bypasses the scarring that

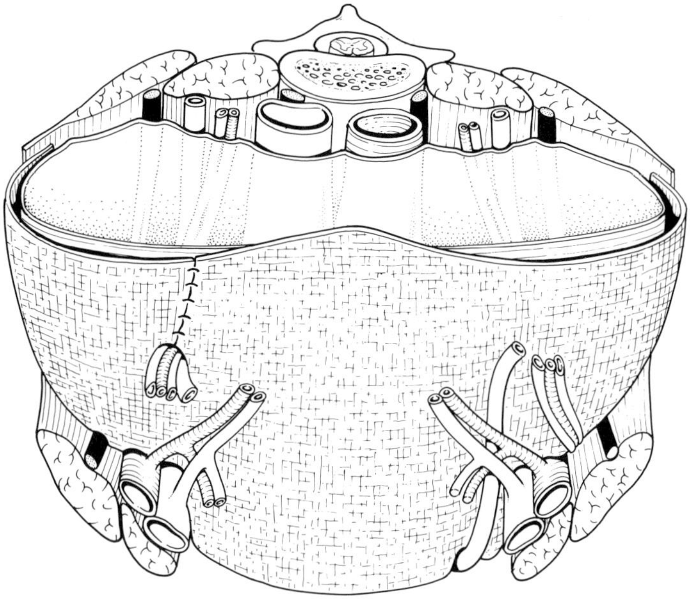

Figure 12.1.6 The Stoppa procedure. No slit is presently made in the mesh (courtesy of Editions Masson, Paris).

would be encountered by an anterior approach and is not marred by the possibility of testicular atrophy.

The Tension-Free Repair

No operation has attracted so many converts and adepts so quickly as the "tension-free repair". The concept originated with Richard Newman[84] (New Jersey), I. Lichtenstein[70] (California) and A. Gilbert[71] (Florida). Several large series are available for comparison and all seem to sing the praises of the procedure. The technique was introduced as early as 1962 and some surgeons have even become cavalier about excluding sutures altogether. Time, the harshest but fairest of judges, has not revealed the failures predicted by the cynics.

Although several variations abound, they all share one thing in common, the application of a prosthetic mesh on the floor of the inguinal canal from the pubic crest to just beyond the internal ring, the mesh bifurcating on either side of the spermatic cord. With direct hernia, the posterior wall is sometimes imbricated. With indirect hernia, the sac is resected. The mesh is held in place with interrupted or continuous sutures. Some[85,86] use no sutures and, marking the mesh with metal clips, they have shown that the prosthesis is not displaced prior to adequate infiltration by scar tissue (Fig. 12.1.7).

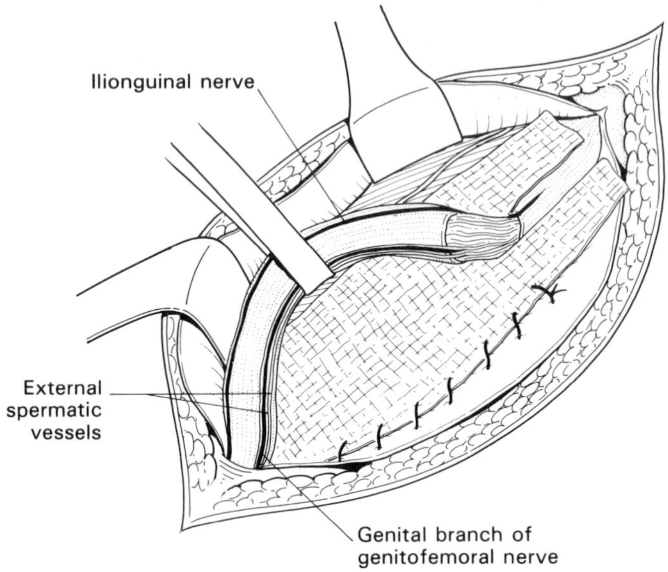

Figure 12.1.7 The tension-free repair (Lichtenstein) (courtesy of the *American Journal of Surgery*).

The "Plug" Technique

The "plug" technique creates some confusion because it is also reported as a tension-free repair. On occasion, the plug technique is simultaneously used with a mesh onlay over the floor of the inguinal canal. Pure "plug" repairs have been reported by Lichtenstein[70] – 1402 cases (1.6% recurrence) – and I. Rutkow[87] – 1563 cases (0% recurrence).

The technique is simple. Once a defect is identified, the fascial edges are defined, the hernia resected or reduced and, whether direct or indirect, a polypropylene plug is used to obliterate the defect. These plugs can be shaped like a cone,[71] a four-flange arrow tip[71,85] or simply a plug made out of a tightly rolled Marlex strip to fit the size of the defect. The cone and arrow tip rely on the tendency of the Marlex to spring back in an open position, deep to the defect and thus obliterate the defect. The rolled plug is sutured into place (Fig. 12.1.8).

These techniques require a minimal amount of dissection, simplify hernia repairs and are easily performed by the novice. They can be done under local anaesthesia and complications are minimal. Testicular atrophy and vascular injuries are practically unknown.

Tension-free repairs obviously would not be adequate for inguinofemoral hernias where the ligament of Poupart is often destroyed.

Table 12.1.11 reveals recurrence rates following primary hernia repairs while Table 12.1.12 represents re-recurrence following repairs of recurrent inguinal hernias.

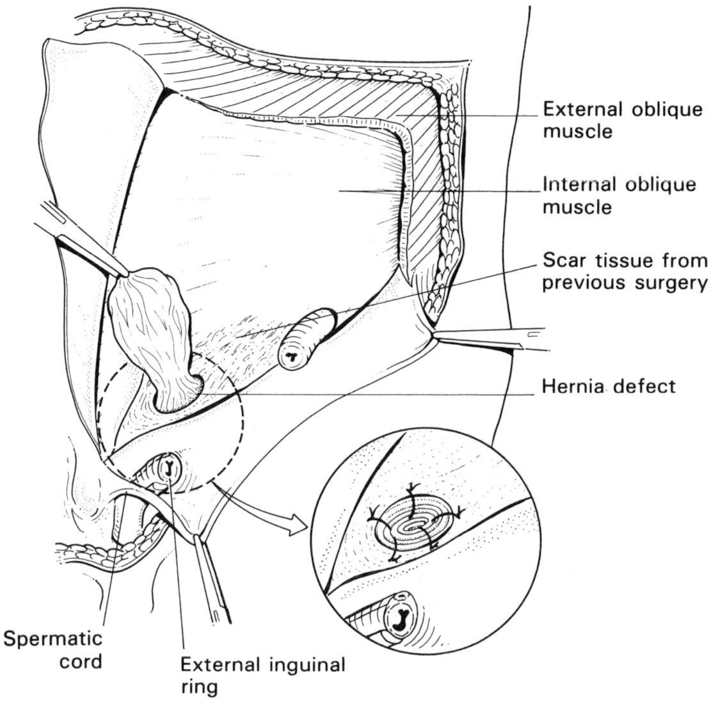

Figure 12.1.8 The plug repair (Lichtenstein) (courtesy of the *American Journal of Surgery*).

Table 12.1.11 Recurrence rate following the use of mesh on primary hernias – tension-free repairs

Author	No. of cases	% follow-up	Years follow-up	Recurrence
Lichtenstein[70]	1000	–	1–5	0.0%
Martin[88]	550	24	6	0.0%
Gruwez[89,90]	111	–	1.5	0.0%
Trabucco[85]	776	98	2.5	0.0%
Corcione[86]	225	–	1.7	0.0%
Gilbert[71]	412	88	2–5	0.24%
Capozzi[91]	745	84	5	0.61%
Tinckler[92]	392	–	1–5	0.77%
Newman[84]	1600	–	35	0.88%
Peyton-Barnes[93]	227	63	1–11	1.65%
Rutkow[87]	1313	–	4	0.0%

Table 12.1.12 Re-recurrence rate following the use of mesh in recurrent inguinal hernia repairs

Author	Technique	No. of cases	% follow-up	Years follow-up	Recurrence
Flament[83]	Rives	586	90	10	1.7%
Shouldice Hospital	Rives	139	–	7	2.16%
Bendavid[5]	Rives	280	–	5	3.2%
Nyhus[53]	Buttress	203	56	10.5	1.7%
Trabucco[85]	Tensionfree	188	98	2.5	0.0%
Gilbert[71]	Tensionfree	29	88	3	3.4%
Kaufman[94]	Tensionfree	57	100	6	1.75%
Gruwez[89,90]	Tensionfree	7	–	1	0.0%
Rutkow[87]	Tensionfree	250	–	4	0.0%
Wantz[69]	UnilStoppa	81	–	–	0.0%
Rignault[82]	UnilStoppa	–	–	–	1.2%
Wantz[29]	Stoppa	108	–	–	8.3%
VanDamme[77]	Stoppa	49	100	1–2	0.0%
Baeten[78]	Stoppa	150	–	1.5–5.5	0.75%
Lichtenstein[70]	Plug	390	–	5	0.5%
Shulman[95]	Plug	1402	–	3–21	1.6%

FEMORAL HERNIA REPAIR BY TRADITIONAL TECHNIQUES

Femoral hernias represent a particular challenge and there are several reasons for this. They are often misdiagnosed (2–25%);[96,97] they incarcerate more frequently than all other abdominal wall hernias combined;[98] they contribute to the highest mortality rate in hernia surgery (6–23%);[96–105] when the first repair fails, re-recurrence rates are highest (up to 75%);[6] the structures needed for repair are rigid and may be distant (Cooper ligament, Gimbernat's ligament, Poupart's ligament, conjoined tendon) or tenuous (iliopubic tract of Thomson); the proximity of the femoral vessels dictates that the operation is always a delicate one.

Reports on femoral hernias are usually of smaller series which do not always distinguish between primary and recurrence. At the Shouldice Hospital, 140–150 patients with femoral hernias are seen yearly, half of whom have a recurrence. Femoral hernias, fortunately, represent the group where the introduction of mesh has radically changed the picture from one of concern to confidence. The traditional repairs for femoral hernias can be divided into three types;

1. the low approach (Bassini, Bassini–Kirschner);
2. the anterior approach (Moschowitz, McVay);
3. the preperitoneal approach (Nyhus).

Table 12.1.13 Recurrence rate in femoral hernia repairs without mesh

Author	Technique	No. of cases	% follow-up	Years follow-up	Recurrence
Ponka[97]	Bassini	44	–	6	2.3%
Bendavid[6]	Bassini–Kirschner	251	84.7	1–8	6.1%
Butters[99]	Bassini–Kirschner	178	–	1–8	3.3%
Ponka[97]	Bassini–Kirschner	44	–	–	2.3%
Glassow[107]	Bassini–Kirschner	1143	–	–	2.0%
Ponka & Bush[96]	Bassini–Kirschner	216	92.0	1–8	6.5%
Ponka[97]	Moschowitz	46	–	6	0.9%
Nyhus & Harkins[3]	Preperitoneal	113	–	–	0.8%
Gaspar & Casberg[49]	Preperitoneal	6	90.0	1–7	0.0%
Bagot & Walters[108]	Preperitoneal	114	79.8	2–21	0.9%
Nyhus & Condon[47]	Preperitoneal	90	–	3	0.0%
Halverson[40]	McVay	96	–	22	3.1%
Barbier[42]	McVay	23	–	12.9	0.0%
Rutledge[39]	McVay	6	–	9.1	0.0%

The Bassini and the Bassini–Kirschner Repairs

Bassini described his femoral hernia repair in 1893.[106] Some confusion has existed since with reference to the tissues approximated in the technique. The more recent descriptions point out that the inguinal ligament is approximated to the pectineal fascia. The latter is a thin, inadequate layer. Bassini, in his text, stated accurately "the pectineal fascia at its *crest*", therefore implying the ligament of Cooper! The Bassini and Bassini–Kirschner operations therefore do not differ.

Success of the repair will depend on the availability of the ligament of Cooper, its angle with reference to Poupart's ligament and the tension generated by the approximation of those two ligaments. These operations are done through a low approach, below the inguinal ligament without disturbing the inguinal canal.

The Moschowitz Repair

This operation represents an anterior approach where the external oblique aponeurosis is split to gain access to the inguinal canal. The transversalis fascia is divided, allowing entry into the space of Bogros. The iliopubic tract of Thomson and/or the inguinal ligament is approximated to the iliopectineal ligament (Cooper's). Here again, tension may be too excessive as one must be left with adequate tissues to carry out the subsequent inguinal repair without tension and distortion of the inguinal ligament.

The McVay (Lotheissen–McVay) Repair

The operation of McVay has given surprisingly good results considering the tension that theoretically could result from the approximation of distant structures. The technique has been dealt with previously. The major drawback is the need for expert hands at performing the operation. The series reported are from Halverson–McVay,[40] Barbier[43] and Rutledge,[39] whose work has been referred to several times. Unusual care must be exercised, as no other repair provides the same potential for vascular compression and injury.

The Nyhus Preperitoneal Approach

Of all groin hernias, femoral hernias have responded best to the Nyhus preperitoneal repair.[47] The technique has been dealt with previously and consists of lowering the iliopubic tract to the ligament of Cooper through a suprapubic, preperitoneal approach. The successful results may be due to the fact that, medially, the iliopubic tract of Thomson is more substantial and consistent than it is more laterally.

FEMORAL HERNIA REPAIRS UTILIZING MESH

The most dramatic improvement resulting from the use of prosthetic mesh has been recorded in the treatment of femoral hernias. Whether the case at hand is a primary or a recurrent femoral hernia, no surgeon should ever hesitate to use mesh. The principles surrounding the repairs are simple enough. Once the hernia is reduced, actual repair of the defect consists in obliterating the defect by a plug from an infrainguinal approach (Fig. 12.1.9);[70,87] by using a large enough segment of mesh through an anterior approach (Fig. 12.1.10);[6,65,66,83] by a preperitoneal approach[29,47] or by a midline infraumbilical, preperitoneal approach.[67] All the techniques report comparable, good results. The choice of the technique would therefore rest with the ease of performance and expertise of the surgeon with that particular technique.

Table 12.1.14 represents recurrence rates following the use of mesh in femoral hernias. It has not always been easy to determine from the literature whether the femoral hernias being treated are primary or recurrences but one lesson has been learned by the hernia expert and that is, to consider all femoral hernias as recurrences or potential recurrences, demanding the utmost skill.

COMPLICATIONS FOLLOWING GROIN REPAIRS

Certain complications (atelectasis, pneumonitis, haematomas, wound infections, thrombophlebitis, urinary retention) will not be discussed since they are not direct complications of hernia surgery. With the trend towards short stay and ambulatory surgeries, some of these complications are becoming unusual.

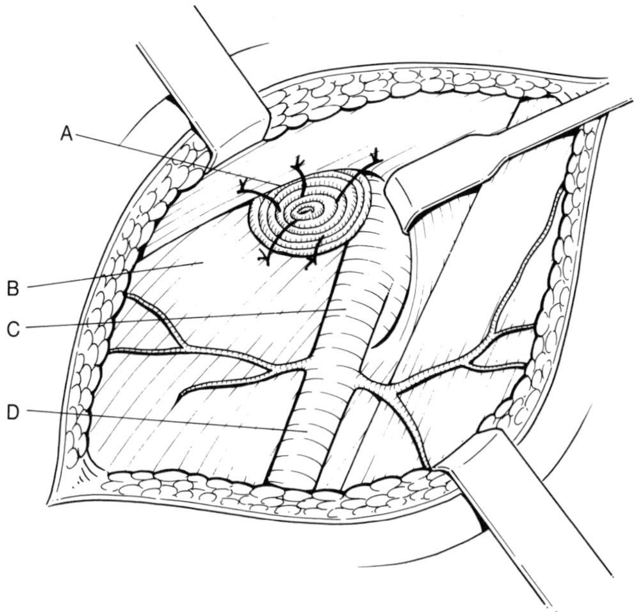

Figure 12.1.9 The femoral plug (Lichtenstein). A: inguinal ligament; B: pectineus muscle; C: femoral vein; D: saphenous vein (courtesy of the *American Journal of Surgery*).

Local anaesthesia has become standard in many institutions, thus eliminating those complications.

Besides recurrences, the relevant direct complications of hernia repairs are ischaemic orchitis, testicular atrophy, vascular compression or laceration, hydrocoeles and seromas.

Ischaemic Orchitis

This is, by definition, swelling and pain of the scrotum and testicle following surgery. This is a common enough complication which resolves without sequelae most of the time, usually within days. Wantz[29] has provided us with figures of 2% and 0.3%. I am convinced that this minor problem is more frequent.

Testicular Atrophy

This unpleasant complication is characterized by an enlarged, firm, painful testicle and low grade fever which can begin within 24–48 hours following surgery. Resolution takes from 6–8 weeks with reference to pain. The testicular atrophy which follows may be partial or total. I have seen this clinical picture

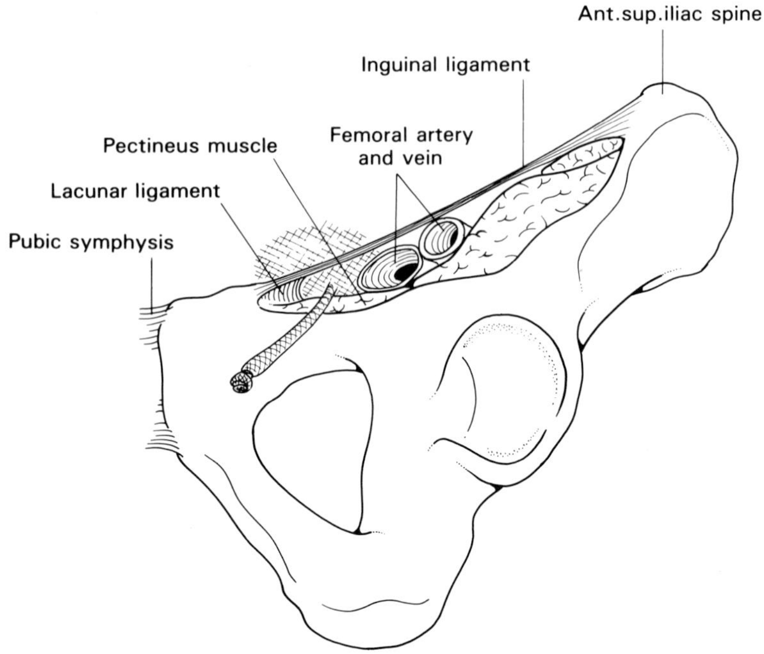

Figure 12.1.10 The "umbrella", inserted from the inferior or anterior approach (courtesy of *Surgery, Gynecology & Obstetrics*).

evolve, however, without a resultant testicular atrophy. Rarely, a testicle may appear completely normal after surgery and, without swelling or pain, the testicle will go on to atrophy. The incidence of testicular atrophy is 0.1 to 1% using the traditional techniques. Proponents of the tension-free repairs never see

Table 12.1.14 Recurrence rate following the use of mesh in femoral hernias

Author	**Technique**	**No. of cases**	**% follow-up**	**Years follow-up**	**Recurrence**
Wantz[69]	Unilateral Stoppa	7	–	–	0.0%
Wantz[29]	Stoppa	16	–	–	0.0%
Lichtenstein[70]	Femoral plug	168	–	14	0.61%
Trabucco[85]	Femoral plug	26p 1r	98	2.5	0.0%
Bendavid[113]	Umbrella	70	–	5–8	0.0%
Shouldice Hospital	Umbrella	280	–	9	1.1%

p = primary
r = recurrence

Table 12.1.15 Complications following inguinal and femoral repairs

Author	Technique	No. of cases	Ischaemic orchitis	Testicular atrophy	Vascular injury	Hydrocoele
Wantz[28,29]	Shouldice	3469p	0.3%	0.06%	–	–
Wantz[28,29]	Shouldice	694r	2.0%	1.7%	–	–
Bendavid[5]	Shouldice	4728p	–	0.1%	–	–
Bendavid[5]	Shouldice	980r	–	0.9%	–	–
Obney[111]	Shouldice	14442	–	–	–	0.9%
Nissen[112]	McVay	230	–	–	6	–
Klausner[115]	McVay	–	–	–	3	–
Brown[110]	McVay	302	–	–	5 (1.6%)	
Barbier[43]	McVay	1140	–	–	4 (0.35%)	
Gilbert[71]	Tensionfree	378	–	–	–	–
Corcione[86]	Tensionfree	225	–	–	–	–
Lichtenstein[70]	Tensionfree	111	–	–	–	–
Stoppa[68]	Stoppa	–	–	–	–	1.5%
VanDamme[77]	Stoppa	100	–	–	–	1.0%
Nyhus[53]	Nyhus buttress	203	–	–	–	0.5%

p = primary
r = recurrence

this complication. Nor do those who use the preperitoneal approach, since no dissection of the cord is carried out.

Vascular Injuries

Every type of herniorrhaphy can be marred by a vascular injury.[109] Fortunately, it is a rare complication. The Lotheissen–McVay repair, however, is the only herniorrhaphy where compression or laceration of the femoral vein is reported with some degree of frequency (Barbier 0.35%;[43] Brown 1.6%[110]). Table 12.1.15 reports 18 cases from four authors.

Hydrocoeles

The largest series was reported by Obney[111] (Shouldice Hospital) – 14,442 operations followed by 0.9% incidence of hydrocoele formation. This complication follows anterior as well as preperitoneal approaches (Nyhus 0.5%;[3] Stoppa 1.5%;[68] VanDamme 1%[77]).

Seromas

In the experience of the Shouldice Hospital, seromas rarely, if ever, complicate the traditional herniorrhaphy.[114] When mesh is used, however, seromas can occur (Bendavid 6.6%[113]). They will usually resorb and rarely require aspiration.

CONCLUSION

Traditional inguinal and femoral herniorrhaphies, properly carried out, yield excellent results. The addition of prosthetics has brought those results near to perfection. The use of local anaesthesia and the spread of short stay and ambulatory surgery have contributed to creating the image that a hernia has become a minor surgical problem.

Is it possible to improve those results without compromising safety and cost? I am not certain...

REFERENCES

1. Casten DF. Functional anatomy of the groin area as related to the classification and treatment of groin hernias. *Am J Surg* 1967; **114**: 894–9.
2. Gilbert AI. An anatomic and functional classification for the diagnosis and treatment of inguinal hernia. *Am J Surg* 1989; **157**: 331–3.
3. Nyhus LM, Harkins HN. *Hernia*, 1st edition. Philadelphia, JB Lippincott, 1964.
4. Obney N, Chan CK. Repair of multiple time recurrent inguinal hernias with reference to common causes of recurrence. *Contemp Surg Dec* 1984, **25**: 25–32.
5. Bendavid R. The Shouldice method of inguinal herniorrhaphy. In: Mastery of Surgery, 2nd edition (eds Nyhus LM, Baker RJ), Little, Brown and Company, Boston, 1992.
6. Bendavid R. Femoral hernias: primary vs recurrence. *Int Surg* 1989; **74**: 99–100.
7. O'Dell A. Personal communication.
8. Ryan EA. An analysis of 313 consecutive cases of indirect sliding inguinal hernia. *Surg Gynecol Obstet* 1956; **102**: 45–58.
9. Welsh DRJ. Sliding inguinal hernias. *Abdominal Surg* 1964; **6**, 4.
10. Welsh DRJ. Repair of indirect sliding inguinal hernias. *Abdominal Surg* 1969; **11**: 204–9.
11. Read RC. Recurrence after preperitoneal herniorrhaphy in the adult. *Arch Surg* 1975; **110**: 666–71.
12. Bassini E. Nuovo Metodo Operativo per La Cura dell'Ernia Inguinale Padova, Prosperini, 1889.
13. Bassini, E. Uber die behandlung des leistenbruches. *Arch Klin Chir* 1890; **40**: 429.
14. Wantz GE. The operation of Bassini as described by Attilio Catterina. *Surg Gynecol Obstet* 1989; **168**: 67–80.
15. Hagan WH, Rhoads JE. Inguinal and femoral hernias, follow-up study. *Surg Gynecol Obstet* 1953; **96**: 226–32.
16. Marsden RJ. Inguinal hernia: a three year review of 2000 cases. *Br J Surg* 1962; **69**: 384–94.
17. Houdard C. Hernies inguinales récidivées de l'adulte. *Rev Prat* 1980; **15**: 701–8.
18. Vayre P, Jost JL. Autoplastic inguinale pour la cure des hernies directes chez l'homme. Communication à la 5e réunion du GREPA, Paris 1983.
19. Callum KG, Doig RL, Kinmouth JB. The results of nylon darn repair for inguinal hernias. *Arch Surg* 1974; **108**: 25–7.
20. Chevrel JP, Duchene P. Sarfati E. L'opération de Bassini. GREPA 1983: **5**: 9–13.
21. Magnusson J, Isaksson B. Recurrence after inguinal hernioplasty. *Acta Chir Scand* 1983; **149**: 157.

22. Berliner S, Burson L, Kate P. An anterior transversalis fascia repair for adult inguinal hernias. *Am J Surg* 1978; **135**: 633–6.
23. Piper JV. A comparison between whole-thickness skin graft and Bassini methods of repair of hernia in men. *Br J Surg* 1969; **56**: 345–8.
24. Bélanger J, Flament JP, Goldstein M. Bilan de 14 années de cures de hernies. *Acta Chir Belg* 1975; **60**: 37–9.
25. Bendavid R. The Shouldice Operation. *Encyclopédie Médico Chirurgicale* (Paris, France), Techniques Chirurgicales, Appareil Digestif 40112, 4.11.12, p. 5.
26. Shearburn EW, Myers RN. Shouldice repair for inguinal hernia. *Surgery* 1969; **66**: 450–9.
27. Volpe L, Galli T. *The Shouldice Repair – Our Experience.* Congress in General and Gastrointestinal Surgery, Hospital San Carlo Borromeo, Milan, March 1991.
28. Wantz G. The Canadian repair of inguinal hernia. In: *Hernia III* (eds Nyhus L, Condon R), pp. 236–52. Philadelphia, JB Lippincott, 1989.
29. Wantz G. *Hernia III* (eds Nyhus L, Condon R), p. 245. Philadelphia, JB Lippincott, 1989.
30. Myers RN, Shearburn EW. The problem of the recurrent inguinal hernia. *Surg Clin Am* 1973; **53**: 555–8.
31. Devlin HB, Gillen PHA, Waxman BP. Short stay surgery for inguinal hernia. Clinical outcome of the Shouldice operation. *Lancet* 1977; **1**: 847–9.
32. Flament JB. Personal communication.
33. Flament JB. *Traitement des Hernies de L'Aine.* International Workshop on Abdominal Wall Hernias, Palermo, Italy, November 1991.
34. Moran MR, Bliek M, Collura M. Double layer of transversalis fascia for repair of inguinal hernia. *Surgery* 1968; **63**: 424–9.
35. McVay CB. The normal and pathological anatomy of the transversus abdominis muscle in inguinal and femoral hernias. *Surg Clin Am* 1971; **51**: 1251.
36. McVay CB. Preperitoneal hernioplasty. *Surg Gynecol Obstet* 1966; **123**: 349.
37. McVay CB, Chapp JD. Inguinal and femoral hernioplasty – the evaluation of a basic concept. *Ann Surg* 1958; **148**: 499–512.
38. Bendavid R. The space of Bogros and the deep inguinal venous circulation. *Surg Gynecol Obstet*; **174**: 355–8.
39. Rutledge RH. Cooper's ligament repair: a 25 year experience with a single technique for all groin hernias in adults. *Surgery* 1988; **103**: 1–10.
40. Halverson K, McVay CB. Inguinal and femoral hernioplasty. A 22 year study of the author's method. *Arch Surg* 1970; **101**: 127–35.
41. Lubeth M. A propos de 1000 cas de hernies de l'aine dont 800 traitées par abaissement au Cooper. Thèse Med (Poitiers) 1979, 13.
42. Barbier J. Traitement des hernies inguinales selon la technique de McVay: A propos de 1000 cas. *Chirurgie* 1984; **100**: 144–9.
43. Barbier J, Carretier M, Richer JP. Cooper ligament repair: an update. *World J Surg* 1989; **13**: 499–505.
44. Asmussen T, Jensen FU. A follow up study on recurrences after inguinal hernia repair. *Surg Gynecol Obstet* 1983; **145**: 353.
45. Jones TP. A comparative study of inguinal herniorrhaphy. *Am Surg* 1975, 20–7.
46. Warlaumont C. Les hernies de l'aine. Doctoral thesis, University of Amiens, 1982.
47. Nyhus LM, Condon RE, Harkins HN. *Preperitoneal Hernioplasty: A Technique for the Repair of All Groin Hernias.* 111th Annual Meeting of the American Medical Association, Chicago, June 1962.
48. Nyhus LM, Klein MS, Rodgers FB. Inguinal hernia. *Curr Prob Surg* 1991; **28**: 417–19.
49. Gaspar MR, Casberg MA. An appraisal of preperitoneal repair of inguinal hernia. *Surg Gynecol Obstet* 1971; **132**: 207–12.

50. Dyson WL, Pierce WS. Changing concept of inguinal herniorrhaphy: experience with preperitoneal approach. *Arch Surg* 1965; **91**: 971.
51. Gregorie HB Jr. Preperitoneal Repair of Groin Hernias. *JS Carolina Med Ass* 1966; **6**: 417.
52. Lindholm A, Nilson O, Tholin B. Inguinal and femoral hernias. *Arch Surg* 1969; **98**: 19.
53. Nyhus LM, Pollack R, Bombeck CT, Donahue PE. The preperitoneal approach and prosthetic buttress repair for recurrent hernia. The evolution of a technique. *Ann Surg* 1988; **208**: 733.
54. Greenburg A. Revisiting the Recurrent Groin Hernia. *Am J Surg* 1987; **154**: 35–40.
55. Ljundahl I. Inguinal and femoral hernia. An investigation of 502 own operated cases. *Acta Chir Scand* 1973; **439**: 81–4.
56. Brogeskov S, Skeie E. Preperitoneal herniorrhaphy. *Acta Chir Scand* 1973; **139**: 45–7.
57. Robertson HT. Preperitoneal approach in the repair of inguinal hernias. *Am J Surg* 1966; **112**: 627.
58. Read RC. A review. The role of protease–antiprotease imbalance in the pathogenesis of herniation and abdominal aortic aneurysm in certain smokers. *Postgrad Gen Surg* 1992; **4**, 161–5.
59. Tugnoli G. *Our Experience in the Treatment of Recurrent Inguinal Hernias*. International Congress on Groin and Incisional Hernias, Padua, November 1991.
60. Cevese PG, Lise M, Spatari V. *La Chirurgia dell'Ernia Inguinale*. International Congress in honour of E. Bassini, University of Padova, November 1986.
61. Kupczyk-Joeris D. *Shouldice Repair in Recurrent Groin Hernia*. Xth Grenslandsymposium, Leuven, Belgium, March 1992.
62. Rotker J. *Recurrence Rate after Inguinal Hernioplasty using the Shouldice Technique*. Xth Grenslandsymposium, Leuven, Belgium, March 1992.
63. Obney N. Shouldice technique for the repair of inguinal hernia. *J Dentist* 1979; **55**: 863–6.
64. Blaisdell FW, Adams DR, Hall AD, Gauder PJ. Preperitoneal hernia repair. Experiences in 101 consecutive cases. *Am J Surg* 1964; **30**: 623.
65. Rives J, Lardennois B, Flament JB, Convers G. La piece en tulle de Dacron, traitement de choix des hernies de l'aine de l'adulte. A propos de 183 cas. *Chirurgie* 1973; **99**: 564–75.
66. Rives J, Stoppa R, Fortesa L, Nicaise H. Les pièces en Dacron et leur place dans la chirurgie des hernies de l'aine. *Ann Chir* 1968; **22**: 159–71.
67. Stoppa R, Petit J, Henry X. Plastie des hernies de l'aine par voie mediane sous peritoneale. *Acta Chir Masson* 1972; **?**: 453–88.
68. Stoppa R, Rives JL, Warlaumont C, Palot JP, Verhaege PJ, Delattre JF. The use of Dacron in the repair of hernias of the groin. *Surg Clin N Am* 1984; **64**: 269–85.
69. Wantz G. Giant prosthetic reinforcement of the visceral sac. *Surg Gynecol Obstet* 1989; **169**: 408–17.
70. Lichtenstein IL, Shulman AG, Amid PK, Montlor HM. The tension-free hernioplasty. *Am J Surg* 1989; **157**: 188–93.
71. Gilbert AI. Sutureless repair of inguinal hernia. *Am J Surg* 1992; **163**: 331–5.
72. Flament JB. *Treatment of Inguinal Hernias*. International Workshop on Abdominal Wall Hernias, Palermo, November 1991.
73. Galeone M, Ferrante F. *Primary Inguinofemoral Hernias of the Adult*. Congress in General and GI Surgery, Hospital San Carlo Borromeo, Milan, March 1991.
74. Zagdoun J, Sordinas A. L'utilisation des plaques de nylon dans la chirurgie des hernies inguinales. *Mem Acad Chir* 1959; **85**: 747–54.
75. Barthes JN. Traitement des hernies et éventrations par une prothèse de nylon: La crinoplaque à propos de 420 cas personnels. Doctoral thesis, Paris, 1971.

76. Rosenthal D, Walters MJ. Preperitoneal synthetic mesh placement for recurrent hernias of the groin. *Surg Gynecol Obstet* 1986; **163**: 285–6.
77. Van Damme JP. A preperitoneal approach in the prosthetic repair of inguinal hernias. *Int Surg* 1985; **70**: 223–6.
78. Baeten CG, Koostra G, van Geldere D. *Stoppa Technique in Bilateral Inguinal Hernias.* Xth Grenslandsymposium, Leuven, Belgium, March 1992.
79. Pailler JL, Vica P. Clinical analysis of expanded PTFE in the treatment of recurrent and complex groin hernias. *Postgrad Gen Surg* 1992; **4**: 168.

79a. Montorsi W. ATTI updating course in general and GI surgery. Milan, March 1991.

80. Gross E. The preperitoneal implantation of Dacron sheet for repair of recurrent repeat and bilateral groin hernia. Xth Grenslandsymposium, Leuven, Belgium, March 1992.
81. Gross E, Kofuncu OA. *Preperitoneal Implantation of Dacron Sheets for Repair of Recurrent, Repeat and Bilateral Groin Hernias.* Xth Grenslandsymposium, Leuven, Belgium, March 1992.
82. Rignault DP. Properitoneal prosthetic inguinal hernioplasty through a Pfannenstiel approach. 1986; **163**: 465.
83. Flament JB, Palot JP. *The Rives Technique.* Congress in General and GI Surgery, Hospital San Carlo Borromeo, Milan, March 1991.
84. Newman R. Personal communication.
85. Trabucco E. ATTI updating course in general and GI surgery. Milan, March 1991.
86. Corcione F. La Tecnica di Trabucco Esperienza Relativa a 225 Casi. International Conference on Inguinal Hernia, Naples, Italy, April 1992.
87. Rutkow I. Personal communication.
88. Martin RE, Max CC. Primary inguinal hernia repair with prosthetic mesh. *Hosp Medica* 1984, **1**, 1–2.
89. Gruwez JA. *Lichtenstein Repair with EPTFE.* Xth Grenslandsymposium, Leuven, Belgium, March 1992.
90. Gruwez JA. *Surgical Diseases of the Abdominal Wall.* Xth Grenslandsymposium, Leuven, Belgium, March 1992.
91. Capozzi JA, Berkenfield JA, Cherry JK. Repair of inguinal hernia in the adult with Prolene mesh. *Surg Gynecol Obstet* 1988; **167**: 124–8.
92. Tinckler LF. Inguinal hernia repair using local anaesthesia. *Ann Roy Coll Surg Eng* 1985; **67**: 268.
93. Peyton-Barnes J. Inguinal hernia repair with routine use of Marlex mesh. *Surg Gynecol Obstet* 1987; **165**: 33–7.
94. Kaufman M, Wiessberg D, Bider D. Repair of recurrent inguinal hernia with Marlex mesh. *Surg Gynecol Obstet* 1985; **160**, 505–6.
95. Shulman A, Amid PK, Lichtenstein IL. The "plug" repair of 1402 recurrent inguinal hernias – a 20 year experience. *Arch Surg* 1990; **125**: 265–7.
96. Ponka JL, Brush BE. The problem of femoral hernia. *Arch Surg* 1971; **102**: 417–23.
97. Ponka JL. *Hernias of the Abdominal Wall*, pp. 243–52. Philadelphia, WB Saunders, 1980.
98. David T. Strangulated femoral hernia. *Med J Aust* 1967; **1**: 258–61.
99. Butters AG. A review of femoral herniae with specific reference to recurrence rate of low operations. *Br Med J* 1948; **2**: 743–5.
100. Cooke RV. Discussion of small bowel obstruction. *Proc R Soc Med* 1958; **51**: 503–8.
101. McClure RD, Fallis LS. Femoral hernia, report of 90 operations. *Ann Surg J* 1939; **109**: 987–1000.
102. Dunphy JE. The diagnosis and surgical management of strangulated femoral hernias. *JAM* 1940; **114**: 394–6.
103. Jens J. Strangulated femoral hernia. *Lancet* 1943; **1**: 705–7.

104. Lawson RS. Strangulated hernia. *Alfred Hosp Clin Rep* 1949; **1**: 51.
105. Temple CO. Incarcerated and strangulated femoral hernias. *J Int Coll Surg* 1958; **30**: 1–11.
106. Bassini E. Nuovo Metodo Operativo per La Cura Radicale dell'Hernia Crurale. Angelo Draghi Libraio Editore, Padova, 1893.
107. Glassow F. Recurrent inguinal and femoral hernias. *Br Med J* 1970; **1**: 215–16.
108. Bagot-Walters GA. A retropubic operation for femoral hernias. *Br J Surg* 1965; **52**: 678–82.
109. Helenon C, Lataste J. Les cures herniaires inguinales et crurales. Leur retentissement veineux. *Presse Med* 1960; **68**: 152–3.
110. Brown R, Kinateder RJ, Rosenberg N. Ipsilateral thrombophlebitis and pulmonary embolism after Cooper's ligament herniorrhaphy. *Surgery* 1980; **87**: 230–2.
111. Obney N. Hydrocoeles of the testicle complicating inguinal hernias. *CMAJ* 1956; **75**: 733–6.
112. Nissen HM. Constriction of the femoral vein following inguinal hernia repair. *Acta Chir Scand* 1975; **141**: 279–81.
113. Bendavid R. A femoral "umbrella" for femoral hernia repair. *Surg Gynecol Obstet* 1987; **165**: 153–156.
114. Welsh DRJ, Alexander MAJ. The Shouldice repair. *Surgical Clinics North America*, June 1993, 493.
115. Klausner JM, Noveck H, Skornick Y, Lelcuk S. Femoral vein occlusion following McVay repair. *Postgrad Med J* 1986; **62**: 301–2.

— 12.2 —

Laparoscopic Hernia Repairs

N. KATKHOUDA and J. MOUIEL

INTRODUCTION

Inguinal hernias in the adult result rarely from a persistent processus vaginali or more often from a defect in the transversalis fascia. Over the years, many different techniques have evolved in order to repair the defect in the abdominal wall[1–6] and all share the same features: they are swift and easy to perform and relatively safe when compared with other abdominal procedures. Thus, the modern approach to hernia repair towards the end of the twentieth century should not only be efficient, with the lowest possible recurrence rate, but also remain simple to perform and safe for the patient. Laparoscopic hernia repair has the potential to fulfil all these requirements and, due to the minimal invasive approach, may also be better tolerated by the patient.

The first published reports of laparoscopic hernia repair in 1982[7] and later suffered from a lack of experimental background to the technique, little or no assessment of the follow-up of the patient and poor reporting of the complications and recurrence rates. Some of the techniques proposed laparoscopically to repair inguinal hernias since then have certainly been innovative[8–10] but unfortunately did not rely on the sound anatomical basis for hernia repairs which had been set by open surgery.[6,11–15] The techniques for laparoscopic inguinal hernia repair which we report in this chapter have evolved with regard both to technique and indication over the last few years and can be safely recommended to most patients.

ANATOMICAL CONSIDERATIONS

It is essential to recognize the anatomical structures of the preperitoneal space as seen through the laparoscope from the inside in order to be able to achieve an efficient hernia repair (Figs 12.2.1–2). Three important landmarks which the surgeon should focus upon are Cooper's ligament, the medial umbilical ligament (embryological remnant of umbilical artery) and the epigastric vessels as they

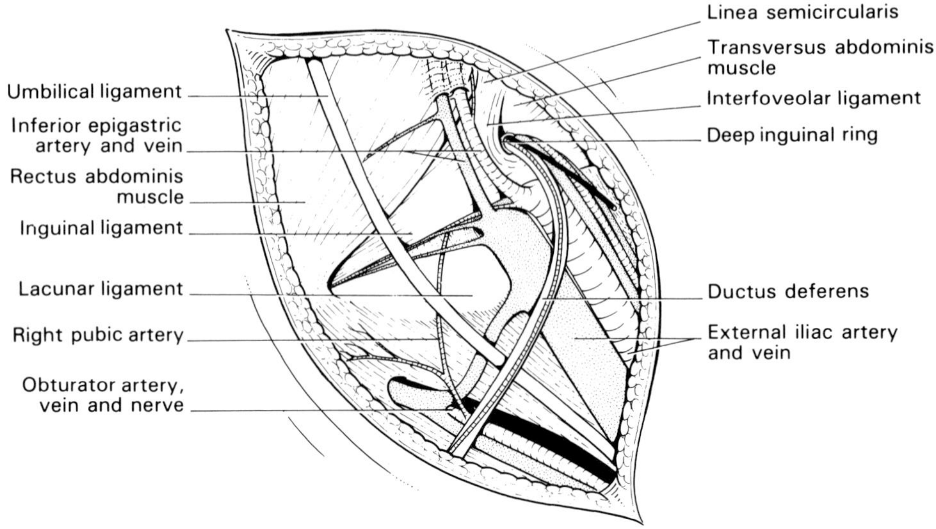

Figure 12.2.1 Anatomy of the right peritoneal space.

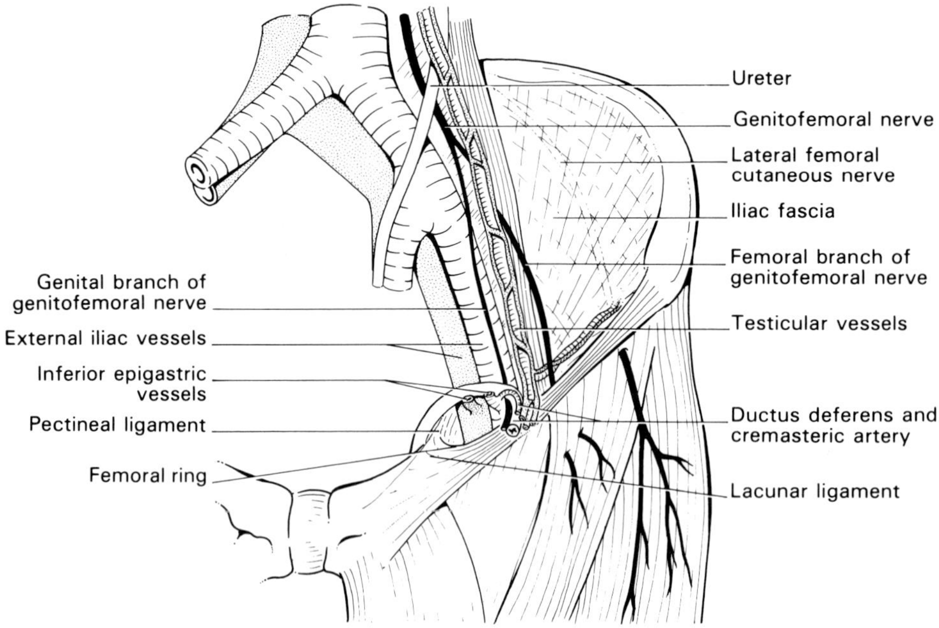

Figure 12.2.2 The lateral nerves on the psoas muscle.

come off the external iliac artery and vein. Along with the ilio-pubic tract, these landmarks define the spaces associated with inguinal hernia: indirect hernias lateral to the epigastric vessels and direct hernias medial to the epigastric vessels but lateral to the medial umbilical ligament within the triangle of Hesselbach.

Following the introduction of laparoscopic hernia repair, a further triangle has been described – the triangle of Doom – located between the vas deferens and the spermatic vessels in which lie the external iliac vein and artery. It is obviously important that no staples or sutures should be placed in this region. If this triangle is extended in the lateral direction to the psoas muscle, the lateral femorocutaneous nerve and the genitofemoral nerve can be found and these should be kept in mind when lateral sutures or staples are placed during laparoscopic hernia repair. One of the complications of laparoscopic hernia repair is damage to either or both of these nerves, producing postoperative paraesthesia or neuromas. The triangle of Doom could therefore be extended laterally to the psoas muscle and incorporates these reserves.

CLASSIFICATION OF GROIN HERNIAS

All operative approaches to hernia repairs must have a precise anatomical basis. Nyhus has developed a new classification with respect to the anatomical aspects of the lower abdominal wall.[11] This classification may be used to select which laparoscopic technique is the most appropriate for any given hernia.

Type I Paediatric type (patent processus vaginalis) with a normal internal ring.

Type II Indirect inguinal hernia with an intact posterior wall of the inguinal canal, but a weakened internal ring.

Type IIIa A direct hernia.

Type IIIb A large indirect hernia with an associated weak posterior wall.

Type IIIc Femoral hernia.

Type IV Any recurrent hernia.

TECHNIQUES[18–28]

Four techniques for laparoscopic hernia repair may be performed;

1. the intraperitoneal onlay mesh (IPOM);
2. the transabdominal preperitoneal mesh (TAM);

3. the total extraperitoneal mesh repair (TEM);
4. closure of the internal ring for types I and II hernias.

The first repair, involving intraperitoneal onlay mesh, is controversial and has not been performed by these authors, but will be described briefly later.

OPERATING ROOM SET-UP

The patient is positioned supine with the bladder catheterized to prevent any obstruction of the dissection of the preperitoneal space due to a full bladder. The patient is then prepared and draped and the two monitors are positioned at the foot of the operating table and the patient's legs remain together. The surgeon stands at the left shoulder of the patient, operating with both hands. This position is adequate for repair of both sides of the groin. A steep Trendelenburg position is usually required in order to remove the small bowel from the pelvic cavity.

INSTRUMENTATION

Three ports are necessary for this operation: a 10 mm umbilical port for the video endoscope; a 10 mm port on the side of the hernia; and a 5 mm port in the opposite iliac fossa (Ethicon Endosurgery, Cincinnati, Ohio) (Fig. 12.2.3). A 30° oblique-viewing laparoscope is to be preferred to the end-viewing laparoscope, if available, particularly for leftsided hernias operated on by righthanded surgeons.

THE TRANSABDOMINAL PREPERITONEAL MESH REPAIR

Following induction of the pneumoperitoneum which is maintained at 12 mmHg, the ports are inserted as described above. The two lateral ports are inserted two fingers medially and inferiorly to each anterior superior iliac spine using grasping forceps and electrocoagulation scissors. The hernia sac in question is reduced and a peritoneal flap incised from lateral to medial (Fig. 12.2.4A). The lateral incision begins over the psoas muscle lateral to the deep inguinal ring and extends medially above the deep inguinal ring to the medial umbilical ligament in order to avoid the genital branch of the genitofemoral nerve.

This peritoneal flap is dissected downwards towards the iliac vessels inferiorly and then on the upwards side towards the anterior abdominal wall muscles

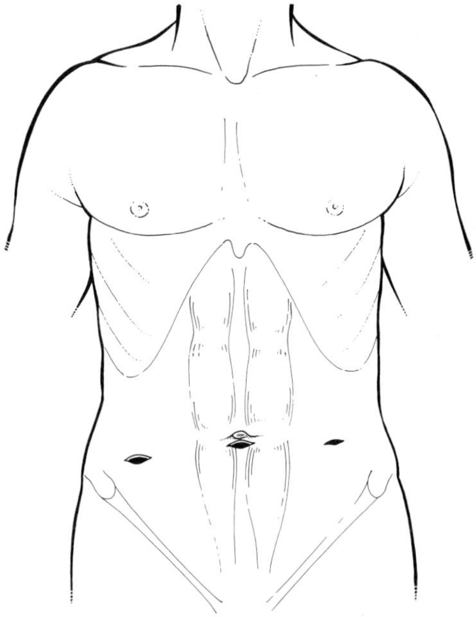

Figure 12.2.3 Trocar placement (Storz, Tuttlingen, Germany).

superiorly. This peritoneal flap includes the hernia sac. This will always be the case for direct hernias, but in the case of very large indirect inguinoscrotal hernias, the distal part of the sac is divided and left within the scrotum.

The preperitoneal space is then dissected using an atraumatic technique with the scissors closed and used to brush the tissue in each direction. This dissection of the areolar tissue can be performed with minimal requirement for haemostasis. The anatomical landmarks around this region can then be demonstrated and when dissection is complete the arch of the transversus abdominal muscle (and conjoint tendon) and the ileopubic tract can be finally recognized. At the most lateral aspect of the dissection the psoas muscle and the two nerves (laterofemorocutaneous nerve and the genitofemoral nerve) may be recognized.

Dissection of the Cord Structures

An important step in the dissection of the inguinal region is the dissection (parietalization technique of Stoppa) of the spermatic cord off the peritoneum. This will allow the cord to be pushed to the side of the pelvic cavity in order to lay the mesh over the hernia defect. This dissection of the cord consists of blunt dissection of the vas deferens from the spermatic vessels just proximal to the deep inguinal ring, mobilizing the peritoneum from this surface. If this is not done, the mesh will need to be split in order to cover the hernia defects and this may predispose to recurrence.

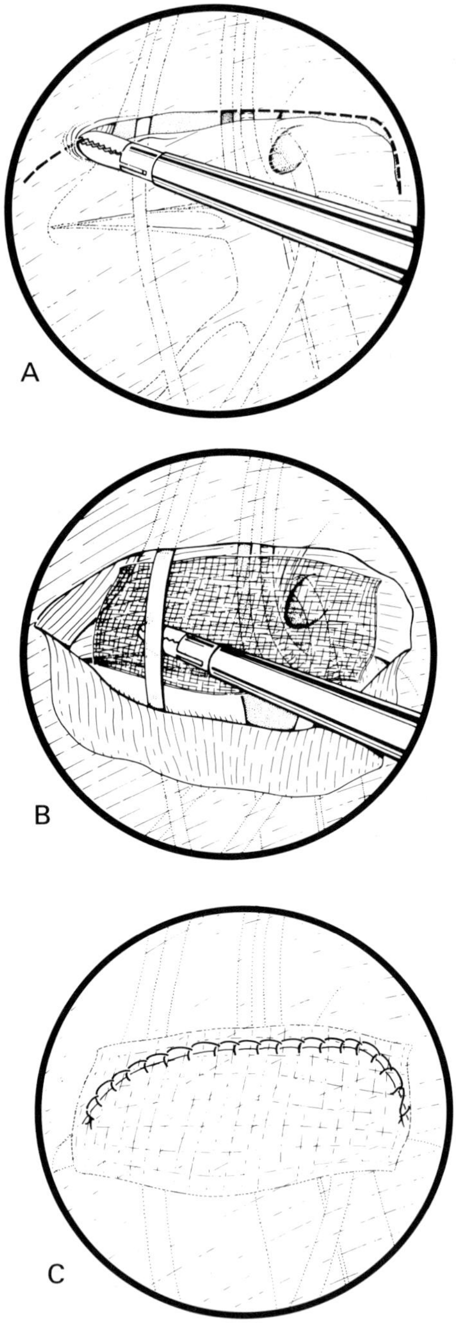

Figure 12.2.4 Transabdominal preperitoneal approach. A: peritoneal incision; B: peritoneal flap and positioning of the mesh; C: closure of the peritoneum using continuous sutures.

Reduction of the Hernia Sac and Placement of the Mesh

Once the hernia sac has been completely reduced and the dissection of the preperitoneal space completed, a mesh is introduced and fixed in place using staples. The mesh used by the authors is a 6 cm × 11 cm polypropylene mesh (Ethicon Inc, Cincinnati, Ohio) and is to be preferred over the other types of mesh because of its transparent structure, allowing visualization of the elements over which it lies before stapling and its relative memory, permitting a perfect anatomical placement. The mesh is rolled up in a cigarette fashion and loaded backwards into one of the trocars protected by a reducing sleeve. Once it is within the peritoneal cavity it is rolled into place and should cover all hernia spaces in their entirety, including indirect, direct and femoral spaces (Fig. 12.2.4B). The mesh is secured in place by staples (Ethicon Inc. Cincinnati, Ohio) starting laterally above the psoas muscle and the iliopubic tract, taking care not to damage the associated nerves and continuing along the upper border to Cooper's ligament medially. If staples are not available, intraperitoneal suturing can be performed using extracorporeal knotting technique.

Once the mesh has been stapled in place, the peritoneal flap is replaced over the mesh and stapled in place. This is facilitated by reducing the pressure of the pneumoperitoneum from 12 mmHg to 9 mmHg. It is thought to be important to completely cover the mesh with the peritoneal flap to prevent any possible exposure of the mesh to the underlying viscera and possible adhesion formation. This is ideally performed in an overlap fashion. Again, if staples are not available, a continuous suture may be used to close the peritoneal flap (Fig. 12.2.4C). No intraperitoneal drainage is required and following removal of the carbon dioxide and ports, the skin incisions are closed with single interrupted sutures after careful closure of the fascia in the 10 mm trocar entry ports.

TECHNIQUE OF TOTAL EXTRAPERITONEAL MESH REPAIR (TEM)

An open laparoscopy is performed around the inferior pole of the umbilicus using a circular incision. Retractors are inserted, the underlying fascia is incised and the peritoneum is demonstrated. The peritoneum should not be entered as the plane of cleavage lies in the extraperitoneal space deep to the rectus muscles. The plane is found using a blunt dissection technique with the help of the laparoscope attached to the camera. It is easy to observe the light from the laparoscope passing in this plane from the umbilicus towards the symphysis pubis. Once at the symphysis pubis the laparoscope is gently moved in a lateral direction to demonstrate Cooper's ligament on the side of the hernia.

The preperitoneal space is then insufflated at low pressure first and subsequently at a slightly higher pressure in order to improve access and this will also help with the dissection. The additional ports for dissection are inserted just medial to the anterior superior iliac spine and just below and lateral to the umbilical port on the opposite side from the hernia. The preperitoneal space is then dissected free as described for the transabdominal preperitoneal repair and the same landmarks are identified. Another elegant technique is the dissection of the preperitoneal space using an inflatable balloon (Origin Inc.).

At this point, it is clear that, using this technique, the space for dissection is small and the freedom for movement is limited accordingly. Furthermore, any perforation of the underlying peritoneum will allow carbon dioxide to escape into the abdominal cavity which subsequently compresses the preperitoneal space. If this occurs, equilibration of pressures must occur before dissection continues and this is facilitated by opening the peritoneal defect widely. There is always the possibility of converting the preperitoneal approach to the transabdominal approach should access prove impossible.

If a large hernia sac is found with an associated lipoma, this must be resected using an Endoloop (Ethicon Inc, Cincinnati, Ohio) and the lipoma removed through one of the trocars. This technique is obviously difficult to perform for inguinoscrotal or sliding hernias. Once the hernia sac has been dissected free, mesh is installed as described in the previous transabdominal technique and stapled in place. The obvious advantage of this approach over the transabdominal approach is that the peritoneum does not have to be closed over the hernia and there are no complications that may be associated with transabdominal laparoscopy as the peritoneum has never been entered.

TECHNIQUE OF INTRAPERITONEAL ONLAY MESH

The only possible theoretical indication for this technique may be presented by the small indirect hernia in the young patient (type I or II). A non-absorbable mesh could be placed over the indirect hernia defect and stapled in place (Fig. 12.2.5). This mesh obviously should be stapled to the underlying muscular structures in addition to the peritoneum, otherwise there is an increased risk of movement and subsequent recurrence. Of all the different types of mesh available, expanded PTFE in theory should be the best, as the least intra-abdominal adhesion formation would be expected. However, we are not aware of any laparoscopic experimental studies which have confirmed or refuted this opinion.

DIRECT REPAIR OF INTERNAL RING USING SUTURE

An ideal indication for this technique is presented by the small indirect hernias in the young patient (types I and II). A transabdominal approach is performed

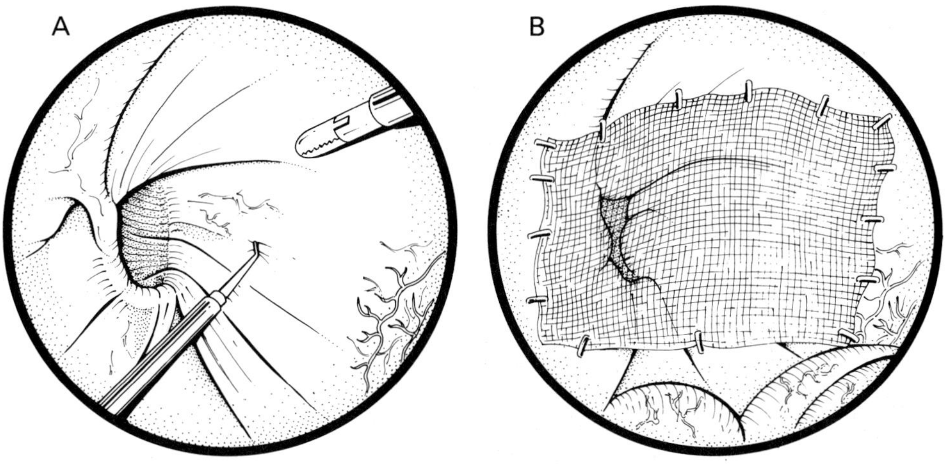

Figure 12.2.5 A: small indirect hernia; B: intraperitoneal onlay mesh.

and once the peritoneal sac has been dissected free the internal ring is approximated using 2–3 interrupted sutures after mobilizing the spermatic cord laterally (Fig. 12.2.6). The use of this ileopubic tract as a solid supporting structure for the sutures is important in this technique and the sutures are most easily tied using an extracorporeal knotting technique (such as Roeder's knot).

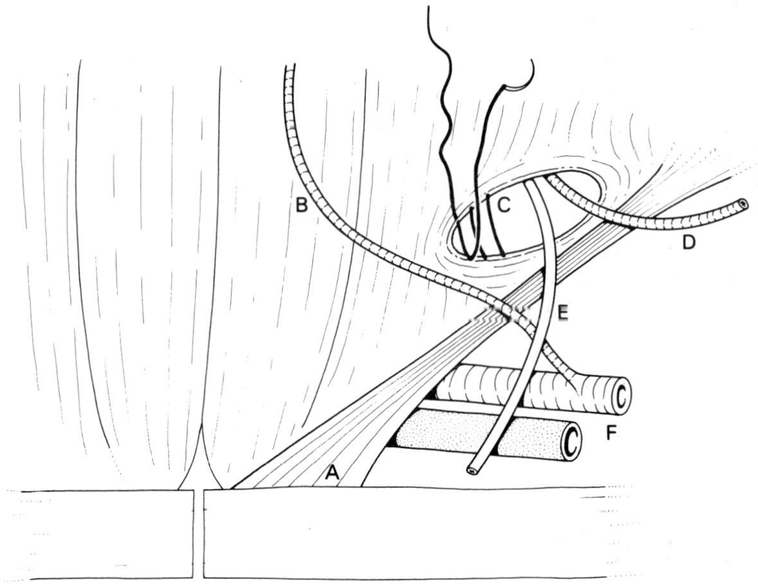

Figure 12.2.6 Closure of the ring for type II hernias (small indirect hernias in the young adult). A: Cooper's ligament; B: epigastric vessels; C: sutures on the internal ring; D: spermatic vessels; E: vas deferens; F: iliac vessels.

INDICATIONS

To date, the best indications for the laparoscopic preperitoneal mesh repair are presented by recurrent inguinal hernias, large hernias in patients with a weak muscular abdominal wall, bilateral hernias, large inguinoscrotal hernias and sliding hernias. There has been no scientific evidence in the literature regarding the morbidity of meshes using this technique. Furthermore, the mesh repair has been extensively investigated during open surgery in several large studies and in our own unit we have performed over 1500 open Stoppa mesh repairs for inguinal hernias. The risk of infection or migration of the mesh into adjacent organs is perhaps more theoretical than real, but care must be taken to completely close the peritoneal flap to avoid this potential complication. For type II hernias (small indirect hernias in the young adult under the age of 18 years), the hernia sac could be reduced and the defect in the internal ring closed with sutures such as might occur during repair of paediatric hernias. Long term problems with mesh and perhaps associated complications regarding sterility are currently under analysis, but no evidence has yet been produced to contraindicate its use.

RESULTS

Between January 1991 and March 1994 we have performed 290 laparoscopic hernia repairs with one recurrence (follow-up 2–25 months). There has been no mortality and 8 complications (two groin pains, one paresthesia of the inguinal canal, three haematomas in the groin, one hypercarbia associated with an elevation of the PCO_2 leading to a conversion from the total extraperitoneal repair to the intraperitoneal preperitoneal repair and one incisional hernia from the 10 mm trocar wound). The total extraperitoneal repair in unpublished multicentre trials has so far shown more pain in the groin area and an increased risk of hypocarbia due to resorption of the CO_2 in the closed preperitoneal space which appears to be higher. The hospital stay in our series has been short (mean 1.3 days) and a quick return to normal activity noted in the majority of patients. Thus, this tension-free repair without any large and painful skin incisions permits an early and pain-free return to normal activities for the patient.

CONCLUSION

Laparoscopic hernia repair is an efficient technique associated with a small morbidity and compares favourably to current open surgical techniques. Patients are relatively pain-free following this procedure and can return to work and normal activities much quicker than following conventional hernia repairs. Although the follow-up of most series is not longer than three years, the initial results show a very low recurrence rate comparable to the mesh repair using Stoppa's technique at open surgery. Stoppa demonstrated that most of the recurrences occurred in the first year and the recurrence rate decreased thereafter, so a technically satisfactory operation will probably prove to be efficient in the long term.

The two real problems of the laparoscopic hernia repair are the cost of the operation, which is higher than for conventional surgery; and the necessity for general anaesthesia. The increased cost should be compared with the gain associated by a quicker and more productive return to work by the majority of patients, and in the future general anaesthesia may not be required for laparoscopic hernia repairs. Laparoscopic surgery without carbon dioxide insufflation using abdominal wall suspension is currently being examined. In the future, this may prove to be the answer to performing laparoscopy under local anaesthesia without a tense pneumoperitoneum.

Among the techniques described here the most reproducible and efficient appears to be the transabdominal preperitoneal mesh repair which has the advantage of being easy to teach to surgeons in training. It also allows a more simple reduction of large hernias and a simultaneous exploration of the intra-abdominal cavity. The total extraperitoneal approach, although more elegant, has a higher incidence of postoperative pain and is more difficult to reproduce and teach. Intraperitoneal onlay mesh is not advocated at the current time. Future trials and prospective randomized studies will be required to establish whether laparoscopic hernia repair can meet the gold standard represented by open hernia surgery.

REFERENCES

1. Bassini E. Sulla cura radicale dell'ernia inguinale. *Arch Soc Ital Chir* 1887; **4**: 380.
2. Halsted WS. The radical cure of inguinal hernia in the male. *Bull Johns Hopkins Hosp* 1893; **4**: 17–24.
3. Marcy HO. A new use of carbolized catgut ligatures. *Boston Med Surg J* 1871; **85**: 315–16.
4. Marcy HO. *The Anatomy and Surgical Treatment of Hernia*. New York, D. Appleton and Co, 1892.
5. Andrews E. A method for herniotomy utilizing only white fascia. *Ann Surg* 1924; **80**: 225–38.
6. McVay CB. Inguinal and femoral hernioplasty. Anatomic repair. *Arch Surg* 1948; **57**: 524–30.
7. Ger R. The management of certain abdominal hernias by intraabdominal closure of the sac. *Ann R Coll Surg Eng* 1982; **64**: 342–4.
8. Corbitt JD Jr. Laparoscopic herniorrhaphy. *Surg Laparosc Endosc* 1991; **1**: 23–5.
9. Schultz L, Graber J, Pietraffitta J, Hickok D. Laser laparoscopic herniorrhaphy: a clinical trial. Preliminary results. *J Laparoendosc Surg* 1991; **1**: 41–5.

10. Popp LW. Improvement in endoscopic hernioplasty: Transcutaneous aquadissection of the musculoskeletal defect and preperitoneal endoscopic patch repair. *J Laparoendosc Surg* 1991; **1**: 83–90.
11. Nyhus LM, Pollack R, Bombeck TC, Donahue PE. The preperitoneal approach and prosthetic buttress repair for recurrent hernia. *Ann Surg* 1988; **208**: 733–7.
12. Stoppa RE, Warlaumont CR. The preperitoneal approach and prosthetic repair of groin hernia. In: *Hernia* (eds Nyhus L, Condon R), pp. 236–52. Philadelphia, JB Lippincott, 1989.
13. Griffith GA. The Marcy repair of indirect inguinal hernia: 1870 to the presnt. In: *Hernia* (eds Nyhus L, Condon R), pp. 106–18. Philadelphia, JB Lippincott, 1989.
14. Lichtenstein IL, Shulman AG, Amid PK, Montlor MM. The tension-free hernioplasty. *Am J Surg* 1989; **157**: 188–93.
15. Shearburn EW, Myres RN. Shouldice repair of inguinal hernia. *Surgery* 1969; **66**: 450–9.
16. Ger R, Monroe K, Duvivier R, Mishrick A. Management of indirect inguinal hernias by laparoscopic closure of the neck of the sac. *Am J Surg* 1990; **159**: 370–3.
17. Ger R. The laparoscopic management of groin hernias. *Contemp Surg* 1991; **39**: 15–19.
18. Katkhouda N, Mouiel J. Traitement laparoscopique des hernies de l'aine de l'adulte. *Chirurgie endoscopique* 1992; **3**: 7–10.
19. Katkhouda N, Mouiel J. Traitement laparoscopique. In: *Actualités Digestives Médico-Chirurgicales*, (ed. Mouiel J), pp. 115–21. Paris, Masson, 1993.
20. Fitzgibbons RJ Jr, Schmid S, Santoscopy R *et al.* Open laparoscopy for laparoscopic cholecystectomy. *Surg Laparosc Endosc* 1991; **2**: 216–22.
21. Philipps EG. Personal communication.
22. McKernan JB. Laparoscopic repair of inguinal hernias using a totally extraperitoneal prosthetic approach. *Surg Endosc* 1983; **7**: 26–8.
23. Arregui ME, Davis CJ, Yucel O, Nagan RF. Laparoscopic mesh repair of inguinal hernia using a preperitoneal approach: a preliminary report. *Surg Laparosc Endosc* 1992; **2**: 53–8.
24. Laparoscopic Surgery: The International Experience. Indianapolis, Ind. 1991; May 20–22.
25. Spaw AT, Ennis BW, Spaw L. Laparoscopic hernia repair: the anatomic basis. *J Laparoendosc Surg* 1991; **5**: 269–77.
26. Franklin ME Jr. Personal communication.
27. Toy FK, Smoot RT. Toy–Smoot laparoscopic hernioplasty. *Surg Laparosc Endosc* 1991; **3**: 151–5.
28. Salerno GM, Fitzgibbons RJ Jr, Filipi CJ. Laparoscopic inguinal hernia repair. In: *Surgical Laparoscopy* (ed. Zucker KA), pp. 281–93. St Louis, QMP, 1991.

Overview

Hernia surgery

The repair of inguinal hernias using the laparoscopic approach initially attracted a wide and enthusiastic surgical audience. However, the high early recurrence rate swiftly dampened down this enthusiasm, until better techniques were developed. There is now general agreement that the best repair is the insertion of a mesh in the pre-peritoneal space, whether approached from within the peritoneal cavity or totally pre-peritoneal. The latter has many attractions but is a much more demanding procedure, and although the former is technically straightforward and has early recurrence rates similar to open repairs, there remain areas for concern. First, a general anaesthetic is required; second, there is an inherent morbidity – and mortality – from laparoscopy (even if the open technique is employed); and, third, additional complications associated with bowel herniation through the peritoneal defect (however well closed) and adhesions of the bowel to the mesh have occurred. Thus a relatively simple and efficient open operation, which can be performed under local anaesthesia, with a low morbidity and almost zero mortality, as a day case procedure, has escalated to an expensive laparoscopic procedure with unknown long-term efficiency and a definite morbidity. This is not to say that long-term data from laparoscopic repair will not produce results every bit as good as those described from the Shouldice clinic by Bendavid (Chapter 12.1), but we must remain wary regarding its application at present. It would seem logical to conclude that bilateral and recurrent hernias might be the best indication at present, but patient demand will undoubtedly broaden these indications.

13.1

Expectations in Emergency Abdominal Surgery

T. T. IRVIN

INTRODUCTION

A recent study of 1190 emergency admissions in Exeter[1] identified 18 different diagnostic categories or causes of an acute abdomen (Fig. 13.1.1). However, two thirds of the patients fell within three categories: non-specific abdominal pain (NSAP); acute appendicitis; and intestinal obstruction. NSAP and acute appendicitis were the most common diagnoses in young patients and intestinal obstruction was most common in the elderly (Fig. 13.1.2).

There were 51 deaths in this study resulting in a hospital mortality of 4.4% and a perioperative mortality rate of 8%. The common causes of perioperative death were laparotomy for inoperable disease (mainly inoperable malignancies and massive mesenteric infarction), ruptured abdominal aortic aneurysm, perforated peptic ulcer and colonic resections (Fig. 13.1.3).

Thirty nine patients had an essentially negative laparotomy, the indication for surgery being suspected appendicitis in 31 cases. The overall incidence of removal of a normal appendix was 15.5% and there was a 22.4% incidence of unnecessary appendicectomy in patients aged 20–29 years.

DIAGNOSIS AND MANAGEMENT OF THE ACUTE ABDOMEN

Diagnostic Aids

Modern aids in the diagnosis of the acute abdomen include structured patient interviews, computer programmes based on Bayesian probability, plain and contrast radiography, abdominal ultrasonography, CT scanning, fine catheter aspiration cytology of the peritoneum and laparoscopy.[2–13] However, the initial clinical decision in the individual patient is based on bedside assessment and the

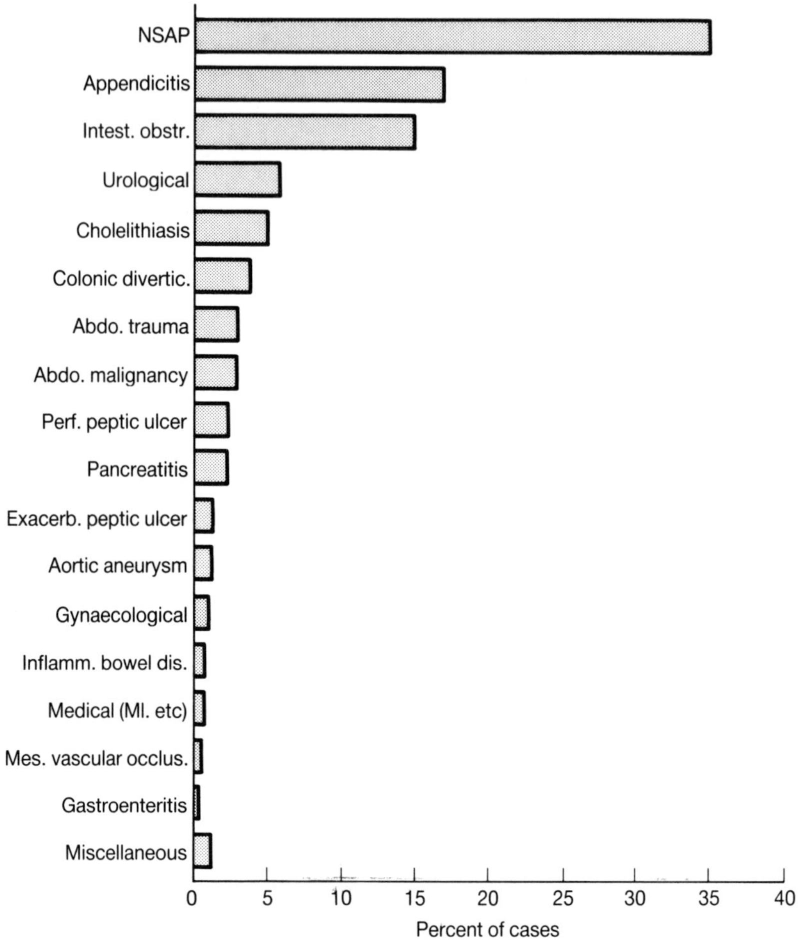

Figure 13.1.1 Causes of the acute abdomen in a series of 1190 emergency surgical admissions.

clinical findings.[14] Clinicians making such decisions require skills which are commensurate with the task. These skills may be enhanced by the use of the structured patient interview and a computer prediction of the probable diagnosis. In practice, few clinicians use computers in the diagnosis of abdominal pain, despite the demonstrable advantages.[15]

Initial Assessment

This bedside assessment should result in a working diagnosis and a policy decision concerning the immediate management of the patient (Fig. 13.1.4). This will mean that the patient falls within one of three management groups:

1. *An urgent or emergency operation is required*: examples include patients with ruptured abdominal aortic aneurysm, those with strangulated external hernias and those with unequivocal evidence of a diffuse or spreading peritonitis. Investigations in these patients mainly relate to an assessment of the general fitness of the patient.
2. *Does not need an operation*: examples include patients with non-specific abdominal pain and those with clinical features of uncomplicated biliary or ureteric

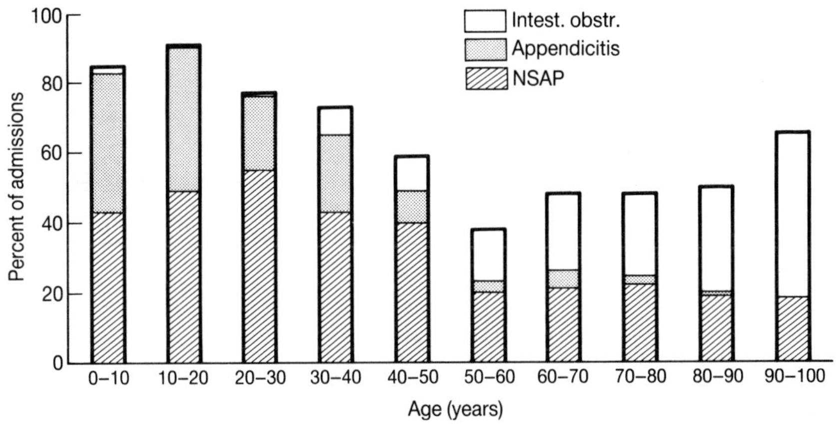

Figure 13.1.2 Age incidence of non-specific abdominal pain (NSAP), acute appendicitis and intestinal obstruction.

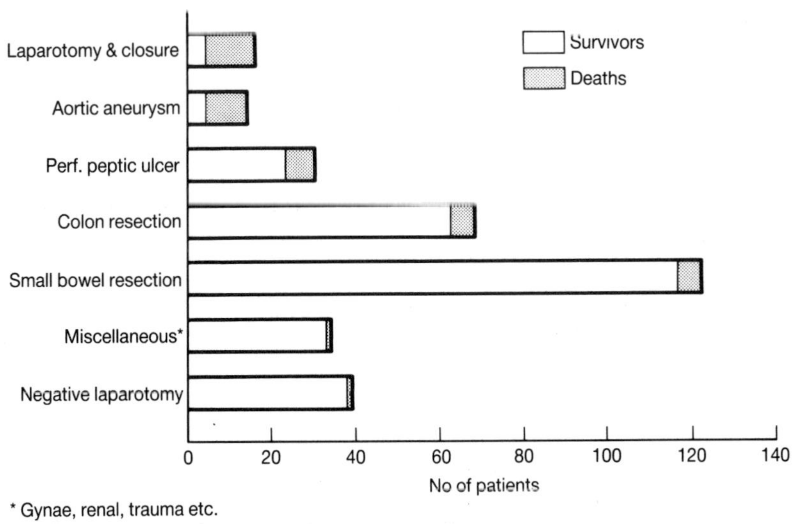

Figure 13.1.3 Acute abdomen: causes of hospital mortality.

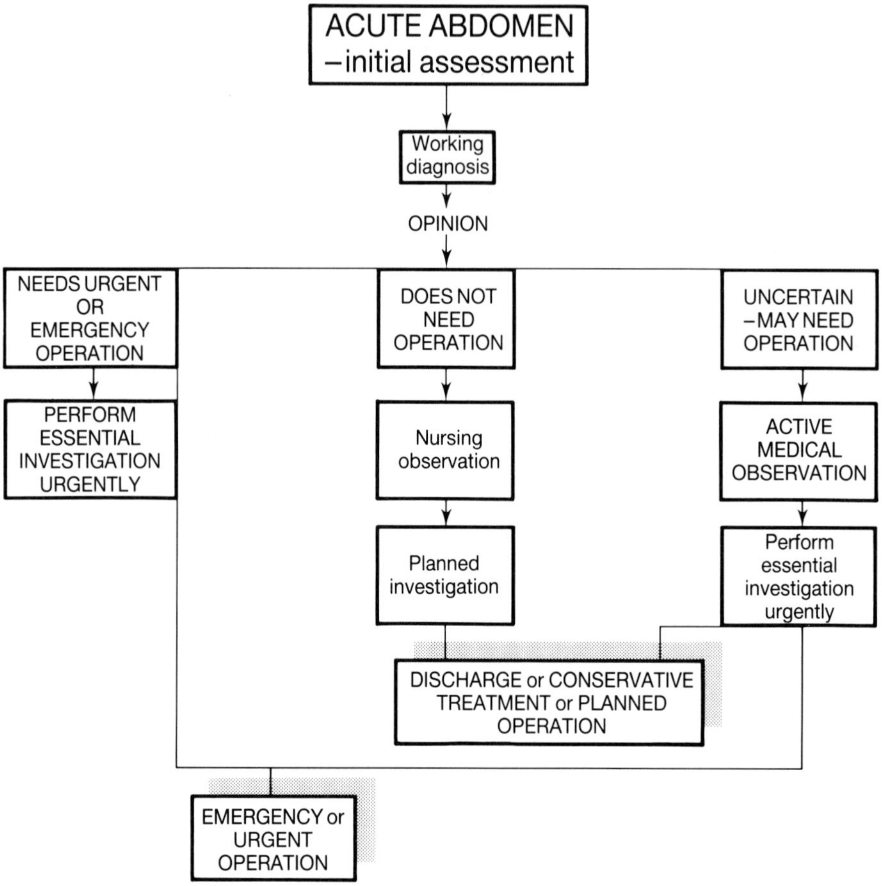

Figure 13.1.4 Algorithm for the initial assessment of the acute abdomen.

colic. Investigations are planned according to the working diagnosis and often require specialist techniques of diagnostic imaging. These investigations are unhurried and are usually performed during the normal office hours of the radiology department.

3. *Uncertain – may need an operation*: examples include patients with equivocal signs of appendicitis; those with localized peritonitis attributable to acute cholecystitis or colonic diverticulitis; and those with signs of incomplete intestinal obstruction. Such cases need active medical observation[14] and, where appropriate, urgent investigations are performed to assist the diagnosis or decision making process. Moreover, the attending surgeon needs to reassess the patient at intervals to determine if the policy decision needs to be altered. Patients in this category are undoubtedly most at risk of surgeon related errors of judgement and avoidable delays in surgical treatment.

A review of all causes of the acute abdomen is beyond our remit. In this chapter only the common causes of abdominal pain are included, those which may present problems in diagnosis and management and those which may be amenable to laparoscopic diagnosis or treatment.

SPECIFIC CAUSES OF THE ACUTE ABDOMEN

Acute Appendicitis

Acute appendicitis is the most common specific cause of emergency presentation. The incidence is age related. Approximately 40% of emergency admissions under 20 years of age have acute appendicitis whereas less than 1% of patients over 80 years of age are suffering from this condition (Fig. 13.1.2).

Diagnosis

The clinical features are influenced by the speed of presentation, the position of the appendix, the presence or absence of appendiceal perforation or gangrene and the age of the patient.

The variable nature of the presenting clinical signs creates a potential for unnecessary delays in diagnosis and treatment. Traditionally, this has resulted in a policy of early surgical exploration based on clinical suspicion and in the knowledge that 8–33% of such operations may prove unnecessary.[16] When the decision to operate is based purely on clinical assessment, the "acceptable" rate for the removal of normal appendices may be around 10%. Below this level, there may be harmful delays in the diagnosis of perforated appendicitis.[17]

Can we do better than this? Are there other tests or investigations which assist the diagnosis in doubtful cases? Setting aside the question of laparoscopy, the most common method is abdominal ultrasonography. In a study of 525 patients with suspected appendicitis Ooms *et al.*[18] found that ultrasonography was accompanied by a 7% incidence of unnecessary appendicectomy. A positive diagnosis of appendicitis was made in 86% of scans although there was a lower success rate in cases of perforated appendicitis. Davies *et al.*[12] reported 95% accuracy in the diagnosis of appendicitis by ultrasonography and they suggested that suspected appendicitis may be one of the few indications for emergency scanning of the acute abdomen. The method has the added value that it may demonstrate causes of the acute abdomen which do not require immediate surgical intervention, particularly in young females in whom the presenting features of pelvic inflammatory disease or other gynaecological pathology may be confused with atypical appendicitis.

An alternative or additional technique for the assessment of doubtful cases is fine catheter aspiration cytology of the peritoneum. Counts of neutrophil leucocytes in the peritoneal aspirate are a guide to the presence or absence of peritoneal inflammation and, in a study of 61 patients with acute abdominal pain, Vipond *et al.*[11] found that the method had a sensitivity of 86% and a specificity of 88%. However, the method is subject to a small incidence of technical failure, particularly in obese subjects, and it is unsuitable in children. Moreover, it does not establish the cause of an acute abdomen. Whilst a positive test might provide additional persuasion to the surgeon to operate in a doubtful case, it seems unlikely that the method will assume great significance in the diagnosis of appendicitis.

Treatment

Appendicectomy is usually performed by junior doctors in training. The operation is carried out through a 4–5 cm grid-iron or transverse incision in the right iliac fossa. Generally, the incision is sited over the point of maximum tenderness but it is possible to place the skin incision in the pubic hairline and, with suitable retraction of the skin and subcutaneous tissue, to enter the abdomen through the standard McBurney approach.[19] However, there are occasions when surgical access is inadequate through small, transverse or low incisions and the wound must be extended before the appendix can be safely delivered and removed. This problem chiefly arises in the removal of high retrocaecal appendices or in obese subjects.

In adults presenting with diffuse lower abdominal peritonitis, when the diagnosis of appendicitis may be in doubt, many surgeons perform a laparotomy through a midline or paramedian lower abdominal incision. Protagonists of this approach claim that it enables better peritoneal toilet than the limited access achieved through an incision in the right iliac fossa.

The standard operation of appendicectomy involves the freeing of the appendix from any inflammatory or congenital adhesions, division of the mesoappendix, ligation of the base of the appendix and inversion of the appendicular stump beneath an absorbable pursestring suture in the caecum. In the difficult case, when the tip of the appendix is relatively inaccessible or adherent, it may be necessary to remove the appendix in retrograde fashion, commencing the dissection at the base of the appendix. In other cases, it may not be possible to invaginate the appendicular stump if the caecum is inflamed and friable. Although this may be a matter of some concern to inexperienced surgeons there is no evidence that inversion of the stump is necessary or that failure to perform this procedure results in long term complications.[20–23]

A minority of patients present late with a localized appendicular mass or an appendicular abscess. The distinction between a mass and an abscess is based on the severity of local tenderness, the extent of the systemic disturbance and the findings on abdominal ultrasonography. Demonstration of an abscess is generally regarded as an indication for surgical drainage and experienced surgeons also remove the appendix. An appendix mass is treated conservatively in the first instance. In most cases the inflammation will resolve and the patient will later undergo an interval appendicectomy. Localization of peritoneal sepsis is generally poor in children and in the very old and it is rarely wise to embark upon conservative treatment of the appendicular mass in these patients.

All abdominal explorations for appendicitis are carried out under broad spectrum antibiotic cover. A single dose of antibiotic may be sufficient when the appendix is not perforated or gangrenous.[24] In patients with severe sepsis, however, it is advisable to perform a peroperative lavage of the wound and peritoneum with tetracycline[25] and systemic antibiotic therapy may be required for 3–5 days.

Outcome

The mortality of appendicitis has fallen from a level of 4% in the early part of the century to a present level of around 0.2%.[26] The median duration of hospital stay after appendicectomy is four days. Patients undergoing laparotomy through a paramedian or midline incision remain in hospital for 7–10 days and the duration of stay is also prolonged in the 4–7% of cases who develop postoperative complications. The most common complication is wound infection. The risks of wound infection are largely related to the severity of the appendicular sepsis. Gangrene or perforation of the appendix occur in 15–50% of cases and are associated with wound infection rates of 33–63%.[27] Systemic antibiotic therapy is only partially successful in preventing postoperative wound sepsis in these cases.

Other early complications include residual intraperitoneal abscesses, prolonged ileus and intestinal obstruction. The late complications of appendicectomy include bowel obstruction due to adhesions, incisional hernia and an increased incidence of a right inguinal hernia. It is frequently stated that the peritoneal sepsis associated with appendicitis may be a potent cause of female infertility but there is little evidence to support this contention.[28]

Intestinal Obstruction

The common causes of intestinal obstruction are shown in Fig. 13.1.5.

External Hernia

This condition remains the most common cause of intestinal obstruction. In a majority of cases an oblique inguinal hernia is responsible and the small intestine is the site of obstruction or strangulation. Femoral hernias are a common cause of intestinal obstruction in female patients and obstruction of the small intestine occasionally occurs in other types of external hernia.

The tender irreducible external hernia requires an urgent operation and this is carried out as soon as the patient can be made fit for a general anaesthetic.

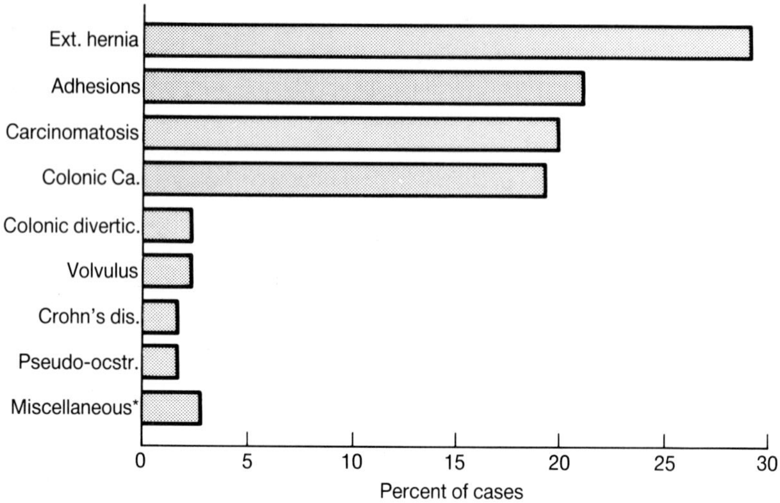

* Cause uncertain (no op.) 3: gallstone ileus 1; cystic fibrosis 1.

Figure 13.1.5 Causes of acute intestinal obstruction.

Occasionally, a strangulated groin hernia is repaired under local anaesthesia when the patient is medically unfit.

In the common type of strangulated inguinal hernia, the surgical approach through the inguinal canal permits a resection of the small intestine, should this prove to be non-viable, and formal repair of the hernia. The Shouldice technique of repair is associated with the lowest risk of recurrence.[29] Obstructed femoral hernias may be explored through the groin (the "low approach") or through the inguinal canal but the best exposure for a bowel resection is obtained in the preperitoneal (McEvedy) approach above the inguinal canal. Approximately one third of the patients with obstructed femoral hernia require a bowel resection.[30] Large obstructed paraumbilical or incisional hernias may contain multiple matted loops of intestine. Gangrene of the intestine is less common in such hernias but a tedious surgical dissection is frequently necessary before the hernia can be repaired.

Operations for obstructed or strangulated external hernias are associated with a perioperative mortality of 2–3%, mainly due to the effects of coexisting medical disorders. Many of these patients are elderly and frail. The median duration of hospital stay is seven days but patients requiring a bowel resection generally stay longer and there is an increased incidence of postoperative wound sepsis compared with elective operations for external hernias.

Adhesions

Peritoneal adhesions are the second most common cause of acute obstruction of the small intestine. In virtually every case the adhesions are a consequence of a previous surgical operation, often following resections of the large intestine. Obstructions due to congenital adhesions are very uncommon.

Three questions arise for the surgeon involved in the initial assessment of such cases:

1. Are there clinical signs of intestinal strangulation?
2. Is it likely that the obstruction is due to adhesions?
3. Is the obstruction complete or incomplete (subacute)?

Clinical suspicion of intestinal strangulation based on persistent pain and abdominal tenderness is an absolute indication for an urgent laparotomy. The diagnosis of adhesional obstruction is supported by evidence of previous abdominal surgery and, in some cases, a history of previous attacks of obstruction. Approximately 30% of the patients with adhesional obstruction may be managed conservatively but it is important to identify the likely candidates for non-operative treatment at an early stage. Plain radiographs of the abdomen are of little value but contrast studies of the small intestine, whilst not foolproof, are helpful in the decision making process in uncertain cases.[2,7,31]

The surgical treatment of adhesive obstruction is often tedious and technically demanding, particularly in recurrent cases. There is a perioperative mortality of 1–2%, chiefly due to coexisting medical disorders, thromboembolic complications and persistent or early recurrence of the obstruction. Prolonged ileus is the principal cause of morbidity after such surgery and the median duration of stay in hospital is eight days.

Carcinomatosis

In a majority of cases there is a history of abdominal malignancy. The site of obstruction is almost invariably in the small intestine but there may be multiple sites of obstruction in advanced cases and the situation may be further complicated by the effects of previous radiotherapy on the small intestine.

The decision making process may be extremely difficult in such cases and needs to take account of the certainty of the diagnosis of abdominal malignancy, the prospects of relieving the obstruction and the potential quality of life thereafter. About 25% of cases will settle with non-operative treatment but nearly half of these patients will return with a recurrence of the obstruction. Most patients undergo a laparotomy either at the first or at a subsequent admission unless they have clear evidence of widespread malignancy. Not infrequently, it transpires that the obstruction is due to adhesions or the effects of radiotherapy and not a recurrent malignancy.[32]

It is rarely possible to resect the abdominal malignancy and the operation usually involves a bypass of the obstruction by enteroenterostomy. In some cases, several bypasses may be required when there are multiple sites of obstruction. The perioperative mortality in these patients is 15–20% and the causes of death include cardiac and pulmonary complications, unrelieved obstruction and faecal fistulae. The median duration of stay of surviving patients is 12 days.

Colorectal Cancer

Cancer of the large intestine ranks fourth in the list of causes of intestinal obstruction. The disease presents with large bowel obstruction in 16% of cases and more than half of the primary tumours are located in the left colon. However, growths of the proximal intestine are associated with a higher incidence of obstruction.[33]

The diagnosis is frequently based on clinical suspicion and the findings in plain radiographs of the abdomen. There is confidence in the clinical diagnosis when the radiograph shows gross distension of the large bowel proximal to the site of obstruction and an absence of gas distal to this point.

In some cases the radiological features are less explicit, particularly if there is gas in the rectum or when there are accompanying features of small bowel obstruction with dilatation and air fluid levels. An emergency contrast enema should be performed in doubtful cases.[6] Otherwise, there is a risk that a colonic pseudo-obstruction will be missed.[34]

The standard treatment for an obstructing tumour of the right colon is a one stage right hemicolectomy with primary ileocolic anastomosis. However, the optimal treatment for tumours of the left colon remains controversial. Most surgeons perform a primary resection of the obstructing tumour but there are differing views on the wisdom of a primary anastomosis in such cases. Primary anastomoses in obstructed cases have been associated with a high incidence of failure[35] and most surgeons use a Hartmann's procedure or, when possible, exteriorize the ends of bowel. However, primary anastomoses may be safely performed if the faecal contents are expelled by intraoperative colonic lavage.[36,37] Alternatively, the anastomosis may be protected by the so-called intracolonic bypass procedure. An intraluminal tube is attached to the bowel wall with absorbable sutures proximal to the suture line and it effectively prevents contact between the anastomosis and the bowel contents until it is expelled after two weeks.[38]

The mortality after emergency surgery for obstructing cancer of the large intestine remains high (17–38%).[39–41] Many of the patients are elderly or unfit and much of the mortality results from complications of coexisting medical diseases. The median duration of hospital stay in surviving patients is 12 days. Unfortunately, the long term prognosis is also poor, only 11–29% surviving five years.[35]

Other Causes of Obstruction

Other causes of intestinal obstruction include colonic diverticular disease, volvulus of the sigmoid colon or caecum, Crohn's disease and gallstone ileus.

Colonic diverticular disease may be clinically indistinguishable from a carcinoma when it presents with large bowel obstruction. The usual finding at operation is an obstructing mass in the sigmoid colon and this is usually treated by primary resection in similar fashion to an obstructing carcinoma.

In the UK and the USA, volvulus of the sigmoid colon occurs predominantly in the elderly and in neuropsychiatric patients. Gross distension of the abdomen and characteristic radiographic appearances should alert the clinician to the diagnosis but the diagnosis may be missed or delayed in up to 40% of cases.[42] An urgent laparotomy is required when abdominal tenderness or signs of peritonism suggest infarction of the twisted loop but 33–90% of cases are treatable by simple sigmoidoscopic decompression of the obstructed loop.[43–45] Unfortunately, recurrence is common and it is generally recommended that elective surgical treatment should follow non-operative decompression of the volvulus. Resection of the sigmoid colon is required if infarction has occurred but opinions differ on the correct course of action when the loop is found to be viable or when the patient undergoes elective surgery. The choice rests between sigmoid resection and an attempt to fix the colon to prevent recurrence of the volvulus. The latter may be achieved by transverse plication of the leaves of the sigmoid mesentery (mesosigmoidoplasty)[45,46] or by banded coloplasty.[47] These techniques have been associated with a low perioperative mortality. Overall, the mortality of sigmoid volvulus is 14–15%.

Volvulus of the caecum is less common than sigmoid volvulus and the diagnosis is more difficult. The presenting clinical features are those of a distal closed loop small bowel obstruction and plain radiographs of the abdomen are diagnostic in less than 20% of cases. An emergency barium enema will provide the diagnosis in 88% of cases.[48] Contrast enemas or colonoscopy are rarely successful in relieving the obstruction and virtually all patients require an urgent laparotomy. Again, the surgical management is controversial. Twenty percent of cases require a resection for gangrene of the caecum. For the remainder, the choice rests between simple untwisting, caecopexy, tube caecostomy or resection. In a study of 568 cases of caecal volvulus, Rabinovici *et al.*[48] found that the highest morbidity and mortality rates followed resection and tube caecostomy and they recommended untwisting and caecopexy for cases not complicated by intestinal gangrene. This method was associated with a perioperative mortality of 10% and recurrence of the volvulus in 13%.

Obstructions due to Crohn's disease usually affect the small intestine or enterocolic anastomoses resulting from previous treatment of the disease. Most obstructions will resolve with conservative management but recurrence is common. Patients with persistent or recurrent obstruction require laparotomy but the surgery of Crohn's disease has become much more conservative in recent years and many patients can be treated by strictureplasty rather than by resection of the diseased bowel.[49]

Gallstone obstruction of the intestine is uncommon. In most cases the gallstone impacts in the ileum but the diagnosis may be elusive and less than half of the cases have the classical radiological sign of air in the biliary tree.[50]

Ultrasonography is helpful in confirming the presence of cholelithiasis.[51] Treatment involves surgical removal of the gallstone by enterotomy but most surgeons leave the biliary–enteric fistula undisturbed. The patients tend to be elderly and unfit and there is a perioperative mortality of around 18%. Late complications include recurrent gallstone ileus, cholecystitis and cholangitis.

Colonic Pseudo-obstruction

This uncommon condition presents with clinical and radiological features of an acute large bowel obstruction. Confusion in diagnosis and inappropriate management are associated with a substantial morbidity and mortality.[52] The pathogenesis of the condition is obscure but there are known associations with cardiovascular diseases, abdominal and skeletal trauma, various types of surgery, malignancies, inflammatory conditions, assisted ventilation, metabolic disturbances, drug therapy and various neurological disorders.[34]

There is usually impressive abdominal distension. Bowel sounds are variable and the rectum is usually empty. Blood analyses may reveal an electrolyte disturbance or uraemia. Plain radiographs of the abdomen characteristically reveal a gas filled colon and a cut off at fixed points but a positive diagnosis is made by a contrast enema using a dilute solution of barium or a water soluble contrast medium.[6]

Pseudo-obstruction should be managed conservatively unless there is suspicion of colonic ischaemia or perforation. Associated factors (e.g. drug therapy or electrolyte disturbances) should be treated if possible. Some cases may respond to combined pharmacological sympathetic blockade and parasympathetic stimulation[53] or treatment with cisapride.[54] Colonoscopic decompression of the colon should be attempted if there is no improvement. Laparotomy is required when conservative treatment or attempted decompression fail and when there is suspicion of intestinal ischaemia or perforation. Surgical decompression of the colon is required and a tube caecostomy is preferable to a transverse colostomy. Patients often fare badly after laparotomy and there is a 15–40% mortality after surgical decompression of the colon.[55]

Acute Complications of Cholelithiasis

The complications of cholelithiasis include severe attacks of biliary colic, acute cholecystitis, pancreatitis, ascending cholangitis, empyema and gangrene or perforation of the gall bladder.

Diagnosis

The presenting signs and symptoms usually enable a confident clinical diagnosis and a strategy for investigation and management. The exceptions are the few patients presenting with a spreading or diffuse peritonitis resulting from perforation or gangrene of the gall bladder. The final diagnosis in these patients is usually made at laparotomy.

Diagnostic errors occur chiefly in patients with atypical biliary pain and in those with other causes of right upper quadrant pain or tenderness. Biliary colic presenting as discomfort in the chest may be confused with myocardial infarction and right upper quadrant pain may be caused by acute duodenal ulceration, pleurisy, pulmonary embolism, herpes zoster or a high retrocaecal appendicitis.

Abdominal ultrasonography is the most useful investigation. Indeed, acute biliary problems account for the majority of urgent scans of the acute abdomen and the diagnostic yield is almost equivalent to that of radionuclide scanning of the biliary system.[56–58] Urgent endoscopic retrograde cholangiography (ERCP) is required when the patient is jaundiced, when there is clinical evidence of cholangitis and in some cases of gallstone pancreatitis.

Treatment

Acute biliary colic is managed by symptom control, cessation of oral intake, intravenous fluids and the development of a treatment plan for the gallstones. Urgent surgical intervention is unnecessary but a surgical strategy is required to prevent further attacks. In elderly or unfit patients the decision may be to withhold surgical treatment because of the associated operative risk.

Cases of acute cholecystitis require a restriction of oral intake, broad spectrum antibiotics and intravenous fluids but the surgical management of this complication remains controversial. The traditional policy is to treat the patient conservatively with an expectation that the inflammation will resolve and the patient is recalled for an interval cholecystectomy. An alternative policy of early cholecystectomy during the acute attack has been advocated in recent years.[59–61] Protagonists of early surgery point to errors in diagnosis associated with conservative treatment, the risk of complications such as abscess formation, perforation or gangrene of the gall bladder and a 25% incidence of recurrent attacks of cholecystitis during the waiting period for elective surgery. Nevertheless, the case for a routine policy of early cholecystectomy is unconvincing. Errors in the diagnosis of acute cholecystitis are unusual with real-time ultrasonography and complications of acute cholecystitis are fortunately uncommon. Moreover, many of the patients are elderly and early cholecystectomy may be accompanied by a 10% perioperative mortality, most deaths being related to the complications of coexisting medical disorders.[62] The duration of stay after early and late cholecystectomy is very similar (13 days). It seems sensible to reserve early cholecystectomy for those who fail to settle with conservative management and those who have clinical or ultrasonographic signs of complications such as empyema, perforation or abscess formation.

Percutaneous cholecystostomy should be considered in patients who are manifestly unfit for major abdominal surgery. In the critically ill, this method can be used for the treatment of acute cholecystitis, empyema and perforation with localized abscess formation.[63,64] Open surgical cholecystostomy is associated with a 5% mortality in such cases. The subsequent management of the gall bladder depends on the fitness of the patient and the presence or absence of symptoms. The treatment options include non-operative management, percutaneous cholecystolithotomy and laparoscopic or open cholecystectomy.[65]

Ascending cholangitis is almost invariably caused by bile duct stones. The patients are often gravely ill with circulatory collapse, jaundice, high fever and positive blood cultures. The immediate treatment involves the use of appropriate intravenous fluids and broad spectrum antibiotics and careful monitoring. Fortunately, most patients respond to these initial measures but urgent investigation by ultrasonography and endoscopic retrograde cholangiography is required. Many of these patients are elderly or relatively unfit for major surgery and surgical exploration of the bile duct is associated with a 21–29% perioperative mortality.[66,67] The treatment of choice is endoscopic sphincterotomy and non-operative extraction of the bile duct stones. Clearance of the stones is achieved in more than 80% of cases with this technique and the mortality of 1–11% is related to specific complications of the procedure such as haemorrhage, duodenal perforation and acute cholecystitis, the complications of coexisting medical disorders and persistence of the cholangitis.[68–70] The management of the gall bladder after successful endoscopic therapy remains controversial. Hansell *et al.*[70] found that 18% of patients had symptoms which were sufficiently troublesome to warrant cholecystectomy.

Pancreatitis

Acute pancreatitis is an increasingly common abdominal emergency. In the UK, cholelithiasis accounts for 30% of cases in males and 53% of cases in females.[71] Alcohol abuse is the next most common cause of pancreatitis and other identifiable causes include carcinoma of the pancreas, drugs, hypothermia, sepsis and ERCP. The mortality is age related: Fan *et al.*[72] reported a mortality of 6% in patients aged less than 50 years and 21% in patients aged more than 75 years.

Diagnosis

The presenting signs and symptoms of pancreatitis are varied and a bedside diagnosis may be difficult even with the help of a computer. However, a serum amylase level greater than 1000 international units is diagnostic of pancreatitis and this investigation should be routine in the assessment of the acute abdomen. Modest elevations of serum amylase are not uncommon in various acute abdominal conditions, such as biliary peritonitis, perforated peptic ulcer, gangrenous intestine, high small bowel obstruction and leaking aortic aneurysm but these conditions are usually excluded by abdominal radiographs, ultrasonography, CT scan and abdominal paracentesis. However, it is safer to proceed to laparotomy when doubt persists. Most of the conditions mimicking pancreatitis are potentially lethal without prompt surgical intervention whereas there is little evidence that pancreatitis is aggravated by exploratory laparotomy.[73,74]

It is important to identify those patients who have gallstones and those who have severe pancreatitis. Attacks of gallstone pancreatitis may be aborted by urgent endoscopic sphincterotomy[75] and patients with severe pancreatitis require aggressive management. Early ultrasonography will detect two thirds of the cases with gallstones and it appears to be more reliable than radionuclide biliary scanning.[76] Only 34–39% of severe attacks of pancreatitis are detected by clinical assessment but scoring systems based on multiple laboratory criteria will detect up to 60% of severe cases.[77–79]

Treatment

The mild attack of pancreatitis is treated by rest of the alimentary tract, intravenous fluids and appropriate analgesia. Patients with gallstones should undergo cholecystectomy as soon as the attack has settled, preferably at the same admission.[80–82] Patients with unexplained or idiopathic attacks of pancreatitis should undergo ERCP. This investigation may reveal unsuspected gallstones or various types of pancreatic pathology.[74]

Patients with severe pancreatitis require careful monitoring and physiological support and are best managed in a high dependency or intensive care unit. The mortality is largely related to the complications of pancreatic necrosis. There is some evidence that severe attacks associated with gallstones may be aborted by endoscopic sphincterotomy[75] but peritoneal lavage has no apparent value.[83] Surgical treatment is required for the complications of pancreatic necrosis. Contrast enhanced CT scans will demonstrate necrotic pancreas but the decision to operate must take into account the general condition of the patient as well as the findings in a scan. There is a poor correlation between scan findings and disease severity.[9] A CT scan is the investigation of choice for pancreatic pseudocysts and abscesses.[74]

Pseudocysts are most common in alcoholic pancreatitis and the treatment of choice remains internal surgical drainage. In most cases the cyst can be treated by the operation of cystgastrostomy. In recent years, pseudocysts have been treated by percutaneous drainage under ultrasound or CT control but recurrence is common.[84] Limited experience with endoscopic transgastric drainage of cysts suggests that this method may be successful in 50% of cases.[85–87]

Pancreatic abscesses are associated with mortality rates of 14–100% and require radical surgical treatment. The operation involves debridement of the pancreatic slough and necrotic fat. Some surgeons then irrigate the pancreatic bed, using a closed drainage system. Others use the technique of laparostomy, leaving the abdomen open and preventing evisceration with moist packs.[88,89] Percutaneous techniques of abscess drainage have been successful in 50% of cases[90] and may avoid the need for repeated laparotomy in selected cases.

Perforated Peptic Ulcer

There has been a reduction in the incidence of perforated peptic ulcer in recent years. This has been accompanied by other significant epidemiological changes: a majority of the patients are elderly; 70% have acute ulcers and surgical treatment has been associated with mortality rates of 18–48%.[91–94] The ratio of pyloroduodenal to gastric ulcers is 4 : 1.

Diagnosis

The classic presentation is a patient with signs of a diffuse peritonitis and evidence of a pneumoperitoneum on erect radiographs of the abdomen or chest. Two thirds of patients have no significant dyspeptic history and more than 50% of elderly patients have a history of treatment with non-steroidal anti-inflammatory drugs or corticosteroids. In a minority of patients, signs of peritoneal irritation are localized to the right upper quadrant or right side of the abdomen and may be confused with other abdominal emergencies such as appendicitis or acute cholecystitis. An urgent water soluble contrast study should be performed when the diagnosis and need for surgical intervention are in doubt.

Treatment

The virtual disappearance of chronic peptic ulcers as a cause of gastroduodenal perforation has resulted in a radical reappraisal of the treatment of perforation. A definitive procedure such as a vagotomy or a partial gastrectomy is rarely appropriate and the choice now rests between non-operative management and simple suture of the perforation.[95–97]

Non-operative management has traditionally been reserved for patients who are manifestly unfit for a surgical operation and, unsurprisingly, the method has been accompanied by high mortality rates. Critics of the method have also pointed to the fact that it may result in errors in diagnosis and delays in appropriate surgical treatment. However, recent studies have suggested that 70% of perforations can be successfully managed by an aggressive regimen of nasogastric suction, intravenous antibiotics and H_2 antagonists.[97] Careful and repeated assessments of such cases are required to identify non-responders and water soluble contrast studies will identify those in whom the perforation fails to seal spontaneously.

Nevertheless, the majority of surgeons advise operative intervention for perforated peptic ulcer. When possible, the perforation is closed with a series of absorbable sutures and an omental patch is used to reinforce the suture line. Gastric ulcers are biopsied to exclude malignancy. Occasionally, the perforation is too large or the tissue too friable to permit suture closure and the defect is closed with an omental "plug". In rare instances, a giant perforation may require treatment by formal gastric resection. Patients treated by simple suture of the ulcer must be given H_2 antagonists or a proton pump inhibitor such as omeprazole for a minimum period of six months after surgery.[95]

The complications of treatment of perforated peptic ulcers include the complications of coexisting medical disorders in the elderly, pulmonary embolism, intraperitoneal abscesses, wound infection and reperforation. The mortality rates reported with the different types of treatment are 2–78% with non-operative treatment, 11–41% after simple suture, 3–13% after vagotomy and drainage and 18–40% after partial gastrectomy.[91,94,96,98] The considerable variation in the mortality rates is undoubtedly linked to case selection, the age of the patients, the presence of coexisting medical disorders, the speed of presentation and the presence or absence of shock on admission. The median duration of stay in surviving patients is 13 days after surgery and eight days after non-operative treatment.

Acute Colonic Diverticulitis

Diverticular disease occurs in 5% of the population but becomes more common with advancing age. The sigmoid colon is affected in 90% of cases. The classical clinical features of acute diverticulitis include pain in the left lower quadrant, nausea, low grade fever, leucocytosis and variable abdominal distension. A mass may be palpable in the left iliac fossa. In other cases, the clinical picture is that of a diffuse lower abdominal peritonitis and a few patients present in a moribund state with a diffuse faecal peritonitis. However, urgent operations are required in less than one third of emergency admissions.[99]

Diagnosis

The incidence of acute diverticulitis may be exaggerated. Patients with signs confined to the left iliac fossa may be suffering from colonic spasm rather than diverticulitis. A contrast enema may assist the diagnosis[100] and a CT scan may show increased density of the pericolic fat and thickening of the colonic wall.[8] However, in the vast majority of cases the diagnosis is made on clinical grounds and definitive investigations are performed after the attack has resolved.

Patients presenting with diffuse peritonitis require urgent surgery and the finding of a large pneumoperitoneum in plain radiographs of the abdomen suggests the presence of colonic perforation. There is a risk of operating unnecessarily on patients presenting with equivocal signs of lower abdominal sepsis. Active observation (Fig. 13.1.4) is required in such cases. An initial impression of widespread tenderness may be modified when the patient is reassessed with adequate analgesia, fluid replacement and antibiotic therapy over a period of two or three hours.[101]

Treatment

All patients are given intravenous fluids and broad spectrum antibiotics and the vast majority of patients with localized inflammation will settle with these measures alone. Less than one third of cases require surgical intervention and the need may be apparent immediately (in cases of generalized peritonitis) or after several hours or days. When operation is necessary, the diseased bowel (usually the sigmoid colon) should be resected. Conservative non-resectional surgery based on colostomy, drainage of the peritoneal cavity or suture of the colonic perforation is accompanied by a higher morbidity and perioperative mortality than resectional techniques.[102] Some surgeons recommend primary anastomosis with or without a temporary colostomy after resections for diverticulitis but most prefer a staged procedure, the first operation involving exteriorization of the bowel or a Hartmann's procedure. The risks of primary anastomosis may be lessened by on-table colonic lavage or by the intracolonic bypass procedure.[37,38]

Patients with localized diverticular sepsis may develop an intraperitoneal abscess. Various surgical strategies have been used in such cases, including resection of the diseased bowel, but non-operative percutaneous drainage of the abscess may be a suitable alternative to emergency surgery in selected cases.[103,104] Frequent reassessment by ultrasonography or CT scanning is essential after percutaneous drainage.[90]

Specific complications after surgery for diverticular disease include continuing peritoneal sepsis, wound infection and intestinal obstruction. The mortality resulting from Hartmann's procedure is 12%[102] and the median duration of stay of surviving patients is 12 days.

Gynaecological Disorders

Various disorders of the female reproductive system may present as an acute abdomen,[105,106] including pelvic inflammatory disease, functional ovarian cysts, ectopic pregnancy and gynaecological neoplasms. In practice, diagnostic errors chiefly occur in young females and the problems which these patients create for the general surgeon are:

1. identification of the cause of the abdominal pain;
2. knowing what to do with the gynaecological condition.

Many acute gynaecological conditions do not require surgical intervention. Moreover, the surgical treatment of non-malignant disorders has become increasingly conservative or specialized. There is therefore a risk that the general surgeon may operate unnecessarily and may undertake an inappropriately radical or destructive surgical procedure. General surgeons should not hesitate to seek the assistance of gynaecologists when faced with gynaecological problems.

Diagnosis

Pelvic ultrasonography is invaluable in the diagnosis of gynaecological disorders.[106] The investigation may reveal free fluid in the pelvis, thickening of the adnexae, adnexal masses or a gestational sac. The investigation should be routine in all young females in whom there is uncertainty concerning the need for laparotomy. Unfortunately, fine catheter aspiration cytology of the peritoneum may be misleading in patients with acute pelvic inflammatory disease.[11] Serum immunoradiometric assays of human chorionic gonadotrophin should be performed in all cases of suspected ectopic pregnancy and high vaginal swabs for microbiological culture in all cases of suspected pelvic inflammatory disease.

Treatment

Pelvic inflammatory disease. Most patients will respond to treatment with antibiotics and analgesia. An increasing proportion of these cases are caused by chlamydia infections. A minority of patients develop tubo-ovarian abscesses, often related to delayed presentation or treatment. The abscess may be treated successfully with antibiotics but rupture or leakage requires urgent laparotomy. Hysterectomy and salpingo-oophorectomy provide the best prospect of freedom from long term problems of pelvic sepsis but may be unacceptable in young patients.

Ectopic pregnancy. Treatment of the condition depends on the general condition of the patient, the operative findings and the patient's desire for future childbearing. The standard treatment (and that which is provided by most general surgeons) is unilateral salpingectomy but some cases may be suitable for treatment by conservative methods including linear salpingotomy, segmental tubal excision or fimbrial expression. It has been estimated that 95% of cases can be treated by conservative methods[107] but these methods are not included in the normal repertoire of most general surgeons. Moreover, small ectopic pregnancies without signs of haemoperitoneum or impending rupture may be aborted by the use of methotrexate.

Functional ovarian cysts. Haemorrhage from a corpus luteum or follicular cyst may present as an acute abdomen. The diagnosis may be made with relative confidence in the case of a corpus luteum cyst by serum gonadotrophin measurements and pelvic ultrasound. The diagnosis of bleeding follicular cysts is more difficult. Surgery is unnecessary unless the haemorrhage is unusually persistent and should be limited to excision of the cyst.

Gynaecological neoplasia. Adnexal torsion may complicate large ovarian lesions. The tumour is usually a benign cyst and the diagnosis is readily made by pelvic ultrasonography.[108] Early diagnosis of adnexal torsion may enable the surgeon to perform conservative surgery. Salpingo-oophorectomy is required if the adnexal mass is infarcted. Occasionally malignant neoplasms (usually of the ovary) present acutely with lower abdominal pain, tense ascites or obstruction of the small intestine. Surgical treatment in such cases is almost invariably palliative but should aim to remove as much of the neoplasm as possible, including excision of the greater omentum. The ultimate prognosis is very poor.

Acute Superior Mesenteric Ischaemia

This lethal condition claims several lives every year in most surgical units (Fig. 13.1.3). Classically, there is massive infarction of the small intestine due to occlusion of the superior mesenteric artery. The occlusion is embolic in 35% of cases and thrombotic in the remainder.[109]

Diagnosis

The diagnosis is notoriously difficult and physical signs may be absent until infarction of the intestine has occurred. Hyperphosphataemia associated with a leucocytosis and metabolic acidosis are strongly suggestive of mesenteric ischaemia.[110–112] Some surgeons recommend emergency angiography when there is clinical suspicion of this condition but there is a 30–50% incidence of negative investigations[113,114] and the angiogram may be misleading if the patient has already suffered a silent visceral arterial occlusion.

Treatment

The diagnosis is made at autopsy in more than half of the cases and there is an 85% mortality in those diagnosed in life.[109] Few patients survive massive resections of the small intestine but earlier diagnosis of the condition would provide more opportunities for surgical restoration of the arterial blood supply before infarction occurs.

NON-SPECIFIC ABDOMINAL PAIN (NSAP)

In reality NSAP is a convenience diagnosis for a large group of acute admissions in whom we are unable positively to identify a physical cause for abdominal pain (Fig. 13.1.1). The diagnosis may be amended if further investigation reveals a physical explanation. Some patients are found to have viral, campylobacter or yersinia infections, worm infestations, the irritable bowel syndrome, or gynaecological abnormalities. Others may have a psychosomatic illness.[115] Ten percent of patients aged more than 50 years are found to have an abdominal malignancy.[116] NSAP is more common in young patients (Fig. 13.1.2), particularly female subjects, and it is frequently difficult to distinguish between this diagnosis and appendicitis or pelvic inflammatory disease.

Diagnosis

Computer techniques are of particular value in the diagnosis of NSAP and ultrasonography may be helpful in excluding gynaecological abnormalities or appendicitis. Unfortunately, a proportion of these patients (9% in our own experience) undergo an unnecessary laparotomy, usually because a diagnosis of appendicitis cannot be excluded.

Treatment

Successful treatment depends on recognition that the patient does not require a surgical operation (Fig. 13.1.4). Patients in the age range 5–50 are usually discharged in 3–4 days. The median duration of stay increases in older patients due to the higher level of suspicion of alternative diagnoses and the perceived need for more invasive investigations.

REFERENCES

1. Irvin TT. Abdominal pain: a surgical audit of 1190 emergency admissions. *Br J Surg* 1989; **76**: 1121–5.
2. Paterson-Brown S, Vipond MN. Modern aids to clinical decision-making in the acute abdomen. *Br J Surg* 1990; **77**: 13–18.
3. DeDombal FT, Leaper DJ, Horrocks JC, Staniland JR, McCann AP. Human and computer-aided diagnosis of abdominal pain: further report with emphasis on performance of clinicians. *Br Med J* 1974; **1**: 376–80.
4. Lawrence PC, Clifford PC, Taylor IF. Acute abdominal pain: computer aided diagnosis by non-medically qualified staff. *Ann Roy Coll Surg Eng* 1987; **69**: 233–4.
5. Campbell JPM, Gunn AA. Plain abdominal radiographs and acute abdominal pain. *Br J Surg* 1988; **75**: 554–6.
6. Stewart J, Finan PJ, Courtney DF, Brennan TG. Does a water soluble contrast enema assist in the management of acute large bowel obstruction? A prospective study of 117 cases. *Br J Surg* 1984; **71**: 799–801.
7. Riveron FA, Obeid FN, Horst M, Sorensen VJ, Bivins BA. The role of contrast radiology in presumed bowel obstruction. *Surgery* 1989; **106**: 496–501.
8. Pillari G, Greenspan B, Vernace FM, Rosenblum G. Computed tomography of diverticulitis. *Gastrointest Radiol* 1984; **9**: 263–8.
9. London NJM, Leese T, Lavelle JM *et al.* Rapid-bolus contrast-enhanced dynamic computed tomography in acute pancreatitis: a prospective study. *Br J Surg* 1991; **78**: 1452–6.
10. Evans C, Rashid A, Rosenberg IL. An appraisal of peritoneal lavage in the diagnosis of the acute abdomen. *Br J Surg* 1975; **62**: 119–20.
11. Vipond MN, Paterson-Brown S, Tyrrell MR, Coleman D, Thompson JN, Dudley HAF. Evaluation of fine catheter aspiration cytology of the peritoneum as an adjunct to decision making in the acute abdomen. *Br J Surg* 1990; **77**: 86–7.

12. Davies AH, Mastorakou I, Cobb R, Rogers C, Lindsell D, Mortensen NJ. Ultrasonography in the acute abdomen. *Br J Surg* 1991; **78**: 1178–80.
13. Paterson-Brown S, Vipond MN, Simms K, Gatzen C, Thompson JN, Dudley HAF. Clinical decision making and laparoscopy versus computer prediction in the management of the acute abdomen. *Br J Surg* 1989; **76**: 1011–13.
14. Jones PF. Practicalities in the management of the acute abdomen. *Br J Surg* 1990; **77**: 365–7.
15. Sutton GC. Computer-aided diagnosis: a review. *Br J Surg* 1989; **76**: 82–5.
16. Lau W, Fau S, Yiu T, Chu K, Wong S. Negative findings at appendectomy. *Am J Surg* 1984; **148**: 375–8.
17. Velanovich V, Satava R. Balancing the normal appendectomy rate with the perforated appendicitis rate: implications for quality assurance. *Am Surg* 1992; **58**: 264–9.
18. Ooms HWA, Koumans RKJ, Ho Kang You PJ, Puylaert JBCM. Ultrasonography in the diagnosis of acute appendicitis. *Br J Surg* 1991; **78**: 315–18.
19. Temple WJ. Bikini appendectomy incision as an alternative to the McBurney approach for appendicitis. *Can J Surg* 1990; **33**: 343–4.
20. Cleland G. Caecocolic intussusception following appendicectomy. *Br J Surg* 1953; **41**: 108–9.
21. Kingsley DPE. Some observations on appendicectomy with particular reference to technique. *Br J Surg* 1969; **56**: 491–6.
22. Sinha AP. Appendicectomy: an assessment of the advisability of stump invagination. *Br J Surg* 1977; **64**: 499–500.
23. Street D, Bodai BI, Owens LJ, Moore DB, Walton CB, Holcroft JW. Simple ligation vs stump inversion in appendectomy. *Arch Surg* 1988; **123**: 689–90.
24. Krukowski ZH, Irwin ST, Denholm S, Matheson NA. Preventing wound infection after appendicectomy: a review. *Br J Surg* 1988; **75**: 1023–33.
25. Stewart DJ, Matheson NA. Peritoneal lavage in appendicular peritonitis. *Br J Surg* 1978; **65**: 54–6.
26. Office of Population Censuses and Surveys. *Mortality Statistics: Causes, England and Wales, 1985*. London, HMSO, 1987.
27. Drumm J, Donovan IA, Wise R, Lowe P. Metronidazole and augmentin in the prevention of sepsis after appendicectomy. *Br J Surg* 1985; **72**: 571–3.
28. Puri P, McGuinness EP, Guiney EJ. Fertility following perforated appendicitis in girls. *J Pediatr Surg* 1989; **24**: 547–9.
29. Devlin HB, Gillen PHA, Waxman BP, MacNay RA. Short stay surgery for inguinal hernia: experience of the Shouldice operation. *Br J Surg* 1986; **73**: 123–4.
30. Nicholson S, Keane TE, Devlin HB. Femoral hernia: an avoidable source of surgical mortality. *Br J Surg* 1990; **77**: 307–8.
31. Dunn JT, Halls JM, Berne TV. Roentgenographic contrast studies in acute small bowel obstruction. *Arch Surg* 1984; **119**: 1305–8.
32. Walsh HPJ, Schofield PF. Is laparotomy for small bowel obstruction justified in patients with previously treated malignancy? *Br J Surg* 1984; **71**: 933–5.
33. Phillips RKS, Hittinger R, Fry JS, Fielding LP. Malignant large bowel obstruction. *Br J Surg* 1985; **72**: 296–302.
34. Dorudi S, Berry AR, Kettlewell MGW. Acute colonic pseudo-obstruction. *Br J Surg* 1992; **79**: 99–103.
35. Irvin TT, Greaney MG. The treatment of colonic cancer presenting with intestinal obstruction. *Br J Surg* 1977; **64**: 741–4.
36. Dudley HAF, Radcliffe AG, McGeehan D. Intraoperative irrigation of the colon to permit primary anastomosis. *Br J Surg* 1980; **67**: 80–1.
37. Koruth NM, Krukowski ZH, Youngson GG *et al*. Intraoperative colonic irrigation in the management of left-sided large bowel emergencies. *Br J Surg* 1985; **72**: 708–11.

38. Ravo B. Colorectal anastomotic healing and intracolonic bypass procedure. *Surg Clin N Am* 1988; **68**: 564–8.
39. Waldron RP, Donovan IA, Drumm J, Mottram SN, Tedman S. Emergency presentation and mortality from colorectal cancer in the elderly. *Br J Surg* 1986; **73**: 214–16.
40. Irvin TT. Prognosis of colorectal cancer in the elderly. *Br J Surg* 1988; **75**: 419–21.
41. Runkel NS, Schlag P, Schwarz V, Herfarth C. Outcome after emergency surgery for cancer of the large intestine. *Br J Surg* 1991; **78**: 183–8.
42. Mangiante EC, Croce MA, Fabian TC, Moore OF, Britt LG. Sigmoid volvulus. A four-decade experience. *Am Surg* 1989; **55**: 41–4.
43. Theuer C, Cheadle WG. Volvulus of the colon. *Am Surg* 1991; **57**: 145–50.
44. Friedman JD, Odland MD, Bubrick MP. Experience with colonic volvulus. *Dis Colon Rectum* 1989; **32**: 409–16.
45. Subrahmanyam M. Mesosigmoplasty as a definitive operation for sigmoid volvulus. *Br J Surg* 1992; **79**: 683–4.
46. Ponticelli A, Mastrobuono I, Matarazzo E *et al.* Mesosigmoidoplasty in the treatment of sigmoid volvulus in children. *S Afr J Surg* 1989; **27**: 105–7.
47. Salim AS. Management of acute volvulus of the sigmoid colon: a new approach by percutaneous deflation and colopexy. *World J Surg* 1991; **15**: 68–72.
48. Rabinovici R, Simansky DA, Kaplan O, Mavor E, Manny J. Cecal volvulus. *Dis Colon Rectum* 1990; **33**: 765–9.
49. Alexander Williams J. Conservative operations for Crohn's disease of the small bowel. *World J Surg* 1985; **9**: 945–51.
50. Clavien P-A, Richon J, Burgan S, Rohner A. Gallstone ileus. *Br J Surg* 1990; **77**: 737–42.
51. Pedersen PR, Petersen KK, Topp SW. Value of ultrasonography in the diagnosis of gallstone ileus. *Radiology* 1988; **28**: 479–80.
52. Dudley HAF, Paterson-Brown S. Pseudo-obstruction. *Br Med J* 1986; **292**: 1157–8.
53. Neely J, Catchpole B. Ileus: the restoration of alimentary tract motility by pharmacological means. *Br J Surg* 1971; **58**: 21–7.
54. Graham J. Cisapride for severe non-ulcer dyspepsia, pseudo-obstruction and constipation. *Med J Aust* 1989; **150**: 667.
55. Vanek VW, Al-Salti M. Acute pseudo-obstruction of the colon. *Dis Colon Rectum* 1986; **29**: 203–10.
56. Worthen NJ, Uszler JM, Funamara JL. Cholecystitis: prospective evaluation of sonography and ^{99m}Tc-HIDA cholescintigraphy. *AJR* 1981; **137**: 973–8.
57. Samuels BI, Freitas JE, Bree RL, Schwab RE, Heller ST. A comparison of radionuclide hepatobiliary imaging and real-time ultrasound for the detection of acute cholecystitis. *Radiology* 1983; **147**: 207–10.
58. Ralls PW, Colletti PM, Lapin SA *et al.* Real-time sonography in suspected acute cholecystitis. *Radiology* 1985; **5**: 767 71.
59. McArthur P, Cuschieri A, Sells RA, Shields R. Controlled clinical trial comparing early with interval cholecystectomy for acute cholecystitis. *Br J Surg* 1975; **62**: 850–2.
60. Archibald SD, Colaponto ND, Frost P. Early surgical management of acute cholecystitis. *Can J Surg* 1979; **22**: 464–6.
61. Van der Lindent W, Sunzel H. Early versus delayed operation for acute cholecystitis. *Am J Surg* 1976; **120**: 7–13.
62. Addison NV, Finan PJ. Urgent and early cholecystectomy for acute gallbladder disease. *Br J Surg* 1988; **75**: 141–3.
63. Van Sonnenberg E, Wittich GR, Casola G *et al.* Diagnostic and therapeutic percutaneous gallbladder procedures. *Radiology* 1986; **160**: 23–6.
64. McGahan JP, Lindfors KK. Percutaneous cholecystostomy: an alternative to surgical cholecystostomy for acute cholecystitis. *Radiology* 1989; **173**: 481–5.

65. Cheslyn-Curtis S, Russell RCG. New trends in gallstone management. *Br J Surg* 1991; **78**: 143–9.
66. Vellacott KD, Powell PH. Exploration of the bile duct: a comparative study. *Br J Surg* 1979; **66**: 389–91.
67. Duron JJ, Dutet D, Imbaud P *et al.* Chirurgie des voies biliaires du sujet age de 75 ans et plus. *Ann Med Int* 1985; **135**: 547–50.
68. Cotton PB, Vallon AG. Duodenoscopic sphincterotomy for removal of bile duct stones in patients with gallbladders. *Surgery* 1982: **91**: 628–30.
69. Davidson BR, Neoptolemos JP, Carr-Locke DL. Endoscopic sphincterotomy for common bile duct calculi in patients with gall bladder in situ considered unfit for surgery. *Gut* 1988; **29**: 114–20.
70. Hansell DT, Millar MA, Murray WR, Gray GR, Gillespie G. Endoscopic sphincterotomy for bile duct stones in patients with intact gallbladders. *Br J Surg* 1989; **76**: 856–8.
71. Thomson SR, Hendry WS, McFarlane GA, Davidson AI. Epidemiology and outcome of acute pancreatitis. *Br J Surg* 1987; **74**: 398–401.
72. Fan ST, Choi TK, Lai CS, Wong J. Influence of age on the mortality from acute pancreatitis. *Br J Surg* 1988; **75**: 463–6.
73. Cooper MJ, Williamson RCN, Pollock AV. The role of peritoneal lavage in the prediction and treatment of severe acute pancreatitis. *Ann Roy Coll Surg Eng* 1982; **64**: 422–7.
74. Poston GJ, Williamson RCN. Surgical management of acute pancreatitis. *Br J Surg* 1990; **77**: 5–12.
75. Neoptolemos JP, Carr-Locke DL, London N *et al.* Controlled trial of urgent endoscopic retrograde cholangiopancreatography and endoscopic sphincterotomy versus controlled treatment for acute pancreatitis due to gallstones. *Lancet* 1988; **ii**: 979–83.
76. Neoptolemos JP, Nerry JM, Carr-Locke DL, Fossard DP. The urgent diagnosis of gallstones in acute pancreatitis; a prospective study of three methods. *Br J Surg* 1984; **71**: 230–3.
77. Ranson JHC, Rifkind KM, Roser DF *et al.* Prognostic signs and the role of operative management in acute pancreatitis. *Surg Gynecol Obstet* 1974; **139**: 69–81.
78. Imrie CW, Benjamin IS, Ferguson JC *et al.* A single centre double-blind trial of Trasylol therapy in primary acute pancreatitis. *Br J Surg* 1978; **65**: 337–41.
79. Corfield AP, Cooper MJ, Williamson RCN *et al.* Prediction of severity in acute pancreatitis: prospective comparison of three prognostic indices. *Lancet* 1985; **ii**: 403–7.
80. Paloyan D, Simonowitz D, Skinner DB. The timing of biliary tract operations in patients with pancreatitis associated with gallstones. *Surg Gynecol Obstet* 1975; **141**: 737–9.
81. Ranson JHC. The timing of biliary surgery in acute pancreatitis. *Ann Surg* 1979; **189**: 654–63.
82. Tondelli P, Stutz K, Harder F, Schuppisser J-P, Allgower M. Acute gallstone pancreatitis: best timing for biliary surgery. *Br J Surg* 1982; **69**: 709–10.
83. Mayer AD, McMahon MJ, Corfield AP *et al.* Controlled clinical trial of peritoneal lavage for the treatment of severe acute pancreatitis. *New Eng J Med* 1985; **312**: 399–404.
84. Bradley EL III. Pancreatic pseudocysts. In: *Complications of Pancreatitis. Medical and Surgical Management* (ed. Bradley EL III), pp. 124–53. Philadelphia, WB Saunders, 1982.
85. Bernardino ME, Amerson JR. Percutaneous gastrocystostomy: a new approach to pancreatic pseudocyst drainage. *AJR* 1984; **143**: 1096–7.
86. Kozarek RA, Brayko CM, Harlan J *et al.* Endoscopic drainage of pancreatic pseudocysts. *Gastroenterol Endosc* 1985; **31**: 322–8.

87. Hancke S, Henriksen FW. Percutaneous pancreatic cystogastrostomy guided by ultrasound scanning and gastroscopy. *Br J Surg* 1985; **72**: 916–17.
88. Mughal MM, Bancewicz J, Irving MH. Laparostomy: a technique for the management of intractable intra-abdominal sepsis. *Br J Surg* 1986; **73**: 253–9.
89. Bradley EL III. Management of infected pancreatic necrosis by open drainage. *Ann Surg* 1987; **206**: 542–50.
90. Lameris JS, Bruining HA, Jeekel J. Ultrasound-guided percutaneous drainage of intra-abdominal abscesses. *Br J Surg* 1987; **74**: 620–3.
91. Watkins RM, Dennison AR, Collin J. What has happened to perforated peptic ulcer? *Br J Surg* 1984; **71**: 774–6.
92. Coleman JA, Denham MJ. Perforation of peptic ulceration in the elderly. *Age Ageing* 1980; **9**: 257–61.
93. Feliciano DV, Bitondo CG, Burch JM *et al.* Emergency management of perforated peptic ulcers in the elderly patient. *Am J Surg* 1984; **148**: 764–7.
94. Irvin TT. Mortality and perforated peptic ulcer: a case for risk stratification in elderly patients. *Br J Surg* 1989; **76**: 215–18.
95. Raimes SA, Devlin HB. Perforated duodenal ulcer. *Br J Surg* 1987; **74**: 81–2.
96. Keane TE, Dillon B, Afdhal NH, McCormack CJ. Conservative management of perforated duodenal ulcer (short note). *Br J Surg* 1988; **75**: 583–4.
97. Crofts TJ, Park KGM, Steele RJC, Chung SSC, Li AKC. A randomised trial of nonoperative treatment for perforated peptic ulcer. *New Eng J Med* 1989; **320**: 970–3.
98. Simpson CJ, Lamont G, Macdonald I, Smith IS. Effect of cimetidine on prognosis after simple closure of perforated duodenal ulcer. *Br J Surg* 1987; **74**: 104–5.
99. Haglund U, Hellberg R, Johns ENC, Hult RNL. Complicated diverticular disease of the sigmoid colon. An analysis of short and long-term outcome in 392 patients. *Ann Chir Gynecol* 1979; **68**: 41–6.
100. Kourtesis GJ, Williams RA, Wilson SE. Acute diverticulitis: safety and value of contrast studies in predicting need for operation. *Aust NZ J Surg* 1988; **58**: 801–4.
101. Krukowski ZH, Koruth NM, Matheson NA. Evolving practice in acute diverticulitis. *Br J Surg* 1985; **72**: 684–6.
102. Krukowski ZH, Matheson NA. Emergency surgery for diverticular disease complicated by generalized and faecal peritonitis: a review. *Br J Surg* 1984; **71**: 921–7.
103. Greco RS, Kamath C, Nosher JL. Percutaneous drainage of peridiverticular abscess followed by primary sigmoidectomy. *Dis Colon Rectum* 1982; **5**: 53–5.
104. Gerzof SC, Johnson WC. Radiologic aspects of diagnosis and treatment of abdominal abscesses. *Surg Clin N Am* 1984; **64**: 53–66.
105. Paterson-Brown S, Eckersley JRT, Dudley HAF. The gynaecological profile of acute general surgery. *J Roy Coll Surg Edinb* 1988; **33**: 13–15.
106. Burnett LS. Gynecologic causes of the acute abdomen. *Surg Clin N Am* 1988; **68**: 385–398.
107. Leach RL, Ory SJ. Modern management of ectopic pregnancy. *J Reprod Med* 1989; **34**: 324–38.
108. Bowen A. Ovarian torsion diagnoses by ultrasonography. *South Med J* 1985; **78**: 1376–9.
109. Wilson C, Gupta R, Gilmour DG, Imrie CW. Acute superior mesenteric ischaemia. *Br J Surg* 1987; **74**: 279–81.
110. Jamieson WG, Marchuk S, Rowsom J, Durand D. The early diagnosis of massive intestinal ischaemia. *Br J Surg* 1982; **69**: S52–3.
111. Ghanem M, Goodale RL, Spanos P, Tsung MS, Wangansteen OH. Value of leukocyte counts in the recognition of mesenteric infarction and strangulation of shorter intestinal lengths. *Surgery* 1970; **68**: 635–45.
112. Brooks DH, Carey LC. Base deficit in superior mesenteric artery occlusion, an aid to early diagnosis. *Ann Surg* 1973; **177**: 352–6.

113. Boley SJ, Sprayregen S, Siegelman SS, Veith FJ. Initial results from an aggressive roentgenological and surgical approach to acute mesenteric ischaemia. *Surgery* 1977; **82**: 848–55.
114. Clark RA, Gallant TE. Acute mesenteric ischaemia: angiographic spectrum. *AJR* 1984; **142**: 555–62.
115. Gray DWR, Collin J. Non-specific abdominal pain as a cause of acute admission to hospital. *Br J Surg* 1987; **74**: 239–42.
116. De Dombal FT, Matharu SS, Staniland JR *et al*. Presentation of cancer to hospital as "acute abdominal pain". *Br J Surg* 1980; **67**: 413–16.

13.2

Laparoscopic Surgery in the Acute Abdomen

S. PATERSON-BROWN, H. J. SCOTT and A. DARZI

INTRODUCTION

In the management of the acute abdomen laparoscopy has both a diagnostic and therapeutic role. The use of diagnostic laparoscopy in patients with acute abdominal pain is not new[1] and many studies have demonstrated an improvement in surgical decision making associated with its use, particularly when the need for operation is uncertain.[2] There is no doubt that laparoscopy is useful in those patients with suspected appendicitis,[3,4] especially in women.[5] Not only may the decision to operate be confirmed or refuted but laparoscopy may allow a more strategically placed incision to be made.

Although laparoscopic procedures such as appendicectomy have been performed by some surgeons for many years,[6] only recently have these become more commonplace. With the increased use of elective laparoscopy by general surgeons which has accompanied the introduction of laparoscopic cholecystectomy, there has been an associated increase in emergency laparoscopic surgery for both diagnostic and therapeutic purposes. In addition to laparoscopic appendicectomy, which has rapidly gained in popularity over the last few years[7–10], many other procedures are now being performed.

TECHNIQUE OF DIAGNOSTIC LAPAROSCOPY IN THE ACUTE ABDOMEN

Laparoscopy is performed under general anaesthesia as described earlier (Chapter 4) with the open technique preferable – and essential if intestinal obstruction is suspected or there have been several previous abdominal operations. The laparoscope and video camera are inserted through the umbilical port and a general inspection of the peritoneal cavity carried out. At this stage a definitive diagnosis may be established or alternatively a second port may be required to assist in the abdominal exploration. If acute appendicitis is suspected this port is best inserted through a lower right or left iliac fossa incision, both of which can be used later if the decision is made to proceed to laparoscopic appendicectomy. A blunt probe or pair of grasping forceps is inserted through this second port in order to manipulate the bowel and improve inspection of the viscera. It is important to be able to employ full Trendelenburg and reverse Trendelenburg positions, in addition to right and left tilt, during inspection to improve visualization of the peritoneal cavity.

TECHNIQUE FOR LAPAROSCOPIC APPENDICECTOMY

Following confirmation of the diagnosis of acute appendicitis at diagnostic laparoscopy, additional ports are inserted as shown (Fig. 13.2.1). The tip of the appendix is grasped by toothed grasping forceps inserted down the right iliac fossa port and drawn up into the port (if a 10 mm port is used). If the appendix is very friable an Endoloop (Ethicon Ltd, UK) may be placed over the tip of the appendix for traction. It is best not to place the right iliac fossa port too close to the appendix and the authors recommend a site inferior to it.

Once the appendix mesentery has been placed on a stretch using the grasping forceps, dissection commences using scissors inserted through the left iliac fossa

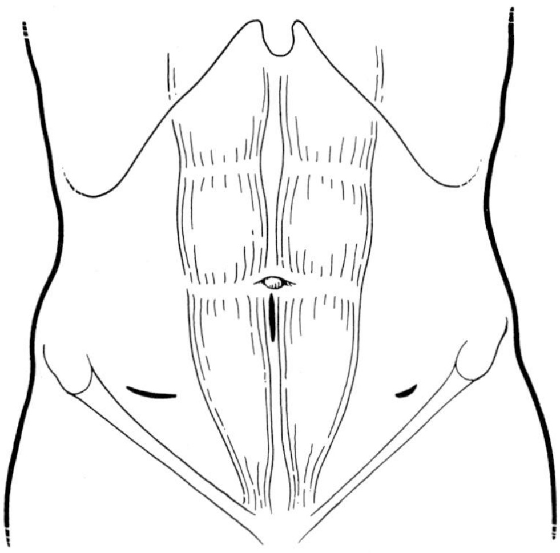

Figure 13.2.1 Position of ports for laparoscopic appendicectomy. The laparoscope is inserted through the umbilical port and the instruments inserted through both iliac fossa ports. In difficult circumstances the laparoscope may need to be moved to the lower left iliac fossa port which should be 10 mm. This will also permit the insertion of metal clips for the appendix mesentery if required.

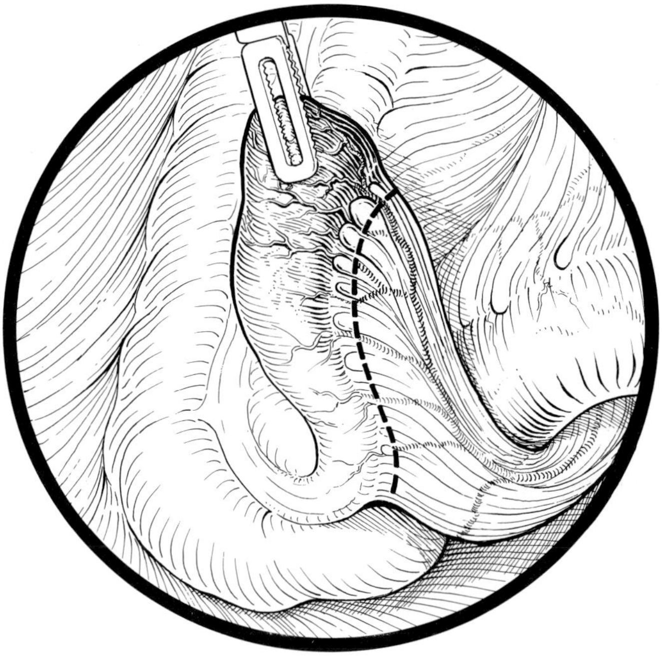

Figure 13.2.2 When the appendix mesentery is divided by electrocoagulation the line of division should be kept close to the appendix wall to avoid the main trunk of the appendicular artery, as demonstrated here.

port. The authors prefer the electrocoagulation technique, first described by Pier and colleagues[8], whereby the appendix mesentery is coagulated and then divided from the tip to the base, keeping very close to the appendix wall (Fig. 13.2.2). The disposable hooked scissors (Endopath, Ethicon Ltd, UK) are ideal for this technique as small bleeding points may be picked up and coagulated with the hooked tips of the scissors. Alternatively the mesentery may be divided between titanium clips, but this leaves a specimen which may be too bulky to remove through the port. If it becomes necessary to clip the appendix mesentery a clip applicator can be inserted down the left iliac fossa 10 mm port.

Once the appendix has been dissected free, three separate catgut Endoloops are placed around the base, which is divided with scissors leaving two Endoloops on the caecal side. The Endoloops are passed down the left iliac fossa port and the grasping forceps inserted through the right iliac fossa port are passed through the loop before grasping the appendix. The Endoloop is then tightened. During dissection it is important to keep up the tension on the appendix mesentery either by moving the grasping forceps or by drawing the appendix tip further into the right iliac fossa port (hence the usefulness of a 10 mm right iliac fossa port).

The authors use unipolar electrocoagulation, taking care not to apply excessive power and to maintain as much distance as possible between the line of dissection and the caecal pole. Other surgeons use bipolar coagulation with specially designed forceps[8] and there is little doubt this is to be preferred where possible.

Once the appendix has been dissected from the caecum it may be removed through the right iliac fossa 10 mm port without contamination of the abdominal wall. If it is too bulky – as is often the case in severe cases of acute appendicitis or when the mesentery has had to be "clipped" – then it may be placed in a small retrieval bag before removal. The right iliac fossa is then thoroughly irrigated with an antibiotic solution which is then removed by suction. In the opinion of the authors both irrigation and suction are important, particularly in cases of severe inflammation and contamination, as the pneumoperitoneum undoubtedly disseminates the intra-abdominal infection. If the surgeon has difficulty completing the suction of the pelvis, a small drain can be left in the pelvis for 4–6 hours postoperatively to ensure complete drainage.

In cases of gross inflammation, initial blunt dissection of the inflammatory mass using a blunt probe will usually reveal the appendix. In patients with retrocaecal appendicitis, grasping forceps inserted through the left iliac fossa port are used to push the caecum (not grasp it) to the patient's left, revealing part of the retrocaecal appendix which may then be grasped with the forceps inserted down the right iliac fossa port. If access is difficult the laparoscope can be transferred from the umbilical port to the left iliac fossa and many surgeons do this as a routine. The dissection may then be carried out using instruments inserted down the umbilical port. Occasionally a fourth access port may need to be inserted in the right upper quadrant, through which a pair of atraumatic bowel holding forceps can be inserted to elevate the caecum.

The authors do not routinely invert the appendix stump and there is good evidence from open surgery that this is not necessary.[11] Although stump inversion may be performed laparoscopically if required,[6] such as following perforation to the base of the appendix, a small extension of the right iliac fossa incision will permit the caecal pole to be drawn into the wound under laparoscopic guidance and formal closure of the stump performed. Before videolaparoscopy became available some surgeons who performed diagnostic laparoscopy in cases of suspected acute appendicitis went on to perform what has been described as "laparoscopic assisted appendicectomy" when an acutely inflamed appendix was seen.[12] A small incision is made directly over the appendix which can then be grasped under laparoscopic guidance. This technique may still be combined with the videolaparoscopy equipment if necessary.[13]

TECHNIQUE FOR CLOSURE OF PERFORATED PEPTIC ULCER

Perforated peptic ulcer is another condition for which the laparoscopic approach has many attractions. Once the diagnosis has been confirmed at laparoscopy a

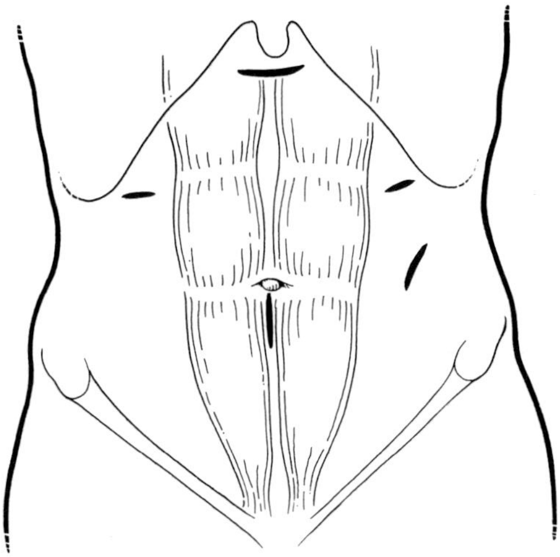

Figure 13.2.3 Position of ports for closure of a perforated peptic ulcer. The laparoscope is inserted through the umbilical port, the bowel holding forceps through the left midabdominal port and the instruments for dissection and repair inserted through the two upper quadrant ports. A fifth epigastric port may be required for additional access.

thorough peritoneal toilet is performed using a 10 mm suction/irrigation device through a second port inserted in an appropriate position, usually in the left upper quadrant area. If the perforation has been well sealed by an omental plug no further treatment is required[14] and confirmation of this can be determined preoperatively by a water soluble contrast meal,[15] or at surgery by insertion of dye or air down the nasogastric tube.

The surgeon may stand on the patient's right side or between the legs and once the perforation has been identified additional ports are inserted as shown in Figure 13.2.3. The secret of exposure lies in the insertion of atraumatic bowel holding forceps through the leftsided 10 mm port which are used to grasp the antrum of the stomach and retract it towards the left iliac fossa (Fig. 13.2.4). In most cases this manoeuvre will suffice but if not, additional exposure can be achieved by elevating the left lobe of liver from the anterior surface of the duodenum using a retractor inserted down an epigastric port. A suitable pedicle of greater omentum is identified and brought up to the perforation using two pairs of grasping forceps inserted through the left and right upper quadrant ports. The omental plug may then be sutured into place using a suture and needle holder passed down the left upper quadrant port (Fig. 13.2.4). If the perforation is small and the omentum thin, a stapled closure may be possible using a hernia stapler. If this is contemplated the left upper quadrant 5 mm port should be replaced by a 12 mm port through which a hernia stapler can be inserted and the omentum stapled over the perforation.

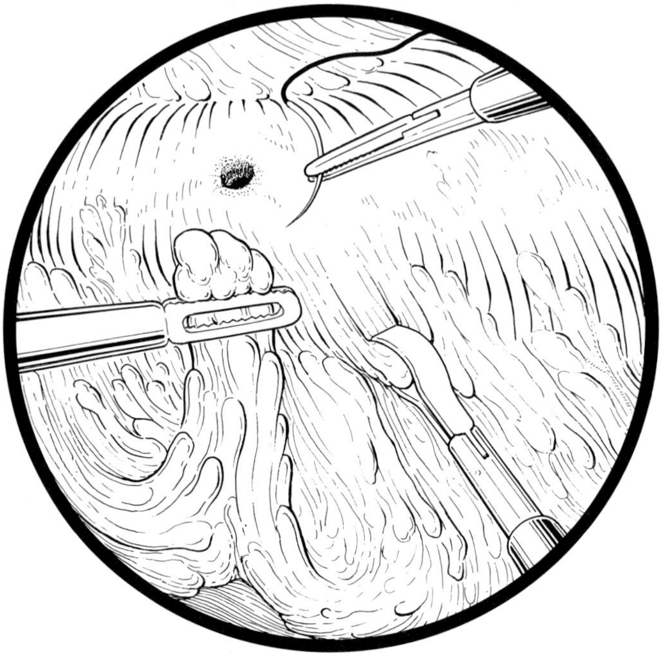

Figure 13.2.4 Part of the greater omentum is brought up to the perforation, using grasping forceps inserted down the right upper quadrant port, and sutured into place using the needle holder and needle inserted down the left upper quadrant port.

TECHNIQUE OF DIVISION OF ADHESIONS FOR INTESTINAL OBSTRUCTION

Laparoscopy is performed using the open technique (Chapter 4) and after initial inspection has confirmed the diagnosis and revealed the area most likely to contain the adhesive band, a second port is inserted under direct vision. This need only be a 5 mm port through which a blunt probe or grasping forceps are inserted. A third port will usually be required to insert the scissors for division of the adhesions once they have been exposed. Before dividing the obstructing band it is important to demonstrate a distal segment of collapsed intestine in order to confirm that this adhesion is the cause of the obstruction. Following division of this band, the distal intestine will rapidly distend making subsequent assessment very difficult.

TECHNIQUE OF LAPAROSCOPIC CHOLECYSTECTOMY FOR ACUTE CHOLECYSTITIS

The approach to urgent laparoscopic cholecystectomy for acute cholecystitis is the same as for the elective operation with the exception that the gall bladder invariably requires decompression. This may be performed by inserting a large bore cannula directly into the gall bladder through the anterior abdominal wall. Once decompressed in this manner, there will be very little leakage through the small hole which remains. If the contents of the gall bladder are too viscous to be removed through this cannula a small hole can be made in the fundus through which a suction tube is inserted. This hole can be closed by suture to prevent spillage of stones or simply grasped by the retracting forceps until the end of the procedure when the whole gall bladder may be placed into a retrieval bag. Thereafter the operation proceeds as for elective cholecystectomy.

RESULTS

The authors have now performed 304 laparoscopies for acute abdominal pain; 186 were diagnostic and in 118, therapeutic procedures were attempted.

Diagnostic Laparoscopy

Of the 186 patients undergoing diagnostic laparoscopy no further procedure was performed in 94 and 92 patients went on to open surgery (Table 13.2.1). Some of these patients have previously been reported in a series of studies performed at

Table 13.2.1 Diagnostic laparoscopy

Diagnosis	n	Open surgery
Acute appendicitis	62	62
Appendix mass	1	0
PID	45	3
NSAP	28	3
Ovarian cysts	25	5
Small bowel obstruction	4	4
Carcinomatosis	3	0
Diverticulitis	3	3
Perforated duodenal ulcer	3	3
Ectopic pregnancy	2	2
Torsion of appendix epiploica	1	1
Retrograde menstruation	1	1
Mesenteric infarction	1	1
Primary peritonitis	1	0
Empyema of gall bladder	1	1
Acute cholecystitis	1	0
Endometriosis	1	0
Torsion of ovary	1	1
Tuberculous peritonitis	1	1
Perforated small bowel tumour	1	1

St Mary's Hospital London[16,17] which examined the influence of laparoscopy on clinical decision making in patients with acute abdominal pain in whom the decision to operate was uncertain. In these studies the surgeon made a preoperative decision as to whether a "look and see" or "wait and see" policy would normally be adopted and then laparoscopy was performed. The potential error rate in this difficult group of patients was reduced by laparoscopy from 37/125 (30%) to 5/125 (4%).[18] Furthermore, without laparoscopy the unnecessary appendicectomy rate in women would have been 39% compared with 15% in men.[19]

In addition to improving management, the overall incidence of non-specific abdominal pain in *all* patients admitted to St Mary's Hospital with an acute abdomen during the period of these studies was only 163/661 (25%) using selective laparoscopy. This contrasts with figures in excess of 40% from other studies.[20]

Therapeutic Laparoscopy

Laparoscopic procedures were attempted in 118 patients (Table 13.2.2). Laparoscopic appendicectomy was attempted in 83 patients and was successful in 70 (84%). In a further two patients with gangrenous appendicitis, direct exposure of the caecal pole for safe closure was performed by extending the right iliac fossa incision at the end of the procedure. The laparoscopic procedure was converted to open appendicectomy in 11 patients due to technical difficulties. One patient who had undergone a successful laparoscopic appendicectomy required a second operation five days later for persistent signs of pelvic sepsis. This was performed through a standard appendicectomy incision and a small amount of infected fluid was removed, following which the patient made a swift recovery. The appendix stump was intact and the pelvic fluid was thought to be the result of inadequate removal of the peritoneal wash-out fluid at the end of the laparoscopic appendicectomy. Two further patients who had undergone successful laparoscopic appendicectomies developed complications: one patient

Table 13.2.2 Therapeutic laparoscopy

Attempted procedure	n	Successful	Conversion
Appendicectomy	83	72	11
Repair perforated duodenal ulcer	14	10	4
Cholecystectomy for acute cholecystitis	11	10	1
Division of adhesions for small bowel obstruction	7	1	6
Excision fimbrial cysts	2	2	0
Reduction and repair incarcerated femoral hernia	1	1	0

with perforated appendicitis continued to demonstrate persistent signs of sepsis for a further five days postoperatively and a second patient developed small bowel obstruction. Both settled without requiring further surgery.

Attempts to repair a perforated peptic ulcer laparoscopically were made in 14 patients and this was successful in all but four. One of these four underwent surgery early on in the series and had a successful suture repair performed laparoscopically but a small laparotomy was carried out to confirm the adequacy of closure.

Laparoscopic treatment of adhesive small bowel obstruction was attempted in seven patients using the open technique for insufflation in all. In only one patient was it possible to identify a single band and this was successfully divided laparoscopically. However, one patient had a small bowel volvulus successfully treated laparoscopically, but because no cause could be identified a laparotomy was performed. At laparotomy no obstructing lesion was identified and the patient made a full recovery.

Laparoscopic Appendicectomy

Reports are now available of large series of laparoscopic appendicectomies in both adults and children with excellent results.[8,9] Pier and colleagues[8] have recently reported 678 patients who underwent appendicectomy; laparoscopic appendicectomy was attempted in 639 and was successful in all but 14. The average operating time was only 15–20 minutes but postoperative stay was surprisingly long, with many patients remaining in hospital for up to seven days. Both acutely inflamed and perforated appendices were included.

The overall advantages of laparoscopic appendicectomy over the open procedure with regard to operating time and postoperative stay remain unclear although recent attempts to answer these questions by prospective study[21,22] do suggest advantages for the laparoscopic technique. Not only is the mean postoperative stay reduced from between 4–7 days after open appendicectomy to around 2–3 days following laparoscopic appendicectomy, but follow-up showed less pain at home and a much faster return to work and sporting activities, an important factor for young, fit, working adults. It has also been suggested that long term complications may be less following the laparoscopic method as early follow-up laparoscopy after both open and laparoscopic appendicectomy reveals a much lower incidence of adhesions in the laparoscopic group (2/20 vs. 16/20).[23]

It might be argued that gangrenous appendicitis with perforation and generalized peritonitis should represent a contraindication to laparoscopic appendicectomy, as an appropriately sited incision can permit swift removal of the diseased organ with minimal contamination. Likewise, the advantages of laparoscopic appendicectomy (as opposed to diagnostic laparoscopy) in children where small strategically placed incisions lead to a swift operation with minimal postoperative morbidity and an early return to normal activities remain debatable.

Repair of Perforated Peptic Ulcer

There have been several reports of successful closure of perforated peptic ulcers using intra-abdominal sutures,[24,25] fibrin sealant[26] or alternatively, peroperative gastroscopic insertion of a Dormia basket may be used to bring a plug of omentum through the perforation.[27] A recent report describes an ingenious method of inserting a gelatin sponge plug and fibrin sealant.[28] Although it may not be possible to treat all patients with a perforated peptic ulcer laparoscopically, there is now a good case for performing laparoscopy and attempting laparoscopic repair in all patients who are cardiovascularly stable following adequate resuscitation. Not only will laparoscopy confirm the diagnosis but a better examination of the peritoneal cavity and a more thorough peritoneal toilet can be achieved, particularly when a 10 mm suction device is used. In the frail and elderly patient the sparing of an upper abdominal incision should allow early mobilization with reduced postoperative complications, although a comparative study has yet to be performed.

Division of Adhesions in Intestinal Obstruction

The problems of using laparoscopy to divide adhesions in the presence of established intestinal obstruction are obvious and pneumoperitoneum should be achieved using the open technique. Although division of widespread intra-abdominal adhesions will not be possible using laparoscopy, selected patients with an isolated band are suitable.[27] With experience this method of treatment may become more popular and a recent study from France reported successful division of an obstructing band adhesion in ten of 20 patients with small bowel obstruction in whom laparoscopy was performed.[29]

Urgent Cholecystectomy for Acute Cholecystitis

In the early period of laparoscopic cholecystectomy many surgeons excluded patients with acute cholecystitis but in line with the changing trends in open surgery towards early cholecystectomy for acute cholecystitis,[30] reports of laparoscopic cholecystectomy for acute cholecystitis are now available. Although some studies show a much higher conversion rate in acute cases (25% vs. 4%), the morbidity and mortality rates do not differ.[31] A recent study from Edinburgh has shown that in a series of 31 patients with acute cholecystitis, laparoscopic cholecystectomy was successful in 29, with only two minor complications and one retained common bile duct stone.[32] The group in Edinburgh had to decompress the gall bladder in ten patients and perform a retrograde dissection in three. Open operation may still be the most appropriate treatment when the gall bladder is frankly gangrenous in order to prevent the much higher risk of rupture associated with the laparoscopic mobilization and dissection.

DISCUSSION

The early recognition of gynaecological conditions such as pelvic inflammatory disease and the Fitz-Hugh – Curtis syndrome[33] following diagnostic laparoscopy is important if prompt treatment is to be started and complications such as infertility are to be reduced.[34] More recently, laparoscopy has been used in the acute abdomen specifically to investigate suspected intestinal ischaemia following aortic reconstruction and may even be performed at the bedside.[35]

The question remains as to whether to proceed to appendicectomy if either the appendix cannot be seen and no other diagnosis can be made at laparoscopy or a normal looking appendix is visualized but no other cause for the patient's symptoms are identified. In the former situation many surgeons would recommend appendicectomy – a view with which the authors concur. In the latter situation appendicectomy for a macroscopically "normal-looking" appendix on the basis that evidence of microscopic inflammation can be found in 19% of specimens[36] is not necessarily generally accepted. In the St Mary's studies no cause for the patient's symptoms was found in 23/125 patients undergoing laparoscopy and in only four was appendicectomy performed, two because the appendix could not be seen, one in whom laparoscopy failed and one in whom the appendix looked inflamed but histology demonstrated serosal inflammation only.[18] Not one of these four appendices removed showed mucosal inflammation and none of the remaining 19 patients in whom no further procedure was performed subsequently required appendicectomy. However, the consequences of removing a "normal" appendix may be much less following laparoscopic appendicectomy than for the open operation and each surgeon will have his or her own views on this. Only one normal-looking appendix removed laparoscopically in our series demonstrated microscopic evidence of acute inflammation.

As diagnostic laparoscopy becomes more popular in the acute abdomen, so the opportunity to perform other emergency laparoscopic procedures will occur. It is now possible to perform appendicectomy, repair of perforated peptic ulcer, division of band adhesions and urgent cholecystectomy for acute cholecystitis using the laparoscopic method and many centres employ this technique as a routine. Other conditions amenable to laparoscopic surgery include acute diverticulitis. Diagnostic laparoscopy provides excellent information regarding the state of the diverticular disease and with current enthusiasm and success for laparoscopic assisted colectomy (Chapter 8.2) it would not be unreasonable to expect similar techniques to be applied to acute diverticulitis in selected cases. Preoperative information regarding a colonic leak can be obtained from a retrograde contrast enema[37] and would help the surgeon plan operative strategy pending laparoscopic inspection. A localized abscess without overt faecal soiling would be amenable to drainage under laparoscopic guidance. In cases of perforation requiring resection, the extent and severity of disease would determine how much is feasible using laparoscopy.

Although these procedures are now possible using laparoscopic techniques their feasibility alone does not yet justify their practice beyond the bounds of prospective studies and tightly controlled audit of results.

REFERENCES

1. Sugarbaker PH, Bloom BS, Sanders JH, Wilson RE. Preoperative laparoscopy in diagnosis of acute abdominal pain. *Lancet* 1975; **1**: 442–5.
2. Paterson-Brown S, Vipond MN. Modern aids to clinical decision making in the acute abdomen. *Br J Surg* 1990; **77**: 13–18.
3. Leape LL, Ramenofsky ML. Laparoscopy for questionable appendicitis – can it reduce the negative appendicectomy rate? *Ann Surg* 1980; **191**: 410–13.
4. Deutsch AA, Zelikovsky A, Reiss R. Laparoscopy in the prevention of unnecessary appendicectomies: a prospective study. *Br J Surg* 1982; **69**: 336–7.
5. Spirtos NM, Eisenkop SM, Spirtos TW, Poliakin RI, Hibbard LT. Laparoscopy – a diagnostic aid in cases of suspected appendicitis. Its use in women of reproductive age. *Am J Obstet Gynecol* 1987; **156**: 90–4.
6. Semm K. Endoscopic appendicectomy. *Endoscopy* 1983; **15**: 59–64.
7. Gangal HT, Gangal MH. Laparoscopic appendicectomy. *Endoscopy* 1987; **19**: 127–9.
8. Pier A, Gotz F, Bacher C. Laparoscopic appendectomy in 625 cases: from innovation to routine. *Surg Laparosc Endosc* 1991; **1**: 8–13.
9. Valla JS, Limmone B, Valla V *et al.* Laparoscopic appendectomy in children: report of 465 cases. *Surg Laparosc Endosc* 1991; **1**: 166–72.
10. Leahy PF. Technique of laparoscopic appendicectomy. *Br J Surg* 1989; **76**: 616.
11. Engstrom L, Fenyo G. Appendicectomy: assessment of stump invagination – a prospective, randomized trial. *Br J Surg* 1985; **72**: 971–2.
12. Fleming JS. Laparoscopically directed appendicectomy. *Aust NZ J Obstet Gynecol* 1985; **25**: 238–40.
13. Byrne DS, Bell G, Morrice JJ, Orr G. Technique for laparoscopic appendicectomy. *Br J Surg* 1992; **79**: 574–5.
14. Walsh CJ, Khoo DE, Motson RW. Laparoscopic repair of perforated peptic ulcer. *Br J Surg* 1993; **80**: 127.
15. Crofts TJ, Park KGM, Steele RJC, Chung SSC, Li AKC. A randomized trial of non-operative treatment for perforated peptic ulcer. *New Eng J Med* 1989; **320**: 970–3.
16. Paterson-Brown S, Eckersley JRT, Sim AJWS, Dudley HAF. Laparoscopy as an adjunct to decision-making in the "acute abdomen". *Br J Surg* 1986; **73**: 1022–4.
17. Paterson-Brown S, Vipond MN, Simms K, Gatzen C, Dudley HAF. Clinical decision-making and laparoscopy versus computer prediction in the management of the acute abdomen. *Br J Surg* 1989; **76**: 1011–13.
18. Paterson-Brown S. The acute abdomen: the role of laparoscopy. In: *Gastrointestinal Emergencies, Part I*, (eds Williamson RCN, Thompson JN), pp. 691–703. London Baillière Tindall, 1991.
19. Paterson-Brown S, Thompson JN, Eckersley JRT, Ponting GA, Dudley HAF. Which patient with suspected appendicitis should undergo laparoscopy? *Br Med J* 1988; **296**: 1363–4.

20. Gray DWR, Collin J. Non-specific abdominal pain as a cause of acute admission to hospital. *Br J Surg* 1987; **74**: 239–42.
21. McAnena OJ, Austin O, O'Connell PR, Hederman WP, Gorey TF, Fitzpatrick J. Laparoscopic versus open appendicectomy: a prospective evaluation. *Br J Surg* 1992; **79**: 818–20.
22. Attwood SEA, Hill ADK, Murphy PG, Thornton J, Stephens RB. A prospective randomized trial of laparoscopic versus open appendectomy. *Surgery* 1992; **112**: 497–501.
23. De Wilde RL. Goodbye to late bowel obstruction after appendicectomy. *Lancet* 1991; **338**: 1012.
24. Nathanson LK, Easter DW, Cuschieri A. Laparoscopic repair/peritoneal toilet of perforated duodenal ulcer. *Surg Endosc* 1990; **4**: 232–3.
25. Sunderland GT, Chisholm EM, Lau WY, Chung SCS, Li AKC. Laparoscopic repair of perforated peptic ulcer. *Br J Surg* 1992; **79**: 785.
26. Mouret P, Francois Y, Vignal J, Barth X, Lombard-Platet R. Laparoscopic treatment of perforated peptic ulcer. *Br J Surg* 1990; **77**: 1006.
27. Perissat J, Collet D, Edye M. Therapeutic laparoscopy. *Endoscopy* 1992; **24**: 138–43.
28. Tate JJT, Dawson JW, Lau WY, Li AKC. Sutureless laparoscopic treatment of perforated duodenal ulcer. *Br J Surg* 1993; **80**: 235.
29. De Watteville JC. *Abord Endoscopique des Occlusions du Grele*. 3rd World Congress of Endoscopic Surgery, Bordeaux, 1992.
30. Addison NV, Finan PJ. Urgent and early cholecystectomy for acute gall bladder disease. *Br J Surg* 1988; **75**: 141–3.
31. Domergue J, Fabre JM, Guillon F *et al*. Laparoscopic cholecystectomy in acute and non-acute cholecystolithiasis. *Res Surg* 1991; **3**: 147–9.
32. Wilson RG, Macintyre IMC, Nixon SJ, Saunders JH, Varma JS, King PM. Laparoscopic cholecystectomy as a safe and effective treatment for severe acute cholecystitis. *Br Med J* 1992; **305**: 394–6.
33. Wood JJ, Bolton JP, Cannon SR. Biliary-type pain as a manifestation of genital tract infection: the Curtis–Fitz-Hugh syndrome. *Br J Surg* 1982; **69**: 251–3.
34. Pearce JM. Pelvic inflammatory disease. *Br Med J* 1990; **300**: 1090–1.
35. Iberti TJ, Salky BA, Onofrey D. Use of bedside laparoscopy to identify intestinal ischaemia in postoperative cases of aortic reconstruction. *Surgery* 1989; **105**: 686–9.
36. Lau WY, Fan ST, Yiu TF, Chu KW, Suen HC, Wong KK. The clinical significance of routine histopathologic study of the resected appendix and safety of stump invagination. *Surg Gynecol Obstet* 1986; **162**: 256–8.
37. Kourtesis GJ, Williams SE. Acute diverticulitis: safety and value of contrast studies in predicting need for operation. *Aust NZ J Surg* 1988; **58**: 801–4.

Overview

Acute abdominal surgery

Some of the early work on laparoscopy in general surgery, reported by Sugarbaker in North America, involved its role in deciding which patient with acute abdominal pain did or did not require laparotomy. Other papers have since followed and it is now generally accepted that all patients with acute abdominal pain in whom the decision to operate is in doubt should be offered laparoscopy. The majority of these patients will be young females and the elderly but, as laparoscopic surgery develops, this group is expanding to engulf all patients whose possible condition can be managed by laparoscopic or laparoscopic-assisted surgery. Data are now available to support the laparoscopic treatment of appendicitis, acute cholecystitis, perforated peptic ulcers and gynaecological conditions. Furthermore, the management of patients with intestinal obstruction from band adhesions, acute diverticulitis and complicated Meckel's diverticulum is also possible laparoscopically and may prove beneficial in selected patients.

At present most emergency procedures are performed by relatively junior staff, and the introduction of laparoscopic techniques will require close and careful supervision if the undoubted benefits are to be realized.

14.1

Early Assessment of Abdominal Trauma

M. OCHSNER, D. BURRIS and H. R. CHAMPION

INTRODUCTION

The treatment of abdominal trauma parallels the development of abdominal surgery. Prior to the advances of the latter part of the nineteenth century (anaesthesia, suturing techniques, abdominal operation and the concept of asepsis), the treatment of abdominal trauma was expectant. Those who sustained massive vascular or solid organ injuries died quickly from haemorrhage; those who sustained hollow viscus disruption died more slowly, from peritonitis and those who did not suffer either of these injuries usually survived, but only if the treatments administered did not prove fatal.[1] Today, advances in prehospital and inhospital trauma management, anaesthesia, blood component therapy and intensive care allow more patients with major abdominal trauma to survive their injuries. An example is the dramatic decrease in mortality from abdominal gunshot wounds since the mid-nineteenth century (Table 14.1.1).[2]

Today's surgeon must manage an increasing number of severely injured patients who require aggressive resuscitation and rapid, accurate evaluation to identify and treat life-threatening injuries. These patients can offer some of the greatest challenges to the general surgeon and the determination of the need for and timing of operative intervention is one of them.

Table 14.1.1 Mortality from abdominal gunshot wounds[2])

Late nineteenth century	98%
World War I	45%
World War II	25%
Korea	12%
Vietnam	8.5%
Today	5.5%

Identification of those patients who need operative intervention to repair their injuries and those who would do as well, if not better, without surgery is the crux of early assessment of abdominal trauma. Most of this chapter is devoted to describing the current means available to the general surgeon to make that distinction.

MECHANISM OF INJURY

The pathophysiology of an injury is related to the mechanism involved in creating the injury. By convention, mechanisms are divided into the two broad categories of blunt and penetrating. The basis of this division is more than epidemiological, as the forces involved and associated injury patterns are markedly different. A fundamental knowledge of the pathophysiology resulting from blunt and penetrating injury is necessary to effectively manage the trauma patient with possible abdominal injuries.

Blunt Trauma

Injuries resulting from a blunt mechanism comprise those due to direct transmissions of force and those related to rapid deceleration or acceleration. With a direct blow, the majority of injury can be related to the amount of force transmitted to the area of the impact. A kick to the right flank, for example, may result in a fractured kidney. Rapid deceleration injuries, such as those resulting from a fall, motorcycle or automobile crash and rapid acceleration injuries such as a pedestrian struck by a motor vehicle, may arise from three additional mechanisms. These are injuries that:

1. relate to the sudden deceleration of a vehicle with the passenger continuing forward to strike various internal components of the vehicle or, if ejected, other stationary objects;
2. result from organs striking the supporting structures of the chest and abdomen (i.e. the spine, lower ribs and abdominal wall);
3. result from points of anatomic fixation (which gives rise to additional forces such as shear and torque). Classic examples of the latter include rupture of the thoracic aorta at the ligamentum arteriosum and renal artery injury associated with sudden vertical deceleration.

One additional mechanism of injury relates to the hydrostatic forces that apply to hollow viscera and large blood vessels; a sudden increase in intraluminal pressures can result in rupture of these structures.[3] The magnitude and direction of force are additional critical factors that determine where and to what degree injury will occur. Injury patterns associated with anterior–posterior directions of force, for example, can be quite different from those generated from the lateral and vertical directions.

Finally, individual characteristics of an organ determine its ability to withstand forces. The lung can withstand a certain amount of force without significant damage, whereas the same amount of force applied to the liver results in massive parenchymal disruption.[4]

Often, injuries resulting from direct blows may be suspected based on an associated contusion or deformity of the torso. In contrast, injuries resulting from deceleration/acceleration may have no associated external evidence of trauma and require an appropriate index of suspicion to establish the diagnosis.

Penetrating Trauma

The two main types of penetrating injuries are stab and gunshot wounds. In evaluating stab wounds, the type of weapon and its length are important. When evaluating patients with gunshot wounds, the type of weapon, the number of shots fired from what direction and distance they travelled and whether the patient had been shot in the past are all portions of the history that may be helpful.

Stab wounds produce low velocity injuries, the severity of which is determined by the size of the object, the depth of penetration and which structures are lacerated or punctured along the object's path. Impaled objects, because they often provide temporary tamponade when major vascular injuries are present, should not be removed prior to vascular control or exsanguination may result.[5]

Gunshot wounds differ from stab wounds in that the former produce relatively high velocity injuries because tissue destruction, to varying degrees, extends beyond the path of the missile and they can also create secondary missiles (i.e. bone fragments) which increase the amount of tissue destruction. Gunshot wounds can be divided in those of high velocity and low velocity, defined according to whether the gun's muzzle velocity exceeded 2000 feet per second. Higher velocity weapons are more likely to cause greater tissue damage radial to the path of the projectile, via a shock wave effect as the projectile dissipates its energy.[6] Therefore, more injury should be suspected radial to the obvious projected path of the path of the projectile.[6] A complicating factor, however, is the tendency of projectiles to deviate from a straight path, especially after striking bone; therefore a straight line connecting entrance and exit wounds may not accurately represent the structures injured.[7]

Shotgun wounds are a subcategory of low velocity wounds with extensive tissue damage. Shotgun blasts, in which a large mass of projectiles is released at one discharge at relatively close range, impart all of their kinetic injury to the tissue. The closer the range, the closer the clustering of the pellets and the greater velocity and destructive power they carry.[8]

OVERVIEW OF RESUSCITATION

The critical factors affecting outcome in abdominal trauma are aggressive resuscitation of shock and early diagnosis of any intra-abdominal injury. Delays in diagnosis directly result in increased morbidity and death.[9] Although physical examination of the abdomen can be extremely reliable in many surgical disease processes, among trauma patients it has a sensitivity and specificity of only 50%, even when the examination is conducted by the most skilled clinicians.[10] Blood is a non-irritating substance in the peritoneal cavity with a physiological pH; therefore, peritoneal signs may be absent or subtle in patients with haemoperitoneum. Pain from injuries such as a fractured femur can obscure subtle, less painful findings of an associated abdominal injury. The presence of other injuries adjacent to the peritoneal cavity, such as fractured lower thoracic ribs, rectus muscle haematomas, pelvic fracture and renal contusion can cause abdominal wall guarding and referred pain in the absence of intra-abdominal injury.

The intention of describing the many confounding factors that can affect the accuracy of physical examination of the abdomen is not to diminish its importance but rather to more clearly elucidate the specific considerations in evaluation of the injured versus other patients with potential surgical disease and to emphasize the need for adjunctive methods for establishing the diagnosis of intra-abdominal injury. A thorough baseline examination is mandatory with frequently repeated exams by the same person at regular intervals to identify conditions that may develop or that were absent or obscured by other injuries upon admission.

All other methods of evaluating the abdomen have inherent shortcomings. Therefore, only with complete, multiple abdominal examinations – with consideration of the mechanism of injury and the judicious use of adjuvant diagnostic resources – can morbidity and mortality associated with delay in diagnosis of abdominal injury be eliminated or reduced.

Assessment

Thorough evaluation of the trauma patient requires progression through the following basic steps: a brief history, primary survey, secondary survey, response to resuscitation and laboratory and radiographic studies. The diagnosis of abdominal injury is often established during the secondary survey, upon which the majority of the text will focus.

Patient History

In trauma, as in other surgical disciplines, patient history is often a critical factor in establishing the diagnosis. By relaying time and mechanism of injury, condition of the patient at the scene and additional descriptive information (e.g. the amount of blood on the pavement or extrication time), emergency medical personnel from the scene provide the surgeon with invaluable information regarding the severity of injury. Additional information, such as allergies, medications, past medical history and when the patient ate last can often be obtained from the patient, relatives or associates. All patient history information should be sought early, particularly that provided by personnel at the scene, whose presence in the resuscitation area is typically of brief duration.

Primary Survey

In discussions of abdominal trauma it is assumed, but should not be taken for granted, that the basic precepts of resuscitation and stabilization have been followed. A patent airway should be assured and supplemental oxygen administered. Those patients with unstable airways or who are in profound shock should be intubated, with simultaneous immobilization of the cervical spine, when indicated.

The patient's ability to breathe should be assessed and if respiratory efforts are inadequate (as manifested clinically by tachypnoea, ineffective respiratory efforts, cyanosis or abnormal arterial blood gas measurements), mechanical ventilation may be required. Many trauma centres and emergency departments currently use pulse oximeters to non-invasively assess oxygenation. Correction of pneumothorax and amelioration of muscular splinting from the pain of rib fractures by adequate analgesia may correct inadequate respiratory efforts without intubation.

The adequacy of circulation should be determined next. The colour and temperature of the skin as well as the rate of capillary refill can provide valuable information regarding cutaneous perfusion and the presence of hypovolaemic shock. Heart rate and rhythm and blood pressure should be determined; however, one should keep in mind that significant intravascular volume loss can be present in young patients with a normal blood pressure due to their remarkable ability to compensate with vasoconstriction. Sinus tachycardia, because it can be caused by pain, anxiety, drugs or hypoxia, is an unreliable indicator of hypovolaemia in the trauma patient. Similarly, a normal or slow heart rate is unreliable for ruling out hypovolaemia because up to 50% of such patients with traumatic injuries may have major intravascular depletion.[2] Large bore intravenous lines should be inserted, with crystalloid solutions or blood products as necessary and any obvious haemorrhage controlled with pressure.

Next, a brief neurological examination should be performed to determine the patient's level of consciousness and to identify any local or lateralizing signs indicative of a major injury to the brain or spinal cord. Pupil size and reactivity should be documented and a quick assessment of mental status can be recorded using the mnemonic device AVPU, which stands for "Awake, responds to Verbal stimuli, responds to Painful stimuli and Unresponsive".[11] These can be repeated rapidly and can identify subsequent neurological improvement or

Table 14.1.2 Glasgow Coma Scale[12]

Best eye opening response	
Spontaneous	4
To voice	3
To pain	2
None	1
Best verbal response	
Oriented	5
Confused	4
Inappropriate words	3
Incomprehensible sounds	2
None	1
Best motor response	
Obeys commands	6
Localizes pain	5
Withdraws (pain)	4
Flexion (pain)	3
Extension (pain)	2
None	1

deterioration. A gross assessment of the motor and sensory status of all four extremities should be documented. Glasgow Coma Scale[12] (Table 14.1.2) scores should be obtained and a more thorough neurological examination should be conducted during the secondary survey.

Finally, the patient should be completely disrobed and the entire body (including the back) examined to identify all injuries. The primary survey should be conducted rapidly, preferably within 2–3 minutes.

Secondary Survey

Resuscitation should be accomplished simultaneously with evaluation. In fact, the response of the patient to resuscitation can identify undiagnosed shock, particularly in the young, otherwise healthy trauma patient. An improvement in vital signs after initial resuscitation with 2 litres of crystalloid, for example, is a good indication that the patient's injuries are not lethal. Persistent signs of shock or secondary deterioration of vital signs after initial improvement with resuscitation suggest serious injuries and in those patients with torsal injury, the presumed source of blood loss should be the chest or abdomen.

The abdomen is inspected for open wounds, abrasions and bruises. Transverse bruises over the lower abdomen and angled bruises over the upper quadrants are classic for both two-point (seat) and three-point (shoulder) restraint injuries in motor vehicle crashes. The presence of these "seat belt" signs is associated with intra-abdominal injury, mainly of the hollow viscera, in as many as one third of patients.[13] A distended abdomen may indicate massive haemoperitoneum, but it is sometimes difficult to differentiate this condition from a chronically distended abdomen or distension secondary to hollow visceral dilatation from air (particularly when mask ventilation has been used prior to arrival in the trauma centre or emergency department by prehospital personnel). Conversely, as much as 2 litres of blood may be present within the peritoneal cavity without remarkable abdominal distension.[14]

Routine auscultation for bowel sounds is seldom useful in the examination of the trauma patient. Bowel sounds may be absent due to the presence of spinal fractures or flank haematomas or they may be missed amid the noise of a busy trauma centre or emergency department. Further, the presence of bowel sounds does not rule out injury.

On palpation, the location and severity of tenderness is assessed. Peritoneal signs may be obvious, as in the classic "board-like" abdomen, or when more subtle, they may be elicited with gentle percussion or shaking of the patient or bed. A bold, deep push with sudden release (rebound tenderness) is rarely necessary. As mentioned previously, abdominal tenderness is not always due to intra-abdominal injury and may instead arise from lacerations or contusions to the abdominal wall or from fractures of the lower rib cage.

Evaluation of the bony pelvis includes firm compression over the pubic symphysis: tenderness elicited in this manner suggests possible pubic ramus fracture and alerts the examiner to the possible presence of urethral injury. Pelvic stability is next assessed by anterior/posterior and medial/lateral pressure over the iliac wings. If free motion of the iliac wings is encountered, then probable disruption of the posterior elements of the pelvis exists and significant retroperitoneal bleeding may be present.

A pelvic examination in female patients is used to assess for blood in the vagina, lacerations of the vaginal wall and possible pregnancy. In all patients, digital rectal examination is used to detect lacerations, protruding fracture fragments and gross blood. While stool occult blood tests tell little about acute injury, they should be performed for complete evaluation of the patient. For example, a relatively minor traumatic blood loss may be compounded by a chronic gastrointestinal blood loss.

In the male, an abnormally high prostate level can signifiy possible urethral disruption. Blood in the urethral meatus, fractured pubic ramus or a scrotal haematoma also suggest urethral injury and require retrograde urethrography prior to catheteriziation of the bladder followed by cystography.[15]

The patient's back should be examined; whenever possible, the patient should be rolled onto one side with the spine kept straight. In addition to obvious signs of injury, the spinous processes of the lower thoracic and lumbar vertebrae should be palpated to detect tenderness that may accompany fractures of the spine. The presence of tenderness of the proximal lumbar spine (L1 through L3) and subsequent diagnosis of a fracture there should raise suspicion for an associated pancreatic or duodenal injury.

A gastric tube should be inserted either nasally or orally to assess for blood in the stomach and remove gastric contents to prevent aspiration into the airways. A urinary catheter should be inserted if there is no evidence of genitourinary injury, to assess for blood in the urine and allow continuous monitoring of the urinary output (a crude index of the adequacy of resuscitation).

As mentioned earlier, the patient should be re-examined frequently, firstly because some physical findings may become more apparent with time than on initial evaluation and secondly so that subtle deterioration in haemodynamic stability may be identified early and precipitous cardiopulmonary collapse may be avoided.

Laboratory Evaluation

Determination of blood type and crossmatch is the only mandatory laboratory examination for the patient with suspected abdominal trauma. Evaluation of haematocrit, haemoglobin and arterial blood gases also can be quite useful, as can urinalysis. Both haemoglobin and heamatocrit levels are valuable as baseline determinations. While haemoglobin levels may more accurately reflect acute haemorrhage than haematocrit levels, both of these tests can document significant blood loss if they reveal abnormally low values after injury. The converse does not hold true, however, because normal haemoglobin or haematocrit levels do not rule out acute blood loss. Arterial blood gas levels provide information regarding oxygenation, ventilation and the presence of metabolic acidosis. A base deficit greater than 5 mmol dl^{-1} in the absence of obvious blood loss from the head, chest or extremities suggests potential occult intra-abdominal bleeding.[16] Urinalysis documents the presence of gross microscope haematuria, which frequently mandates further evaluation.

Other laboratory tests of less urgency include determinations of electrolytes, serum amylase, white blood cell count, liver function, toxicology and blood alcohol levels. All of these may give clues as to the type and extent of abdominal injury, but none is sensitive or specific enough to pinpoint injury to any particular abdominal organ.

DIAGNOSTIC INTERVENTIONS

Radiographic Studies

Plain X-Ray

In blunt trauma, the most useful radiographs for evaluation of the abdomen are those of the chest and pelvis, to rule out the presence of injury to these areas. Occasionally, diaphragmatic hernia can be diagnosed on chest X-ray if the nasogastric tube or an airfilled hollow viscus is seen in the chest. Free air under the diaphragm on an upright chest X-ray, although rarely seen, suggests intra-abdominal hollow viscus injury. The flat abdominal film for evaluating the kidney, ureter and bladder, known as a KUB, may reveal non-specific, subtle signs of injury such as widening of the stripes between bowel loops, the presence

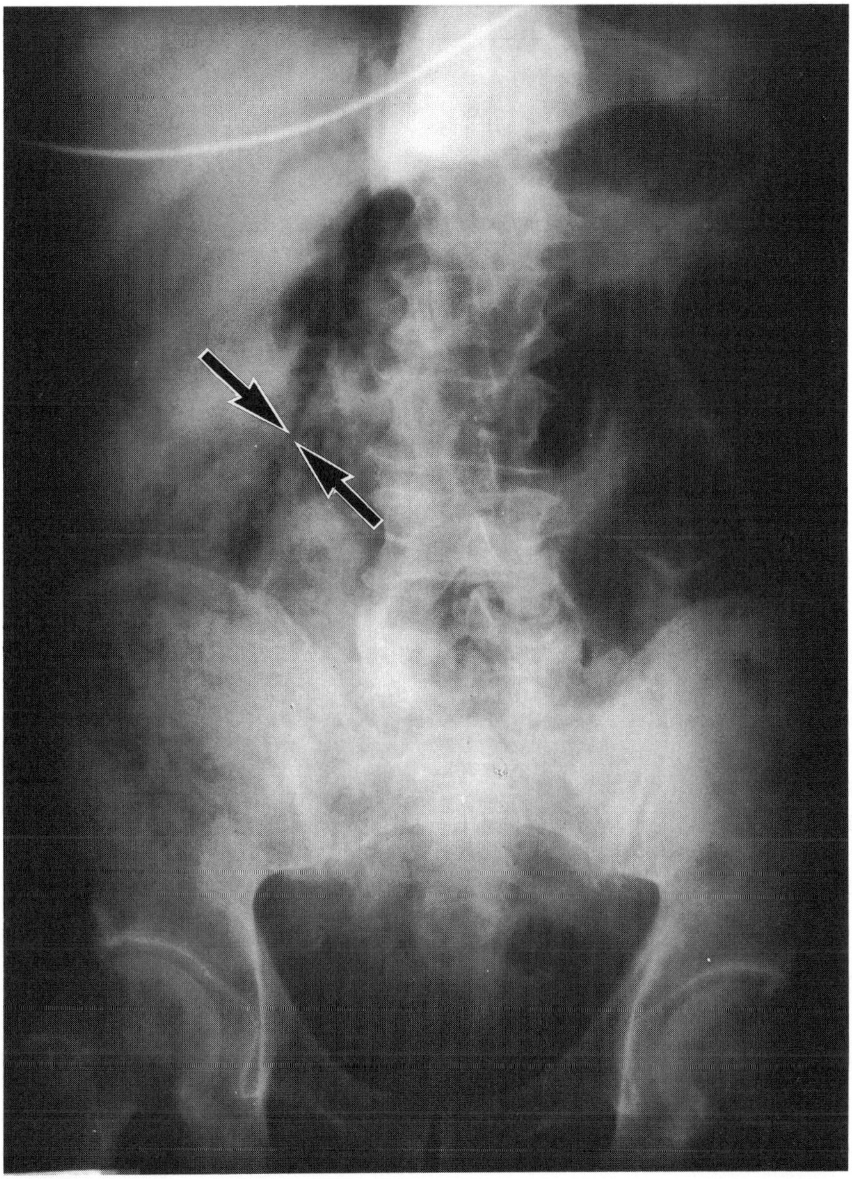

Figure 14.1.1 Retroperitoneal air from perforated duodenum, evidenced as air along a right psoas margin.

of retroperitoneal air around the duodenum (Fig. 14.1.1) or loss of psoas margin. For the most part, however, the KUB is of limited practical value for detecting blunt abdominal injuries.

In penetrating trauma, abdominal wounds should be marked with radiographic opaque markers, such as paper clips. The KUB may then provide useful

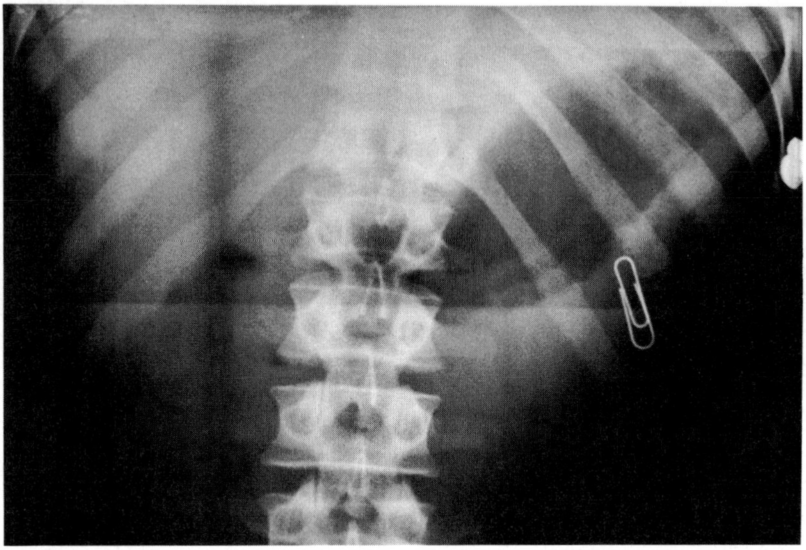

Figure 14.1.2 Bullet in abdomen with entrance wound marked by paper clip.

information regarding the possible trajectory of the projectile and organs injured. Gunshot wounds, in particular, should be marked as the number of missiles seen provides valuable information (Fig. 14.1.2). For example, a patient with two penetrating wounds to the abdomen may have sustained either a through-and-through single gunshot wound, two separate gunshot wounds with both bullets lodged in the abdomen or one bullet in the abdomen and another in the chest or thigh, or as a bullet embolus in the distal lower extremity. Occasionally, more missiles are found than predicted by the number of external wounds, which prompts a repeat, more thorough search for additional entrance sites. In the absence of fresh wounds, the presence of old scars or further questioning of the patient may reveal a prior history of an abdominal gunshot wound. Although the KUB can be extremely useful in diagnosing abdominal injury in patients with penetrating injuries, obtaining KUB results should never delay the patient in extremis from going to the operating threatre.

Contrast Radiographic Studies

Contrast radiography has an important role in the diagnosis of injury to intra-abdominal organs. While most of these studies can be performed after acute, life-threatening injuries have been identified or excluded, the one exception is the intravenous pyelogram (IVP).

Patients presenting in shock from ongoing intra-abdominal haemorrhage due to either blunt or penetrating trauma, with gross haematuria, should have a rapid IVP performed. The purpose of the IVP is to document the number and presence of functioning kidneys, prior to laparotomy, to enable the surgeon to better decide whether to remove or aggressively attempt salvage of an injured kidney. The patient is given 2 ml kg^{-1} contrast material and a KUB is obtained at 3–5 minutes after injection and again at 10–15 minutes if time allows. The patient in extremis may need to proceed to laparotomy prior to IVP. Once major haemorrhage has been controlled, however, an IVP should be performed on the operating table, if possible, prior to definitive management of renal injuries.

In the haemodynamically stable patient without urgent indications for laparotomy, further evaluation of the kidneys is indicated in all patients with gross haematuria and in those with microscopic haematuria of greater than 50 red blood cells (RBC) per high-powered field. Ideally, a formal IVP with tomograms should be performed in the radiological suite, which increases the accuracy of the test. However, many of the findings on formal IVP are non-specific and CT scan with contrast is more sensitive, specific and allows staging and non-operative management of the majority of renal injuries, including selected injuries from penetrating trauma.[17]

Other radiological studies that can be performed less urgently include the retrograde urethrogram and contrast cystogram. When the physical examination suggests urethral disruption, blood at the urethral meatus, scrotal haematoma, high-riding prostate or pubic symphysis fracture, a retrograde urethrogram must be performed before placement of a Foley catheter. If urethrogram results are normal, a cystogram should then be performed.[17]

Whenever there is suspicion of bladder injury, urethral injury or gross haematuria (blunt trauma), a cystogram should be performed. Cystograms are often routinely performed in patients with pelvic fracture, even in the absence of gross haematuria, because the degree of distortion of the bladder provides useful information regarding the size of the associated retroperitoneal haematoma (Fig. 14.1.3). An adequate cystogram requires 300 ml of contrast material instilled by gravity and two films, one with the bladder distended and one with the bladder empty. If 300 ml will not flow by gravity, then the contrast material should be gently infused with a syringe. Inadequate distension of the bladder can lead to missed injuries.[17]

While rarely indicated, abdominal arteriography may be useful in certain patients with isolated abdominal trauma. This procedure is frequently performed following studies such as aortic arch and pelvic arteriography for aortic rupture and severe pelvic fracture, respectively.[18] The coeliac and both renal arteries are cannulated and suitable arterial bleeders in the liver, spleen and kidney can be embolized.[18]

Computed Tomography

Computed tomography (CT) with oral and intravenous contrast is a non-invasive, relatively accurate method of delineating intra-abdominal injury, both

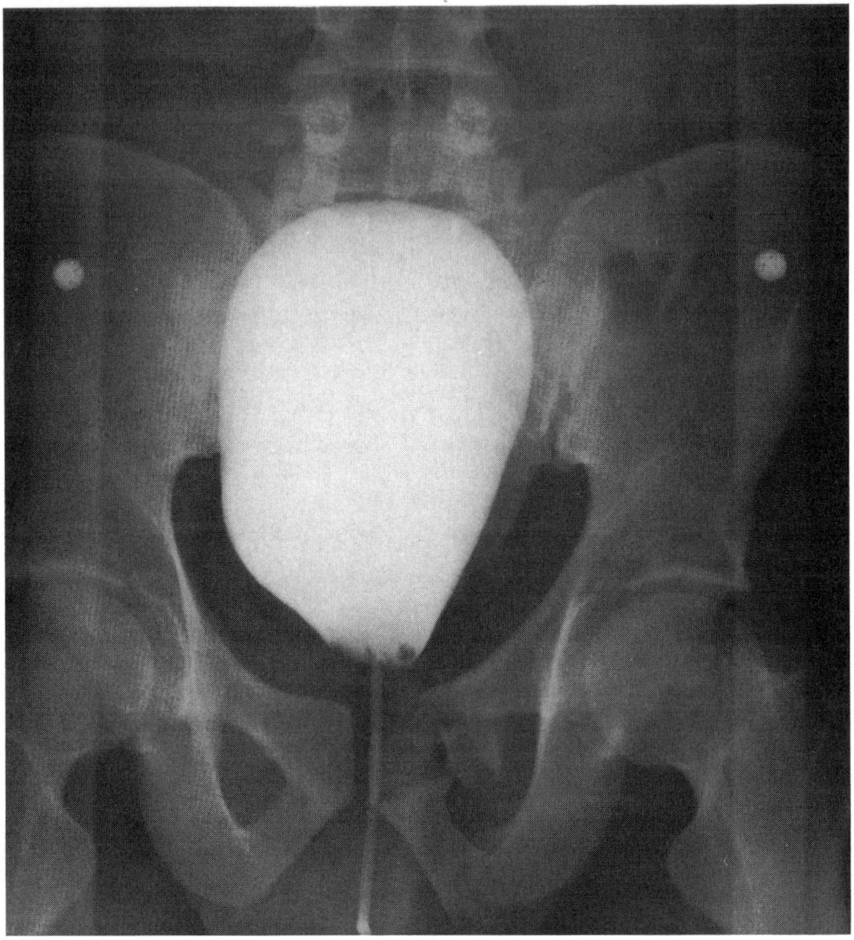

Figure 14.1.3 Retrograde cystogram in patient with pelvic fracture demonstrating "teardrop" distortion of bladder by the retroperitoneal haematoma.

by direct visualization of intra-abdominal solid and retroperitoneal organs and indirectly by demonstrating haemoperitoneum (Fig. 14.1.4).[19] CT scans are used for staging of renal, hepatic and splenic injuries, which allows selection of appropriate patients for non-operative management, although specific criteria for selection remain varied and controversial.

The fact that CT is not reliable for evaluating acute, hollow viscus injuries precludes its use in most penetrating trauma patients.[20] The exception is the possible retroperitoneal hollow viscus injury. Unlike diagnostic peritoneal lavage (DPL), the diagnostic accuracy of the CT scan is very dependent on the experience of the person interpreting the films.[21] Other drawbacks include the length of time required to perform and interpret the test, the fact that personnel must be diverted from the resuscitation area to transport and monitor the

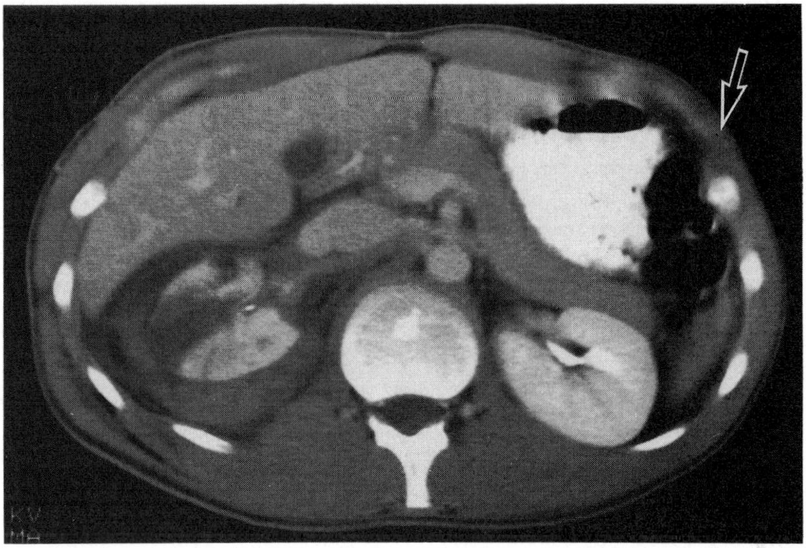

Figure 14.1.4 CT scan of the abdomen demonstrating a fractured right kidney, managed non-operatively with good results.

patient during the procedure and the problems that arise when a rapidly deteriorating trauma patient needs to be resuscitated in the CT suite.[22]

Use of the CT scan should be reserved for the haemodynamically stable patient with suspected intra-abdominal solid organ or retroperitoneal injury. The CT scan is particularly useful, and better than DPL, for identifying suspected retroperitoneal injury. CT scans are also indicated for stable patients in whom a relative contraindication to DPL exists, such as previous surgery.

Ultrasonography

Ultrasonography offers a rapid, non-invasive method of evaluating the abdomen for haemoperitoneum. While it can offer fairly sophisticated structural evaluations of many organs, this ability is very operator- and experience-dependent. In a recent study of use of ultrasonography by surgeons, the pericardium, the pouch of Douglas and the right and left upper abdominal quadrants were examined for the presence of fluid (Fig. 14.1.5).[23] Results of the study indicate that these four views are rapidly learned by surgeons and surgical residents, who may quickly, accurately and at the patient's bedside diagnose free fluid in these areas, thereby predicting intra-abdominal bleeding.[23] Sonograms are used extensively for abdominal evaluation in Europe, especially Germany,[24] and also in Japan[25] but they have not been widely adopted for this use in the United States because they fail to reliably identify hollow organ injuries with minimal bleeding; are highly dependent on operator ability and experience; and are

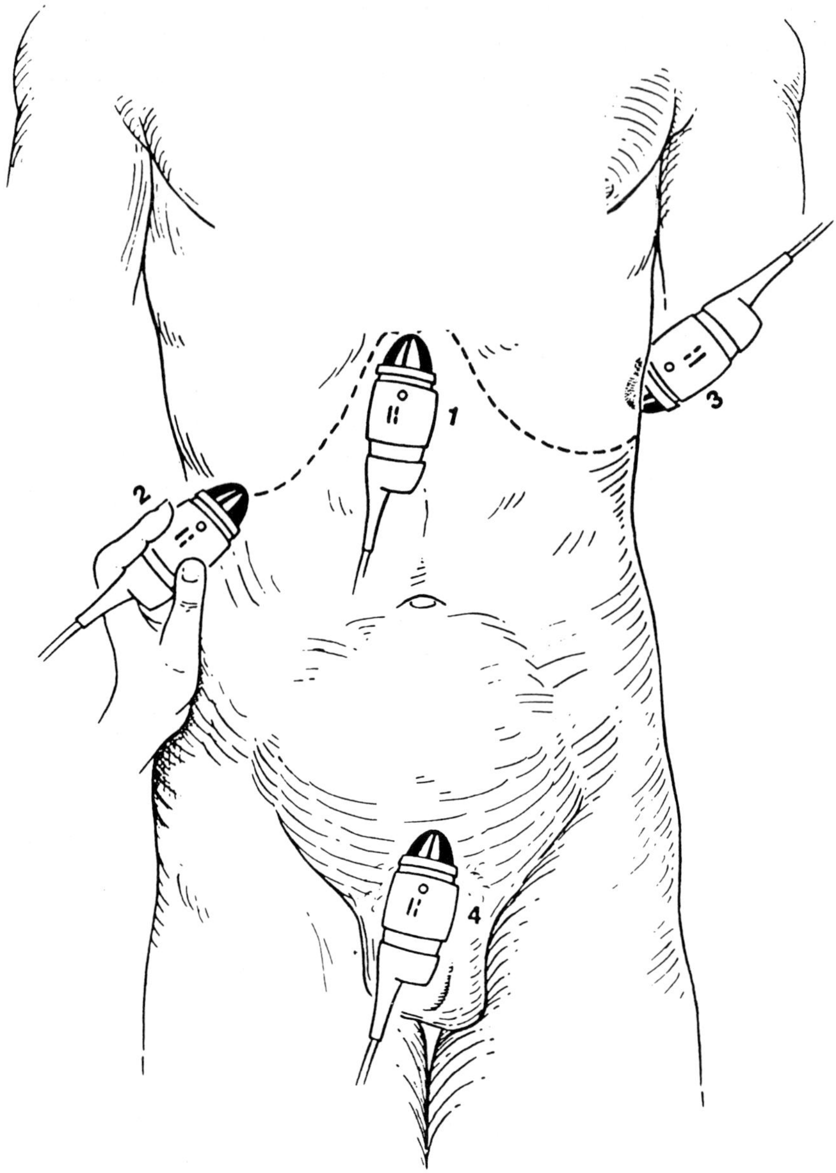

Figure 14.1.5 The four transducer positions for sonographic evaluation of the trauma patient.[23]

costly and not widely available in the resuscitation area of most trauma centres.[23]

One of the most useful roles for ultrasonography is in the patient with multiple injuries, either blunt or penetrating, with chest and abdominal wounds who presents in shock. Ultrasound enables the surgeon quickly to determine the site of the most severe blood loss. The absence of free fluid in the abdomen, for example, may allow the surgeon to concentrate first on the chest wounds, while detection of a large volume of fluid in the abdomen may prompt immediate laparotomy.

Diagnostic Peritoneal Lavage

Diagnostic peritoneal lavage (DPL) is rapid, reproducible and relatively easy to perform. It has become the cornerstone of the evaluation of abdominal trauma since it was popularized by Root[26] in 1965. DPL is indicated when the patient has a potential for abdominal injury due to mechanism, with no obvious indications for surgical exploration. This may occur when the patient is unconscious or performance of a reliable abdominal examination is not possible due to head or spinal injury or the presence of alcohol or drugs. DPL is also indicated if the physical examination cannot be repeated for an extended period (e.g. the patient must be anaesthetized for treatment of other injuries). DPL has a limited role in penetrating trauma, particularly in evaluating stab wounds where evidence of peritoneal violation is inconclusive. Patients who present in shock with no obvious source of blood loss should routinely undergo DPL to determine if the abdomen is the source.

Preparation for any DPL technique requires placement of urinary and gastric drainage catheters. Operation of the catheters should be verified and the bladder and stomach emptied prior to placement of the lavage catheter so that these organs are not injured.

To perform a DPL, a catheter is inserted into the peritoneal cavity by the open, semiopen or percutaneous technique. In adults, one litre (20 $ml\ kg^{-1}$ in children) of warmed crystalloid solution is instilled into the abdomen and allowed to return through the closed system. Evaluation of the return fluid may give evidence of an intra-abdominal injury that requires surgical intervention.

Open Technique

The open method usually requires a surgeon and assistant, and sterile preparation and draping. After placement of local anaesthesia, a 1–2 cm incision is made in the skin below the umbilicus (Fig. 14.1.6A) (unless there is an associated pelvic fracture that requires placement of the incision immediately above the umbilicus to avoid entering a preperitoneal haematoma that may be associated with the fracture). The incision is oriented vertically and such a distance from the umbilicus as to be easily incorporated into a midline incision if necessary. The incision is carried through to the peritoneum, which is tented, sharply opened and the catheter inserted oriented downward and posteriorly into the pelvis. This is the lowest portion of the abdominal cavity in the supine patient, so the lavage fluid will collect there for removal. A pursestring suture

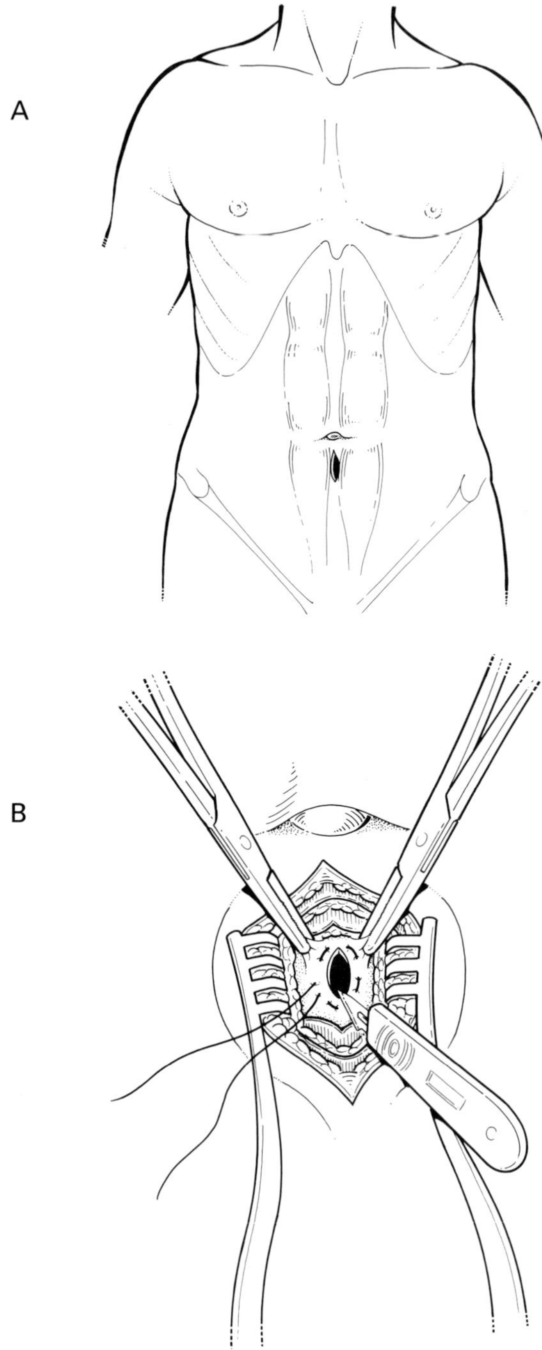

Figure 14.1.6 A: location of incision for DPL (open technique); B: Pursestring suture readied for placement of catheter.[54]

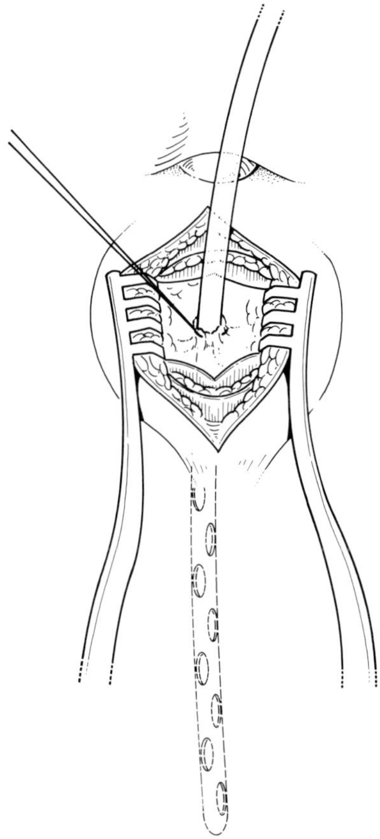

Figure 14.1.6 C: Pursestring suture secures catheter and closes the peritoneum.

secures the catheter into place and closes the peritoneum (Fig. 14.1.6B and C). The fluid is instilled by hanging the bag above the patient and allowing it to run in through standard intravenous tubing. While it is infusing, the rest of the incision is closed in layers around the catheter. When all of the fluid has been instilled, it is allowed to drain by gravity into the bag, which has been placed on the floor. Usually, once the incision is closed, the fluid has returned and the catheter can be withdrawn.

While the fluid is being instilled, the patient should be gently rocked from side to side and the bed tilted head up and head down to allow the fluid to wash freely through the abdomen; this ensures that there is no area of isolated bleeding that is not sampled. Return of all the fluid is the goal, which is seldom obtained, although returns of over 700 ml are common. If less than 300 ml returns, the catheter should be manipulated or replaced to obtain more fluid. The amount of urine return, drainage from chest tubes and gastric tubes should be monitored closely, because return of the fluid through these avenues indicates the need for surgery.

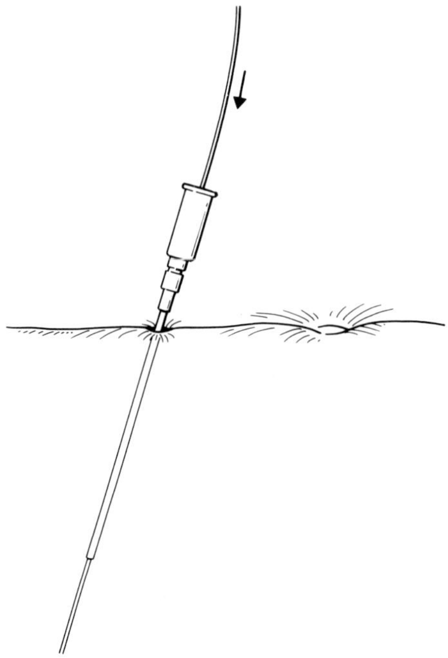

Figure 14.1.7 A: percutaneous placement of flexible-tipped wire through 18 gauge needle; B: placement of DPL catheter over flexible-tipped wire through skin nick.[54]

Percutaneous Technique

The percutaneous approach as described by Lazarus[27] involves placement of an 18 gauge needle through the abdominal wall into the peritoneal cavity in the same location as the other lavage methods. A guide wire with a flexible tip is placed through this needle and the needle is withdrawn (Fig. 14.1.7A). The lavage catheter is then placed over the wire through a small nick in the skin (Fig. 14.1.7B). This technique is *not* to be confused with a previous technique of placing the catheter *over* a larger, percutaneous trocar. The trocar method was associated with a higher complication rate than the open technique and has largely been abandoned. In contrast, the newer percutaneous DPL technique has been shown in several studies to have a low complication rate.[27,28] The percutaneous method offers the additional benefits of being faster, requiring a smaller sterile field and only one surgeon. If return of the fluid is slow with this method and does not respond to manipulation of the catheter, the original can be removed and a second placed, usually with prompt return of the fluid.

Semiopen Technique

The semiopen technique may incorporate portions of both other methods. It is essentially the same as the open method, except for the depth of the incision. The

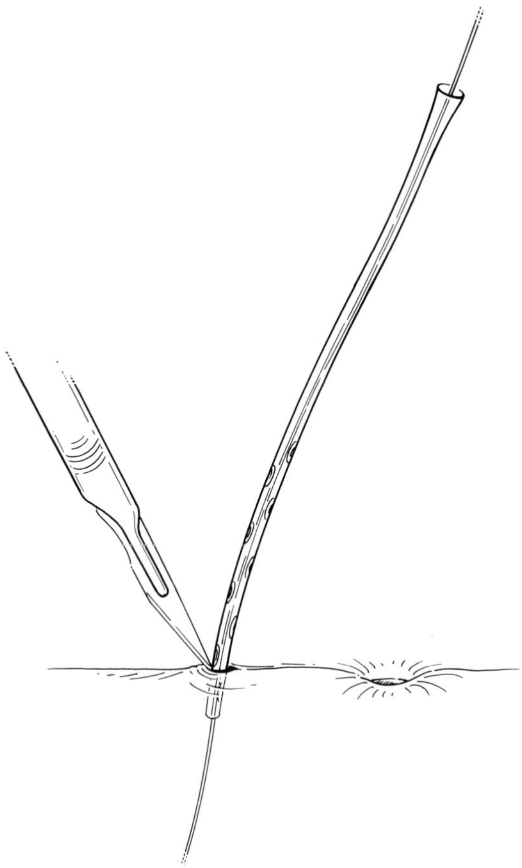

Figure 14.1.7 (B)

operator may stop at the fascia or the peritoneum, then use the needle and guide wire method to introduce the catheter. This is sometimes useful for a very obese patient for whom the small gauge needle is not long enough to penetrate through the peritoneum.[29]

For all techniques, return of more than 10 ml of gross blood on aspiration of the catheter is indication for abdominal exploration. The presence of more than 100 000 RBC/mm^3, more than 500 white blood cells/mm^3 or any amylase, bile, bacteria or food particles also may indicate the need for surgery (Table 14.1.3).

Some intestinal injuries do not bleed very much and may actually produce a "negative" lavage. Use of alkaline phosphatase (AP) as another marker for intestinal trauma has shown some promise in dog studies.[30] A recent evaluation of DPL fluid for AP levels greater than 10 ul^{-1} may predict intestinal injuries that would not otherwise have been suspected using the usual criteria for the evaluation of the lavage fluid.[31] These findings, however, have not been universal.[32] Currently, evaluation of AP should be limited to patients who have a high

Table 14.1.3 Evaluation of diagnostic peritoneal lavage fluid

Positive
Aspiration of 200 ml gross blood
$\geq$100 000 RBC ml^{-1} ($\geq$10 000 for penetrating)
$\geq$500 WBC ml^{-1}
Amylase higher than serum normal ($\geq$175 IU/100 ml)
Bile
Food particles
Bacteria on Gram stain
Intermediate
Aspiration of pink fluid
50 000–100 000 RBC ml^{-1}
100–500 WBC ml^{-1}
Amylase 75–175 IU/100 ml
Negative
Aspiration of clear fluid
$\leq$50 000 RBC ml^{-1}
$\leq$100 WBC ml^{-1}
Amylase $\leq$75 IU/100 ml

probability of intestinal injury, such as those with seatbelt bruises or stab wounds, in whom the lavage is otherwise negative.[31]

Use of DPL is absolutely contraindicated only in patients with other indications for immediate abdominal surgery. Relative contraindications include pregnancy and previous abdominal surgery with potential for adhesions. The open technique can still be used at other sites on the abdomen to avoid the uterus or previous surgical scars. This should be performed only by a very experienced member of the team. Computed tomography (CT) might be a better diagnostic method for patients with evidence of previous abdominal surgery.

Complications of DPL are reported in the range of 1–2%, depending on the technique, and include laceration of hollow viscera, bleeding from the abdominal wall, infusion of the fluid extraperitoneally and laceration of large and small vessels of the abdomen.

Accuracy is greater than 98%, with a false-negative rate in the range of 0.5–2% and a false-positive rate of about 1%.[33]

While the role of DPL in blunt trauma is well accepted, its role is less well defined in penetrating trauma. Penetrating trauma is more likely to cause hollow viscus injuries without much bleeding than is blunt trauma, so reliance on the same red blood cell (RBC) count for both types of injuries may lead to some missed injuries. There are reports that the accuracy of DPL for penetrating wounds of the abdomen has been improved by lowering the threshold from 100 000 RBC/mm^3 to anywhere from 50 000 to 2000 RBC/mm^3.[3,34] The concept of lowering the absolute number of RBCs that constitutes a positive DPL has been challenged in a prospective study that shows a low false-negative rate and a low non-therapeutic laparotomy rate using 100 000 RBC/mm^3.[35] The use of DPL in penetrating trauma must be coupled with an evaluation of the type of wound and an assessment by local exploration of its location and depth of penetration. These factors will be discussed more fully later in the chapter.

DPL results must be evaluated in the context of the entire clinical picture, especially for patients in the "indeterminate" lavage category who don't quite reach a "positive" level, but whose return fluid is not crystal clear.

While DPL accurately detects certain types of abdominal injury and has lowered the rate of missed injuries, some of the injuries detected require no surgical repair at exploration. These injuries are usually solid organ injuries that may, in fact, be extensive but have stopped bleeding by the time surgery is performed. It is to lower this rate of "non-therapeutic" laparotomies, which may be as high as 15%,[36] that other methods of ruling out injuries are sought.

Laparotomy

In some instances, the clinical suspicion of an occult injury is high enough that operative diagnostic techniques are mandated. The most thorough evaluation of the abdomen is still accomplished by the gold standard of the exploratory laparotomy. Only at open exploration may the surgeon see and palpate. The surgeon's decision to perform an open exploration, however, must weigh individual experience and the potential for delay associated with other, non-invasive methods. Although laparotomy may prolong the patient's recovery time by three to five days, this is preferable to missing a serious injury.

One argument against laparotomy has been the complication rate associated with negative explorations. Weigelt and Kingman[37] report complication rates of 22% in patients with no other injuries and 37% in those with other injuries for negative exploratory laparotomy. Over half of these were atelectasis. In those with no other injury, serious complications were only in the order of 5%, including a 2% wound infection rate. Long term follow-up revealed a 5% rate of small bowel obstruction, most of which were related to those patients who required extensive retroperitoneal dissection to exclude injury. The risk of significant complications from a negative laparotomy, therefore, is low and insignificant when compared with the complications that arise from missed injuries.

When the suspicion of injury is high enough with equivocal findings, abdominal exploration becomes an important part of the trauma surgeon's armamentarium.

Video Endoscopy

Due to major technological advances and the overwhelming international success of laparoscopic cholecystectomy, video assisted endoscopic surgical techniques are being applied to many traditionally open surgical procedures, including the diagnosis of torsal intracavitary injury. Although recently published reports describe mostly diagnostic, and some therapeutic, applications of this new technology, the exact role of laparoscopy and thoracoscopy in the trauma patients remains to be defined.

Laparoscopy

Laparoscopy was first described as a diagnostic modality in the injured patient by Gazzaniga in 1976.[38] Despite several subsequent reports of the efficiency of laparoscopy for evaluating the abdomen for injury,[39,40] this procedure was not seriously considered practical by the majority of surgeons until the breakthrough with laparoscopic cholecystectomy. Numerous reports have appeared in the literature in the past two or three years describing the experience of several individual institutions with diagnostic laparoscopy (DL).[41–44]

Most of the reported laparoscopic experience in trauma is anecdotal and there are few well-designed protocols that accurately compare this new technology with current standards of care. DL has been used in blunt and penetrating trauma patients,[39,41–44] under local[39,41,42] and general[43,44] anaesthesia, in the emergency department[39,41,42] and main operating suite,[43,44] acutely[39–43] and delayed[45] and as a diagnostic[39,41–45] and therapeutic[39,42,43,45] modality. Most authors report favourable results and cite reductions in the negative and non-therapeutic laparotomy rate at their institutions when DL was used in place of, or in addition to, conventional diagnostic modalities. Only one study has prospectively compared DL with DPL as a diagnostic modality in a mixed blunt/penetrating trauma population.[41] The authors demonstrated that DL could be performed safely under local anaesthesia, in the emergency department, in the majority of their patients, although they concluded that DL offered no advantages over DPL as a primary diagnostic tool for abdominal trauma except for patients with anterior abdominal stab wounds. This experience emphasizes the need for well-designed clinical trials to determine the role of DL in the evaluation of the patient with abdominal trauma.

Complications associated with DL in trauma patients include tension pneumothorax, iatrogenic bowel injury, insufflation of the preperitoneal space and missed injuries.[39,41–44] Reported theoretical concerns include respiratory difficulty with insufflation in awake, non-intubated patients, increased PCO_2, increased risk of deep venous thrombosis secondary to impaired venous return from the pneumoperitoneum, gas embolus via lacerated intra-abdominal vessels and increased intracranial pressures in head injured patients (again from the pneumoperitoneum).[42]

Based on review of the current literature, indications for DL in the trauma patient include:

1. documentation of the presence of peritoneal penetration in selected patients with stab wounds to the anterior abdomen and flanks;

2. documentation of the presence of peritoneal penetration in selected patients with tangential gunshot wounds to the abdomen;
3. blunt trauma with equivocal DPL or CT scan findings;
4. evaluation of the diaphragm in blunt and penetrating trauma.

Reported therapeutic uses of DL that show promise for the future include diaphragmatic repair, haemostasis of minor hepatic and splenic injuries and salvage and reinfusion of intra-abdominal blood from patients undergoing non-operative management of solid organ injury.[39,42,43,45]

Thoracoscopy

Although thoracoscopy was developed by Swedish surgeon Jacobaeus in 1910[46], the first use of the technique in trauma patients was documented by Branco in 1946.[47] Prior to the advent of video assisted thoracoscopy (VAT), there were only five series reported in the literature of experience with thoracoscopy in the trauma patient. In 1993, Ochsner *et al.* reported on the use of thoracoscopy in the diagnosis of diaphragmatic injury in penetrating trauma patients.[48] Further, VAT has been used recently to evacuate retained haemothoraces following blunt and penetrating trauma.[48,49]

Complications reported with VAT in trauma patients include ventricular ectopy with manipulation of the heart, empyema and postoperative bleeding from a non-iatrogenic lung laceration.[48] Concerns include the preference for a double lumen tube, the requirement for general anaesthesia and the risk of gas embolus if insufflation is used to accelerate lung collapse.

At the present time, diagnosing injury to the diaphragm and evacuation of retained haemothoraces are established indications for VAT in the trauma patient. While VAT does provide a better view of the posterior recesses of the diaphragm than DL, VAT requires tube thoracoscopy drainage, which could represent an additional source of morbidity in patients without a haemo/pneumothorax from the injury.

Future applications of VAT include control of chest wall bleeding, diaphragmatic repair, evaluation of the mediastinum in penetrating trauma patients and endoscopic stapling of lung lacerations. As in DL, well-designed clinical trials to evaluate and compare VAT with current conventional diagnostic and therapeutic modalities are necessary before the exact role of VAT can be established.

DECISION POINT

The process of initial assessment and resuscitation, as described above, often reveals the need for abdominal exploration. Patients in shock with obvious abdominal injury should have abdominal surgery without delay, as should those with peritoneal signs, gross gastrointestinal blood loss or rectal or vaginal disruption on examination. In blunt trauma, patients in extremis without other apparent sources of blood loss, even without obvious abdominal injury, should undergo exploration without delay. In penetrating trauma, those with obvious entry into the abdomen from a gunshot wound should undergo exploratory laparotomy.

Of these patients who remain, there are some who may require abdominal operation but the indications are not clear. These include unstable blunt trauma patients that have other potential sources of blood loss (pelvic fractures, long bone fractures) and an equivocal examination; and stable patients with potential abdominal injury (based on mechanism) who, due to head injury, alcohol or drugs, have an unreliable examination or who will be lost to examination by having to undergo anaesthesia for repair of other injuries.

In the penetrating trauma group, there are stable patients in whom the trajectory and location of the wound suggest that there may not have been penetration of the abdomen. Some stab wounds, while penetrating the abdomen, may cause no intra-abdominal injury. However, approximately half of the patients who are stable and have intra-abdominal injuries from stab wounds will have a normal abdominal examination.[50]

Some areas of the abdomen offer special challenges in diagnosis. The thoracoabdominal region is that region protected by the ribs but is variably abdomen and thorax depending on the motions of the diaphragm. Injuries in this area (from the nipple line to the umbilicus anteriorly and from the tip of the scapula to the rib margin posteriorly), especially penetrating injuries, may damage organs of either or both areas. The retroperitoneal organs are separated from the rest of the abdomen and may be injured without peritoneal findings, leading to delayed diagnosis with catastrophic results. Pancreatic injuries, for example, may be quite severe and present with no obvious peritoneal findings due to the retroperitoneal position of that organ. The sequelae of a missed pancreatic injury can be devastating.

To determine which patients require abdominal exploration, further tests must be performed.

AUTHORS' APPROACH

In an effort to avoid missing injuries and performing negative or non-therapeutic laparotomies, we use the following approaches that combine experience and clinical data.

Any patient who presents with abdominal trauma and is haemodynamically unstable, despite initial efforts to resuscitate according to the "ABC" approach elucidated in the Advanced Trauma Life Support (ATLS) curriculum,[11] should be taken directly to the operating room for abdominal exploration.

Blunt Trauma

Haemodynamically stable blunt trauma patients with obvious peritoneal signs should undergo exploratory laparotomy. Those at risk for abdominal injury and an equivocal examination due to unconsciousness or the presence of drugs or alcohol, or who will be lost to examination because they will receive anaesthesia for another reason, usually undergo DPL to rule out other injuries. Ultrasonography also may prove to be a reliable method in this situation. If the DPL is negative, but there is still a high suspicion for retroperitoneal injury (e.g. gross haematoma), a CT scan may be obtained, otherwise the patient remains under observation in the hospital. CT scans generally are substituted for DPLs when there is evidence of previous abdominal surgery or retroperitoneal injury. A CT scan demonstrating free fluid or an injury is a clear mandate for exploration. Occasionally, CT will demonstrate a solid organ (liver, kidney or spleen) injury, which may be followed non-operatively provided there is no other evidence of injury.

A difficult subset of blunt trauma patients with multiple injuries are those with pelvic fractures. While these patients may have significant ongoing bleeding from their fractures, they may not have an intra-abdominal injury requiring surgery. Whether their continued blood loss originates from the fracture or from an abdominal injury must be rapidly determined. If there is evidence of urethral injury, a retrograde urethrogram can be quickly accomplished; if the results are normal, then a cystogram is performed. If the cystogram reveals an intraperitoneal bladder injury, then laparotomy is performed for repair, if urethral or extraperitoneal bladder injuries are identified or placement of a suprapubic catheter is necessary. If both results are normal, an IVP can be quickly obtained while a sonogram or supraumbilical DPL is performed. Should these show no evidence of injury, then the fracture is stabilized. If bleeding continues subsequent to fracture stabilization, then an arteriogram with embolization of bleeding vessels is performed.

Using such a combined approach, the non-therapeutic laparotomy rate for blunt trauma patients may be as low as 5%.[36]

Penetrating Trauma

Patients with obvious injury manifested by peritoneal signs, protruding abdominal contents, gastrointestinal bleeding from nasogastric tube or rectum or bleeding from the vagina or urinary tract should undergo exploratory laparotomy. If there is evidence, from urinary bleeding or wound trajectory, that suggests the kidneys may have been injured, a rapid IVP should be obtained.

Gunshot Wounds

Patients with gunshot wounds to the abdomen should undergo exploratory laparotomy.

Some abdominal gunshot wounds may be tangential, with the physical examination revealing a low probability that the peritoneum was entered; these may be evaluated with local wound exploration. If lack of penetration cannot be demonstrated, then those with anterior wounds should have exploratory laparotomy. Because DPL is inaccurate in these patients,[51] laparoscopy may be used, with exploratory laparotomy following evidence that the projectile penetrated the peritoneum. Tangential flank and back wounds may be evaluated with contrast CT, including colonic contrast, to evaluate for retroperitoneal injury. Often, the path of the projectile may be traced by the injured tissue seen on the CT scan and shown to clearly avoid any major structures. Flank wounds anterior to the posterior axillary line may be evaluated with laparoscopy. The patient should undergo exploratory laparotomy if injury cannot be absolutely excluded by these methods. Patients sustaining high velocity wounds to the abdomen should have abdominal exploration regardless of evidence of penetration due to the shock waves that may cause intraperitoneal injury without actually penetrating the peritoneum.

Stab Wounds

Patients with stab wounds and peritoneal signs, prolapse of abdominal contents or obvious organ injury (such as blood in the urine) should undergo operative exploration. Those who are asymptomatic should undergo a local exploration of the wound under local anaesthesia to ascertain if there is entry into the peritoneal cavity. If the end of the tract can be clearly visualized and does not enter the abdomen, then the patient may be observed overnight and discharged. The approach to those patients in whom the end of the tract cannot be seen should be determined somewhat by the location of the stab wound.

A selective approach, as outlined below, can be expected to reduce the non-therapeutic laparotomy rate to about 7%, with minimal morbidity.[52]

Anterior Abdominal Wounds

DPL may be used to determine that there is no major internal injury, using either the standard red blood cell count[50] or a number in the range of 1000–50 000 RBC ml^{-1}.[34] While each of these reports suggests a low negative exploration rate (approximately 5%), a missed injury rate of about 4% and minimal morbidity (about 2%), some hollow viscus injuries still may be missed with potentially devastating results. We use a cut-off level of 10 000 RBC ml^{-1}; above this level, we perform operative exploration of the abdomen. Laparoscopy has been useful in some of these cases to demonstrate whether the peritoneum was penetrated, followed by exploration for those with penetration.

Flank Wounds

Flank wounds are treated in much the same way as anterior abdominal wounds. The major exception is that, because the retroperitoneal portions of the colon may be injured more easily without any indication in DPL, there is a lower threshold to explore these patients. Mobilization of the colon via laparoscopy may adequately expose the site of potential injury without formal laparotomy and CT with colonic contrast can also be used safely in these patients.[53]

Back Wounds

Back wounds are less likely to enter the abdomen than other types of wounds but when they do, they are more likely to cause retroperitoneal injuries without positive findings on abdominal examination or DPL. Back wounds, based on location, the size of the wound and the weapon, may be observed or further evaluated via CT with colonic contrast.

Thoracoabdominal Wounds

Thoracoabdominal wounds may cause injury to the diaphragm with minimal bleeding. The suspicion must be high to detect these injuries. If left unrepaired, the associated long term morbidity may be considerable. In patients with pneumothorax, we have found thoracoscopy very useful in evaluating the diaphragm. If there is an injury to the diaphragm, we proceed to laparotomy.[48]

If the patient does not have a pneumothorax, we perform a laparoscopy to exclude a diaphragmatic injury. If such an injury is present, a formal laparotomy is performed unless we can demonstrate a single injury in an underlying solid organ that is not bleeding.

SUMMARY

Many diagnostic means are at the disposal of the surgeon to evaluate patients with abdominal trauma. Because there is no one method that will always help the surgeon know when and when not to operate, the surgeon must always be aware of the strengths and weakness of each. Patient history, physical examination and the results of each adjunctive test must be taken into account. While objective criteria need to be used and carefully considered, a rigid application of the "cut-off" numbers of certain tests cannot be universally applied. A thoughtful application of the above methods to the trauma patient should lead to a non-therapeutic laparotomy rate of about 7%, with minimal missed injuries and morbidity.

Video laparoscopy and thoracoscopy may soon offer new ways of determining when and when not to operate. These advances will probably be in the areas of indeterminate lavage and thoracoabdominal injuries. Laparoscopy/thoracoscopy is very operator-dependent, however, so care will have to be taken when defining the areas in which it may be used, to avoid inadequate evaluation fuelled by positive reports of its use.

REFERENCES

1. Mullins RJ, Trunkey DD. Samuel D. Gross: pioneer academic trauma surgeon of 19th century America. *J Trauma* 1990; **30**: 528 38.
2. Wisner DH. General assessment of penetrating and blunt abdominal trauma. In: *Abdominal Trauma*, 2nd edition (eds Blaisdell FW, Trunkey DD.), pp. 1–12. Stuttgart, Thieme; 1993.
3. Geoghegan T, Brush B. The mechanism of intestinal perforation from non-penetrating abdominal trauma. *Arch Surg* 1957; **73**: 455.
4. Salander JM, Bingham R. Mechanisms of force in trauma. In: *Current Therapy of Trauma* (eds Trunkey DD, Lewis FR.), pp. 44–6. Philadelphia, BC Decker, 1991.
5. Horowitz MD, Dove DB, Eismont FJ, Green BA. Impalement injuries. *J Trauma* 1985; **25**: 914–16.
6. Demuth WE. Bullet velocity and design as determinants of wounding capability: an experimental study. *J Trauma* 1966; **6**: 222.
7. Jorden GL, Beall AC. Diagnosis and management of abdominal trauma. *Curr Prob Surg* 1971; 5–7.
8. Sherman RT, Parrish RA. Management of shotgun injuries: a review of 152 cases. *J Trauma* 1963; **3**: 76.
9. Trunkey DD, Hill AC, Schecter WP. Abdominal trauma and indications for celiotomy. In: *Trauma* (eds Moore EE, Mattox KL, Feliciano DV.), p. 416. Norwalk, Appleton and Lange, 1991.
10. Olsen WR, Hildreth OH. Abdominal paracentesis and peritoneal lavage in blunt abdominal trauma. *J Trauma* 1971; **11**: 824.
11. Advanced Trauma Life Support Course, p. 15. American College of Surgeons, 1989.
12. Teasdale G, Jennett B. Assessment of coma and impaired consciousness. A practical scale. *Lancet* 1974; **2**: 81.
13. Asbun HJ, Irani H, Roe EJ, Bloch JH. Intra-abdominal seatbelt injury. *J Trauma* 1990; **30**: 189–93.
14. Trunkey DD, Sheldon DF, Collins JA. The treatment of shock. In: *The Management of Trauma* (eds Zuidema GD, Rutherford RB, Ballinger WF.), p. 106. Philadelphia, WB Saunders, 1985.
15. Dixon CM, McAninch JW, Carroll PR. Urethral and bladder injuries. In: *Abdominal Trauma*, 2nd edition (eds Blaisdell FW, Trunkey DD.), p. 280. Stuttgart, Thieme, 1993.
16. Shackford SR. Initial management of patients with multiple injuries. Prob Crit Care 1987; **1**: 550–8.
17. Carroll PR, Dixon CM, McAninch JW. The management of renal and ureteral trauma. In: *Abdominal Trauma*, 2nd edition (eds Blaisdell FW, Trunkey DD.), pp. 250–76. Stuttgart Thieme, 1993.
18. Ben-Menachem Y, Fisher RG. Radiology. In: *Trauma* (eds Moore EE, Mattox KL, Feliciano DV.), Norwalk, Appleton and Lange, 1991. 195–217.
19. Peitzman AB, Makaroun MS, Slasky BS, Ritter P. Prospective study of computed tomography in initial management of blunt abdominal trauma. *J Trauma* 1986; **26**: 585–92.
20. Marx JA, Moore EE, Jorden RC, Eule J. Limitations of computed tomography in the evaluation of acute abdominal trauma: a prospective comparison with diagnostic peritoneal lavage. *J Trauma* 1985; **25**: 933–7.

21. Fabian TC, Mangiante EC, White TJ, Patterson CR, Boldreghini S, Britt LG. A prospective study of 91 patients undergoing both computed tomography and peritoneal lavage following blunt abdominal trauma. *J Trauma* 1986; **26**: 602–8.
22. Wisner DH, Danto LA. Peritoneal lavage, computerized tomography, angiography, ultrasound and magnetic resonance imaging. In: *Abdominal Trauma* 2nd edition (eds Blaisdell FW, Trunkey DD.), pp. 32–56. Stuttgart, Thieme, 1993.
23. Rozycki GS, Ochsner MG, Jaffin JH, Champion HR, Dinsmore BJ, Maxwell D. Prospective study of ultrasound evaluation in trauma patients. *J Trauma* 1993; **34**: 516–27.
24. Röthlin MA, Näf R, Amgwerd M, Candinas D, Frick T, Trentz O. Ultrasound in blunt abdominal trauma and thoracic trauma. *J Trauma* 1993; **34**: 488–95.
25. Kimura A, Otsuka T. Emergency center ultrasonography in the evaluation of hemoperitoneum: a prospective study. *J Trauma* 1991; **31**: 20.
26. Root HD, Hauser CW, McKinley CR, LaFave JW, Mendiola RP Jr. Diagnostic peritoneal lavage. *Surgery* 1965; **57**: 633–7.
27. Lazarus HM, Nelson JA. A technique for peritoneal lavage without risk or complication. *Surg Gynecol Obstet* 1979; **149**: 889–92.
28. Lopez-Viego MA, Mickel TJ, Weigelt JA. Open versus closed diagnostic peritoneal lavage in the evaluation of abdominal trauma. *Am J Surg* 1990; **160**: 594–7.
29. Ochsner MG, Herr D, Drucker W, Champion HR. A modified Seldinger technique for peritoneal lavage in trauma patients who are obese. *Surg Gynecol Obstet* 1991; **173**: 158–60.
30. Marx JA, Moore EE, Bar-Or D. Peritoneal lavage in penetrating injuries of the small bowel and colon: value of enzyme determinations. *Ann Emerg Med* 1983; **12**: 68–70.
31. Jaffin JH, Ochsner MG, Cole FJ, Rozycki GS, Champion HR. Alkaline phosphatase levels in diagnostic peritoneal lavage as a predictor of hollow visceral injury. Louisville, Abstracts of the American Association for the Surgery of Trauma, 1992, p. 32.
32. Megison SM, Weigelt JA. The value of alkaline phosphatase in peritoneal lavage. *Ann Emerg Med* 1990; **19**: 503–5.
33. Fischer RP, Beverlin BC, Engrave LH, Benjamin CI, Perry JF. Diagnostic peritoneal lavage. Fourteen years and 2586 patients later. *Am J Surg* 1978; **136**: 701–4.
34. Oreskovich MR, Carrico CJ. Stab wounds of the anterior abdomen: analysis of a management plan using local wound exploration and quantitative peritoneal lavage. *Ann Surg* 1983; **198**: 411–19.
35. Thal ER. Evaluation of peritoneal lavage and local wound exploration in lower chest and abdominal stab wounds. *J. Trauma* 1977; **17**: 642–650.
36. Sorkey AJ, Farnell MB, Williams HJ, Mucha P, Ilstrup DM. The complementary roles of diagnostic peritoneal lavage and computed tomography in the evaluation of blunt abdominal trauma. *Surgery* 1989; **106**: 794–801.
37. Weigelt JA, Kingman RG. Complications of negative laparotomy for trauma. *Am J Surg* 1988; **156**: 544–7.
38. Gazzaniga AB, Stanton WW, Bartlett RH. Laparoscopy in the diagnosis of blunt and penetrating injuries to the abdomen. *Am J Surg* 1976; **131**: 315.
39. Berci G. Elective and emergent laparoscopy. *World J Surg* 1993; **17**: 8–15.
40. Carnevale N, Baron N, Delaney HM. Peritoneoscopy as an aid in the diagnosis of abdominal trauma: a preliminary report. *J Trauma* 1977; **17**: 634–41.
41. Salvino CK, Esposito TJ, Marshall WJ, Dries DJ, Morris RC, Gamelli RL. The role of diagnostic laparoscopy in the management of trauma patients: a preliminary assessment. *J Trauma* 1993; **34**: 506–15.
42. Sackier JM. Laparoscopy in the emergency setting. *World J Surg* 1992; **16**: 1083–8.
43. Fabian TC, Croce MA, Stewart RM, Pritchard FE, Minard G, Kudsk KA. A prospective analysis of diagnostic laparoscopy in trauma. *Ann Surg* 1993; **217**: 555–565.

44. Ivatury RR, Simon RJ, Weksler B, Bayard V, Stahl WM. Laparoscopy in the evaluation of the intrathoracic abdomen after penetrating injury. *J Trauma* 1992; **33**: 101–9.
45. Smith RS, Meister RK, Tsoi EKM, Bohman HR. Laparoscopically guided blood salvage and autotransfusion in splenic trauma: a case report. *J Trauma* 1993; **34**: 313–14.
46. Jacobaeus HC. Possibility of the use of the cystoscope for investigation of serous cavities. *Munch Med Wochenschr* 1910; **57**: 2090.
47. Branco JMC. Thoracoscopy as a method of exploration in penetrating injuries of the chest. *Dis Chest* 1946; **12**: 330.
48. Ochsner MG, Rozycki GS, Lucente F, Wherry DC, Champion HR. Prospective evaluation of thoracoscopy for diagnosing diaphragmatic injury in penetrating thoracoabdominal trauma: a preliminary report. *J Trauma* 1993; **34**: 704–10.
49. Mancini M, Smith LM, Nein A, Buechter KJ. Early evacuation of clotted blood in hemothorax using thoracoscopy: case reports. *J Trauma* 1993; **34**: 144–7.
50. Feliciano DV, Bitondos CG, Steed G, Mattox KL, Burch JM, Jordan GL. Five hundred open taps or lavage in patients with abdominal stab wounds. *Am J Surg* 1984; **148**: 772–7.
51. Thal ER, May RA, Beesinger D. Peritoneal lavage. Its unreliability in gunshot wounds of the lower chest and abdomen. *Arch Surg* 1980; **115**: 430–433.
52. Jackson GL, Thal ER. Stab to back and flank. *J Trauma* 1979; **19**: 660–667.
53. Phillis T, Sclafani SJA, Goldstein A, Scalea T, Panetta T, Shaftan G. Use of the contrast-enhanced CT enema in the management of penetrating trauma to the flank and back. *J Trauma* 1986; **26**: 593–601.
54. Rozycki GS, Paul BK. Diagnostic peritoneal lavage. In: *Rob & Smith's Operative Surgery, Part 1*, 4th edition (eds Champion HR, Robbs JV, Trunkey DD.), pp. 27–33. London, Butterworths, 1989.

14.2

Laparoscopy in Abdominal Trauma

A. NAGY and M. SUTTER

INTRODUCTION

Since its introduction in 1901 by Kelling,[1] laparoscopy has not enjoyed widespread acceptance in the general surgical community but with the advent of laparoscopic cholecystectomy and other minimally invasive procedures, diagnostic laparoscopy has become more popular in the last few years.[2] It is therefore not surprising that laparoscopy is now being considered by more general surgeons for the evaluation of the patient with abdominal trauma, whether sustained by blunt or penetrating forces. It seems likely that the role of diagnostic and therapeutic laparoscopy in trauma patients will be subjected to close scrutiny in future years but we must be careful that the enthusiasm generated by other laparoscopic techniques does not lead to a promotion of laparoscopy in trauma patients in an unsafe and unreasonable way.[3,4] Laparoscopy must undergo prospective study to enable comparison with existing and established methods of evaluation.

The goals of this chapter are to provide an overview of the controversies surrounding the evaluation of the traumatized abdomen, to discuss the technique of laparoscopy as applied specifically to the evaluation of abdominal trauma, to outline the indications and contraindications of the procedure and to discuss the published data promoting laparoscopy as a safe alternative for evaluating the injured abdomen.

HISTORY AND CONTROVERSIES

The assessment of the injured abdomen is one of the most challenging tasks that the general surgeon faces and is particularly difficult in blunt injury of the multiply injured patient, in whom the clinical picture may be clouded by mental obtundation, alcohol or drugs. Such patients face a number of potentially life-threatening injuries and almost 10% of the injuries in civilian practice that require operative exploration are the result of blunt abdominal trauma.[5] Initial assessment must be followed by quick diagnostic procedures and prompt therapy to correct potentially life-threatening problems. The situation differs from penetrating trauma where the decision to operate may be easier to make. Many surgeons in the past decided on the "safe course" and proceeded to exploratory laparotomy when there was a strong suspicion of major intra-abdominal injuries following blunt abdominal trauma.

Due to the excessive number of negative laparotomies in this setting, Root *et al.*[6] promoted diagnostic peritoneal lavage (DPL) and the technique has become firmly established in the armamentarium of the general surgeon. If peritoneal lavage yielded a frankly bloody fluid, it was recommended that surgical exploration be undertaken. If the fluid had a red blood cell count in excess of 100 000/mm^3 and a white blood cell count over 5000/mm^3, the patient required laparotomy. It is, however, possible that the use of these criteria may lead to exploration in a significant number of patients whose intra-abdominal injuries are stable and in whom bleeding has stopped. The patient may therefore undergo an unnecessary laparotomy which adds further to the overall morbidity, particularly when there are associated multiple injuries.

In an attempt to reduce the negative exploration rate at laparotomy, a handful of surgeons worldwide began to employ laparoscopy for diagnosis of intra-abdominal injuries. Notably, Tostivint[7] in France and Heselson[8] in South Africa promoted laparoscopy for evaluation of trauma in the 1960s. Gomel, a gynaecologist in Vancouver, Canada, recommended its use in general surgery and also specifically for blunt abdominal trauma and multiple trauma victims in the 1970s.[9] Gazzaniga[10] of California echoed the recommendation for the use of laparoscopy in the diagnosis of blunt and penetrating injuries to the abdomen. Berci[11] also enthusiastically promoted this technique and modified the procedure by undertaking it in the emergency room with a minilaparoscope. Cohen[12] employed laparoscopy for diagnosis in six patients who sustained abdominal trauma from penetrating injury in three and blunt injury in the remainder. It must be recognized that there are few contraindications to diagnostic peritoneal lavage and complications are extremely rare.[13]

In the 1980s, the less invasive techniques of ultrasonography and CT scans were introduced. The criteria for the use of these techniques were similar to those of peritoneal lavage, being employed in the stable patient with possible intra-abdominal injuries from blunt trauma. The advantages of these techniques were that they were non-invasive, they could assess the organs suspected of being injured and some degree of quantitation of free fluid within the peritoneal cavity could be inferred. They could also be repeated without any apparent harm to the patient if non-operative management was chosen.[14]

During this era of enthusiasm for CT scanning, ultrasound and peritoneal lavage, laparoscopy was not under serious consideration by most surgeons. Indeed, during this period any attempt to promote laparoscopy as a valuable tool in the evaluation of abdominal trauma met with considerable criticism and scepticism.[15] Critics of the laparoscopic technique stated that laparoscopy was an incomplete examination which did not allow the surgeon to assess accurately the retroperitoneum and incompletely assessed possible pancreaticoduodenal injuries. In addition, the monocular vision obtained with a small laparoscope confused most general surgeons who were used to wide exposure and handling of the intra-abdominal organs.

With the arrival of video laparoscopy and the successful introduction of laparoscopic cholecystectomy, some surgeons were willing to reconsider this modality of diagnosis. Other surgeons in smaller centres had continued to use laparoscopy throughout this period. (Pereles, Thunder Bay, Ontario, personal communications). These surgeons did not often have the benefit of expert radiologists to interpret CT findings, if CT scanners were available. In a recent publication of the *Surgical Clinics of North America* (Vol. 71, No. 2. 1992), devoted to a discussion of "contemporary problems in trauma surgery", no mention is made of the use of laparoscopy, so the proponents of the technique will have considerable difficulty in collecting enough data to persuade centres of its value in the evaluation of abdominal trauma.

TECHNIQUE OF LAPAROSCOPY IN ABDOMINAL TRAUMA

The technique of laparoscopy is fully discussed in an earlier chapter in this book. Certain points which are applicable to abdominal trauma deserve emphasis and close attention to detail is mandatory if the examination is to prove fruitful.

Laparoscopy must be performed under full sterile precautions. The patient must be haemodynamically stable and an airway must be secured. A nasogastric tube and a Foley catheter should be in place, although this is common practice in the multiply injured patient arriving in our trauma unit. Adequate intravenous lines must be in place and the patient must be co-operative and cannot be combative. This is particularly important if the examination is to be carried out under local anaesthetic and with intravenous sedation. The patient must lie on an operating table that affords mobility to facilitate the positioning of the patient for the various aspects of the examination. To examine the left upper quadrant, a right side decubitus position is desirable. A head down position may be more useful to examine the pelvis.

The safe establishment of pneumoperitoneum is of paramount importance for a successful completion of the examination. Irrespective of whether the Veress needle or the open Hasson method is employed, previous abdominal scars must be carefully avoided. Nitrous oxide may be more desirable for insufflation if the examination is to be performed under local anaesthesia since carbon dioxide is more irritating to the peritoneal lining. Instrumentation and equipment must be in good working order. An adequate light source, suction apparatus and accessory instrumentation are essential.

Perhaps the major reason for the unpopularity of laparoscopy in the past was the unavailability of video laparoscopic equipment. The surgeon was required to hold the laparoscope in one hand and use a palpating probe or grasping forceps or suction device in the other to achieve adequate exposure. With the older technique the surgeon often had to infer possible injury by accumulation of blood in the vicinity of an organ without actual visualization of the site of injury. With the introduction of the video laparoscope both hands of the surgeon are freed and grasping forceps can be applied through accessory ports to manipulate loops of bowel and evaluate possible solid organ injuries by elevating those organs.

It is our own belief that laparoscopic examination is better carried out in the operating room with full sterile preparation, under general anaesthesia and adequate muscle relaxation. This approach gives the surgeon the opportunity to induce pneumoperitoneum without discomfort to the patient and achieve this with less insufflation of gas and, as a result of the muscle relaxation, afford a better space to carry out the examination. This approach also provides the surgeon with an opportunity to immediately open the patient's abdomen if this is indicated without the need for further transfer of the patient from the emergency room to the operating theatre.

We prefer to use an 11 mm port to accommodate a 10 mm laparoscope which provides adequate lighting for the entire abdominal cavity. It is also preferable to use a 30° forward oblique laparoscope which gives the examining surgeon better access to recesses of the abdominal cavity; in particular, a more thorough evaluation of the liver surface, diaphragmatic surfaces and the splenic and hepatic flexures of the colon can thus be carried out. Although most grasping instruments and suction probes can be adequately introduced through 5 mm accessory ports, it is our recommendation that the accessory 10 mm ports are employed. With this approach, the surgeon can move the telescope to various locations in order to improve visualization. In addition, larger calibre suction can be introduced from various directions to clear blood, thereby improving visualization. The location for the placement of these ports is depicted in Figure 14.2.1. Accessory instrumentation (Fig. 14.2.2) includes the Endoshear (United States Surgical, Norwalk, CT) which may help in division of peritoneal reflections of the colon to visualize possible injuries in the retroperitoneal portion of these structures. The Endograsp (United States Surgical, Norwalk, CT) and the Endoclinch (United States Surgical, Norwalk, CT) aid the surgeon in the "running" of the small bowel which is systematically examined from the ileocaecal junction.

An adequate examination of the entire small bowel can be carried out if there is no major haemoperitoneum present. If an excessive amount of blood interferes with adequate visualization, the safest approach is to avoid further manipulation and to proceed to immediate laparotomy. Unnecessary prolongation of the examination in this situation puts the patient at risk and may delay corrective measures. Methylene blue should be available for instillation through the nasogastric tube to evaluate the duodenum for possible injury. Methylene blue staining in the peritoneal cavity will indicate perforation. An adequate suction device must be available and the suctioned blood or intestinal contents

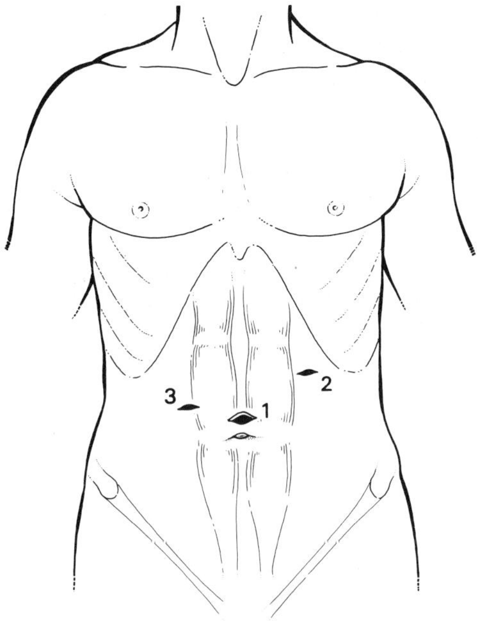

Figure 14.2.1. Port sites.

sent for culture and sensitivity studies. If intestinal perforation is diagnosed, laparotomy should be undertaken since most surgeons are not yet adequately trained to repair perforations laparoscopically in this situation. Careful attention to detail in the performance of laparoscopy will yield a satisfactory examination.

INDICATIONS

Blunt Trauma

Blunt abdominal trauma can be extremely difficult to evaluate when the patient arrives in the emergency department and the effects of the injury may only be evolving. Thus, an abdomen which presents a relatively benign picture initially may, in a very short period of time, become a major concern. The clinical picture is often further confused due to the associated injuries, such as limb fractures, thoracic or head trauma, mental obtundation and the effects of alcohol or drugs, all of which contribute to confusion in clinical assessment. Blood loss is difficult to gauge due to the associated injuries and the abdomen becomes the prime suspect for the source of blood loss.

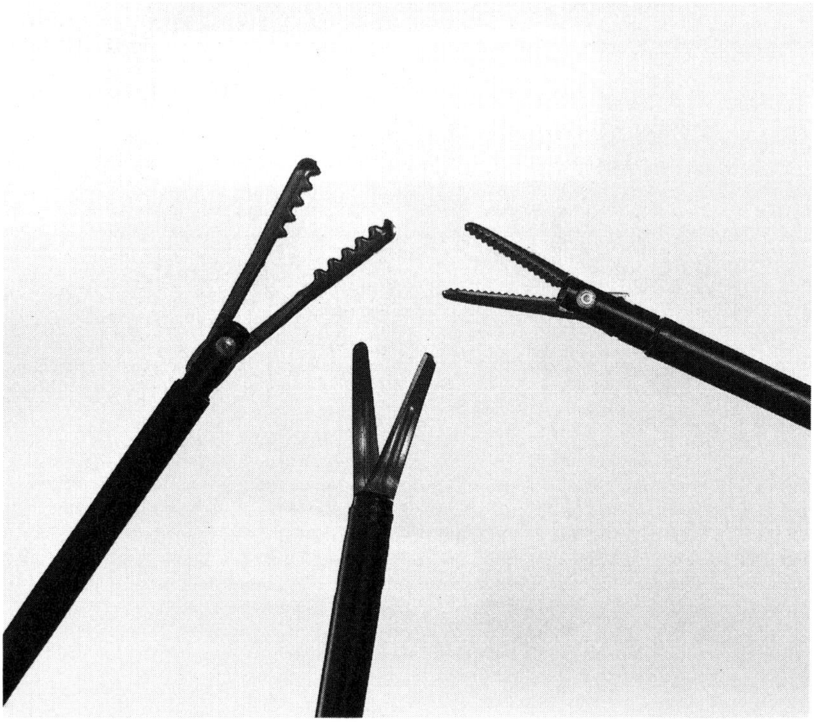

Figure 14.2.2. Accessory instruments: Endoclinch, Endoshear, Endograsp.

If following initial survey and assessment, abdominal signs continue to be equivocal, laparoscopy provides the most definitive early evaluation technique. The general surgeon should promote diagnostic laparoscopy as a primary procedure before surgery is embarked upon, since it will remove the dilemma, often faced by the anaesthetist, when a patient suddenly becomes hypotensive during lengthy non-abdominal procedures. In that clinical situation, the abdominal surgeon has little choice but to proceed with an often non-therapeutic exploratory laparotomy on a distended abdomen.

Prolonged resuscitation with crystalloids during lengthy procedures may be associated with intra-abdominal oedema, ileus and abdominal distension. The blood loss during lengthy orthopaedic or neurosurgical procedures is frequently underestimated and the abdomen is suspected as a source of blood loss. Early exploratory laparoscopic evaluation reassures the entire operating team involved with the patient's care that the abdomen is indeed not the source of trouble. If, at the time of laparoscopy, an unstable abdominal injury is identified (such as bleeding liver laceration, mesenteric tear or splenic laceration), expeditious laparotomy is undertaken. Exploratory laparoscopy may add little morbidity to the multiply injured patient. However, exploratory laparotomy based on a positive lavage but associated with a stable intra-abdominal injury

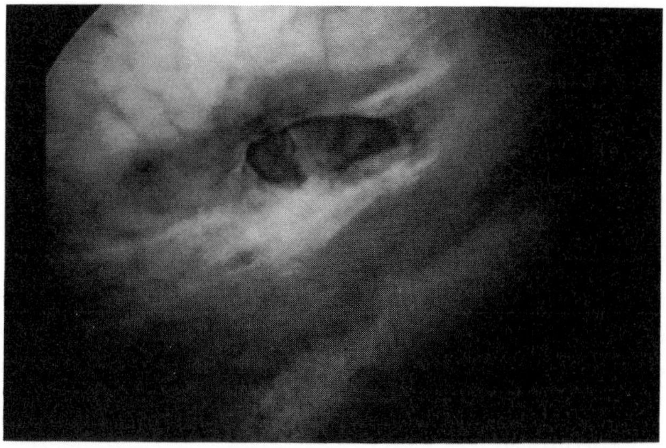

Figure 14.2.3. Abdominal stab wound penetrating peritoneum.

would add major morbidity to an already multiply injured patient. Exploratory laparotomy, even with a positive diagnostic peritoneal lavage, leads to negative laparotomy in a significant number of patients.[16,17]

Penetrating Trauma

Abdominal Stab Wounds

Not all abdominal stab wounds either penetrate the peritoneum or, even if the peritoneum has been violated, cause intra-abdominal organ damage (Figs 14.2.3 and 4). These injuries are therefore ideally evaluated by laparoscopy.

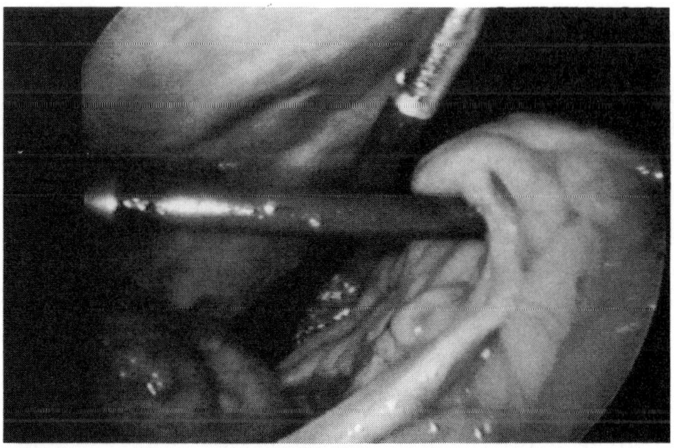

Figure 14.2.4. No corresponding intra-abdominal injury identified.

Indirect methods to try to diagnose peritoneal penetration, such as local wound exploration or sinograms, are often inconclusive.[18] Laparoendoscopic evaluation will most definitely establish if peritoneal penetration has taken place and also whether significant intra-abdominal injury has occurred which may require laparotomy.[3,16] The stab wound must be closed in case penetration has taken place and leakage of gas would interfere with adequate establishment of pneumoperitoneum. The site of the injury must be indented with a finger following the placement of the laparoscope in order to examine the parietal peritoneum with care. A 30° forward oblique laparoscope is useful, especially for screening the diaphragmatic surface. If penetration has taken place, systematic non-traumatic evaluation of the underlying viscera can be carried out with the aid of further ports and manipulating instruments.

Gunshot Wounds

The use of laparotomy in penetrating trauma due to gunshot wounds has, in the past, been considered as a contraindication for laparoscopy.[19,20] However, laparoscopic evaluation of tangential abdominal gunshot wounds have been reported to be quite successful in avoiding laparotomy.[21,22] In this situation, the mechanism of injury seems to justify the initial approach by exploratory laparoscopy. In these cases, the entrance and exit wounds and the inferred trajectory of the bullet leave sufficient doubt as to peritoneal penetration. The patient is often quite tender on abdominal examination due to the soft tissue injury induced by the path of the bullet. The critical question is, however, whether peritoneal penetration has actually occurred. Often such penetration is not found at laparoscopy. These patients, therefore, will avoid unnecessary exploratory laparotomy.

CONTRAINDICATIONS AND COMPLICATIONS

The mortality of laparoscopy has been reported to be around 0.1–0.2%.[23] Major complications should occur in less than 1% of procedures and are usually due to the establishment of pneumoperitoneum or insertion of the port.[24] During establishment of pneumoperitoneum, gas embolization can occur. If so, the patient must be turned to the left lateral decubitus position which will reduce the obstruction of the outflow of the right heart. To avoid such complication, it is good practice to begin insufflation at a very low rate. The anaesthetist thus will have a chance to monitor the patient and be alert to early signs of this extremely rare complication,[25] but one which is a reality in trauma patients in whom any torn vein may be open to the high pressure of carbon dioxide in the abdominal cavity.[24]

If laparoscopy is performed under local anaesthesia a vasovagal response may occur which will lead to hypoxaemia.[26] Pneumothorax, another rare complication of laparoscopy, can occur due to the need for increased positive pressure ventilation to counteract the effects of pneumoperitoneum. Traumatic, congenital or hiatal defects in the diaphragm may contribute to the development of this complication.[3] Any emphysematous bullae may also rupture as a result of the positive pressure ventilation. Fortunately, these complications are extremely rare and maintaining low insufflation pressures will reduce their occurrence.[27] Injuries due to the insufflating Veress needle and port insertion are usually traceable to faulty technique and have been reported to occur in up to 2.7/1000 patients.[28]

There are few contraindications to laparoscopy, but previous abdominal incisions may give rise to multiple intra-abdominal adhesions and laparoscopy would be a less fruitful examination in this setting. Although adhesions can be lysed through the laparoscope, such additional manoeuvres in the trauma setting can complicate and unduly prolong the procedure. An evaluation of the patient's coagulation status should also be sought prior to the evaluation of the traumatized abdomen. Uncorrected prolonged bleeding tendency would contraindicate laparoscopic evaluation as well as possible ensuing laparotomy.

Laparoscopy is an invasive surgical procedure and the surgeon must pay great attention to detail before embarking upon it. However, in spite of the inherent risks associated with laparoscopy, such as cardiopulmonary compromise, the results of abdominal overdistension and the potential for viscus and vascular perforation, the overall risks are less than the potential morbidity associated with exploratory laparotomy.[29]

LITERATURE REVIEW

The use of laparoscopy for the assessment of abdominal injuries is not a new concept and there are numerous reports in the English literature reporting the results of the technique. Heselson compared the results of laparoscopy to management without laparoscopy for both blunt and penetrating abdominal trauma as early as the 1960s.[8] In 68 laparoscopies for trauma only one false-positive examination resulted and there were no known false-negative examinations. The use of laparoscopy in his series resulted in a decreased hospital stay for both blunt and penetrating trauma victims. Heselson believed that laparoscopy was the most valuable single investigation in the diagnosis of abdominal injury. Gazzaniga in 1976 reported on 39 laparoscopies; 24 in patients suffering from blunt trauma and 11 in patients with penetrating trauma.[10] Among the blunt trauma victims in his series, 42% had a negative laparoscopy and they were thus saved a laparotomy. Interestingly, in these ten patients (42%), three had a positive diagnostic peritoneal lavage. In the blunt trauma group of patients, there was one unnecessary laparotomy, i.e. no injury was identified requiring a surgical correction, for a rate of 7% (one in 14), whereas in the penetrating injury group, the unnecessary laparotomy rate was 39% (five in 13), with one false-negative examination in the penetrating trauma group, a missed colonic perforation.

In a study by Carnevale,[16] laparoscopy was performed prior to laparotomy in 20 patients with abdominal trauma in whom laparotomy was indicated, either by physical examination, radiological results, laboratory data or the results of diagnostic peritoneal lavage. Carnevale and his group were able to avoid laparotomy in 60% of the patients as a result of the laparoscopic findings. Only one patient in this series had an unnecessary laparotomy, for a rate of 13%.

A new technique for minilaparoscopy for blunt abdominal trauma using a 5 mm port which can be employed in the emergency department was first reported by Sherwood and Berci in 1980.[30] This initial series of 15 patients has been expanded by Berci[31] to a total of 150 patients and is the largest recorded series of laparoscopy in blunt abdominal trauma. With this technique, laparoscopies were performed in the emergency room under intravenous sedation and with the use of local anaesthetic. This is in direct contrast to all other series in which laparoscopy was performed in the operating room or, in one instance, in the intensive care unit.[10] Berci reported a negative laparoscopy with no evidence of haemoperitoneum in 84 of the patients (56%). Of the remainder, 38 patients (25%) had a positive laparoscopy, i.e. minimal to moderate haemoperitoneum, but no injury or only minimal lacerations and thus did not require an exploratory laparotomy. A total of 28 patients (19%) had a severe haemoperitoneum and required emergency laparotomy. There was no unnecessary laparotomies but there was one missed injury, a sigmoid perforation, for a false-negative rate of 75%.

At present, diagnostic peritoneal lavage is still considered as the gold standard for investigation of blunt abdominal trauma. Unfortunately, to date in the English literature, there is only one prospective randomized study comparing diagnostic peritoneal lavage to laparoscopy for evaluation of blunt abdominal trauma. In a multicentre trial, Cuschieri *et al.*[32] randomized 55 patients suffering blunt abdominal trauma to two groups. One group was evaluated by peritoneal lavage, while the other group was assessed using minilaparoscopy as described by Berci. Both tests were 100% sensitive in detecting intra-abdominal injury; however, peritoneal lavage had a specificity of 83% while minilaparoscopy had a specificity of 94%. The positive predictive value was also higher for minilaparoscopy than for peritoneal lavage (92% and 72% respectively). In addition, the unnecessary laparotomy rate was lower in the minilaparoscopy group (8%) than in the peritoneal lavage group (27%). Following the publication of these data, the study was continued to a total of 80 patients and the minilaparoscopy group continued to have a significant reduction in the number of unnecessary laparotomies.[33]

With the present popularity of laparoscopy, there has been a resurgence of interest in the literature in use of the technique in trauma. Sosa[21] used laparoscopy to evaluate the integrity of the peritoneum following tangential abdominal gunshot wounds in eight patients. He was able to avoid laparotomy in six patients since there was no peritoneal perforation identified. The intrathoracic abdomen is a difficult area to evaluate following penetrating trauma. Ivatury[3] recently assessed the role of laparoscopy in this anatomical area, extending from the nipple line to the umbilicus. Of 40 patients undergoing laparoscopy, 20 (50%) had no penetration of the peritoneum while one other patient had a non-bleeding liver laceration with no evidence of other injury. Twenty one of the 40 patients in this study avoided laparotomy. The unnecessary laparotomy rate in Ivatury's series was 47% (nine of 19 patients). However, this may be falsely high due to the protocol to perform laparotomy on all patients with peritoneal perforation and significant haemoperitoneum. Laparoscopy was successful in detecting injuries to the diaphragm in seven patients. It is important to note that there is a risk of life-threatening pneumothorax if laparoscopy is performed on patients with occult diaphragmatic injuries and this occurred in one patient. Despite this risk, Ivatury feels that laparoscopy is a superior method of detecting isolated occult injuries to the diaphragm.

The retroperitoneum and the retroperitoneal duodenum is another area which is difficult to assess. Gazzaniga reported on the successful identification of a duodenal rupture[10] while Livingston[4] was able to diagnose a retroperitoneal haematoma with the use of the laparoscope in five of six patients. However, Livingston and his colleagues were only able to visualize the spleen in one of the 39 patients, although three patients in their series were found to have splenic injuries. All three of these patients had a substantial amount of blood visualized in the left upper quadrant; however, the diagnosis of definite splenic trauma was not made until laparotomy. Both Gazzaniga and Berci agree that complete visualization of the spleen is not possible laparoscopically,[10,31] but the specific signs indicating a splenic injury on laparoscopy include blood in the pericolic gutter, above the tip of the spleen or under the omentum, giving it a bluish tint.

The ability of laparoscopy to detect hollow viscus injury is controversial. In the study by Livingston,[4] four patients had a total of 20 small bowel injuries. At laparoscopy, two of these patients had a significant haemoperitoneum with clot obscuring the bowel injuries, while in the other two patients small bowel injuries were not actively sought due to the presence of other organ injuries requiring laparotomy. This is in direct contrast to Gazzaniga who found that the diagnosis of small bowel perforation was obvious due to the presence of small bowel contents along the gutters and small bowel serosal inflammatory changes.[10] It is of note that both the missed injuries in the literature were perforations of a hollow viscus, specifically in colonic perforations. The instillation of methylene blue via the nasogastric tube and subsequent laparoscopy is one method to further assess the integrity of the small bowel.[3]

Livingston was also concerned about the inability to reliably evacuate blood and clot from the peritoneal cavity, thus preventing him from adequately assessing the abdominal contents. He felt that this was one of the major limiting factors to the use of laparoscopy in abdominal trauma.[4] This problem is not discussed by other authors. Interestingly, laparoscopy tends to overestimate the amount of blood in the peritoneal cavity. In a study using cadavers, Gazzaniga found that 50 cc of blood in the peritoneal cavity appeared through the laparoscope to represent major bleeding.[10]

Review of the literature has yielded no deaths attributable to laparoscopy and few complications occurred. Therefore, the advantages of laparoscopy are quite evident. The ability to distinguish active bleeding from self-limited bleeding is a clear advantage over other diagnostic modalities. This results in fewer laparotomies which, in turn, results in decreased patient morbidity and decreased hospital stay.[4,8,10,16]

DISCUSSION AND FUTURE CONSIDERATIONS

The widespread acceptance of laparoscopic cholecystectomy and other laparoscopic procedures[2] will give surgeons new skills, the use of which will be translated into everyday surgical practice including the evaluation of abdominal trauma. It is evident that more surgeons are using exploratory laparoscopy to advantage in evaluation of abdominal trauma.[34] Exploratory laparoscopy in trauma patients will undergo further evaluation by comparing it with established techniques such as diagnostic peritoneal lavage and computed tomography. A video laparoscope and new instrumentation will be much more attractive to surgeons than the older techniques of laparoscopy.

Irrespective of whether laparoscopy is performed under local anaesthetic or under general anaesthesia, it is an invasive technique. It is no panacea for the evaluation of abdominal injuries, but it is hoped that its judicious application will improve the avoidance of negative laparotomy especially in the multiply injured patient. Diagnostic peritoneal lavage, although widely accepted as a highly sensitive indicator of intra-abdominal injury, may in fact be too sensitive. In addition, its use in diagnosing suspected penetrating abdominal stab wounds may be unreliable. Muckart and MacDonald reported a 31% failure to identify significant injury in their series of 35 patients.[35]

However, laparoscopy may not afford a complete assessment of the retroperitoneum to which CT scan, combined with contrast, would draw attention. Diagnostic laparoscopy does not need to be a passive observation technique, but with the help of accessory instruments introduced through extra ports, hollow organs can be more thoroughly examined. CT scan will not diagnose diaphragmatic rupture in most instances but laparoscopy will do so.[36]

It is important to realize that laparoscopy has little to offer in situations where clear violation of the peritoneal cavity has occurred due to through-and-through gunshot wounds or high velocity missiles. These patients require urgent exploratory laparatomy. Eventually, perhaps, laparoscopic techniques and skills can be developed to deal with these injuries through the laparoscope but for the present time, the use of laparoscopy in the traumatized abdomen can only be recommended in the diagnostic sphere. A weakly positive diagnostic peritoneal lavage in a stable patient should also be followed by diagnostic laparoscopy as a significant number of these positive "taps" are followed by negative laparotomies.[37] Sandy (personal communication) in our institution has found a significant number of patients who underwent negative laparotomy following a positive diagnostic peritoneal lavage in a current review. We are currently conducting a study to identify patients who do not require laparotomy following a positive diagnostic peritoneal lavage by performing laparoscopy prior to laparotomy. Laparoscopy, however, is contraindicated in patients who, following blunt abdominal trauma, exhibit haemodynamic instability, abdominal distension or frank peritonitis. In these instances, definitive clinical signs must override any desire to employ a multitude of diagnostic techniques such as diagnostic peritoneal lavage, CT scanning and ultrasound as well as laparoscopy. Efficient, quick, exploratory laparotomy is indicated.

In patients with gunshot wounds or penetrating stab wounds where indications for laparotomy clearly exist (peritonitis and/or hypotension) no further useful information will be afforded by diagnostic laparoscopy. If plain films of the abdomen show free air or diaphragmatic rupture, exploration is in order. Evisceration of abdominal organs also is best managed by exploratory laparotomy.

Last, but not least, surgeons unfamiliar with the details of laparoscopic evaluation should not undertake laparoscopy in patients with abdominal trauma. For the success of laparoscopy, one must have adequate instrumentation and equipment, a stable patient *and* an experienced surgeon.

Acknowledgement

The authors would like to acknowledge Fern Rushton, Gayle Uthoff, Vicki Chor and Shirlee Wallace of the Department of Surgery, University of British Columbia, for preparation of this manuscript.

REFERENCES

1. Kelling G. Über oesophagoskopie, gastroskopie und colioskopie. *Munch Med Wochenschr* 1901; **49**: 21–24.
2. Zucker K. Perceived future of laparoscopic general surgery. *Can J Surg* 1992; **35**: 297–304.
3. Ivatury RR, Simon RJ, Weksler B, Bayard V, Stahl WM. Laparoscopy in the evaluation of the intrathoracic abdomen after penetrating injury. *J Trauma* 1992; **33**: 101–8.
4. Livingston DH, Tortella BJ, Blackwood J, Machiedo GW, Rush BF. The role of laparoscopy in abdominal trauma. *J Trauma* 1992; **33**: 471–5.
5. McAnena OJ, Moore EE, Marx JA. Initial evaluation of the patient with blunt abdominal trauma. *Surg Clin N Am* 1990: **70**: 495.
6. Root HD, Hauser CV, McKinley CR, LaFave JW, Mendiola RP. Diagnostic peritoneal lavage. *Surgery* 1965; **57**: 633.
7. Tostivint R, Rozenberg H, Chauveinc L, Sanchez MF. Laparoscope dans les traumatismes abdominaux. *J Chir (Paris)* 1971; **102**: 77–84.

8. Heselson J. Peritoneoscopy in abdominal trauma. *S Afric J Surg* 1970; **8**: 53–60.
9. Gomel V. Laparoscopy in general surgery. *Am J Surg* 1976; **131**: 319–23.
10. Gazzaniga AB, Stanton WW, Bartlett RH. Laparoscopy in the diagnosis of blunt and penetrating injuries to the abdomen. *Am J Surg* 1976; **131**: 315–18.
11. Berci G, Dunkelman D, Michel SL, Sanders G, Wahlstrom E, Morgenstern L. Emergency minilaparoscopy in abdominal trauma. *Am J Surg* 1983; **146**: 261–5.
12. Cohen MM. Peritoneoscopy in general surgery. *Can J Surg* 1981; **24**: 490–3.
13. Powell DC, Bivins BA, Bell RM. Diagnostic peritoneal lavage. *Surg Gynecol Obstet* 1982; **155**: 257.
14. Trunkey D, Federle MP. Editorial. Computed tomography in perspective. *J Trauma* 1986; **26**: 660.
15. Nagy AG. Diagnostic laparoscopy. *Am J Surg* 1989; **157**: 490–3.
16. Carnevale N, Baron N, Delaney HM. Peritoneoscopy as an aid in the diagnosis of abdominal trauma: a preliminary report. *J Trauma* 1977; **17**: 634–41.
17. Olsen WR, Hildreth DH. Abdominal paracentesis and peritoneal lavage in blunt abdominal trauma. *J Trauma* 1971; **11**: 824.
18. Feliciano DV. Diagnostic modalities in abdominal trauma. *Surg Clin N Am* 1991; **71**: 244–5.
19. Berci G, Sackier JM, Pas MP. Emergency laparoscopy. *Am J Surg* 1991; **161**: 332–5.
20. Robinson HB, Smith GW. Applications for laparoscopy in general surgery. *Surg Gynecol Obstet* 1976; **143**: 829–33.
21. Sosa JL, Sims D, Martin L, Zeppa R. Laparoscopic evaluation of tangential abdominal gunshot wounds. *Arch Surg* 1992; **127**: 109–10.
22. Cohen MM. Letter to the Editor. *Arch Surg* 1992; **127**: 747.
23. Vilardell F, Seres I, Merti-Vincente A. Complications of peritoneoscopy: survey of 1455 examinations. *Gastrointest Endosc* 1968; **14**: 178–80.
24. Cali RW. Laparoscopy. *Surg Clin N Am* 1980; **60**: 420–2.
25. Scott DB, Julian DG. Observation on cardiac arrhythmias during laparoscopy. *Br Med J* 1972; **1**: 411–13.
26. Peterson EP. Anaesthesia for laparoscopy. *Fertil Steril* 1971; **22**: 695–8.
27. Doctor WH, Hussain Z. Bilateral pneumothorax associated with laparoscopy: a case report of a rare hazard and review of the literature. *Anaesthesia* 1973; **28**: 75–81.
28. Phillips JM. Complications of laparoscopy. *Int J Gynecol Obstet* 1977; **15**: 157–62.
29. Ayers JWT, Ansbacher R. Laparoscopy: applications in general surgical practice. In: *Surgical Endoscopy Yearbook* (eds Dent TL, Strodel WE, Turcotte JG.), p. 454. Chicago: Year book Medical Publishers Inc, 1985.
30. Sherwood R, Berci G, Austin E, Morgenstern L. Minilaparoscopy for blunt abdominal trauma. *Arch Surg* 1980; **115**: 672–3.
31. Berci G, Sackier JM, Paz-Partlow M. Emergency laparoscopy. *Am J Surg* 1991; **161**: 332–5.
32. Cuschieri A, Hennessy TPJ, Stephens RB, Berci G. Diagnosis of significant abdominal trauma after road traffic accidents: preliminary results of a multicenter clinical trial comparing minilaparoscopy with peritoneal lavage. *Ann Roy Coll Surg Eng* 1988; **70**: 153–5.
33. Cushieri A. Personal communication.
34. Olgin HA. Surgery alert (commentary). 1992; **9**: 21.
35. Muckart DJJ, MacDonald MA. Unreliability of standard quantitative criteria in diagnostic peritoneal lavage performed for suspected penetrating abdominal stab wounds. *Am J Surg* 1991; **162**: 223–7.
36. Adamthwaite DN. Traumatic diaphragmatic hernia: a new indication for laparoscopy. *Br J Surg* 1984; **71**: 315.
37. DuPriest RW, Rodriguez A, Khaneja SC *et al.* Open diagnostic peritoneal lavage in blunt abdominal trauma victims. *Surg Gynecol Obstet* 1979; **148**: 890–4.

Overview

Abdominal trauma

The contribution by Champion's group (Chapter 14.1) clearly charts the optimal method of assessing patients with blunt and penetrating abdominal and chest injury. Although laparoscopy may contribute considerable information in the management of such conditions, it has yet to be established how this will affect patient management and outcome. The potential role of laparoscopy is clearly stated, but continuing prospective evaluation will be required before it is generally adopted by trauma specialists.

15.1

The Non-Operative Assessment of Intra-Abdominal Malignancy

G. PLANT, N. O'ROURKE and M. REES

INTRODUCTION

The preoperative work-up of patients with cancer is dependent on thorough clinical assessment together with specific investigations designed to identify the type of malignancy and the extent of spread. Although the findings of distant nodal spread or ascites confirm non-resectability on clinical grounds, most patients with abdominal malignancy need specific investigation to decide on the most appropriate course of action. In particular, the increasing sophistication of radiology has enabled clinicians to avoid subjecting patients to an unnecessary operative procedure. This review concentrates on the use of modern radiological techniques in identifying the likelihood of an abdominal tumour being resectable. It is not our intention to repeat the basic literature but to expand on the process of identifying the malignancies, their nature, extent and operability. Much of this is performed radiologically and we will concentrate on this aspect. In the first part of this review we have outlined basic radiological principles that will help in understanding which is the most appropriate investigation.

IMAGING TECHNIQUES

When considering a sequence of imaging techniques it is conventional to consider plain films, contrast investigations, nuclear medicine studies and cross-sectional imaging, i.e. ultrasound (US), computed tomography (CT) and magnetic resonance imaging (MRI). While this is convenient in a descriptive sense it is not ideal as a diagnostic process. Selection of the diagnostic technique may be sequential based on a series of findings on an increasingly complex (and more expensive) sequence of tests or it may be sensible to go directly to the most sensitive test. In the abdomen, particularly when looking for the extent of spread of a malignancy, CT is likely to be the investigation of choice.

Individual cases will determine the diagnostic pathway taken but consideration should also be given to inter-reactions between examinations; in particular it is best to avoid performing barium examinations before CT as residual barium may produce artefacts. Following assessment of the primary neoplasm there will be a need to identify distant metastases. Taking into account the likelihood of these being present and the bearing this will have on the decision to operate, a variety of tests may need to be performed.

Chest radiographs will demonstrate lung metastases in the majority of cases in which these are present. A single posteroanterior chest radiograph will reveal 99% of lesions which may be visualized with plain films and a lateral projection is not necessary.[1] Although CT scanning is able to identify lung lesions in approximately 13% more cases, 80% of these lesions will be benign.[2,3] It is therefore not recommended as a screening investigation. Bony metastases are reliably detected by isotope scanning which is worthwhile in a patient with bone pain who is about to undergo extensive surgery for intra-abdominal malignancy. US will detect 50% of liver metastases or approximately 85% of patients with cancer in the liver. This high pick-up rate has encouraged many clinicians to use US as a screening investigation. Positive findings may then be mapped out more accurately by CT examination (see below).

There are a number of factors pertaining to the investigations which are general to all the body areas and these are discussed below.

Plain Films

Plain films are readily available and often ordered as an automatic reaction on admission. In common with many radiological tests the ability to identify a structure depends on its X-ray density or the radiographic contrast between it and surrounding structures. Most abnormalities will not be identified on plain films, but evidence of obstruction to the bowel will at least attest to the direct involvement of the bowel and the need to expedite the decision process.

Contrast Studies and Endoscopy

Contrast investigations are designed to introduce the maximum amount of difference in density between the structure in question and the surrounding tissues. They may produce exquisite detail but may be associated with morbidity or discomfort.

For the upper intestine more information may be forthcoming by endoscopy when the true extent of mucosal spread is more readily appreciated and confirmed by biopsy. An impression of the degree of fixation to surrounding tissues may be apparent and the use of an endoscopic ultrasound probe provides direct evidence of fixation to surrounding vital structures or lymph node status. This new modality is operator-dependent and only available to a few centres; however, in time its role may increase.

Colonoscopy in experienced hands will identify a high percentage of primary colonic lesions but may be incomplete in patients with a very tortuous colon, sigmoid diverticular disease of in the presence of partial obstruction when the bowel cannot be cleared. Both endoscopy and contrast studies of the bowel are useful in establishing the diagnosis of malignancy but are poor contributors to the decision on operability.

Ultrasound

Ultrasound examination is the safest, cheapest and most available of the cross-sectional imaging modalities. The examination is usually quick and simple and there is no associated morbidity. Because ultrasound uses a different modality, the transmission of sound, it has the ability to demonstrate differences between tissues that may not be readily apparent using X-rays. It particularly excels in detecting the difference between solid and cystic lesions.

In common with many imaging techniques a positive result from ultrasound is likely to be reliable; however, a negative result has a much lower level of certainty. There are technical problems associated with ultrasound. The major ones are degradation of the image quality due to the thickness of soft tissue to be traversed. Air or bone causes complete obstruction to the ultrasound beam and this limits visualization of organs deep to these structures. One of the skills of the ultrasonographer is in positioning the patient to open windows between organs to permit visualization of deep structures. The examination is, therefore, very operator-dependent.

Computed Tomography

Computed tomographic images are obtained by the passage of X-rays through the body which are picked up by a series of detectors rotating around the patient. Since its introduction there has been a steady improvement in the technology employed to increase the speed of image acquisition, processing and the spatial resolution. The current developments in this field are a change from the conventional method of imaging one slice at a time to imaging a volume of the patient by spiralling the X-ray tube and detectors around and along the patient. The images are then mathematically generated at any point or in any plane that is desired.

One way of improving the contrast resolution is by administration of radiographic contrast agents which may be ingested or injected. Intravenous contrast agents in particular produce startling changes in the differential density of adjacent structures. This is a dynamic process and if the patient is not scanned during the phase of maximal differential enhancement it is possible for lesions to be obscured by the use of contrast agent. This has led to a number of strategies for imaging parts of the body. Some of these are mutually contradictory and it may not be possible to image optimally for several different organs at one examination.

Magnetic Resonance

Magnetic resonance imaging uses the differences in radio frequency produced by inducing movement in the patient's molecules whilst these molecules are aligned by a strong magnetic field. The technique is developing rapidly and much of the research is directed towards decreasing the time taken to acquire the image to diminish patient movements. These result in loss of spatial resolution so that at present MRI cannot match CT in the abdomen in this respect.

The operator can choose to alter various parameters of the investigation. T_1 and T_2 weighting reflect differences in the relaxation process (the term used for the molecules realigning themselves). In general the T_1 weighted images appear more anatomical and have a higher spatial resolution. T_2 weighted images reflect differences in chemical composition and are more specific in differentiating between different tissue types. A variety of protocols to measure these parameters are designed to speed image acquisition and go under names such as spin echo, gradient echo or echo planar.

Huge advances are being made in gating and other technologies and this will continue to improve. The ability of MRI to identify changes in molecular chemistry means that there is potential for identifying even small morphological changes and this aspect holds great promise. MRI is one of the fastest developing fields of medical technology and the companies are producing new machines at an astonishing rate. Each new scanner incorporates significant advantages and as a result MRI images, even from the newest machines, appear dated within a short time. MRI will be the cross-sectional imaging technique of choice before the end of the decade.

BIOPSY TECHNIQUES

Percutaneous biopsy with guidance by screening, ultrasound and CT has been performed in innumerable cases. A variety of needle sizes have been employed from 14 to 22 French. Most of the finer needles obtain cytology by suction and the larger needles usually use some form of cutting system. These cutting systems may be manually operated such as the Tru-Cut or be mechanical or spring-loaded such as the Biopty device.

Expert cytological services can significantly alter the success rate of diagnostic biopsies. The ability to obtain histological confirmation with minimal morbidity and often on an outpatient basis allows a confident preoperative diagnosis, may prevent the need for surgery and allow more accurate follow-up. Individual practitioners will have their own preferences regarding the modality used and factors of expense, availability and the individual lesions will affect this choice.

Complication rates from guided biopsy have been surprisingly low in nearly all series in which radiological guidance was used. Historically there has been a significant incidence of complications using the 14 gauge needles but a number of recent series comparing the use of 18 gauge and 14 gauge needles in the renal tract have shown that with imaging guidance there is no significant difference in the complication rate between these two sizes and an extremely low complication rate overall.[4]

When morbidity does occur the three main problems that may arise are from bleeding, pancreatitis and tumour seeding. Bleeding is most likely in hepatic biopsies and is diminished when an approach is chosen so that normal hepatic parenchyma is traversed prior to entering even a superficial lesion. Pancreatitis may complicate any intervention in the region of the pancreas. In a series of 185 pancreatic biopsies for tumour, the incidence of severe pancreatitis was 3%.[5] The risk appears greater when smaller lesions or an area of normal pancreas are biopsied when the liberation of pancreatic enzymes is more likely.

One of the contentious issues is that of seeding of tumour along the biopsy track. Seeding of the renal track or peritoneal cavity by tumour cells is reported as rare in large surveys. The incidence of less than 0.01% may be much smaller than the real situation because of reporting problems and the usual patient characteristics of poor prognostic disease.[6] The principal problem for surgeons with needle biopsy is that it can render an operative lesion irresectable by intraperitoneal and abdominal spread of tumour. Needle track seeding has been reported for all major intra-abdominal malignancies.[7] Though this is uncommon, when a patient is clearly operable, the "knee-jerk" progression to biopsy should be curtailed. However, in the patient who is borderline due to age, cardiac disease, etc., the extra information of the tumour type may justify biopsy. Our current policy is to resist preoperative biopsy in patients who are clearly resectable, but in patients in whom the situation is unclear, or who may have a condition amenable to other treatments such as lymphoma, to consider it.

Care and perhaps specific premedication should be considered for hormone containing tumours. Severe and fatal reactions have been reported after fine needle biopsy of both phaeochromocytoma and carcinoid tumours.[8]

GENERAL PRINCIPLES

When considering any patient with a view to resection some general principles are applied:

1. What is the nature of the tumour?
2. Is it involving local structures?
3. Can it be resected without jeopardizing the rest of that organ or that patient?
4. Is there evidence of spread to lymph nodes or distant metastases?
5. Is it oncologically sensible to resect?
6. Does the patient need surgery anyway to alleviate symptoms such as gut obstruction?

In the descriptions that follow we have attempted to give an indication as to the imaging techniques that are used in the day-to-day management of these malignancies. An indication of the sensitivity of each technique has been given where possible. These figures are changing all the time with improvements in the protocols used, the equipment and increasing experience, particularly in CT and MRI.

Where a technique is not mentioned in relation to an anatomical area it is because currently it has little part to play in the non-operative assessment of that group of intra-abdominal malignancies.

LIVER

The majority of liver tumours are metastases, particularly from gut primaries. Other metastases, primary hepatic tumours and a variety of benign conditions make up the rest of the lesions identified. Advances in hepatic surgical techniques have significantly increased the number of lesions that may be resected and made greater calls on the ability to assess these lesions accurately preoperatively. Although the presence of a mass, right hypochondrial pain, abnormal liver function tests and a rise in the carcinoembryonic antigen may indicate possible liver involvement and hence the need for further assessment, most patients with a liver secondary are asymptomatic with normal biochemistry.

Ultrasound, safe, readily available and cheap, tends to be used as the initial investigation or as a screening investigation in patients at risk. Dynamic CT scanning is usually considered a satisfactory imaging technique but as one quarter of lesions in the liver may not be appreciated by this modality there has been a search for other, more sensitive techniques. The dual blood supply to the liver creates opportunities for differential enhancement of lesions. Some lesions, particularly metastases, take their blood supply primarily from the hepatic artery and may be preferentially enhanced by a contrast injection into this system. Alternatively the normal liver parenchyma, receiving 80% of its blood supply from the portal system, may be enhanced by computed arterial portography (CTAP) leaving the metastases as hypodense areas. Magnetic resonance scanning can differentiate tissue types and holds great promise. It is already better than dynamic CT in detecting lesions and will improve.[9]

The use of preoperative percutaneous biopsy may be associated with a significant number of false results. In one series the diagnosis made based on clinical, biochemical and radiological findings was correct in 93%; however, in 25% of cases the histological diagnosis was incorrect,[10] and this together with the morbidity decreases its usefulness.

Ultrasound

Ultrasound is the most widely available, cheap and non-invasive examination. Percutaneously it will detect approximately 50% of liver masses. US is particularly useful with haemangiomas which may have a typical hyperechogenic appearance. The appearance may be sufficiently characteristic in patients in whom neoplasia is not suspected to warrant a presumed diagnosis of haemangioma and a follow-up scan after a period of three to six months.

Although CT does have a higher sensitivity for liver masses there are patients in whom US identifies tumours where CT does not, particularly in the left half of the liver and especially the left lateral segments. These sensitivity figures appear poor on a lesion-by-lesion basis but due to the nature of the metastatic disease the sensitivity of identifying at least one of several lesions in patients with multiple hepatic tumours is very much higher.

Intraoperative ultrasound (IOUS), freed from the constraints of imaging through the abdominal wall and with the ability to use transducers of a higher frequency and sensitivity, has been demonstrated to identify 95% of intrahepatic tumours.[11]

Nuclear Medicine

The use of nuclear medicine for liver imaging has diminished steadily following improvements in other cross-sectional imaging. Technetium (^{99}Tc) sulphur colloid is taken up by the Kupffer cells of the liver and imaged on a Gamma camera. The poor spatial resolution of the system means that small lesions are unlikely to be detected and this technique has been superseded for the initial investigation of malignant disease. Isotope scanning may be useful in the differential diagnosis of intrahepatic lesions. Focal nodular hyperplasia may be difficult to distinguish from neoplasia using other modalities; however, the masses contain normal Kupffer cells which will take up isotope. When the patient is imaged, normal activity will be observed instead of the expected defect in the liver, enabling the diagnosis to be made.

Positron emission tomography (PET) has been described for the diagnosis of haemangiomas. Limited availability of this test and the large number of haemangiomas suggest that it will not be widely used, at least in the United Kingdom.

Computed Tomography

Increasingly sophisticated CT scanners have led to improvements in the identification of small lesions in the liver. Evolution of the protocols used, particularly the amount and timing of intravenous contrast, has optimized differentiation of lesions. Currently dynamic CT scanning during the injection of a bolus of intravenous contrast is the method of choice. Lesion-by-lesion analysis of the results in many series has demonstrated that dynamic CT scanning will identify approximately 75% of intrahepatic tumours.[12]

The difficulties that lead to lack of identification of tumours are lack of spatial resolution, artefacts induced by patient movement and insufficient differentiation between the density of the normal liver and the abnormal area. This difference in density is usually increased by the use of intravenous contrast enhancement; however, occasionally tumours that were hypodense before injection may become isodense following the administration of contrast agents. This may be a problem particularly with metastasis from carcinoma of the breast[13,14] or with neuroendocrine tumours.

Haemangiomas may cause difficulties with all forms of imaging including CT. Many of them have a characteristic appearance on CT as an initial hypodense area followed by peripheral enhancement and slow centripetal infilling over many minutes. This appearance is, however, only seen in approximately 80% and in very large or small haemangiomas the characteristic changes may not be seen. In our first 100 liver resections there was one patient resected for a colorectal secondary in whom the histology proved to be a haemangioma and a second patient with an apparent haemangioma that increased in size during follow-up and, when resected six months later, was confirmed to be a secondary deposit.

Features suggesting that resection will be technically possible include:

1. a plane or capsule around the tumour (Fig. 15.1.1):
2. following resection, sufficient functioning liver will be present;
3. the portal supply to the remaining liver is not involved by tumour;
4. the hepatic veins required for the remaining liver are uninvolved (Fig. 15.1.2).
5. the resection should be oncologically sensible;
6. distant metastases should be absent.

Angiography

Angiography has a reported sensitivity of approximately 52%.[15] The identification of small lesions remains problematical and accurate identification of segmental anatomy can be difficult. Some lesions, e.g. haemangioma, focal nodular hyperplasia and hepatic adenoma, may exhibit characteristic angiographic appearances. Approximately 20% of the tumours, however, will not

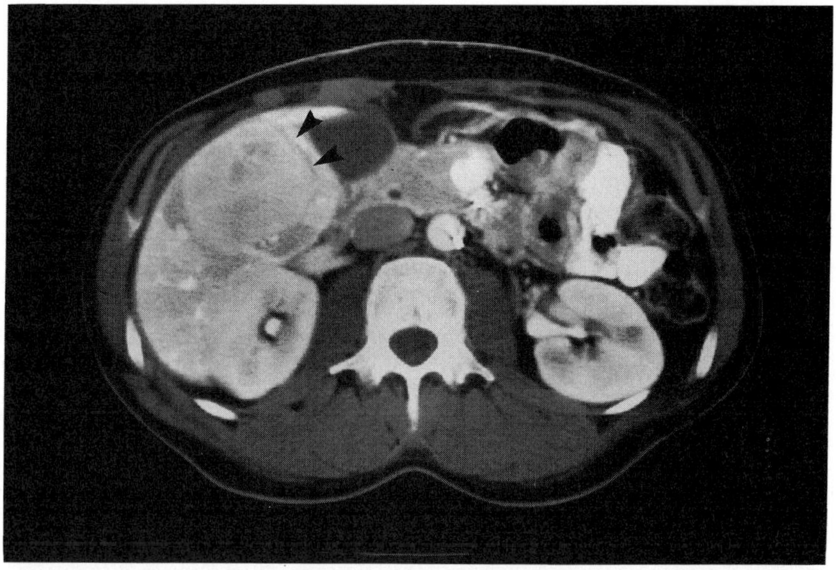

Figure 15.1.1 CTAP study showing a metastatic sarcoma in segment IV, demonstrating a well-defined capsule (arrowheads) which suggested resectability. This finding was confirmed at laparotomy.

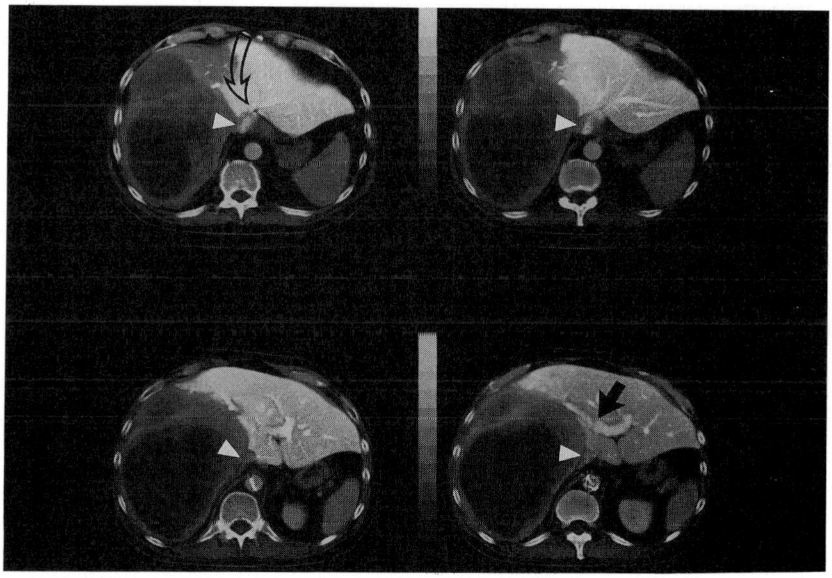

Figure 15.1.2 Histamine secreting haemangioendothelioma of the liver. CTAP demonstrating (1) the tumour does not invade the portal bifurcation (arrow); (2) there is a plane of cleavage between the tumour and the IVC (arrowheads); (3) the middle and left hepatic veins are not involved by this tumour (open arrow).

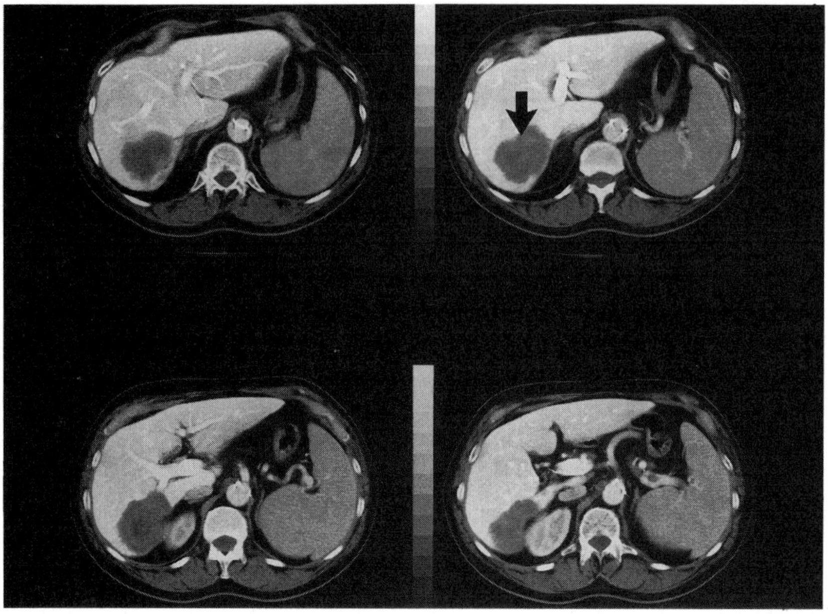

Figure 15.1.3 CTAP demonstrating the typical appearances of a colonic metastasis (arrow) in the liver.

exhibit these appearances and there is significant overlap. Angiography is being used less frequently in the assessment of hepatic tumours although some surgeons like to have an angiogram as a road map.

Complex CT Investigations

The use of alternative complex methods of administration of contrast does lead to an improvement in the sensitivity of CT examinations.

Computed Arterial Portography

Computed arterial portography (CTAP) is a technique in which an angiographic catheter is inserted into the superior mesenteric artery and contrast injected during a CT scan. The contrast passes through the portal system and returns to the liver. Many liver tumours, particularly metastases, take their blood supply from the hepatic artery rather than the portal vein. Therefore, by enhancing the portal supply, normal liver is markedly enhanced and tumours are left as "black holes" within the parenchyma (Fig. 15.1.3). In the diagnosis of intrahepatic metastases CTAP has a sensitivity of 88–95%.[12,16] In our series of 60 patients with hepatic tumours, mainly metastases, in whom resection was performed and the presence of masses confirmed histologically, by palpation

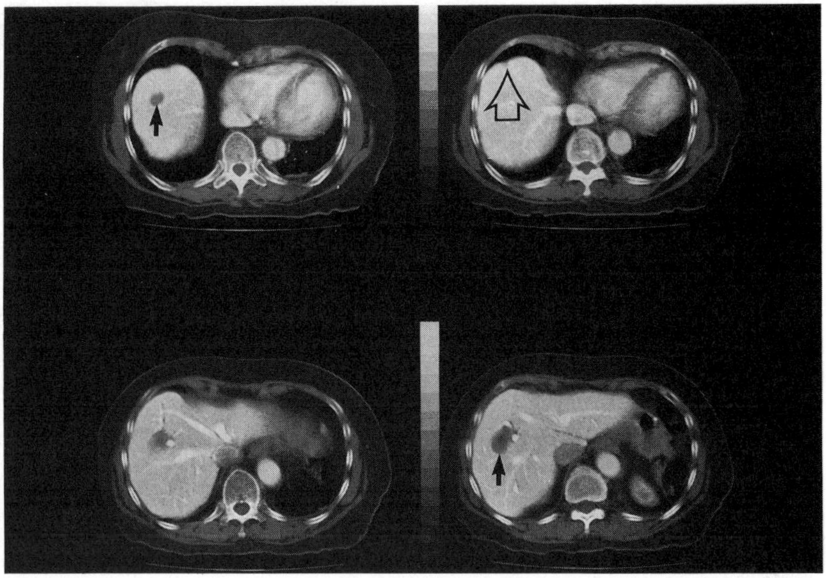

Figure 15.1.4 CTAP study in a patient who had previously had a leiomyosarcoma of the stomach excised. She returned with recurrent pain and had been found on CT to have a locally recurrent tumour. The CTAP study demonstrated multiple deposits (arrowed) including one small superficial metastasis (open arrow).

and IOUS and who have been followed up with CT, the sensitivity of CTAP was 95%. In the diagnosis of hepatocellular carcinoma the reported sensitivity of CTAP (and of other techniques) is lower.

Due to the marked enhancement the ability to identify small lesions is considerably improved and lesions down to 5 mm in size may be seen (Fig. 15.1.4). The price of this sensitivity is the number of other abnormalities that will be identified. In particular small cysts may produce false-positive results. In practice this is usually not a problem because these additional abnormalities may be identified with either late phase scanning, percutaneous or, occasionally, intraoperative ultrasound. The advances in hepatic surgical techniques and the relatively small number of these artefacts that cannot be identified preoperatively means that it is very rare for a lesion to be identified in such a critical position that it alone would determine whether it is possible to perform resection. In these cases laparotomy with intraoperative ultrasound will determine the course taken.

One artefact that is seen fairly commonly is an unenhanced area in the posterior part of segment IV. We have seen it in 13% of 100 CTAP examinations, in patients who have no evidence of tumour involving this area. A similar incidence has been reported in 14% of 50 patients from the group at Emory.[17]

The balance between the proportion of blood supplied by the hepatic artery and the portal vein is a variable one. Pressure from a mass may alter the relative

A

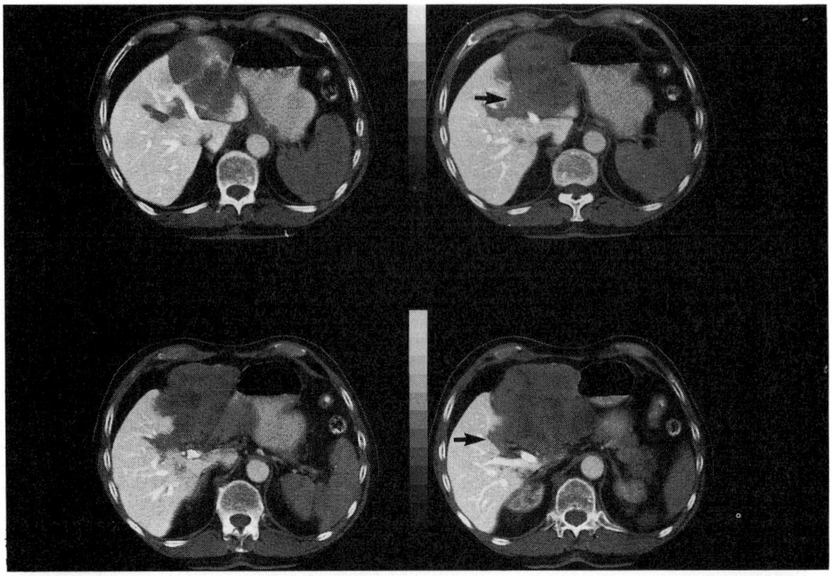

B

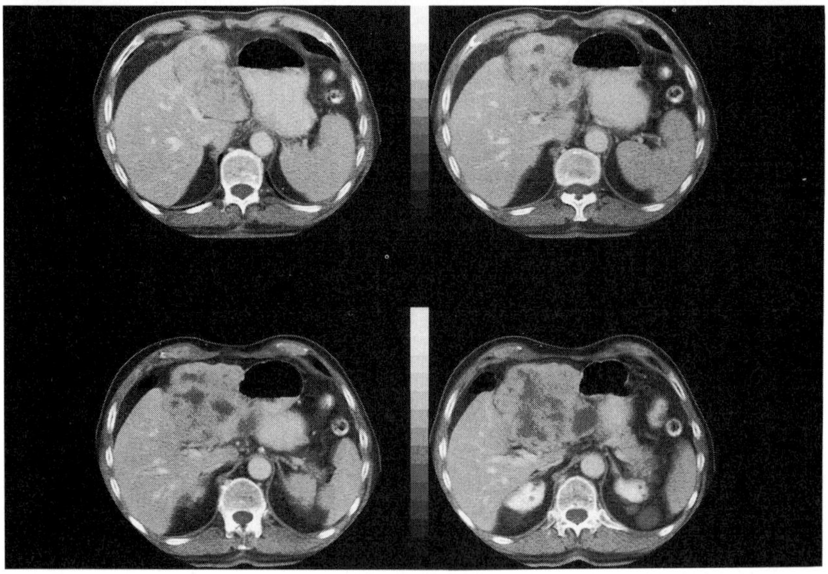

Figure 15.1.5 CTAP study demonstrating a large leiomyosarcoma of the stomach. A: compressing the portal vein and producing a perfusion defect (arrow), mimicking involvement of the liver on the first phase; B: the second phase study suggested the liver was uninvolved, a finding confirmed at surgery.

balance and because of the lower pressure in the portal system it is not uncommon for the portal supply particularly to be reduced by a tumour compressing one of the branches (Fig. 15.1.5). During arterial portography this leads to an area of non-perfusion which has been described as the "straight line sign".[18] This undervisualized area will be well demonstrated by the use of a second phase examination technique, scanning the liver again immediately after the first pass, and we have found this useful for solving this problem.

Specificity remains a problem with arterial portography, particularly with small lesions and when it is not possible to characterize an abnormality on clinical or other grounds. Some tissue types, particularly the neuroendocrine group, may take a significant blood supply from the portal system. Considerable care should be exercised when examining these patients as the expected difference in density between the mass and surrounding liver may not be seen or may only be present for a very short time. Unfortunately dynamic CT may be even more affected and it may not be possible to identify the lesions at all.

In our series the addition of CTAP to the preoperative assessment has reduced the number of patients who had a laparotomy performed with a view to hepatic resection but who proved unresectable on operative examination and intraoperative ultrasound. Of the last 60 patients undergoing laparotomy for hepatic resection and deemed resectable by CTAP, only 3% proved inoperable by palpation and IOUS.

The patients who were inoperable had extrahepatic disease, one had small portal nodes and the other had peritoneal seedlings. In our experience this is such a small number that it does not justify the routine use of laparoscopy especially in patients who often have dense adhesions from the resection of a colorectal primary. When we used dynamic CT scanning and percutaneous preoperative ultrasound only, 25% of patients were found to be unresectable. This inoperability rate was also widely reported by other centres and in one series was as high as 60% for primary hepatocellular carcinoma.[19]

Delayed CT Scanning

Performing a CT scan approximately four hours after the administration of a large dose (75 gm of iodine) of intravenous contrast is a technique that has been used to detect liver masses. It relies on uptake of contrast agent by normal Kupffer cells in the liver. The majority of tumours do not contain these cells and so they will be demonstrated as defects amidst a generally denser liver parenchyma.

The timing of the investigation is not critical and this technique has considerable attraction for convenience of scheduling. Various studies have reported a sensitivity of approximately 90%. The degree of enhancement is not as great as with arterial portography and as a result there is a lower pick-up rate.

Liver-Specific Agents

Various centres have used an intravenous emulsion of oily contrast agent which will be taken up by Kupffer cells and leave tumour unenhanced on scanning. Unfortunately, although this technique holds great promise, centres using the agents have found a significant morbidity with fevers, rigours and malaise being experienced by a large percentage of patients despite pretreatment with steroids and antihistamines. As a result the technique is no longer widely used but there is ongoing research into the development of specific agents.

Oily agents have also been used in patients with hepatoma by injecting Lipiodol contrast agent directly into the hepatic artery and then performing a CT scan (Fig. 15.1.6). The scan may be repeated days or weeks later. This demonstrates rims of Lipiodol around the tumours and may be of particular use in identifying the small daughter tumours of hepatoma.

Magnetic Resonance

MRI scanning of the liver is improving dramatically. The ability to image more rapidly has led to an improvement in spatial resolution although small lesions are still a problem. Despite this, sensitivities of 88% have been reported;[20] in this series the combination of arterial portography and MRI scanning had a sensitivity of 97%. At higher magnet strengths, T_2 weighted spin echo (SE) sequences appear more sensitive (78%) than T_1 SE (47%) and similar to dynamic (71%) or delayed (72%) CT scanning.[21]

MRI using gadolinium-diethylenetriamine penta-acetic acid (Gd-DTPA) intravenously allows utilization of vascular enhancement during scanning. There is improved capacity to differentiate the histological type of tumours with these techniques and it has been applied to hepatic masses. One area where it may be useful is for the differentiation of haemangiomas and metastases. On a scan performed during and shortly after contrast, haemangiomas are seen as hyperintense, homogeneous masses on T_1 weighted images whilst metastases have mixed intensity and relatively low signal. Statistically all the haemangiomas in one series had a higher signal to noise ratio than all metastases and this technique may help differentiate these difficult lesions.[22]

There is no doubt, with improvements in technology, that non-invasive MRI scanning will become more and more useful although problems of availability will continue to thwart some centres.

BILIARY SYSTEM

In its normal state the biliary system, with the exception of the gall bladder, is only marginally visible without the injection of contrast agents. When obstructed, however, the dilated ducts lead directly to the site of the abnormality and the ducts and the lesion are often visualized on US, CT or MRI.

Care should be taken in patients who have had previous duct dilatation as this may remain for the rest of their life despite relief of the obstruction.[23] Biochemical assays will remain normal in these cases and isotope scanning with ^{99}Tc-

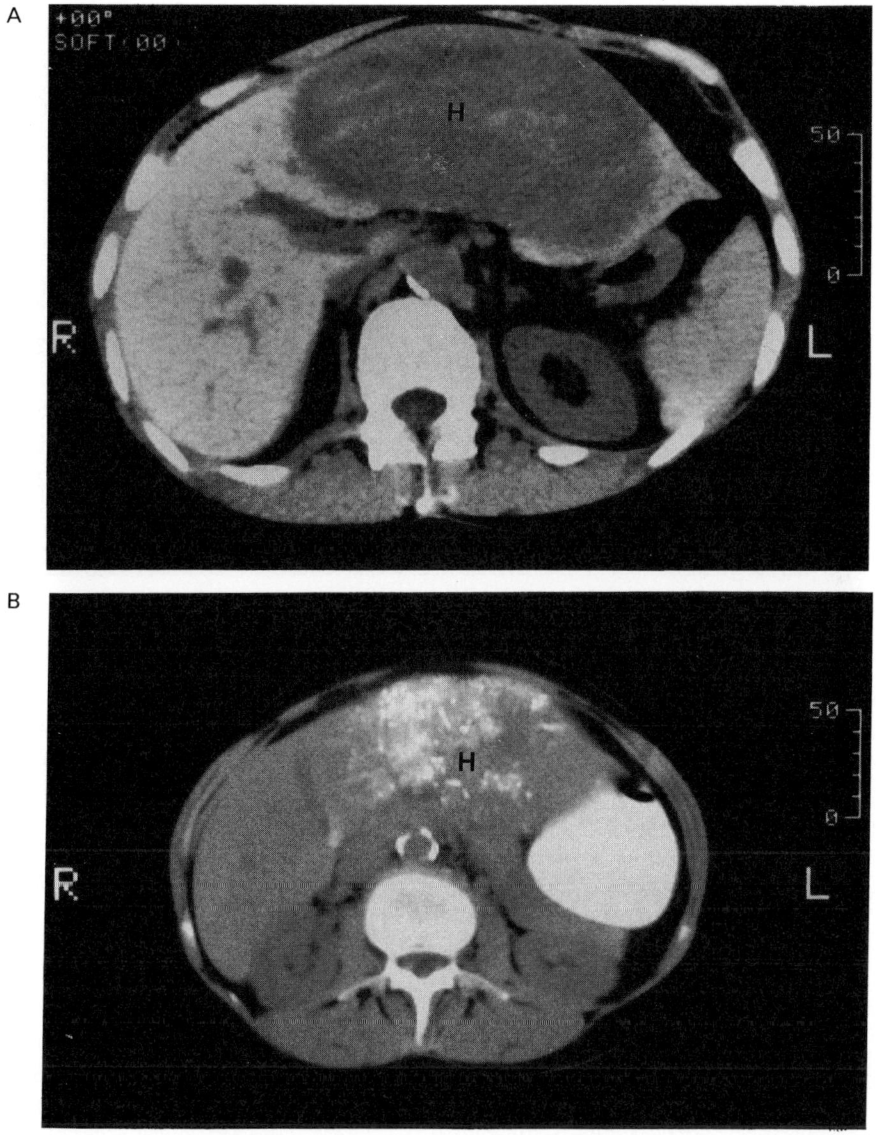

Figure 15.1.6 A: emulsified ethiodol (IOE) enhanced CT scan and B: CT scan following intra-arterial Lipiodol, showing hepatocellular carcinoma (H) (courtesy of Dr D. Redhead, Royal Infirmary, Edinburgh).

HIDA will demonstrate free flow of bile into the gut. However, patients with a treatable cause of biliary obstruction may have ducts of normal diameter.

Cholangiocarcinomas may occur anywhere within the duct system although half occur at the duct bifurcation or distal to it. Klatskin tumours are cholangiocarcinomas arising at the junction of the right and left ducts (Fig.15.1.7).[24] The

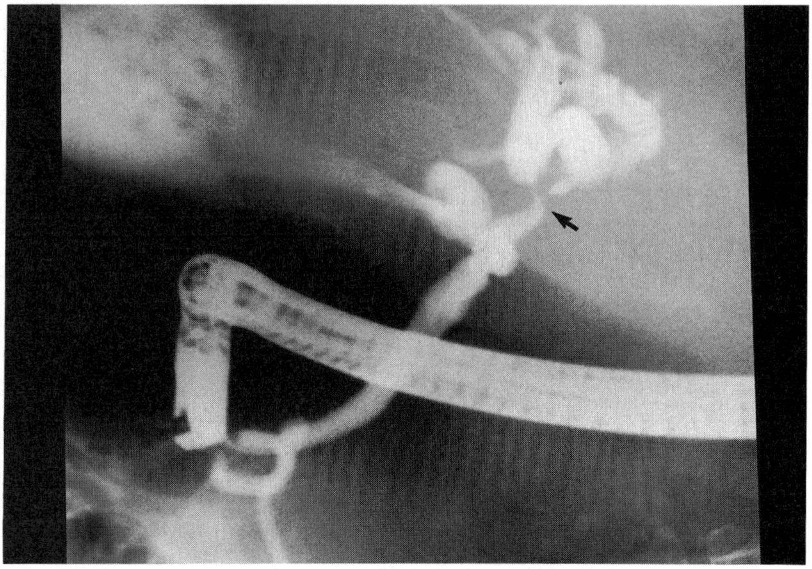

Figure 15.1.7 ERCP showing a typical Klatskin tumour involving the junction of the intrahepatic bile ducts and the common bile duct (arrowed).

resection rate for hilar cholangiocarcinoma is increasing worldwide with a corresponding fall in morbidity and mortality when performed in specialist units.[25] A median survival of two years is expected and the five year survival in recent series has reached a creditable 17%.[26] Despite detailed imaging of the Klatskin tumour the final decision of operability may rest with a trial of dissection.[27] Moreover, intraoperative frozen section may be required to confirm the radicality of resection (Fig. 15.1.8).

Ultrasound

Ultrasound should be the first line of diagnostic examination in most patients and will often indicate the site of obstruction by defining the point where the bile ducts become dilated. If only the intrahepatic ducts are dilated the possibility of a Klatskin tumour is higher.

Cholangiography

Opacification of the biliary tree by injection of contrast, either by percutaneous transhepatic cholangiogram (PTC) or endoscopic retrograde cholangiopancreatogram (ERCP), can produce extremely accurate information for planning resection. As well as allowing the determination of biliary obstruction from non-

A

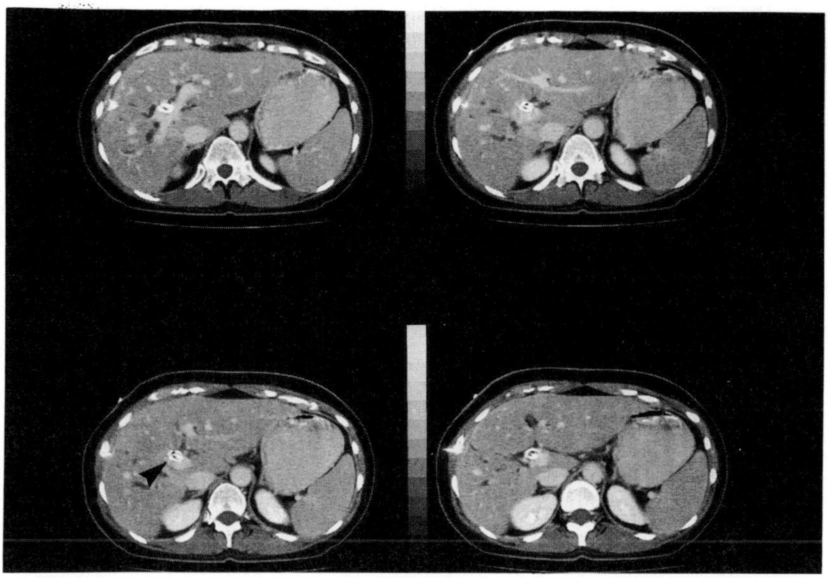

B

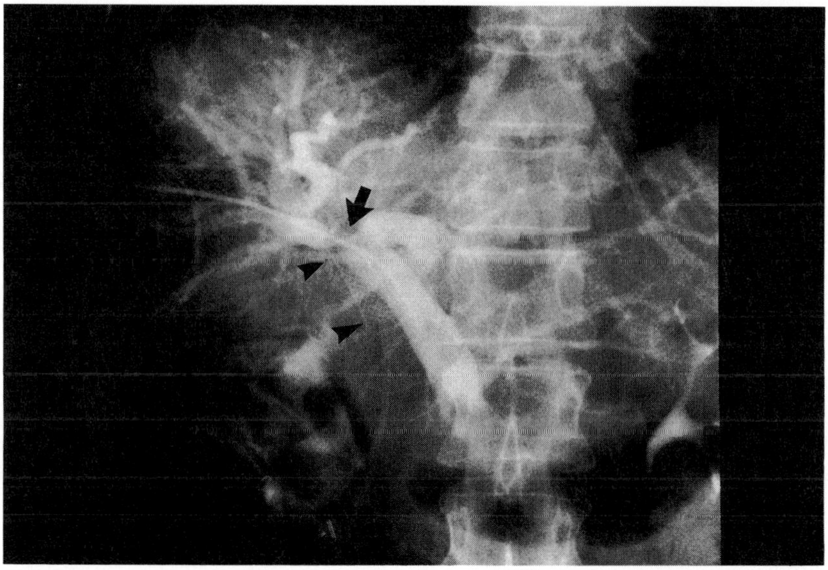

Figure 15.1.8 This patient was referred for a second opinion on a cholangiocarcinoma which had been stented with a Wallstent (arrowheads). A: the CT scan demonstrated a mass lesion which seemed to be involving mostly the right lobe of the liver but sparing the left side. B: A portal venogram demonstrated indentation of the portal vein bifurcation (arrow). At operation the tumour was abutting the junction of the portal vein and so a bypass graft was inserted between the main portal vein and the left portal vein. The tumour was resected with the right lobe, with biliary reconstruction to segments II and III.

neoplastic causes it may be possible to determine the type of lesion with high specificity. A cholangiocarcinoma will produce a characteristic appearance which can usually be distinguished from the obstruction caused by external compression or by conditions such as sclerosing cholangitis. The choice between PTC and ERCP will often reflect local expertise. PTC is more useful if a high obstruction such as a Klatskin tumour is suspected as it may give a clearer indication as to the extent of involvement of the hepatic ducts. In contrast, ERCP allows tumours of the ampulla to be biopsied under direct vision. At ERCP or PTC it is possible to obtain tissue by passing cytology brushes into the biliary ducts.

Following the cholangiogram an indwelling stent may be inserted to palliate the patient's symptoms or to alleviate jaundice to allow a planned resection at a later date.[28,29]

Computed Tomography

Computed tomography can identify biliary obstruction in the majority of cases, 96% in one series.[23] In the diagnosis of the cause of obstruction it is less specific, identifying 70% in a series including biliary calculi.

Cholangiocarcinoma may be difficult to visualize on CT although some lesions may enhance. Others may appear as an intrahepatic mass without specific features. The appearance of duct dilatation with a sudden transition to non-dilated ducts without an obvious mass should suggest the diagnosis, which may need confirmation with cholangiography. CT may indicate extension of the tumour to the right or left half of the liver and help in planning whether the resection should include a hemihepatectomy. If a resection is contemplated then the likelihood of involvement of the portal veins must be clarified and we find the early phase of CTAP useful for this.

Magnetic Resonance

Cholangiocarcinomas may show high signal intensity on T_2 weighted images and low or normal intensity on T_1. MRI may be better than CT at demonstrating the tumour although CT shows the duct dilatation better.[30]

GALL BLADDER

Neoplasms of the gall bladder are rare and may present at a late stage due to their occult nature. They may be demonstrated during routine scanning for gallstones or non-specific abdominal pain. Gall bladder carcinoma (Fig. 15.1.9)

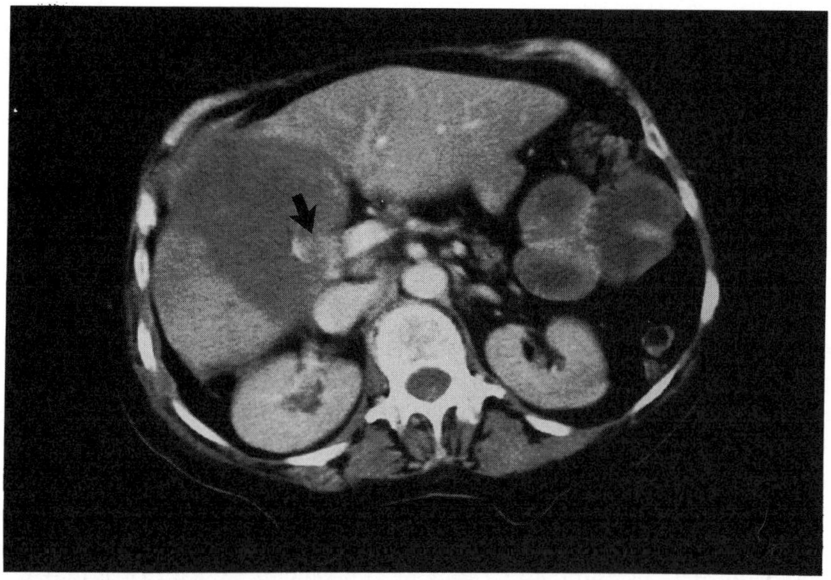

Figure 15.1.9 CT scan showing carcinoma of the gall bladder completely surrounding the portal vein bifurcation (arrow) and hence rendered inoperable.

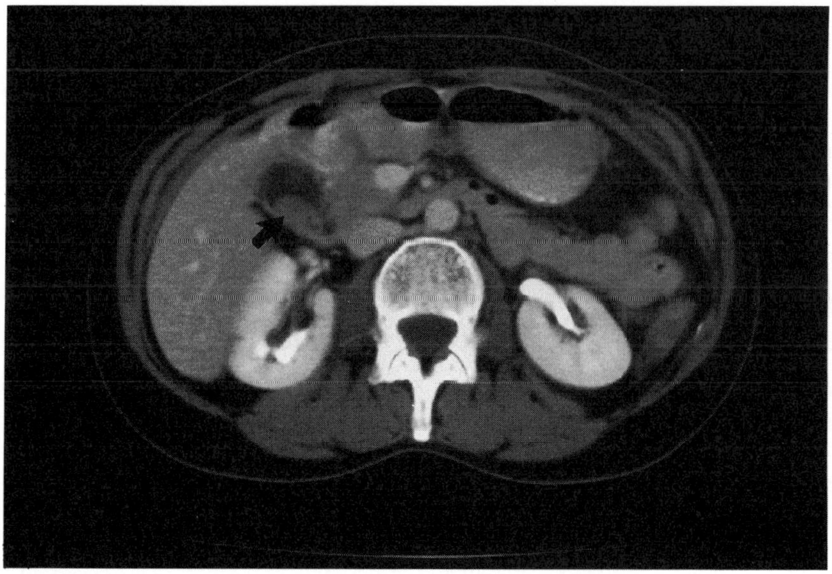

Figure 15.1.10 CT scan of gall bladder demonstrating a discrete mass (arrow) in the wall of the gall bladder without liver involvement. On resection it proved to be a secondary deposit from malignant melanoma.

or metastases, most commonly from melanoma (Fig. 15.1.10),[31] form the majority of lesions. The appearances may suggest malignancy or in a significant minority of cases may be confused with chronic cholecystitis. Gallstones are seen in 45% of patients with carcinoma of the gall bladder and discrete hepatic metastases in 15%.[32]

The treatment of adenocarcinoma of the gall bladder is controversial but it is possible that some patients will benefit from aggressive surgical management.[33,34]

Ultrasound

Ultrasound is the examination of choice for the gall bladder and many patients with gall bladder cancer will be imaged first by US. If the patient is examined at a stage in which the gall bladder carcinoma is involving part of the wall and extending into the lumen of the gall bladder, it is easily visualized. Intrahepatic invasion will be seen in the same way as other intrahepatic lesions. If the tumour is more extensive the gall bladder may be contracted. In this case it may not be possible to distinguish a mass involving the gall bladder from the contracted gall bladder of chronic cholecystitis if local extension is not seen. The extent of the lesion extending outside the gall bladder wall and into the surrounding extra-hepatic structures is very difficult to assess with US.

Computed Tomography

Computed tomography is the most sensitive method of determining the presence, extension and spread of gall bladder cancer. Extra and intrahepatic components can be demonstrated by dynamic CT or, more accurately, by arterial portography (see under Liver).

PANCREAS

Pancreatic malignancies are relatively common, especially in the elderly. Traditionally imaging of the pancreas has been difficult, but cross-sectional imaging techniques have revolutionized diagnosis. Differences in presentation between lesions in the head of the pancreas, often producing biliary obstruction, and those in the body and tail mean that the latter group tend to present later.

Pancreatic adenocarcinoma in its various forms accounts for 80% of the neoplasms of the pancreas and 65% of these occur in the pancreatic head. Differentiation of neoplasm from pancreatitis may be difficult or impossible. In cases without evidence of metastases elsewhere, the presence of peripancreatic inflammatory changes suggests pancreatitis as this is rarely seen with tumours.[35]

Islet cell tumours may be functioning or non-functioning. In 10% of cases insulinomas are multiple or due to islet cell dysplasias and due to metastases in another 10%.[36] The problems associated with accurate localization of insulinomas may be overcome to a large extent by the use of intraoperative ultrasound. This allows precise identification of the tumours and the ability to examine the whole of the gland. Sensitivities of 90% have been reported for this technique.[37]

Contrast Studies

ERCP is an excellent technique for demonstrating neoplasms which affect the pancreatic duct and may be the only way to demonstrate a small ampullary lesion. Direct visualization and biopsy are highly sensitive and specific. There is a small technical failure rate and the morbidity is not insignificant. If a lesion cannot be directly visualized then specificity decreases, particularly in young patients.

Angiography

Until recently the most sensitive technique for defining the resectability of pancreatic neoplasms was a combination of angiography and CT. Occlusion of the vessels precludes resection and encasement is associated with non-resectability in the majority of patients.

In a series of 88 consecutive pancreatic carcinomas 87% were unresectable as determined on CT (Fig. 15.1.11) and angiography. Neither technique sufficed alone in making this determination and MRI did not differ significantly from CT. Small peritoneal metastases were present in 27% of the tumours of the head and 65% of the body and tail of the pancreas. Nearly all these deposits were missed on preoperative imaging.

Transhepatic venous sampling localized 94% of 36 insulinomas in one series[36] compared with CT (26%) and angiography (44%).

Venous sampling during stimulation by selective angiographic injection of calcium has been reported. Angiography combined with CT may be helpful in insulinoma with contrast injected through a selectively positioned catheter.[38]

Ultrasound

Ultrasound is good at demonstrating the effects of a lesion obstructing the biliary tree, which may lead on to the diagnosis of malignancy involving the pancreatic head. However, overlying bowel gas, particularly in patients who

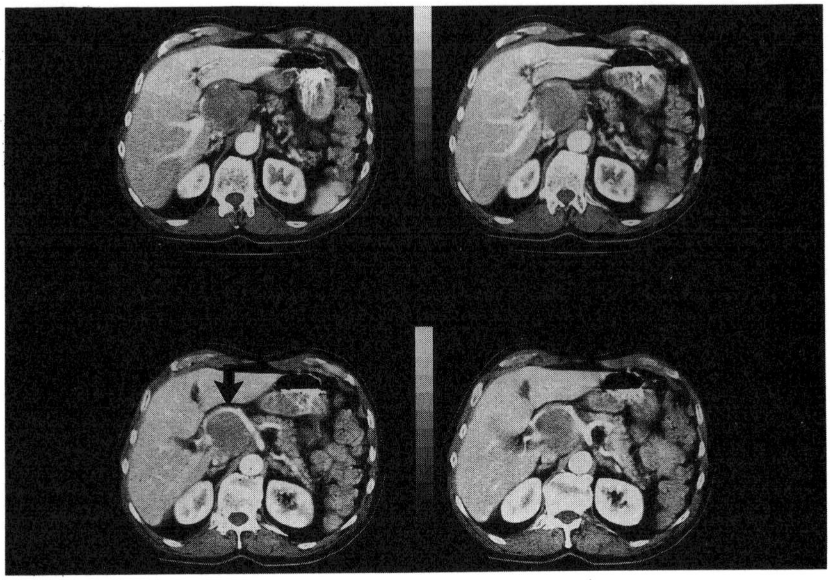

Figure 15.1.11 CT demonstrating a carcinoma of the pancreas involving the portal vein (arrow) and hence non-resectable.

have had previous surgery, may obscure all or parts of the pancreas. As a result, the ability to visualize smaller lesions will be impaired.

Endoscopic Ultrasound

The use of endoscopic techniques to introduce the ultrasound transducer into the stomach and duodenum allows direct contact of a high frequency, high sensitivity transducer with the pancreas without intervening bowel gas. This has proved particularly useful in the localization of islet cell tumours.[39] It has been shown to be superior to angiography and computed tomography in predicting resectability of pancreatic cancer. In a series of 60 patients who underwent all three procedures and subsequent surgery, five patients with surgically proven portal venous involvement were identified by endoscopic ultrasound but not by angiography.[40] The technique is highly operator-dependent and not yet widely available.

Computed Tomography

Dynamic computed tomography is the mainstay of imaging of the pancreas. Because of the small volume of the gland, spatial resolution is at a premium and

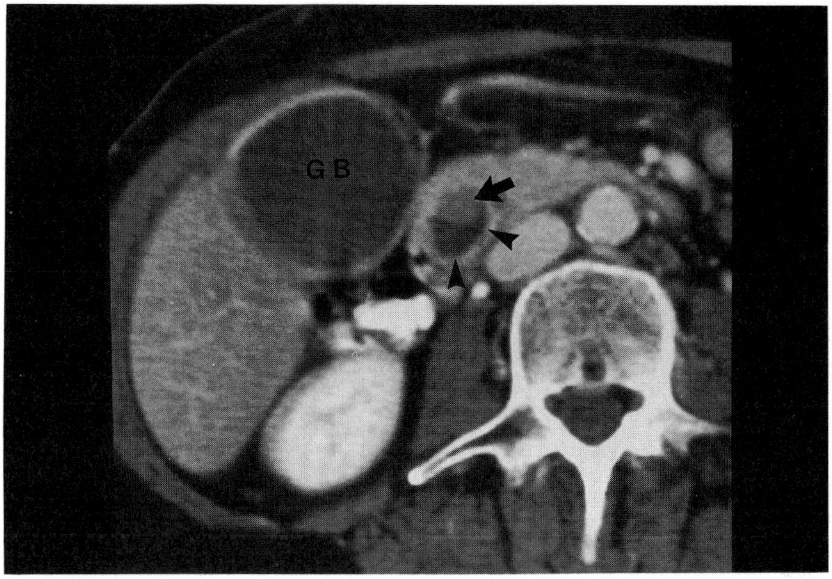

Figure 15.1.12 CT showing an ampullary carcinoma (arrow) in the head of the pancreas invading and obstructing the dilated common bile duct (arrowhead) and gall bladder (GB). Resected by Whipple's procedure.

modern scanners can produce high definition thin slice contiguous scans with short scan times to obtain high spatial resolution without blurring due to patient movement (Fig. 15.1.12). The ability to obtain good images is important as some tumours are only identified by changes in the shape and size of the gland.

Many tumours, particularly those containing cystic elements or necrosis, are hypodense on the unenhanced images. Most of the non-islet cell tumours will become hypodense relative to the normally enhancing tissue during intravenous enhancement. High doses of contrast enhancement will permit visualization of the pancreatic duct outlined by the surrounding tissue and this may detect subtle dilatation as a result of obstruction by tumour. The improved sensitivity for CT when combined with angiography has been referred to previously.

Even with these techniques there are problems with small lesions, particularly ampullary ones, and although cystic abnormalities may be identified it is much harder to identify small solid lesions. Adenocarcinoma of the ampulla accounts for a relatively small number of pancreatic malignancies and is well demonstrated with ERCP. Conventional CT does not usually demonstrate these lesions; however, when combined with hypotonic duodenography CT may show a mass at the ampulla.[41] The sensitivity of this has not yet been analysed but the technique adds to the ability of CT to identify the causes of biliary obstruction.

Islet cell tumours may be functioning or non functioning. The latter tend to enhance following contrast administration, may contain calcification and grow slowly. Insulinomas are almost always hyperdense following enhancement but may be so small as to be difficult to image during the phase of enhancement. Some small tumours, in particular insulinomas, may be multiple. Other islet cell tumours may be situated in or near the pancreas; CT will demonstrate 60–85% of these lesions. Preoperative CT is essential to identify that the tumour is likely to be operable. It may not be possible to identify all of the lesions preoperatively, but they are demonstrated well on endoscopic or intraoperative ultrasound and lesions that are impalpable at laparotomy may be identified via the use of direct contact probes.

RENAL TRACT

Malignancies in the Renal Tract

The malignancies affecting the renal tract can be divided into the mass lesions affecting the renal parenchyma, predominantly renal cell carcinoma which accounts for 85% of all renal neoplasms, and the neoplasms of transitional cell endothelium, which will be treated separately. A small number of benign lesions may also be discovered and some of these may have the capability to become malignant. Some adenomas show oncocytic features with a central scar visible on angiography, CT or MRI. Papillary carcinoma may also show this appearance. Renal cell carcinoma may be bilateral and transitional cell lesions may be multiple so it is important to assess the whole renal tract before surgery.

Mass Lesions

Contrast Studies

Intravenous urography/pyelography (IVU) was for a long time the mainstay for renal imaging. While careful pyelography with tomograms will identify many lesions there is always a potential problem with lesions on the front or back of the kidney which may not be readily appreciated, especially if there is overlying bowel gas. Larger lesions are relatively easy to identify due to distortion of the collecting system and abnormalities in the nephrogram. IVU with tomography will identify 85% of lesions greater than 3 cm, 52% of those 2–3 cm in size, 21% between 1–2 cm and 10% below this size.[42]

Angiography

The use of angiography has become much less common since the advent of CT and MRI. They have proved more sensitive in the detection and staging of tumours and are equally sensitive at detecting venous involvement. Angiography may have a role for tumour embolization in selected cases.

Ultrasound

Although technical problems may make it difficult to get good visualization of the whole of the parenchyma, particularly on the left side, the ready availability of US makes it the most commonly used technique in identifying or confirming the presence of renal masses. While cystic lesions are demonstrated well with ultrasound, small solid lesions are less easy to appreciate. US will detect 85% of renal masses above 2 cm, 60% between 1–2 cm and 26% below 1 cm.[42] Some benign lesions such as oncocytoma may contain fat and calcification and these specific appearances may be identified with ultrasound.

Computed Tomography

Computed tomography is a sensitive discriminator of renal masses using high definition contiguous scans following contrast injection to accurately define lesions. Solid lesions are seen well because of the kidneys' ability to concentrate contrast. CT has a sensitivity of better than 95% for mass lesions. Contrast agents and high definition scanning enables smaller lesions in the walls of cysts to be identified.

Not surprisingly, these smaller lesions are less specific and confusion may be induced by the presence of clot or other irregularities on the wall of the cyst itself. CT allows the detection of the primary tumour, its local spread and any lymphadenopathy and demonstrates tumour thrombus in the renal vein and IVC (Fig. 15.1.13).

One third of patients with hypernephroma will have metastases at diagnosis, though this may be confined to a single site.[43,44] CT is able to image all these sites and provides a simple way to stage these patients. Curry, in a study of atypical renal masses, found a positive predictive value of over 96%.[45]

CT will identify local spread of the tumour with thickening of the connective tissue septa within the perinephric fat. As spread progresses there may be thickening or breaching of Gerota's fascia and invasion of nearby organs. Lymphadenopathy, venous invasion and distant metastases may be visualized. Interestingly the detection of enlarged nodes in patients with renal carcinoma does not necessarily indicate spread. Fifty eight percent of enlarged regional nodes (1–2.2 cm in diameter, median 1.4 cm) were due to inflammatory changes or follicular hypoplasia in a study from Berne.[46]

In a series of patients scanned between 1986 and 1987 using CT, MRI and angiography, CT and MRI correctly T-staged the tumours in 63% and 64% respectively and angiography in 54%. MRI was superior to CT in the detection of nodal disease with an overall accuracy of 89% compared with 77% by CT.[47]

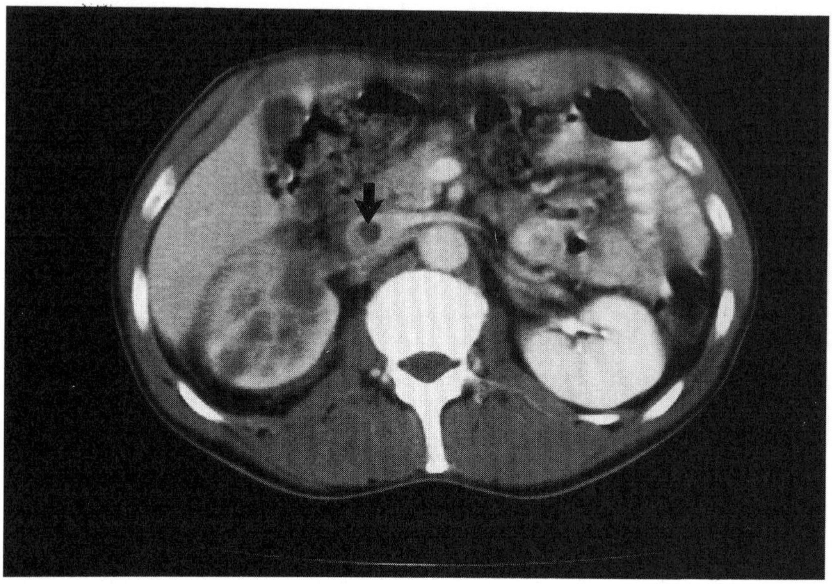

Figure 15.1.13 CT scan of hypernephroma with thrombus extending into the inferior vena cava (arrow).

Angiomyolipomas contain vessels, smooth muscle and fat in varying quantities and this last feature enables a confident diagnosis of this condition to be made. These tumours metastasize very rarely but may invade local structures. Lymphoma or metastases involving the kidney and xanthogranulomatous pyelonephritis may mimic hypernephroma and lead to confusion.

Magnetic Resonance

MRI has an increasing role in the diagnosis of renal mass. In addition to information about the tumour itself it may be possible to identify complications. In a series of 26 patients with renal carcinoma, Roubidoux identified renal vein thrombus in 88% of those with clot, all patients who had clot in the cava and 80% of those with right atrial thrombus. This group used a gradient recalled echo sequence to demonstrate the vascular structures.[48]

MRI is less accurate than CT in the diagnosis of small renal cell carcinomas. Angiomyolipomas are well demonstrated though if they contain only tiny amounts of fat, initial diagnosis may be difficult.

Transitional Lesions

The lesions taking origin from transitional cell endothelium are often small and can sometimes only be identified with certainty when outlined by iodinated contrast agents. They account for 5–10% of renal tumours. A variety of other tumour types can rarely affect the urothelium and are indistinguishable.

Contrast Studies

These lesions may be identified with IVU but their presence often needs confirmation with a direct injection of contrast, most usually by a retrograde pyelogram from the bladder or from percutaneous antegrade nephrostogram. There may be technical problems due to the use of over-concentrated contrast agent obscuring small lesions and specificity is decreased by the presence of filling defects from other causes such as non-opaque stone, blood clot or fungal infections.

Computed Tomography

Computed tomography is used to assess patients with transitional cell carcinoma (TCC). It may differentiate between tumour and other causes such as stone or clot and can assess and stage tumour preoperatively. Despite problems with the size of some of these lesions, CT identifies 90% of primary transitional cell carcinomas of the upper urinary tract.[49] Local and distant spread may be identified but it is not possible to differentiate between lesions limited to the urothelium and those with muscle involvement.

Indeterminate Masses

Some lesions are very difficult to assess despite the use of all imaging techniques. In many series approximately 5% of lesions will be in this group. Once technically adequate examinations have been obtained there may still be doubt over "complicated" cysts with abnormal features in the walls or lumen, thick-walled cysts or lesions that may or may not be solid. Percutaneous guided biopsy with US or CT control or operative inspection should be performed readily in this group. In one series, if three or more "non-cystic" criteria were present, the chance of the lesion being neoplastic was 95%[45] (Fig. 15.1.14).

ADRENAL GLANDS

Primary neoplasms of the adrenal gland vary considerably in size at presentation. Depending on their effects on the hormonal status of the patient they may be occult or may produce symptoms leading to their detection. Adrenal carcinoma and metastatic disease may produce very large masses. These may be

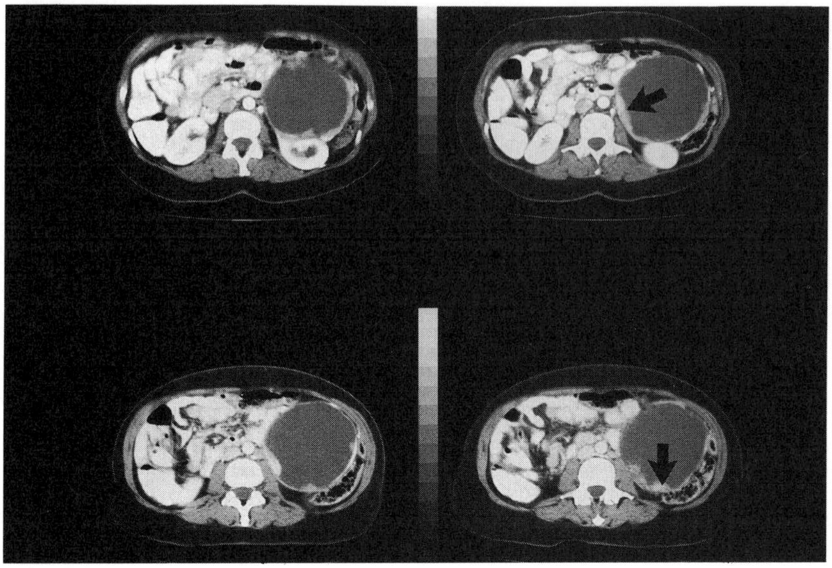

Figure 15.1.14 CT scan of left kidney showing a large cystic lesion of the kidney with irregular and thickened cyst walls (arrows). This identifies it as an atypical or complicated renal cyst and therefore likely to be neoplastic.

locally invasive and CT or MRI is used to identify spread to adjacent organs, in addition to the identification of distant metastases.

Symptomatic phaeochromocytoma will nearly invariably be associated with raised urinary catecholamine, vanillylmandelic acid and metanephrine levels.[50] Ten percent of these lesions lie outside the adrenal medulla, of which 40% will be malignant compared with 6–10% of those in the adrenal.[51] Patients with multiple endocrine adenomatosis type II may develop asymptomatic phaeochromocytomas which may be bilateral though rarely extra-adrenal.

Contrast Examination

Selective adrenal venography with venous sampling may rarely be useful in identifying aldosteronomas if CT and MRI are normal.

Ultrasound

Although US may identify lesions in the adrenal gland its sensitivity is low. It can be used, however, to characterize lesions particularly by distinguishing between cysts and fatty adenomas that on CT have a similar appearance. US guided biopsy is also useful.

Computed Tomography

Computed tomography is the backbone of imaging of the adrenals. High definition contiguous enhanced scans will demonstrate changes in the shape of the adrenal glands, facilitated by the fact that they are surrounded by fat which produces excellent contrast resolution. Problems may be experienced because of the heterogenicity of normal appearances of the adrenal glands. Because the glands are normally very small, it is usually possible to detect lesions down to 0.5 mm in diameter. These tumours may be detected by subtle changes in the contour of the gland. The presence of fluid or fat within the tumour or marked enhancement following intravenous contrast administration increases the pick-up.

Although the appearances of the tumours themselves are normally non-specific, when considered with the clinical and biochemical evidence it is often possible to correctly classify these lesions. The accuracy of CT in identifying adrenal masses exceeds 90%.[52] Adenomas are reliably identified as homogeneous well-defined masses although they may appear of low density or contain calcium. Aldosteronomas are usually smaller than cortisol secreting tumours and so are harder to detect. Phaeochromocytomas may contain central necrosis or calcification and enhance following IV contrast. CT will detect 90% of phaeochromocytomas providing the area containing them is scanned including the bladder, mediastinum and organ of Zuckerkandl. Alpha-adrenergic blockade should be considered when IV contrast is being used as hypertensive crisis has been reported following administration.[53] With the larger adrenal mass, CT is useful in identifying involvement of the liver to alert the surgeon to what may be required. This avoids the need for a bloody trial of dissection in inexperienced hands. The key points are whether the IVC and/or the right hepatic vein are involved. Although it is technically possible to resect both it usually requires specialist surgical skills.

With these large adrenal masses the resectability is best defined preoperatively by CT. At laparotomy it is impossible to tell the degree of invasion until the dissection is well advanced.

Nuclear Medicine

MIBG (^{131}I labelled metaiodobenzylguanidine) scanning has been reported as similar to CT in sensitivity to phaeochromocytomas and allows visualization of the whole body. It is, however, expensive and time consuming.[54]

Magnetic Resonance Imaging

Magnetic resonance imaging is also helped by the presence of fat, especially when using T_1 weighted images when adenomas will be visualized as low signal areas surrounded by the high signal fat. Carcinoma may have a mixed signal on T_1 and on T_2 produce a higher signal than the surrounding fat.

MRI has been reported as comparable to CT in the detection of adrenal masses.[55,56] Scanning of the adrenal should be considered in patients with carcinoma elsewhere who are discovered on CT to have what appears to be a solitary adenoma and no other evidence of metastatic disease. This form of imaging may distinguish between metastasis and adenoma and if equivocal then guided biopsy can be performed.

SPLEEN

Neoplasms of the spleen such as lymphoma and leukaemia produce generalized diffuse increase in size and discrete neoplasms such as metastases produce abnormal areas within normal parenchymal tissue. With all cases of generalized splenic enlargement, the results of imaging are poor although the increase in size may be appreciated.

Plain Films

If the spleen is markedly enlarged then plain films may detect the presence of a mass in the left upper quadrant. In conditions such as myelofibrosis the increase in size may be considerable and may be associated with other changes such as generalized bony sclerosis. If the degree of splenic enlargement is small then plain films have very little place.

Ultrasound

Ultrasound may detect either generalized enlargement or discrete masses in the splenic bed. Discrete lesions within the spleen may be seen as well or better than with CT.

Nuclear Medicine

Isotope scanning of the spleen may show focal defects or generalized enlargement and although there is reasonable sensitivity, specificity is very low.

Computed Tomography

Computed tomography can provide an accurate determination of splenic pathology, but only with focal lesions. In addition it may show other abnormalities such as para-aortic lymphadenopathy or hepatic lesions which may increase the specificity of the diagnosis. In conditions producing lesions less than 1 cm in diameter, particularly when the gland is diffusely involved, CT may be unable to identify discrete lesions and only diffuse enlargement may be identified. It should be remembered that in Hodgkins disease, for example, one third of patients may have splenomegaly without histological involvement of the spleen.[57,58]

Metastases to the spleen are uncommon, occurring in only 4% of patients with cancer, usually with disseminated deposits.[59] One third of splenic metastases seen at autopsy are not visible on CT. Care has to be taken particularly during dynamic CT as there is normally an irregular enhancement pattern during the early stage of dynamic enhancement; this may produce an irregular pattern which may be mistaken for multiple metastases.

Although it is often possible to detect enlargement of the spleen without using specific volume calculations, it may be difficult to determine whether mild splenomegaly is present; up to a 50% increase in size may not be appreciated.

STOMACH AND SMALL BOWEL

Neoplasms of the stomach include adenocarcinoma, leiomyosarcoma, lymphoma and involvement by metastases. The small bowel may be involved by similar disease and there is a higher incidence of primary conditions such as carcinoid which may produce liver metastases.

Endoscopic Examination

Endoscopy has overtaken barium studies as the major way of identifying neoplasms in the stomach. The advantage of gastroscopy is that the true extent of mucosal spread can be identified and confirmed by biopsy. However, endoscopy will not reliably indicate resectability and in the case of linitis plastica, may be difficult to diagnose. The latter may be better seen on a barium meal in the early stages.

Barium Examination

Endoscopy of anything apart from the upper part of the small bowel is not routinely possible. Visualization of the small bowel, therefore, is usually by barium studies. The concept of the "barium meal and follow through" examination has largely been abandoned and has given way to the concept of the small bowel meal as a dedicated small bowel investigation or the rather more invasive small bowel enema which requires intubation of the upper jejunum usually via a transnasal route.

This intubation is more unpleasant for the patient but the proponents of the small bowel enema suggest that the greater distension of the small bowel and the use of a double contrast technique improves the sensitivity of the study.

Computed Tomography

Increasingly CT, with the ability to image the whole of the wall of the viscera, may be used to identify and stage neoplasms of the gut. There may be problems in identification of the site of the involved segment particularly in the small bowel. CT can identify liver secondaries and also demonstrate nodal spread outside the scope of surgical endeavour. However, as with all bowel tumours, there may still be a case for palliative resection for obstruction and therefore the need for extensive preoperative tests is less clear.

In the stomach, CT has the ability to demonstrate thickening of the wall. Enhancement may be seen with scirrhous tumours or in cases of linitis plastica. Neoplasms near the gastro-oesophageal junction may be demonstrated and their extent may be better appreciated by preoperative CT. In one series 76% of patients were not suitable for curative resection due to local or distant spread.[60] In patients with gastric lymphoma CT correctly stages 90% and allows simple follow-up.[61]

It must be remembered that peritoneal seeding is common but unlikely to be identified radiologically.

COLON

Colonic neoplasms may present at an early or late stage. Rectal bleeding may focus diagnostic attention at a very early stage to a tiny adenoma whereas very large lesions may go unnoticed if they do not produce obstruction or change in bowel habit.

Endoscopy

Colonoscopy is becoming increasingly common with its ability to identify and treat; however, it usually contributes little to knowledge about the operability of the tumour.

Contrast Examination

Double contrast barium enema has for many years been the mainstay of diagnostic effort in the proximal colon. The high quality examination has a very high pick-up rate but overlapping of the bowel loops, diverticular disease in the sigmoid region and faecal soiling around the caecum and ileocaecal valve produce areas of diagnostic confusion and possible missed diagnoses.

Ultrasound Examination

Although there is some interest in the use of ultrasound it has not yet gained wide acceptance. The presence of bowel gas makes it difficult and complete examination of the bowel cannot be guaranteed. There has been some interest in the use of ultrasound following administration of a very large fluid enema to distend the bowel and displace air but although high sensitivity has been reported, enthusiasm has been tempered by the technological difficulties involved.

Endosonography

The spread of rectal cancers can be defined by endorectal ultrasound where both the depth of invasion and pararectal lymph node enlargement can be seen. Transanal US has been shown to be more accurate than CT and clinical examination combined.[62] US may thus help define those patients with irresectable rectal cancers more suited to preoperative radiotherapy. Endorectal US is also useful in defining those patients who may be suitable for a peranal excision.[63] MRI may be better but is far more expensive and not yet used routinely.

Computed Tomography

There has been increasing interest in the use of computed tomography, particularly in elderly and frail patients, for the diagnosis of colonic neoplasms. It is relatively non-invasive and provides information about the primary lesion and its spread.

RETROPERITONEAL TISSUES

The tissues of the retroperitoneum may contain a variety of neoplasms. Lymph nodes may be involved with many different neoplasms, major vessels are rarely affected and the musculoskeletal tissues may be involved by any local tumour. The retroperitoneal compartments such as the perinephric space contain fat and other connective tissues which may be affected by primary neoplasms masquerading as lesions of the local organs.

Contrast Studies

Lymphangiography is an extremely sensitive determinant of involvement of small lymph nodes. It is significantly more sensitive than computed tomography in determining whether nodes of less than 15 mm are abnormal and small volume nodal disease can only be detected with this technique. The technical difficulties of performing the test and the time involved, together with the moderate morbidity and the increasing effectiveness of computed tomography, have lead to almost complete abandonment of lymphangiography.

Angiography is exquisitely sensitive in abnormalities involving the blood vessels and will demonstrate any associated thrombus within them.

Ultrasound

Ultrasound examination of the retroperitoneum is hampered by the presence of overlying structures and particularly bowel gas. The results of ureteric obstruction are well demonstrated and this forms the main indication for its use.

Computed Tomography

Computed tomography is very sensitive in determining the presence of neoplasms involving the retroperitoneum. Much of the retroperitoneum is outlined by tissue planes containing fat which improves the sensitivity. Other abnormalities such as lymphadenopathy can be accurately identified although the general CT criteria for lymphadenopathy is nodes measuring more than 10 or 15 mm in diameter. This is obviously a statistical diagnosis and one which has inherent problems. CT will display distant metastases and may give a better definition of local tissue invasion than can be found at laparotomy (Fig. 15.1.15).

There are some specific CT features that may point to surgical diagnoses in retroperitoneal tumours. The presence of fat in the mass suggests a liposarcoma; large regions of necrosis, although non-specific, are commonly found in leiomyosarcoma; calcification is a prominent feature in malignant fibrohistiocytoma.[64,65]

CONCLUSION

One of the most disappointing tasks for any surgeon is to have to tell a patient that nothing could be done at the time of laparotomy. This places great

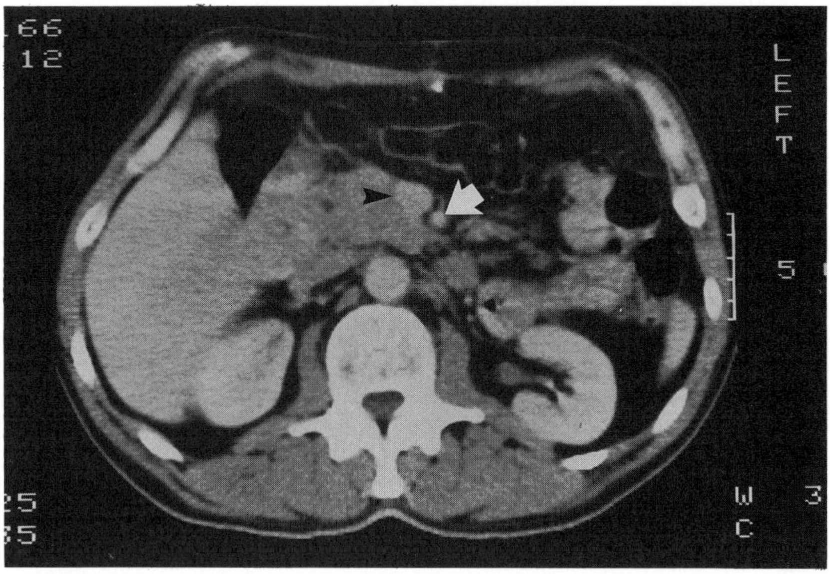

Figure 15.1.15 This patient with fibromatosis had a laparotomy and was assessed as unresectable at this stage. Surgical clips were inserted to mark the extent of the lesion for possible radiotherapy. A subsequent CT demonstrated that the vital structures, the mesenteric artery (arrow) and vein (arrowhead) were discrete from the mass or had a resectable plane and the patient was returned to theatre for a successful curative resection.

importance on making an accurate diagnosis and assessment of tumour spread at a preoperative stage. We have highlighted areas where modern radiological techniques enable patients to undergo laparotomy with a reasonable expectation of a successful outcome and to avoid unnecessary or inappropriate surgery.

The one remaining area where modern radiology may fail to make a correct diagnosis is in the detection of early intraperitoneal seedlings of tumour. In cases where this is likely the next step should be a laparoscopic assessment either as a preliminary or as a planned separate procedure.

It is our view that laparoscopy is a useful adjunct to the preoperative work-up and should not be viewed as a competitor.

REFERENCES

1. Collins CD, Padley SP, Greenwell F, Phelan M. The efficacy of a single posteroanterior radiograph in the assessment of metastatic pulmonary melanoma. *Br J Radiol* 1993; **66**: 117–19.
2. Keogan MT, Tung KT, Caplan DK, Goldstraw PJ, Hansell DM. The significance of pulmonary nodules detected on staging CT for lung cancer. *Clinical Radiology* 1993; in press.

3. Chalmers N, Best JJK. The significance of pulmonary nodules detected by CT but not by chest radiography in tumour staging. *Clin Radiol* 1991; **44**: 410–12.
4. Tung KT, Downes MO, O'Donnell PJ. Renal biopsy in diffuse renal disease–experience with a 14-gauge automated biopsy gun. *Clin Radiol* 1992; **46**: 111–13.
5. Mueller PR, Miketic LM, Simeone JF *et al.* Severe acute pancreatitis after percutaneous biopsy of the pancreas. *AJR* 1988; **151**: 493–4.
6. Smith EH. Complications of percutaneous abdominal fine needle biopsy. *Radiology* 1991; **178**: 253–8.
7. Quaghebeur, Thompson JN, Blumgart LH, Benjamin IS. Implantation of Hepatocellular Carcinoma after Percutaneous Needle Biopsy. *J Roy Coll Surg Edinb* 1991; **36**: 127–8.
8. Bissonnette RT, Gibney RG, Berry BR, Buckley AR. Fatal Carcinoid Crisis after Percutaneous Fine-Needle Biopsy of Hepatic Metastasis: Case Report and Literature Review. *Radiology* 1990; **174**: 751–2.
9. Nelson RC, Chezmar JL, Sugarbaker PH, Bernardino ME. Hepatic tumours: comparison of CT during arterial portography, delayed CT and MR imaging for preoperative evaluation. *Radiology* 1989; **172**: 27–34.
10. Pain JA, Karani J, Howard ER. Pre-operative radiological and clinical assessment of hepatic tumours–is biopsy necessary? *Clin Radiol* 1991; **44**: 181–2.
11. Makuuchi M, Hasegawa H, Yamasaki S. Ultrasonically guided subsegmentectomy. *Surg Gynecol Obstet* 1985: **161**: 346–50.
12. Soyer P, Levesque M, Elias D, Zeitoun G, Roche A. Preoperative assessment of resectability of hepatic metastases from colonic carcinoma: CT portography vs sonography and dynamic CT. *AJR* 1992; **159**: 741–4.
13. DuBrow RA, David CL, Libshitz HI, Lorigan JG. Detection of Hepatic Metastases in Breast Cancer: The Role of Non-enhanced and Enhanced CT Scanning. *Comp Assist Tomog* 1990; **14**: 366–9.
14. Bressler EL, Alpern MB, Glazer GM, Francis IR, Ensminger WD. Hypervascular hepatic metastases: CT evaluation. *Radiology* 1987; **162**: 49–51.
15. Clarke MP, Kane RA, Steele G Jr *et al.* Prospective comparison of preoperative imaging and intraoperative ultrasonography in the detection of liver tumours. *Surgery* 1989; **106**: 849–55.
16. Steves MA, Vidal-Jove J, Sugarbaker PH *et al.* Preoperative radiological evaluation of the liver by computerized tomographic portography in patients with hepatic tumours. *Am Surg* 1989; **58**: 608–12.
17. Del Pilar FM, Bernardino MR. Hepatic pseudolesion: appearance of focal low attenuation in the medial segment of the left lobe at CT arterial portography: *Radiology* 1991; **181**: 809–12.
18. Tyrrell RT, Kaufman SL, Bernardino ME. Straight line sign: appearance and significance during CT portography. *Radiology* 1989; **173**: 635–7.
19. Bismuth H, Castaing D, Garden OJ. The use of operative ultrasound in the surgery of primary liver tumours. *Br J Surg* 1987; **74**: 324–6.
20. Zeman RK, Dritschilo A, Silverman PM *et al.* Dynamic CT vs 0.5 T MR imaging in the detection of surgically proven hepatic metastases. *J Comp Assis Tomog* 1989; **13**: 637–44.
21. Vassiliades VG, Foley WD, Alarcon J *et al.* Hepatic metastases: CT versus MR imaging at 1.5T. *Gastrointest Radiol* 1991; **16**: 159–63.
22. Hamm B, Fischer E, Taupitz M. Differentiation of Hepatic Haemangiomas from Metastases by Dynamic Contrast-Enhanced MR Imaging. *Comp Assist Tomog* 1990; **14**: 205–16.
23. Baron RL, Stanley RJ, Lee JKT *et al.* A prospective comparison of the evaluation of biliary obstruction using computed tomography and ultrasonography. *Radiology* 1982; **145**: 91–8.

24. Carr DH, Hadjis NS, Banks LM, Hemingway AP, Blumgart LH. Computed tomography of hilar cholangiocarcinoma: a new sign. *AJR* 1985; **145**: 53–6.
25. Cameron JL, Pitt HA, Zinner MJ, Kaufman SL, Coleman J. Management of proximal cholangiocarcinoma by surgical resection and radiotherapy. *Am J Surg* 1990; **159**: 91–7.
26. Beorma EG. Research into the results of resection of hilar bile duct cancer. *Surgery* 1990; **108**: 572–80.
27. Cotton PB. Management of malignant bile duct obstruction. *J Gastroenterol Hepatol* 1990; **5**: 63–77.
28. Speer AG, Cotton PB, Russell RCG *et al.* Randomised trial of endoscopic versus percutaneous stent insertion in malignant obstructive jaundice. *Lancet* 1987; **i**: 57–62.
29. Dowsett JF, Vaira D, Hatfield ARW *et al.* Endoscopic Biliary Therapy Using the Combined Percutaneous and Endoscopic Technique. *Gastroenterology* 1989; **96**: 1180–7.
30. Dooms GC, Kerlan RK Jr, Hricak H, Wall SD, Margulis AR. Cholangiocarcinoma: imaging by MR. *Radiology* 1986; **159**: 89–94.
31. Daunt N, King DM. Metastatic melanoma in the biliary tree. *Br J Radiol* 1982; **55**: 873–4.
32. Itai Y, Araki T, Yoshikawa K, Furui S, Yashiro N, Tasaka A. Computed tomography of gallbladder carcinoma. *Radiology* 1980; **137**: 713–18.
33. Scott Jones R. Carcinoma of the gallbladder. *Surg Clin N Am* 1990; **70**: 1419–23.
34. Carty NJ, Johnson CD. Carcinoma of the Gallbladder: a survey of cases in Wessex 1982–1989. *J Roy Coll Surg Edinb* 1991; **36**: 238–41.
35. Haaga JR. *Computed Tomography of the Whole Body*, 2nd edition. Washington, C.V. Mosby 1988.
36. Pasieka JL, McLeod MK, Thompson NW, Burney RE. Surgical approach to insulinomas. Assessing the need for preoperative localization. *Arch Surg* 1992; **127**: 442–7.
37. Grant CS, van Heerden J, Charboneau JW, James EM, Reeding CC. Insulinoma: the value of intraoperative ultrasonography. *Arch Surg* 1988; **99**: 671–8.
38. Krudy AG, Doppman JL, Jensen RT *et al.* Localization of islet cell tumours by dynamic CT: comparison with plain CT, arteriography, sonography and venous sampling. *AJR* 1984; **143**: 585.
39. Glover JR, Shorvon PJ, Lees WR. Endoscopic Ultrasound for Localisation of Islet Cell Tumours. *Gut* 1993; **33**: 108–11.
40. Rosch T, Braig C, Gain T *et al.* Staging of Pancreatic and Ampullary Carcinoma by Endoscopic Ultrasonography. *Gastroenterology* 1992; **102**: 188–99.
41. Pandolfo I, Scribano E, Blandino A *et al.* Tumours of the Ampulla Diagnosed by CT Hypotonic Duodenography. *Comp Assist Tomog* 1990; **14**: 199–200.
42. Warshauer DM, McCarthy M, Street L *et al.* Detection of Renal Masses: Sensitivities and specificities of excretory urography/linear tomography, US and CT. *Radiology* 1988; **169**: 363–5.
43. McClennan BL. Computed tomography in the diagnosis and staging of renal cell carcinoma. *Semin Urol* 1985; **3**: 111–31.
44. McClennan BL, Balfe DM. Oncologic imaging of the kidney and ureter. *Int J Radiat Oncol Biol Phys* 1983; **9**: 1683–704.
45. Curry NS, Reinig J, Schabel SI, Ross P, Vujic I, Gobien RP. An evaluation of the effectiveness of CT vs. other imaging modalities in the diagnosis of atypical renal masses. *Invest Radiol* 1984; **19**: 447–52.
46. Studer UE, Scherz S, Scheidegger J *et al.* Enlargement of regional lymph nodes in renal cell carcinoma is often not due to metastases. *J Urol* 1990; **144**: 243–5.
47. Constantinides C, Recker F, Bruehlmann W *et al.* Accuracy of magnetic resonance imaging compared to computerized tomography and renal selective angiography in pre-operatively staging renal cell carcinoma. *Urologia Internationalis* 1991; **47**: 181–5.

48. Roubidoux MA, Dunnick NR, Sostman HD, Leder RA. Renal carcinoma: detection of venous extension with gradient-echo MR imaging. *Radiology* 1992; **182**: 269–72.
49. Badalament RA, Bennett WF, Bova JG *et al.* Computed tomography of primary transitional cell carcinoma of upper urinary tracts. *Urology* 1992; **40**: 71–5.
50. Cryer PE. The adrenergic nervous system. In: *Diagnostic Endocrinology*, 2nd edition (ed. Cryer PE), pp. 117–34. New York, Oxford University Press, 1979.
51. Hume DM. Phaeochromocytoma in the adult and in the child. *Am J Surg* 1960; **99**: 458–96.
52. Abrams HI, Sieglman SS, Adams DF *et al.* Computed tomography versus ultrasound of the adrenal gland: a prospective study. *Radiology* 1982; **143**: 121–8.
53. Raisanen J, Shapiro B, Glazer GM, Desai S, Sisson JC. Plasma catecholamines in phaeochromocytoma: effect of urographic contrast media. *AJR* 1984; **143**: 43–6.
54. Quint LE, Glazer GM, Francis IR, Shapiro B, Chenevert TL. Phaeochromocytoma and paraganglioma: comparison of MR imaging with CT and 1–131 MIBG scintigraphy. *Radiology* 1987; **165**: 89–93.
55. Reining JW, Doppman JL, Dwyer AJ, Johnson AR, Knop RH. Adrenal masses differentiated by MR. *Radiology* 1986; **158**: 81–4.
56. Schultz CL, Hagga JR, Fletcher BD, Alfidi RJ, Schultz MA. Magnetic resonance imaging of the adrenal glands; a comparison with computed tomography. *AJR* 1984; **143**: 1235–40.
57. Pilepich MV, Rene JB, Munzenrider JE, Carter BL. Contribution of computed tomography to the treatment of lymphomas. *AJR* 1978; **131**: 69–73.
58. Zadin ME, Glatstein E, Dorfman RF. Clinicopathologic studies of 117 untreated patients subjected to laparotomy for the staging of Hodgkin's disease. *Cancer* 1971; **27**: 1277–94.
59. Bernardino ME, Thomas JL, Barnes PA, Lewis E. Diagnostic approaches to liver and spleen metastases. *Rad Clin N Am* 1982; **20**: 469–85.
60. Freeny PC, Marks WM. Patterns of Contrast Enhancement of Benign and Malignant Hepatic Neoplasms during Bolus Dynamic and Delayed CT. *Radiology* 1986; **160**: 613–18.
61. Sharma S, Singhal S, Dixit S *et al.* Primary gastric lymphoma: role of computed tomography. *Tropic Gastroenterol* 1991; **12**: 31–6.
62. Beynon J, Mortensen NJMcC, Foy DMA, Channer JL, Virjee J, Goddard P. Preoperative assessment of local invasion in rectal cancer: digital examination, endoluminal sonography or computed tomography. *Br J Radiol* 1986; **73**: 1015–17.
63. Mortensen N. Rectal and Anal Endosonography. *Gut* 1992; **33**: 148–9.
64. Lane RH, Stephens DH, Reiman HM. Primary Retroperitoneal Neoplasms: CT findings in 90 cases with clinical and pathological correlation. *AJR* 1989; **152**: 83–9.
65. Alvarenga JC, Ball AB, Fisher C, Fryatt I, Jones L, Thomas JL. Limitations of Surgery in the Treatment of Retroperitoneal Sarcoma. *Br J Surg* 1991; **78**: 912–16.

15.2

Laparoscopic Staging of Intra-Abdominal Malignancy

B. A. SALKY

The abdominal cavity is ideally suited for examination by laparoscopy as the laparoscope has the ability of visualizing approximately 85% of the greater sac and a significant portion of the retroperitoneal space. Although previous surgery can limit the complete examination of the abdominal cavity, it is, in itself, not a contraindication to laparoscopy. The more experienced the laparoscopic surgeon, the less of a problem are adhesions, as laparoscopic adhesiolysis is a straightforward procedure. Laparoscopic examination should always be used in conjunction with non-operative (preoperative) investigations, as discussed in Chapter 15.1.

In general, abdominal malignancy is categorized as either intra-abdominal or retroperitoneal and laparoscopic staging has a major role in both. As will be discussed later under each heading, there are many malignant processes which are not amenable to surgical resection. Laparoscopy is successful in obtaining material for histological examination and defining the extent of the disease process in over 95% of cases. In many instances, the patient will be spared an unnecessary exploration by the judicious use of laparoscopy before laparotomy and this is especially true for retroperitoneal lymphomatous malignancy.

The author prefers to use local anaesthesia for the alert and co-operative patient. In more than 800 diagnostic laparoscopic procedures, local anaesthesia was used 92% of the time. When local anaesthesia is used, the insufflation gas should be nitrous oxide instead of carbon dioxide. Carbon dioxide combines with fluid in the abdomen to form carbonic acid which is irritating to the parietal peritoneum and uncomfortable to the patient, whereas nitrous oxide is inert and does not cause parietal peritoneal pain. The abdominal cavity should be insufflated slowly or the patient will experience discomfort. Insufflation is commenced and continued at 1 litre per minute. Overdistension of the parietal peritoneum can cause a reflex bradycardia in the conscious patient and although pretreatment with atropine will decrease its occurrence, it will not eliminate it. The best way to avoid this problem is to prevent overinflation of the abdomen. In fact, the author rarely exceeds 2 litres of gas insufflation in the conscious patient. As a result, reflex bradycardia has not

Table 15.2.1 Indications for laparoscopy

Focal liver disease	104
Second look/prelaparotomy	56
Abdominal mass	55
Ascites	47
Abdominal pain	4

occurred in this series. If the patient is young or unco-operative, general anaesthesia is required. The reader is referred to other references for a more complete review of the use of local anaesthesia in laparoscopy.[1,2]

INTRA-ABDOMINAL MALIGNANCY

Intra-abdominal malignancies frequently present with metastatic liver disease, ascites, mass, pain or obstruction. Intestinal obstruction is a relative contraindication to the performance of laparoscopy, as most of these patients will require open surgery for relief of the obstruction. Laparoscopy has a place in the evaluation of which patients should have traditional resectional surgery. It also has a role as a "second look" procedure in the evaluation of patients who have been treated previously for malignant disease with either surgery or chemotherapy (Table 15.2.1).

METASTATIC LIVER DISEASE

Non-invasive imaging methods are accurate in the detection of liver masses but histological proof is often required to decide on future therapy. The false-negative rate of percutaneous liver biopsy varies between 10% and 45%. There are few studies comparing CT scan biopsy to laparoscopic biopsy. However, the specificity appears greater with the laparoscopic approach.[3,4] Other important staging data may also be obtained with direct visualization of the abdominal cavity. In the author's personal experience, small capsular deposits, not appreciated on non-invasive scanning, are identified 30% of the time. As lesions smaller than 8 mm are rarely seen with CT scanning, it is not surprising that the laparoscopic identification of surface disease will be significant. In the specific case of metastatic colon carcinoma, formal hepatic resection has been precluded by the laparoscopic findings. Table 15.2.2 lists the confirmed histological diagnoses obtained using directed laparoscopic biopsy techniques. Forty eight of the 104 patients (47%) had at least one failed percutaneous attempt at liver biopsy before the laparoscopic procedure. Laparoscopic biopsy was positive in all of the 48 patients.

Table 15.2.2 Focal liver disease

Malignant*	No. of pts	Malignant*	No. of pts
Adenocarcinoma 1° unknown	29	Leiomyosarcoma	2
Hepatocellular cancer	17	Adrenocorticoid cancer	1
Colon cancer	14	Melanoma	1
Pancreatic cancer	10	Histiocytic medullary reticulosis	1
Breast cancer	7	Mesothelioma	1
Lung cancer	4	Epitheloid haemangioendothelioma	1
Gall bladder cancer	4	Prostate	1
Lymphoma	3	Multiple myeloma	1
Carcinoid	3		
Squamous cell cancer	2		
Gastric cancer	2		

*49 patients had failed percutaneous biopsy, all were positive after laparoscopic biopsy

As discussed earlier in this chapter, the laparoscopic procedure is performed under local anaesthesia using a closed, blind technique unless a specific reason for open laparoscopy exists. Coagulation parameters should be studied before laparoscopy and all coagulation defects must be corrected before biopsy is attempted. A vertical, 1 cm incision is made 2.5 cm above and to the left of the umbilicus (transrectus) for insertion of the Veress needle and the laparoscopic trocar (Fig. 15.2.1). The umbilical area is avoided, as prominent collateral vessels may be present in the face of malignant disease of the liver and laceration of these collaterals can be difficult to control. The epigastric vessels are located 3 cm lateral to the midline, so it is important to stay between the midline and the epigastric vessels. The left side of the abdominal wall is preferred because the abdominal wall is thicker on the right, secondary to the fat in the round ligament. The author's personal preference is for a 0° telescope, but familiarity with an angled (30° or 45°) telescope will be helpful at times. A 3 mm or 5 mm second puncture is always placed to allow insertion of additional instruments to manipulate the liver and viscera. The undersurface of the left lobe frequently harbours pathology and it cannot be seen unless the lateral segment is lifted superiorly. Directed liver biopsy is obtained with either a lancet-shaped biopsy forceps or a Tru-cut biopsy needle (Fig. 15.2.2). Haemostasis is maintained by applying pressure to the biopsy site. Rarely, the administration of topical thrombin is needed to supplement pressure. This can be placed percutaneously under direct laparoscopic control. Electrocautery has never been needed to control bleeding in the author's experience. All laparoscopic ports are removed under direct vision to ensure haemostasis in the abdominal wall and this includes the telescope port as well.

The contraindications to directed biopsy are haemangiomata and benign looking liver cysts. The diagnosis of haemangioma is made by its visual appearance. In cases in which the haemangiomata are partially sclerosed, a

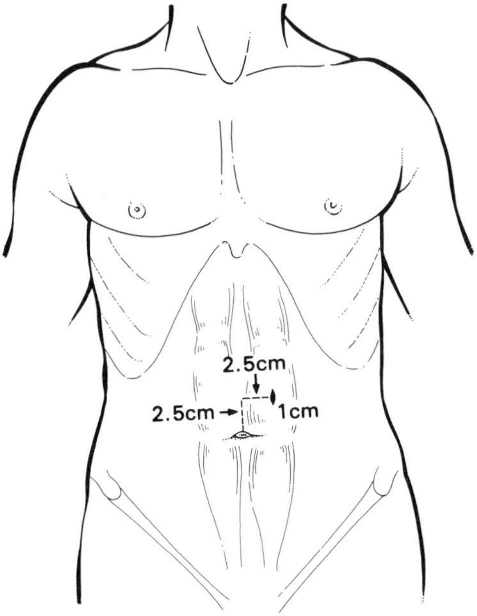

Figure 15.2.1 Trocar locations in diagnostic laparoscopy.

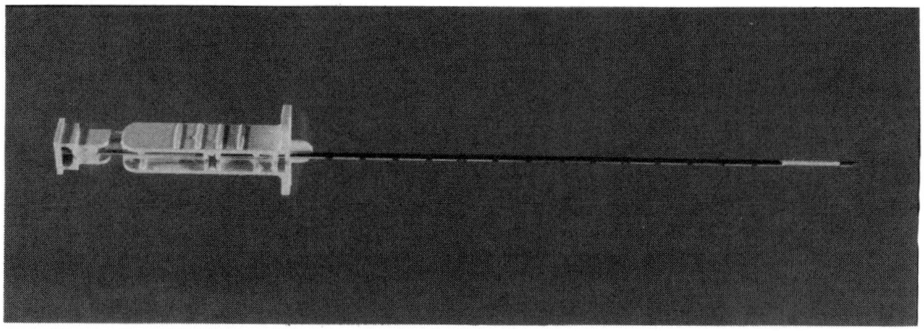

Figure 15.2.2 Biopsy needle which allows core tissue to be removed.

visual diagnosis can be difficult. These lesions tend to be much firmer on laparoscopic palpation than non-sclerosed types. If biopsy is essential, contingency plans for open laparotomy for haemostasis should be made if bleeding cannot be controlled by laparoscopic techniques. Bile containing communicating cysts should not be biopsied, as bile peritonitis may occur afterwards.

A firm histological diagnosis was obtained in 98% of the author's patients in whom it was attempted. The author routinely obtains a frozen section diagnosis before removing the instrumentation. The reason for this is to allow for additional sampling if the pathologist is not confident in the diagnosis. Early in the author's series, a metastatic colon carcinoma was missed when the biopsy needle went through the lesion. This required a repeat laparoscopy. Thereafter, all lesions have been confirmed at the time of the original procedure.

There have been two complications in the author's series. There was one epigastric artery laceration which was not recognized at the time of laparoscopy and subsequently required a laparotomy for diagnosis and treatment. Thereafter, all trocar sites have been visualized from the abdominal side while the laparoscope is still in place. Significant bleeding from these has been identified 0.8% of the time. Haemostasis was maintained with simple pressure in all cases. Bleeding from the original puncture site has been identified in 1.0% of the patients. Suture ligation may be necessary here. There was one delayed bleed from the liver biopsy site in a patient with disseminated intravascular coagulation and liver failure secondary to massive tumour replacement of the liver.

ASCITES

Ascites is a common manifestation of intra-abdominal malignancies[5] and the ascitic fluid is always exudative in its composition. All patients undergo abdominal paracentesis with cytological examination before laparoscopy. The paracentesis is necessary to define the exudative nature of the fluid and to obtain material for cytological examination. If a positive diagnosis is made on cytology, laparoscopic examination of the abdomen is not required. However, if the cytological smear is negative for tumour, the laparoscopic approach is the most direct method to obtaining histology. All patients referred for laparoscopy have had either CT scanning or sonography. If the primary pathology is thought to be ovarian in origin (based on the presence of a pelvic mass), laparoscopy is not indicated as formal exploration is required. The reason is that direct implantation of tumour into the laparoscopic incisions have been reported in ovarian carcinoma and has occurred in the presence of curative resections.

Tense ascites presents a special problem in the performance of laparoscopy, as pneumoperitoneum is difficult to establish. Paracentesis is therefore begun more than 24 hours in advance of the procedure. Approximately 1000–1500 cc are removed every eight hours by a small (5 F) multiholed, polyethylene catheter placed into the abdominal cavity percutaneously. The abdomen should no longer be tense when laparoscopy is performed but it does not have to be flat.

Table 15.2.3 lists the confirmed histological diagnoses found in the patients presenting with ascites and malignant disease. None of the patients with ovarian carcinoma had a pelvic mass which would have precluded the examination. The diagnosis was confirmed on histological examination post procedure. In many of the patients with carcinomatosis, the aggressive pattern of the tumour precluded an absolute histological cell of origin based on pathological review. The most common cause of exudative ascites in non-malignant disease is cirrhosis and this is easily identified by laparoscopy.

Table 15.2.3 Ascites

	No. of patients
Carcinomatosis	22
Ovarian cancer	11
Mesothelioma	3
Hepatoma	3
Myelofibrosis, liver	2
Pancreatic cancer	2
Squamous cancer	1
Chronic lymphatic leukaemia	1
Breast cancer	1
Lymphoma	1

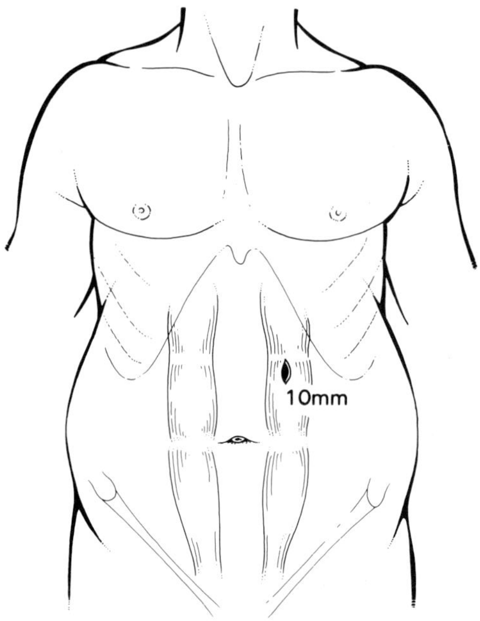

Figure 15.2.3 The protuberant abdomen requires a higher placement of incision.

The procedure is performed under local anaesthesia, but the protuberant, ascitic abdomen does require some deviation from the usual placement sites. Figure 15.2.3 demonstrates the high positioning of the incision for initial trocar placement. If the incision is placed in the normal location, visualization of the upper abdomen will be limited. The Veress needle should be placed parallel to the abdominal wall after entry into the greater sac (Fig. 15.2.4). Insufflation should remain on low flow ($1\ l\ min^{-1}$) throughout the procedure. A cupola of gas must be formed before the Veress needle can be moved into the usual

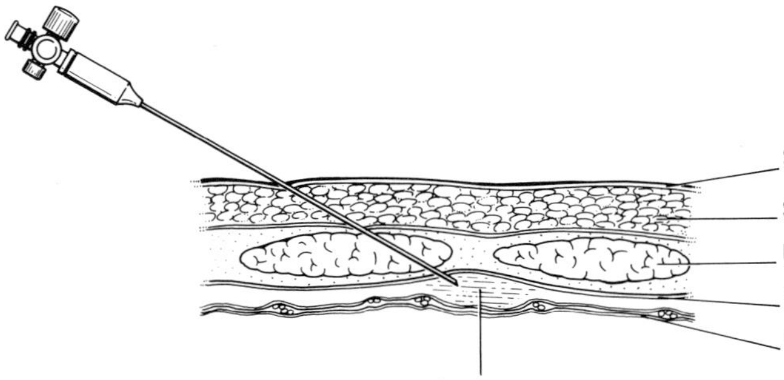

Figure 15.2.4 Pneumoperitoneum needle inserted on angle parallel to abdominal wall to prevent "bubbles" (courtesy of Barry A. Salky MD from *Laparoscopy for Surgeons*, Igaku-Shoin Medical Publishers, New York, 1990).

perpendicular position. If the gas is allowed to flow into the ascitic fluid, large soaplike bubbles will form which will obscure visualization of the peritoneal cavity and the procedure will have to be terminated.

The preferred entry point into the abdomen using the blind puncture technique is transrectus as discussed in the section above. It is uncommon to require more than two punctures when evaluating ascites. The author uses a 5 mm telescope whenever possible and a 3 mm second puncture to minimize the leakage of ascitic fluid after the procedure. While distinctly uncommon to have leakage from the second puncture site, the main trocar site is routinely closed with absorbable suture material to prevent leakage. If leakage does occur, it will always stop on its own over a period of days. There have been no complications related to the laparoscopy in the author's series.

In the author's experience, the diagnostic accuracy of laparoscopy in the evaluation of malignant disease presenting as ascites has been 100%.

MASS

Laparoscopy has a role in the evaluation of malignant abdominal masses to provide histological diagnosis, to assess resectability and to determine chemotherapeutic response. Used in conjunction with preoperative scanning, laparoscopy can decrease the unnecessary laparotomy rate[6] and as technology and instrumentation improve, the therapeutic role of laparoscopic resection of malignant masses may also increase. Table 15.2.1 lists the documented histology obtained by directed biopsy. Twelve patients had blind CHIBA (skinny needle) aspiration attempts which were non-diagnostic. All were positive using laparoscopic control. Included in this group were two patients with pancreatic carcinoma. Early in the author's experience (1980), there were nine patients in whom adhesions did not allow adequate visualization of the malignant mass.

Table 15.2.4 Abdominal mass*

	No. of patients
Non-Hodgkin's lymphoma	18
Adenocarcinoma	18
Pancreatic cancer	5
Carcinoma gall bladder	3
Ovarian carcinoma	2
Lymphosarcoma	2
Spindle cell carcinoma	1
Transitional cell cancer	1
Anaplastic cancer	1
Mesothelioma**	1
Appendiceal carcinoma	1
Liposarcoma	1
Melanoma	1

* 12 patients had failed CHIBA aspirations – all were positive after laparoscopic biopsy
** Perforation
Note: Laparoscopy failed to visualize in 9 patients secondary adhesions

This would not have been a problem now, as lysis of adhesions is relatively straightforward.

Local anaesthesia is preferred, as described earlier in the chapter. The choice of incision site is based on the location of the mass. It is easier to approach the mass from a distance; therefore, the pararectus incision is made on the opposite side. A blind puncture technique is routine but, depending on the number and extent of previous incisions, open laparoscopy may be required. A second puncture is always needed for insertion of additional instruments to manipulate the viscera or biopsy the mass. Occasionally, a third puncture will be needed in order to improve exposure. The author will frequently use 3 mm instrumentation in this setting to minimize patient discomfort.

In the author's experience, the use of laparoscopy as a diagnostic tool in this setting will be greater than 95%.

RETROPERITONAL MASSES

Staging malignant disease which originates in the retroperitoneum is frequently possible using diagnostic laparoscopy.[7] This is especially true if the disease process displaces viscera on preoperative radiological studies or the mass is palpable on abdominal examination. Typically, the CT scan or a barium contrast study will give the information necessary to evaluate the relationship of the mass to other viscera. It is the author's preference to utilize local anaesthesia

Table 15.2.5 Retroperitoneal mass

Non-Hodgkin's lymphoma	14
Carcinoma pancreas	3
Hodgkin's lymphoma	1
Spindle cell sarcoma	1
Transitional cell carcinoma	1
Cystadenoma pancreas	1
Paraganglionoma	1

Table 15.2.6 "Second look"

Indication	No.	Positive explorations	Negative explorations
Chemotherapy	7	3	4
Rising CEA	5	2	3
Colon carcinoma	2	2	0
Ovarian carcinoma	2	2	0
Melanoma	1	1	0
Hepatoma	1	1	0
Mesothelioma	1	1	0
Gastric carcinoma	1	1	0

in the diagnostic mode of laparoscopy. However, general anaesthesia may also be used. More than two accessory ports are commonly needed; therefore, 3 mm ancillary instrumentation is preferred. Movement of adjacent viscera is facilitated by the ancillary ports and the judicial use of a tilt table. Retroperitoneal lymphadenectomy in conjunction with gynaecological and prostatic malignancies are beyond the scope of this chapter. Table 15.2.5 lists the pathology obtained by directed biopsy. A firm diagnosis was possible approximately 80% of the time. Several of the early patients had adhesions which precluded visualization of the mass. Again this would not be a problem now. In fact, the diagnostic rate would be close to 100% today. If non-Hodgkin's lymphoma can be confirmed, laparotomy for diagnosis will not be necessary.

PRELAPAROTOMY, "SECOND LOOK"

Diagnostic laparoscopy is useful in "second look" procedures and in the selection of patients with malignant disease who do not need formal laparotomy.[8] In non-gynaecological "second look" procedures, a thorough evaluation of the abdomen is frequently possible (Table 15.2.6). This is especially valuable in evaluating a patient's response to chemotherapy. It has been much less useful in the evaluation of a rising carcino-embryonic-antigen (CEA) with colon carcinoma. If adhesions preclude a thorough examination, formal laparotomy may

Table 15.2.7 Prelaparotomy*

Indication	No.	Positive explorations	Negative explorations
Colon carcinoma	18	7	11
Pancreatic carcinoma	7	2	5
Gastric carcinoma	2	2	0
Esophageal carcinoma	1	1	0
Hepatocellular carcinoma	1	0	1
Lung carcinoma	1	0	1
Renal carcinoma	1	1	0
Adrenal carcinoma	1	1	0
Klatskin	1	0	1
Leiomyosarcoma	1	0	1

*All positive examinations precluded laparotomy

be required. However, in the author's experience, this has been uncommon as lysis of adhesions laparoscopically can be performed. Prelaparotomy laparoscopy will exclude approximately 25% of the patients with carcinoma of the pancreas from formal laparotomy.[9] The author believes that laparoscopy should precede laparotomy in all patients with carcinoma of the pancreas. In the elderly, frail patient who is at high risk, laparoscopy may exclude some who would not benefit from laparatomy. Table 15.2.7 lists the indications for laparoscopy in these patients.

REFERENCES

1. Boyce HW Jr, Palmer E. *Techniques of Clinical Gastroenterology*. Springfield, Illinois, Charles C Thomas, 1975.
2. Brady PG, Peebles M, Goldschmid S. Role of laparoscopy in the evaluation of patients with suspected hepatic or peritoneal malignancy. *Gastrointest Endosc* 1991; **37**: 27.
3. DeGroen PC, Rakela J, Moore SC *et al.* Diagnostic laparoscopy in gastroenterology. A 14-year experience. *Dig Dis Sci* 1987; **32**: 677.
4. Greene FL. Laparoscopy in oncology cases. *Gastroendosc Clin N Am* 1993; **2**: 205–14.
5. Kriplani AK, Kapur BM. Laparoscopy for pre-operative staging and assessment of operability in gastric carcinoma. *Gastrointest Endosc* 191; **37**: 441.
6. Salky BA, Bauer JJ, Gelernt IM *et al.* The use of laparoscopy in retroperitoneal pathology. *Gastrointest Endosc* 1988; **34**: 227.
7. Salky BA, Bauer JJ, Gelernt IM, Kreel I. Laparoscopy for gastrointestinal diseases. *Mt Sinai J Med* 1985; **52**: 228–32.
8. Salky BA. *Laparoscopy for Surgeons*. New York, Igaku-Shoin Medical Publishers, 1990.
9. Warshaw AL, Gu Z-Y, Wittenberg J *et al.* Preoperative staging and assessment of resectability of pancreatic cancer. *Arch Surg* 1990; **125**: 230.

15.3

Laparoscopic Ultrasonography for Staging of Abdominal Malignancy

T. G. JOHN and O. J. GARDEN

INTRODUCTION

The incorporation of the principles of intraoperative contact ultrasonography into the laparoscopic evaluation of abdominal disease has been inevitable.[1,2] Although the rationale for the use of laparoscopy in the assessment of intra-abdominal malignancies is convincing, both in a diagnostic and, as described in the preceding chapter, a staging role, its potential is limited by a number of factors. Although laparoscopy provides an extensive view of the surface of the abdominal viscera, it is often unable to examine adequately the interior of solid organs, the hollow viscera and inaccessible areas such as the retroperitoneum. Pathological processes within these tissues will therefore remain unseen unless they cause visible surface changes or deform the shape of the organ.

The development of high resolution ultrasound probes which may be passed through standard laparoscopy ports and placed in direct contact with the intra-abdominal organs now allows the laparoscopic surgeon to overcome some of these limitations. In the same way that intraoperative ultrasound "extends the eye and hand of the surgeon" at open surgery, evidence is accumulating to indicate that the same may be said for laparoscopic procedures assisted by intracorporeal ultrasound. Although laparoscopic ultrasonography is still at a relatively early stage in its development, its current primary applications in surgical oncology are in the staging of pancreatic and periampullary cancers and in the preoperative assessment of primary and secondary liver tumours. It is in the management of these conditions that the use of laparoscopic ultrasound will be primarily directed in this chapter.

BACKGROUND AND HISTORICAL PERSPECTIVES

Intracorporeal Contact Ultrasonography

The principles and practice of intraoperative contact ultrasonography (IOUS) have become well established in the fields of hepatobiliary and pancreatic

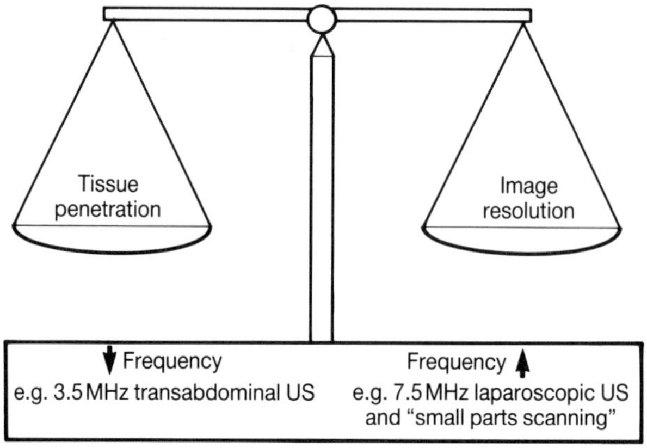

Figure 15.3.1 The principle underlying high resolution contact ultrasound scanning.

surgery over the last ten years.[3] The fundamental advantage of this technique over conventional transabdominal ultrasound is that the ultrasound probe is placed directly upon the surface of the organ to be examined, thus avoiding the need to scan through the interposed tissues. The lower frequency ultrasound probes (e.g. 3.5 MHz) normally required to overcome the ultrasound attenuation and interference caused by the subcutaneous tissues of the abdominal wall, costal margin and bowel gas may consequently be abandoned in favour of probes with higher resolution transducers (i.e. 5 MHz and above) which provide highly detailed, real-time B-mode images of the underlying structures (Fig. 15.3.1).

Assessment of Pancreatic Tumours

In the operative assessment of pancreatic cancers, Rifkin and colleagues[4] described the success of IOUS in detecting impalpable tumours in the head of the pancreas, while Sigel and colleagues reported IOUS to have aided the diagnosis of pancreatic cancer in 25% of operations.[5] In describing their experience with 22 patients undergoing operation for suspected pancreatic cancer, Plainfosse and his coworkers reported that supplementary diagnostic information had been provided by IOUS in 18% and that surgical decision making had been helped in 50% when tumour resectability had been assessed by examining for liver metastases, regional lymphadenopathy, local invasion and major vascular involvement.[6] Serio and colleagues recently reported a similar experience with IOUS in assessing resectability at operation in 32 patients with pancreatic cancer,[7] although the difficulty in differentiating the diagnosis of malignancy from pancreatitis was also highlighted. Despite the enthusiasm shown by some surgeons for this technique, others have preferred at open operation to assess resectability following a trial dissection,[8] and IOUS has thus found limited application in pancreatic surgery.

Nevertheless, the ability of IOUS to "interrogate" the whole pancreas at high resolution has resulted in its adoption for operative localization of neuroendocrine tumours by some,[5,9–12] although its precise value is debatable since the majority of such tumours can be localized at operation following mobilization and careful palpation of the gland. Furthermore, excellent results have now been reported using endoscopic ultrasonography in the preoperative localization of occult pancreatic neuroendocrine tumours.[13]

Assessment of Liver Tumours

It is in the assessment of the liver that IOUS has been shown to be particularly useful,[3,14] as most notably popularized by Bismuth and Castaing.[15] The normal segmental hepatic anatomy and its variants (as described by Couinaud[16]) can be readily identified using the intrahepatic portal pedicles and hepatic veins as landmarks and it is therefore possible to accurately localize lesions within the liver, to facilitate guided biopsy and to determine the extent of liver resection. In this way, Bismuth and colleagues demonstrated that IOUS of the liver was superior to conventional preoperative investigations in assessing potentially resectable liver lesions, conferring additional information in a third of patients and modifying the intended surgical procedure in over a half.[17] Similarly, Makuuchi and colleagues[18] reported the superior sensitivity of IOUS in detecting primary liver tumours, a large proportion of which consisted of small hepatocellular carcinomas concealed within cirrhotic livers. They were able to define characteristic tumour thrombi within portal venous radicles and described novel liver sparing subsegmental resections based upon the new information. More recently, Li and colleagues have reconfirmed these observations and furthermore, report a significantly diminished incidence of tumour infiltration of the liver resection margins in those patients in whom IOUS guided resection of hepatocellular carcinoma was performed.[19] Other workers have illustrated the ability of IOUS to enhance the information available to the surgeon undertaking resection of colorectal liver metastases, underlining its role in achieving a more complete clinical staging and in the appropriate selection of patients for curative major hepatic resection.[20–22]

Other Applications

Intraoperative ultrasound has also been shown to be useful during operations for oesophagogastric malignancies, accurately demonstrating the extent of intramural tumour spread, extramural local invasion and lymph node metastases better than either preoperative imaging studies or operative palpation.[23] This technique has consequently now gained widespread popularity, especially within specialist hepatobiliary centres, and many would now consider IOUS to be an indispensable part of their surgical practice.

DEVELOPMENT OF THE TECHNIQUE

The potential benefits of intra-abdominal contact ultrasonography in staging abdominal malignancies are thus indubitable and in concert with the resurgence in laparoscopic practice witnessed in recent years, it is unsurprising that efforts have been made to develop ultrasound probes that might be passed through small laparoscopic ports and applied directly upon the abdominal organs. However, the first reference to a technique combining laparoscopy with ultrasonography was in the early 1960s when Japanese workers reported success in performing A-mode scanning of gallstones and gall bladder cancer under laparoscopic guidance,[24–26] followed by similar attempts to image gallstones by Look *et al.*, in 1974.[27] Nevertheless, it was not until the later development of prototype "echolaparoscopes", incorporating B-mode ultrasound transducers within the telescope body itself, that more easily interpretable laparoscopic ultrasound images were described.[28] These first generation echolaparoscopes employed mechanical sector scanners and initial reports demonstrated their ability to detect small intrahepatic lesions, some of which could not be seen using standard transabdominal ultrasound scanners.[29–32] Other workers from Japan subsequently reported diagnostic "accuracies" for the sonolaparoscopic detection of intrahepatic lesions in the order of 90%,[26,33] while Bönhof and colleagues[34] described how laparoscopic ultrasound could facilitate guided biopsy of liver tumours. Fornari and colleagues have similarly demonstrated the ability of laparoscopic ultrasound to define and biopsy small hepatocellular carcinomas within cirrhotic livers, lesions which had not been detected during transabdominal ultrasound scanning.[35]

A further important refinement has been the development of probes incorporating linear array ultrasound transducers. In a preliminary report, Frank and co-workers reported the ability of such a system to provide highly detailed and readily interpretable images of the upper abdominal organs,[36] although another Japanese group using a similar system had already described its use in demonstrating both hepatocellular carcinomas in the liver and a pancreatic cancer not visualized during laparoscopy.[37]

Our initial experience with laparoscopic ultrasonography in Edinburgh involved the development of a large bore laparoscopic cannula which was introduced into the peritoneal cavity using a purpose built guide rod and dilator, through which existing 5 or 7.5 MHz linear array ultrasound probes, used for transanal rectal ultrasonography, could be passed.[38] Using this system, seven patients with primary or secondary liver tumours, thought on the basis of conventional preoperative investigations to be potentially resectable, underwent laparoscopy and laparoscopic ultrasound examination. Laparoscopy demonstrated extrahepatic dissemination of disease in two cases whilst laparoscopic ultrasound provided additional useful information in four of the remaining five patients in the form of unsuspected bilobar spread of tumour (two patients), portal venous invasion of tumour (one patient) and a less widespread tumour distribution than expected (one patient).[38] This somewhat cumbersome technique has now been superseded following refinements in probe design. The current commercial availability of a variety of laparoscopic ultrasound probes incorporating ultracompact transducers which may be used with standard 10 mm laparoscopic ports seems certain to be accompanied by the more widespread use of this technique.

There are two fundamental types of laparoscopic ultrasound probe, each with inherent advantages and limitations. In our experience with both sectoral probes (employing a mechanically driven, single crystal, convex sector scanner) and the more sophisticated multi-element linear array laparoscopic ultrasound probes, excellent high resolution images of the underlying structures are immediately obtainable. The ultrasound probe is used independent of the standard laparoscopic telescope and inserted through a separate port, unlike some earlier prototypes in which the two instruments were combined (see "echolaparoscopes" above). The rectilinear image produced by linear array probes undoubtedly renders the scanning plane easier to orientate, with tissue depth indicated on the vertical axis and linear probe movement displayed on the horizontal axis. The advantages of sectoral probes lie with their increased versatility in varying the scanning plane (albeit at the expense of easy orientation to the inexperienced operator) and, depending upon the sectoral scanning angle, a wide area of tissue penetration. Nevertheless, the position of the linear array probe may be adapted for scanning both lobes of the liver, the extrahepatic biliary system and the pancreas. By advancing and withdrawing the probe between alternate ports and by subtle rotatory movements, a full range of scanning between sagittal, oblique and transverse planes may be achieved.[39]

LAPAROSCOPIC ULTRASOUND ASSESSMENT OF PANCREATIC AND PERIAMPULLARY CANCERS

For the majority of patients presenting with ductal pancreatic cancer the outlook is bleak with an overall prognosis of less than 1% five year survival.[40] Nevertheless, "cautious optimism" has accompanied the increasing body of evidence for improved survival in that select minority of patients presenting with small tumours confined to the head of the gland and in whom curative pancreatoduodenectomy (Whipple operation) may now be performed with negligible morbidity and mortality in expert hands.[8,41,42] Ideally, accurate preoperative staging should allow therapeutic decisions to be made without recourse to empirical surgical exploration, an approach which is increasingly being recognized as unjustified in a substantial proportion of patients.[43] The natural history of pancreatic cancer is such that despite preceding radiological investigations such as ultrasound and computed tomography, unsuspected small metastatic deposits in the liver and on the peritoneal surfaces are discovered at laparoscopy or laparotomy in 30–40% of cases.[44–46] The unique role performed by laparoscopy in detecting these hitherto unsuspected distant metastases, and in averting unnecessary laparotomy, thus makes the rationale for its use in the staging of ampullopancreatic cancers compelling (see preceding chapter).

Nevertheless, in the laparoscopic assessment of patients with potentially resectable tumours of the pancreatic head or ampulla, it is rarely possible to visualize the primary tumour and virtually impossible to define accurately locoregional invasion of the contiguous retroperitoneal structures, particularly the peripancreatic and para-aortic lymph nodes and major vascular structures (the portal, superior mesenteric and splenic veins, and coeliac and superior mesenteric arterial trunks). The potential of high resolution contact ultrasound in fulfilling this role is supported in principle by the excellent results achieved in the staging of "ampullopancreatic cancers" using endoscopic ultrasonography (EUS). This is a technique whereby ultrasound probes have been incorporated into the tips of fibreoptic endoscopes permitting detailed scanning of the retroperitoneal structures through the stomach and duodenal wall. In a prospective study assessing 60 patients with ampullopancreatic cancers, Rösch and colleagues reported superior accuracy for EUS over conventional investigations (ultrasound, CT scanning and angiography) in determining tumour size, lymph node metastases and involvement of the portal venous system.[47] Nevertheless, it is not possible to examine the peritoneal cavity for evidence of peritoneal tumour dissemination using this technique, nor is it able to satisfactorily assess the liver for metastases. Indeed, in approximately one third of cases, tumours within the liver may not even be apparent during a laparoscopic examination.[48,49] Laparoscopic ultrasound is now able to address these inherent limitations, thus optimizing the opportunity afforded by the laparoscopic examination to perform a complete staging assessment.

STAGING ASSESSMENT OF LIVER TUMOURS USING LAPAROSCOPIC ULTRASOUND

Aggressive treatment by curative liver resection represents the only realistic hope of survival in the long term for some patients presenting with primary or metastatic liver tumours. However, careful patient selection is important if this exercise is to be worthwhile and early recurrence of disease avoided. Contraindications to liver resection include multiple and extensive bilobar tumour deposits, extrahepatic spread of tumour to the adjacent peritoneal, diaphragmatic and omental surfaces and particularly to the regional lymph nodes, the involvement of which has been shown to be associated with a poor outcome following resection.[50,51] Despite the availability of non-invasive radiological investigations such as ultrasound, enhanced CT scanning, magnetic resonance imaging and visceral angiography, the discovery of irresectable disease at the time of open operation is not uncommon.[1] This outcome represents poor palliation for the patient in whom an exploratory laparotomy may not only be unnecessary, but also associated with significant physical and psychological morbidity. This sequence of events also holds important health economic implications, since more accurate preoperative staging permits more efficient deployment of surgical resources.

In the diagnosis of patients presenting with liver tumours, there is good evidence that laparoscopy with laparoscopic guided biopsy can effectively complement radiological investigations[49] and is superior to "blind" percutaneous needle biopsy.[48] However, its application for the specific purpose of staging potentially resectable lesions has not been widely embraced. In one report testifying to the potential benefits of this approach, Lightdale and colleagues[52] determined during laparoscopy that seven out of eight patients with hepatocellular carcinoma had irresectable disease due to peritoneal metastases, malignant ascites, bilobar tumour or diffuse cirrhosis. Prior to the adoption of staging laparoscopy and laparoscopic ultrasonography as routine staging investigations for patients presenting with potentially resectable liver tumours, our own experience over a three year period was of 16 out of a total of 38 patients (42%) proving irresectable at laparotomy for the aforementioned reasons. In an attempt to address the apparent inadequacies of the existing investigative code, laparoscopy with laparoscopic ultrasound was incorporated into the staging algorithm.

TECHNIQUE OF LAPAROSCOPIC ULTRASONOGRAPHY

A systematic approach has been adopted to the laparoscopic ultrasound assessment of patients with diseases of the hepatobiliary system and pancreas. Under general anaesthesia, two 10 mm laparoscopic ports are inserted as shown in Figure 15.3.2 and a thorough laparoscopic inspection of the peritoneal cavity is performed. The ultrasound probe is introduced via the umbilical or a right lateral abdominal port and may be useful in "palpating" mass lesions, providing retraction of bowel loops and omentum and for tamponade of bleeding biopsy puncture sites.

Liver (Figs 15.3.3–5)

A systematic examination of the liver is performed initially searching for evidence of metastases, which may be typically echo-poor or demonstrate a

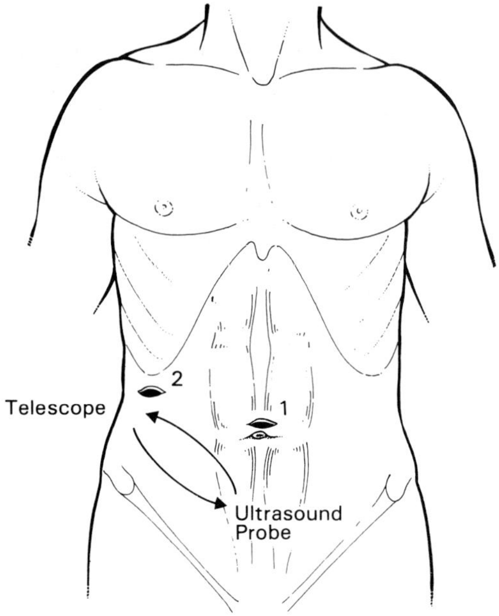

Figure 15.3.2 Laparoscopic cannula placement for patient undergoing staging laparoscopy with laparoscopic ultrasonography in the assessment of hepatobiliary and pancreatic disorders.

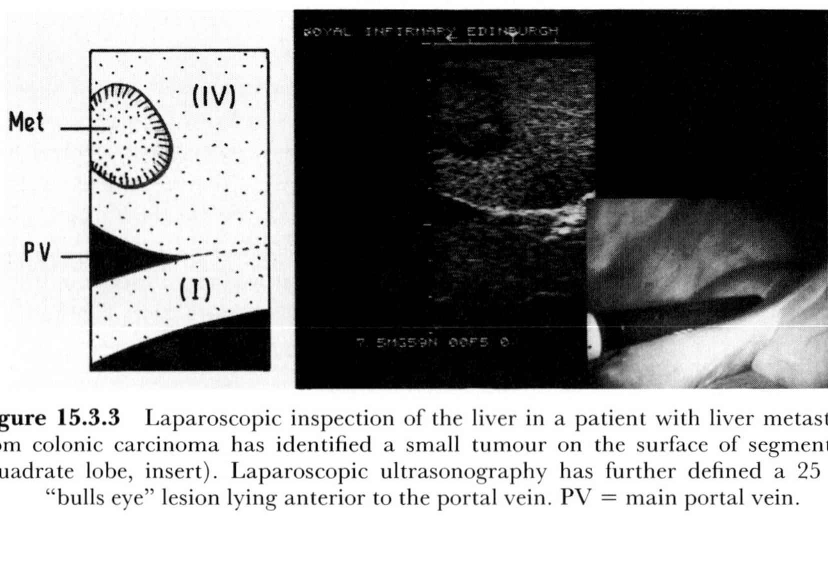

Figure 15.3.3 Laparoscopic inspection of the liver in a patient with liver metastases from colonic carcinoma has identified a small tumour on the surface of segment IV (quadrate lobe, insert). Laparoscopic ultrasonography has further defined a 25 mm "bulls eye" lesion lying anterior to the portal vein. PV = main portal vein.

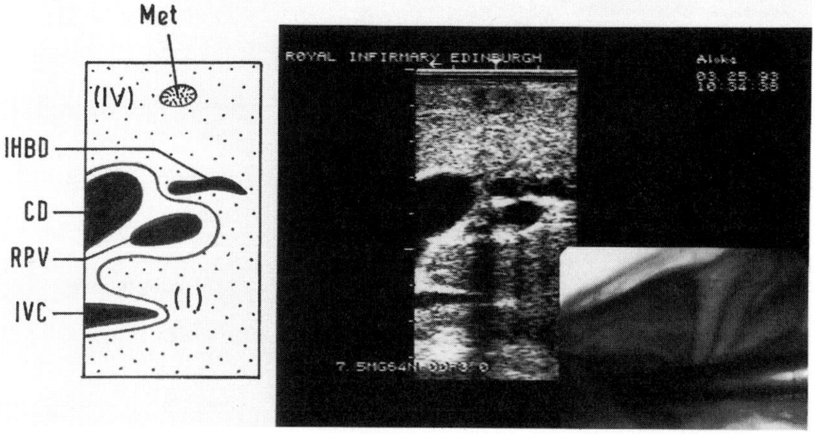

Figure 15.3.4 Laparoscopic inspection of the liver and peritoneal cavity in a patient thought to have resectable pancreatic cancer has revealed no evidence for metastatic disease. The laparoscopic sonogram of hepatic segment IV (quadrate lobe) has demonstrated a previously unsuspected 10 mm metastatic lesion. Note the dilated common hepatic (18 mm) and intrahepatic ducts. CD = common hepatic duct; RPV = right branch of portal vein; IVC = inferior vena cava; Met = metastatic tumour deposit; IHBD = intrahepatic bile duct.

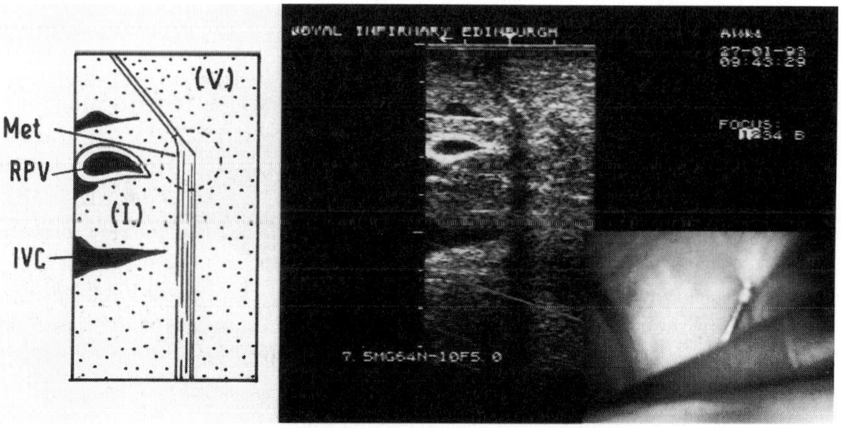

Figure 15.3.5 Laparoscopic ultrasonography has revealed an isoechoic lesion measuring 10 mm deep within the right liver (more obvious during real-time scanning). Laparoscopic ultrasound guided Tru-cut biopsy confirmed the diagnosis of secondary adenocarcinoma. RPV = right branch of portal vein; IVC = inferior vena cava; Met = metastatic tumour deposit.

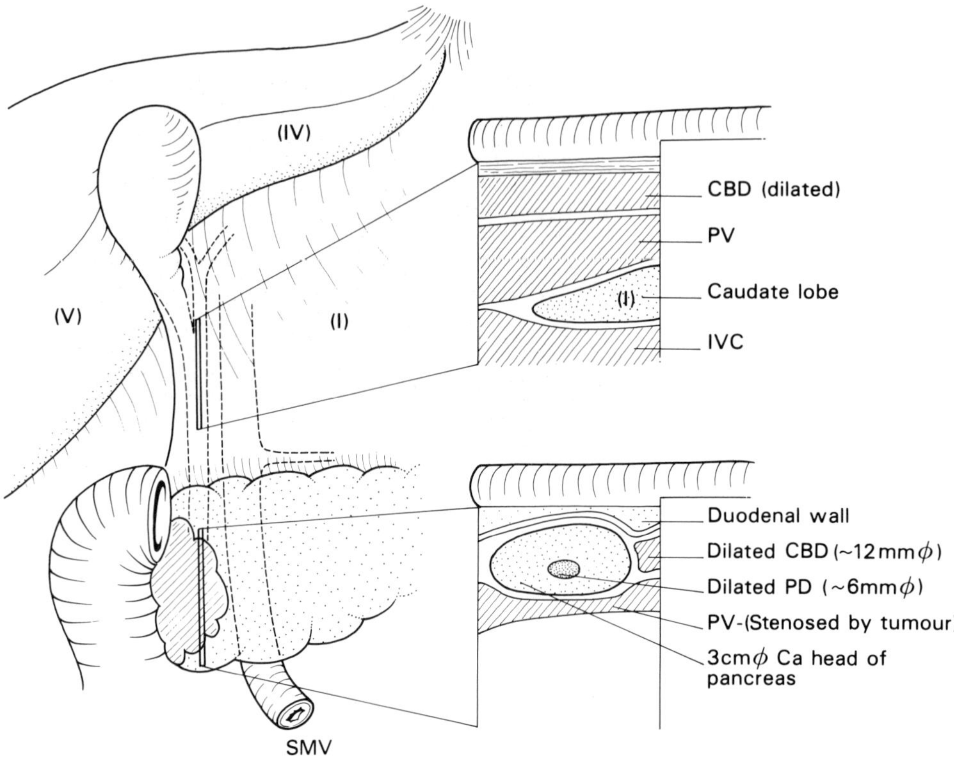

Figure 15.3.6 Schematic depiction of anatomical relationships of the structures of the hepatoduodenal ligament and head of pancreas in a patient with carcinoma of the pancreatic head, and their typical appearances on sagittal cut laparoscopic sonograms obtained using a linear array probe placed through the umbilical cannula. CBD = common bile duct; PV = portal vein; IVC = inferior vena cava; PD = pancreatic duct.

characteristic "bulls eye" or "halo" appearance when hyperechoic or iso-echoic.[53–55] The segmental anatomy of the liver can be defined using the portal and hepatic venous radicles as landmarks as described by Bismuth and colleagues[15,56] and the site of any tumour mass and its relation to the adjacent venous structures documented accurately. Extrahepatic biliary obstruction may be evidenced by intrahepatic duct dilatation (the intrahepatic bile ducts are not normally obvious). Percutaneous biopsy of suspicious lesions may be performed by introducing the needle tip through the liver parenchyma into the plane of the ultrasound beam and then under guidance into the target lesion[34] (see Fig. 15.3.5).

Porta Hepatis (Figs 15.3.3–6)

With the linear array probe placed upon the quadrate lobe (segment IV) of the liver, the common duct, the proper hepatic artery and portal vein may be

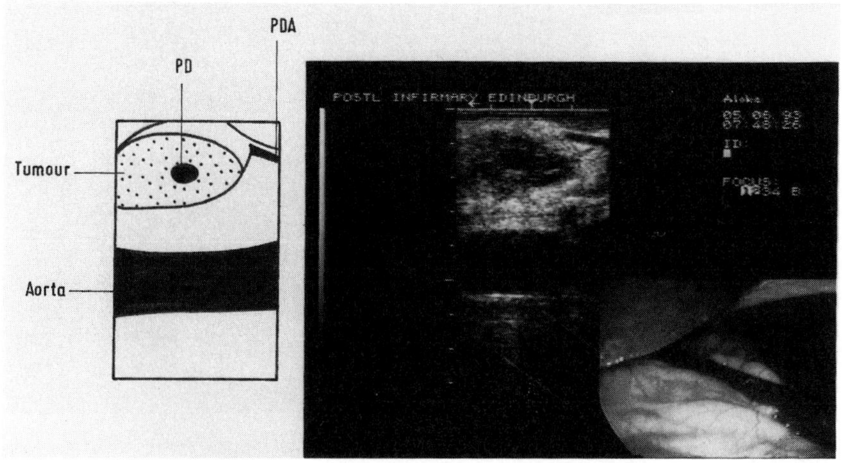

Figure 15.3.7 Laparoscopy identified no evidence of tumour in a patient presenting with malignant obstructive jaundice. Laparoscopic ultrasonography revealed a 3 cm carcinoma of the head of the pancreas (note the well-circumscribed echo-poor tumour with a dilated pancreatic duct measuring 8 mm in diameter). This slightly oblique and medially directed cut passes through the aorta. PD = pancreatic duct; PDA = pancreaticoduodenal artery.

identified as parallel tubular structures lying in front of the inferior vena cava and caudate lobe (segment I). These structures may be distinguished by their positional relationships, the common duct lying anterolateral to the hepatic artery, with the portal vein lying behind. The common duct is also identified by its hyperechoic wall and the absence of pulsation or visible blood flow within its lumen. In cases of biliary obstruction, its diameter often exceeds 10 mm. This landmark is easily identified if a biliary endoprosthesis has already been introduced, although the associated scanning artefact and pneumobilia may cause some interference with the image. The portal vein is characterized as a thinwalled structure displaying laminar venous blood flow, whereas the hepatic artery is smaller and typically pulsatile. The unequivocal identification of these structures is facilitated by the use of Doppler ultrasound sampling when ultrasound systems equipped with this facility are used.[57] The gall bladder is easily visualized from this position and the number and size of any contained gallstones (typically echogenic foci casting dense acoustic shadows) can be observed.

Pancreas (Figs 15.3.6–8)

The hilar structures may also be examined with the ultrasound probe placed beneath the quadrate lobe of the liver (segment IV) directly upon the hepatoduodenal ligament. The clinician may experience some difficulty in satisfactorily imaging the hilar structures whilst using the liver as an "acoustic window" in

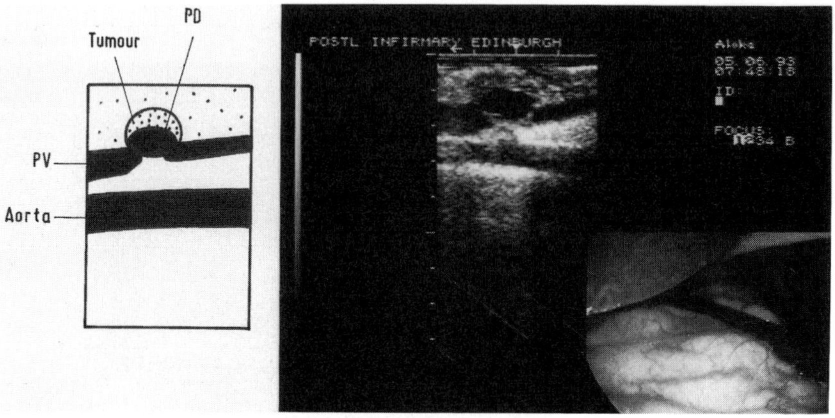

Figure 15.3.8 Same patient as Figure 15.3.7. By sliding the probe medially, the dilated pancreatic duct may be traced into the body of the pancreas. In this laparoscopic sonogram, the pancreatic duct is seen passing through an atrophic neck of pancreas surrounded by a cuff of tumour. The portal vein appears stenosed by invading tumour, which was therefore considered locally irresectable. PV = superior mesenteric–portal vein; PD = pancreatic duct.

patients with enlarged fatty livers or in those with pneumobilia due to a preceding endoscopic sphincterotomy or biliary stent insertion. Having identified the bile duct and portal vein, the probe is gradually withdrawn, simultaneously tracing these structures distally behind the first part of the duodenum to the head of the pancreas, which normally measures no more than 2.5 cm anteroposteriorly. Laparoscopic ultrasound scanning can be performed in a full range of directions about the transverse and sagittal planes by alternating the ports used and withdrawing, advancing or rotating the probe. In this way a linear array ultrasound probe may be used to examine the pancreas in both its long axis and transversely.[39]

The typical ultrasonic features associated with pancreatic cancer are listed in Table 15.3.1. The primary tumour is usually a heterogeneous, predominantly echo-poor mass, often well demarcated from the surrounding tissues. The pancreatic duct, which normally measures less than 3 mm diameter, is often dilated proximal to the tumour and may be associated with atrophy of the body of the pancreas. The superior mesenteric vein, its confluence with the splenic vein, and the portal vein are important landmarks that should be defined as they pass posterior to the neck of the pancreas. Evidence for displacement or invasion by tumour should be sought and leashes of venous collaterals may be identified in cases of venous occlusion. The coeliac and superior mesenteric arterial trunks can be traced from their origins with the aorta, although in our experience we have found detection of arterial tumour encasement difficult. However, an aberrant common or right hepatic artery may be detected arising from the

Table 15.3.1 Features of pancreatic cancer at laparoscopic ultrasonography

Primary tumour	Focal mass (Complex echo texture–predominantly hypoechoic)
Metastatic spread	Liver metastases Regional lymph node metastases (hypoechoic, well demarcated)
Direct invasion	Duodenum/stomach Retroperitoneum Portal, mesenteric, splenic veins/venous collaterals
Secondary effects	Common duct dilatation (>10 mm) Intrahepatic duct dilatation Pancreatic duct dilatation (>3 mm) Atrophy of distal pancreas

superior mesenteric trunk or directly from the aorta and which may characteristically be observed passing behind the head of the pancreas and posterior to the portal vein.

In the assessment of patients with liver tumours, lymph node metastases should be sought in the hepatoduodenal ligament and para-aortic area. In addition, peripancreatic nodal enlargement is of obvious significance in those with pancreatic tumours. Descriptive criteria for distinguishing malignant from reactive nodes based upon their ultrasound appearance have emerged from the work of those in the field of endoscopic ultrasonography. Malignant lymph nodes are typically greater than 5 mm in diameter and are said to have a smooth, well-demarcated hypoechoic appearance, in contrast to benign inflammatory lymphadenopathy where the enlarged nodes are more commonly hyperechoic with less distinct borders.[58,59] However, the EUS experience with these descriptive criteria suggests reliability only in staging oesophageal and gastric carcinomas and that alone they may not be sufficiently specific to make a definitive diagnosis of malignant lymphadenopathy in pancreatic cancer, probably due to the inflammatory reaction which is frequently associated with these tumours.[59,60] Pathological confirmation by fine needle aspiration cytology (laparoscopic ultrasound guided or otherwise) must therefore be recommended before a diagnosis of irresectability can be made with confidence based on these criteria.

RESULTS

Staging of Patients with Pancreatic and Peri-ampullary Cancer

Using a 7.5 MHz linear array probe (Aloka UST-5521-7.5, Keymed Ltd, Southend-on-Sea, UK), our initial experience with 12 patients under consideration for resection of their suspected carcinoma of the head of the pancreas was

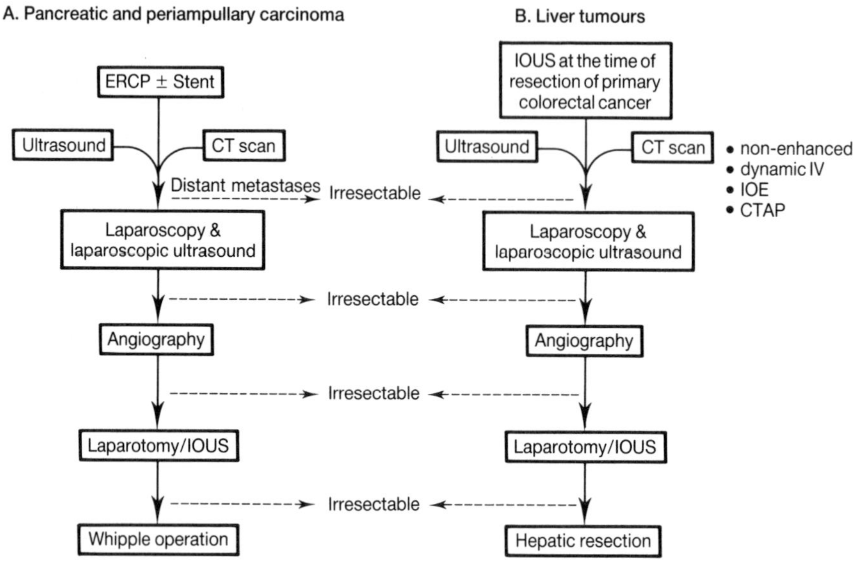

Figure 15.3.9 Investigative algorithms used in the diagnosis and staging of patients with (A) suspected pancreatic and periampullary carcinoma; and (B) liver tumour. IOUS = intraoperative ultrasonography; IOE = iodized oil emulsion; CTAP = CT arterial portography; ERCP = endoscopic retrograde cholangiopancreatography.

encouraging: having detected unexpected advanced disease in four of 12 patients by laparoscopy (malignant ascites, peritoneal dissemination and hepatic metastases), laparoscopic ultrasound demonstrated irresectability in a further two patients (liver metastases, retroperitoneal invasion, portal vein invasion and regional lymphadenopathy). Thus, an unnecessary laparotomy was avoided in six of these 12 patients.[2,39]

Encouraged by this early experience, laparoscopy with laparoscopic ultrasound was performed in 28 patients with histologically proven carcinoma of the head of the pancreas or periampullary region. All were under consideration for curative pancreatic resection, the majority having presented with a clinical picture of malignant obstructive jaundice. All patients were assessed according to an investigative algorithm incorporating ultrasonography, intravenous contrast enhanced CT scanning, laparoscopy with laparoscopic ultrasonography and selective visceral angiography, further investigations or progression to operation being undertaken only when the preceding stage had failed to indicate irresectability unequivocally (see Fig. 15.3.9A).

A prediction of resectability or irresectability was determined both for laparoscopy alone and for the combined laparoscopy/laparoscopic ultrasound examination in the remaining 28 patients. The following factors were taken as criteria for irresectability: peritoneal tumour dissemination, liver metastases, primary tumour ≥5 cm, portal vein involvement (as evidenced by apparent venous occlusion or displacement), regional lymphadenopathy ≥5 mm and invasion of the retroperitoneum or adjacent viscera. These findings were corroborated with the results of selective visceral angiography and in patients without biopsy proven peritoneal and hepatic metastases, by laparotomy and assessment of resectability by palpation, intraoperative ultrasonography and trial dissection of the tumour. Of these 28 patients assessed laparoscopically, ten (36%) ultimately underwent a "curative" pancreatic resection (Whipple pancreatoduodenectomy).

Irresectability due to unsuspected liver and peritoneal tumour was demonstrated by laparoscopy alone in eight patients, in addition to which these findings were missed during two false-negative laparoscopies. Ten out of 28 patients (36%) in our series therefore demonstrated the small peritoneal and liver metastases said to be so characteristic of this disease,[45] 80% of which (eight of ten patients) had been detected by laparoscopy at this stage of the investigative protocol. Laparoscopic ultrasound examination failed to define portal vein invasion by tumour in one patient and produced one false-positive result in another, having misdiagnosed duodenal infiltration and liver metastases. For this reason, the sensitivity of combined laparoscopy and laparoscopic ultrasonography in determining tumour resectability was only 90%, compared with 100% for laparoscopy alone. However, the specificity of the combined procedure was clearly superior, determining tumour irresectability in 88% of patients compared with 44% for laparoscopy alone, giving an overall accuracy of 64% for staging laparoscopy compared with 88% when laparoscopic ultrasonography was also used. Based upon this experience, for patients with suspected tumours of the pancreatic head or periampullary region who are under consideration for resection, we would recommend the incorporation of staging laparoscopy with laparoscopic ultrasonography into a standardized investigative algorithm such as that depicted in Fig. 15.3.9A.

Staging of Patients with Liver Tumours

In our own unit, 52 consecutive patients referred with suspected neoplastic liver disease underwent staging investigations including laparoscopy and laparoscopic ultrasound as outlined in Fig. 15.3.9B. The tumours had been considered potentially suitable for treatment by liver resection in all cases, the preceding radiological investigations undertaken prior to referral indicating no extrahepatic tumour dissemination or bilobar tumour distribution. Laparoscopic assessment was also undertaken when operative assessment with intraoperative ultrasound examination would ultimately have been required to evaluate tumour resectability following equivocal scan results. Colorectal liver metastases were the most common pathology (54%), with primary hepatocellular carcinoma in eight patients and cholangiocarcinoma in one. The sites of primary lesions included gall bladder, ovary, cervix, stomach, leiomyosarcoma of the stomach and colon, were unknown in three patients and were ultimately shown

Table 15.3.2 Additional information obtained by laparoscopic ultrasound in 43 patients under consideration for liver resection

Liver tumour visualized	41 (95%)
Additional staging information	18 (42%)
Multiple/bilobar tumour	12 (28%)
Lymphadenopathy	5 (12%)
Major venous invasion	5 (12%)

to be benign in four (focal nodular hyperplasia, adenoma, cavernous haemangioma and a regenerating nodule within a cirrhotic liver). In two patients the absence of demonstrable liver tumour was demonstrated, preceding investigations having provided false-positive results.

Although 37 patients (73%) demonstrated abdominal scars following previous operations, a direct cutdown approach was frequently employed to gain access to the peritoneal cavity. Access to the peritoneal cavity failed in only two cases due to adhesions (4% failure rate) and there were no laparoscopy associated complications. Additional staging information confirming the irresectable nature of the liver tumour was obtained during laparoscopy in 23 patients (46%). Extrahepatic spread of tumour to involve the peritoneal cavity was observed in 18 cases (36%) and bilobar dissemination was seen in 11 (22%). Laparoscopic ultrasonography was performed in 43 patients (83%), having been deferred because of multiple adhesions and an obvious irresectable tumour load encountered with laparoscopy alone in seven instances. Laparoscopic ultrasonography was able to provide staging information in addition to that obtained by laparoscopy in 18 patients (42%) as shown in Table 15.3.2.

Overall, the adoption of laparoscopy and laparoscopic ultrasonography was seen to have made a considerable impact upon the selection of patients for exploratory laparotomy. Of the 50 patients in whom laparoscopic staging had been undertaken, 14 underwent operative assessment. The only unnecessary laparotomy in this series was performed following a false-positive laparoscopy, where a nodule of fibrous connective tissue situated at the base of the falciform ligament had been mistaken for a solitary colorectal metastasis, and 13 patients thus underwent liver resection with curative intent. This resection rate of 93% in those selected for exploratory laparotomy following staging laparoscopy/laparoscopic ultrasound was significantly superior than a resectability rate of 58% defined for the 38 patients subjected to operative assessment of resectability before laparoscopic staging procedures were employed at our hospital.

CONCLUSIONS

Laparoscopic ultrasonography has a unique role to play in complementing the laparoscopic assessment of abdominal malignancy. The application of its fundamental principles by surgeons performing intracorporeal operative ultrasound, and by endoscopic ultrasonographers, illustrates the potential of this technique and an expansion in the indications for its use will surely accompany continuing refinements in probe design and ultrasound technology. Other applications already include the accurate localization of pancreatic neuroendocrine tumours,[61] the detection of occult liver metastases in patients undergoing laparoscopic resection of primary abdominal malignancies and pelvic lymph node assessment in patients with urological and gynaecological malignancies. Possible therapeutic applications for laparoscopic ultrasonography, such as the direction of laparoscopic interstitial laser therapy or brachytherapy, remain to be evaluated. In the staging of hepatobiliary and pancreatic malignancies, no single investigations are alone satisfactory. Rather, their unique but complementary roles are better appreciated when incorporated into investigative algorithms. We believe there is now good evidence to support the inclusion of laparoscopy, augmented by the innovative technique of laparoscopic ultrasonography, within such a management strategy.

REFERENCES

1. Cuesta MA, Meijer S, Borgstein PJ. Laparoscopy and the assessment of digestive tract cancer. *Br J Surg* 1992; **79**: 486–7.
2. Windsor JA, Garden OJ. Laparoscopic ultrasonography. *Aust NZ J Surg* 1993; **63**: 1–2.
3. Garden OJ. Operative ultrasonography. *Hospital Update* 1992; **18**: 470–9.
4. Rifkin MD, Weiss SM. Intraoperative sonographic identification of nonpalpable pancreatic masses. *J Ultrasound Med* 1984; **3**: 409–11.
5. Sigel B, Machi J, Ramos JR, Duarte B, Donahue PE. The role of imaging ultrasound during pancreatic surgery. *Ann Surg* 1984; **20**: 486–93.
6. Plainfosse MC, Bouillot JL, Rivaton F, Vaucamps P, Hernigou A, Alexandre JH. The use of operative sonography in carcinoma of the pancreas. *World J Surg* 1987; **11**: 654–8.
7. Serio G, Fugazzola C, Iacono C *et al.* Intraoperative ultrasonography in pancreatic cancer. *Int J Pancreatol* 1992; **11**: 31–41.
8. Trede M, Schwall G, Saeger HD. Survival after pancreatoduodenectomy. 118 consecutive resections without an operative mortality. *Ann Surg* 1990; **211**: 447–58.
9. Klotter HJ, Rückert K, Kümmerle F, Rothmund M. The use of intraoperative sonography in endocrine tumours of the pancreas. *World J Surg* 1987; **11**: 635–41.
10. Angelini L, Bezzi M, Tucci G *et al.* The ultrasonic detection of insulinomas during surgical exploration of the pancreas. *World J Surg* 1987; **11**: 642–7.
11. Norton JA, Cromack DT, Shawker TH *et al.* Intraoperative ultrasonographic localisation of islet cell tumours: a prospective comparison to palpation. *Ann Surg* 1988; **207**: 160–8.
12. Van Heerden JA, Grant CS, Czako PF, Service FJ, Charboneau JW. Occult functioning insulinomas: which localizing studies are indicated? *Surgery* 1992; **112**: 1010–15.
13. Rösch T, Lightdale CJ, Botet JF *et al.* Localization of pancreatic endocrine tumors by endoscopic ultrasonography. *New Eng J Med* 1992; **326**: 1721–6.

14. Charnley RM, Hardcastle JD. Intraoperative abdominal ultrasound. *Gut* 1990; **31**: 368–9.
15. Bismuth H, Castaing D. *Operative Ultrasound of the Liver and Biliary Ducts.* Berlin, Springer-Verlag, 1987.
16. Couinaud C. *Le Foie: Etudes Anatomiques et Chirurgicales.* Paris, Masson, 1957.
17. Bismuth H, Castaing D, Garden OJ. The use of operative ultrasound in surgery of primary liver tumours. *World J Surg* 1987; **11**: 610–14.
18. Makuuchi M, Hasegwa H, Yamazaki S, Takayasu K, Moriyama N. The use of operative ultrasound as an aid to liver resection in patients with hepatocellular carcinoma. *World J Surg* 1987; **11**: 615–21.
19. Lau WY, Leung KL, Lee TW, Li AKC. Ultrasonography during liver resection for hepatocellular carcinoma. *Br J Surg* 1993; **80**: 493–4.
20. Gozzetti G, Mazziotti A, Bolondi L *et al.* Intraoperative ultrasonography in surgery for liver tumours. *Surgery* 1986; **99**: 523–9.
21. Brower ST, Dumitrescu O, Rubinoff S, McElhinney JA, Aufses AH Jr. Operative ultrasound establishes resectability of metastases by major hepatic resection. *World J Surg* 1989; **13**: 649–57.
22. Parker GA, Lawrence W, Horsley SJ *et al.* Intraoperative ultrasound of the liver affects operative decision making. *Ann Surg* 1989; **209**: 569–77.
23. Machi J, Takeda J, Kakegawa T *et al.* The detection of gastric and esophageal tumour extension by high-resolution ultrasound during surgery. *World J Surg* 1987; **11**: 664–71.
24. Hayashi S, Wagai T, Miyazawa R *et al.* Ultrasonic diagnosis of breast tumor and cholelithiasis. *West J Surg Obstet Gynecol* 1962; **70**: 34.
25. Yamakawa K, Wagai T *et al. LapUS. Proc Jap Soc Ultrasonics* 1963; **5**: 41.
26. Fukuda M, Mima S, Tanabe T, Suzuki Y, Hirata K, Terada S. Endoscopic sonography of the liver–diagnostic application of the echolaparoscope to localize intrahepatic lesions. *Scand J Gastroenterol* 1984; **19** (suppl. 102): 24–8.
27. Look D, Henning H, Yano N. Direkte ultraschallechographie der gallenblasse unter laparoskopischer sicht. *Forschritte der Gastro-Enterologischen Endoskopie.* Baden-Baden, Witzstrock, 1975 (Lindner H, ed.; vol VI).
28. Fukuda M, Hirata K, Saito K *et al. Studies on Intraluminal Echography in Abdominal Diseases: Echolaparoscopy.* 4th European Conference in Ultrasonics in Medicine, Amsterdam, 1981.
29. Ota Y, Sato Y, Takatsui K *et al.* New ultrasonic laparoscope. Improvement in diagnosis of intraabdominal disease. *Scand J Gastroenterol* 1982; **78** (suppl. 17): 194.
30. Fukuda M, Mima F, Nakano Y. Studies on echolaparoscopy. *Scand J Gastroenterol* 1982; **78** (suppl. 17): 186.
31. Furukawa Y, Sakamoto F, Kanazawa H *et al.* A new method of B-mode ultrasonography under laparoscopic guidance. *Scand J Gastroenterol* 1982; **78** (suppl. 17): 186.
32. Amaraki N, Yoshida K, Yamashiro Y *et al.* Ultrasonic laparoscopy. *Scand J Gastroenterol* 1982; **78** (suppl. 17): 185.
33. Hirata K, Mima S, Fukuda M. High resolution ultrasonography in cancer diagnosis–advances and indications of intraluminal sonography. *Gan To Kagaku Ryoho* 1986; **13**: 1661–7.
34. Bönhof JA, Linhart P, Bettendorf U, Holper H. Liver biopsy guided by laparoscopic sonography. A case report demonstrating a new technique. *Endoscopy* 1984; **16**: 237–9.
35. Fornari F, Civardi G, Cavanna L *et al.* Laparoscopic ultrasonography in the study of liver diseases: preliminary results. *Surg Endosc* 1989; **3**: 33–7.

36. Frank K, Bliesze H, Bönhof JA, Beck K, Hammes P, Linhart P. Laparoscopic sonography: a new approach to intraabdominal disease. *J Clin Ultrasound* 1985; **13**: 60–5.
37. Okita K, Kodama T, Oda M, Takemoto T. Laparoscopic ultrasonography. Diagnosis of liver and pancreatic cancer. *Scand J Gastroenterol* 1984; **19** (suppl. 94): 91–100.
38. Miles WFA, Paterson-Brown S, Garden OJ. Laparoscopic contact hepatic ultrasonography. *Br J Surg* 1992; **79**: 419–20.
39. Murugiah M, Paterson-Brown S, Windsor JA, Miles WFA, Garden OJ. Early experience of laparoscopic ultrasonography in the management of pancreatic carcinoma. *Surg Endosc* 1993; **7**: 177–81.
40. Gudjonsson B. Cancer of the pancreas. *Cancer* 1987; **60**: 2284–303.
41. Carter DC. Cancer of the pancreas. *Gut* 1990; **31**: 494–6.
42. Cameron JL, Pitt HA, Yeo CJ, Lillemoe KD, Kaufman HS, Coleman J. One hundred and forty-five consecutive pancreatoduodenectomies without mortality. *Ann Surg* 1993; **217**: 430–8.
43. Warshaw AL, Fernández del Castillo C. Pancreatic carcinoma. *New Eng J Med* 1992; **326**: 455–65.
44. Cuschieri A. Laparoscopy for pancreatic cancer: does it benefit the patient? *Eur J Surg Oncol* 1988; **14**: 41–4.
45. Warshaw AL, Gu ZY, Wittenberg J, Waltman AC. Preoperative staging and asessment of resectability of pancreatic cancer. *Arch Surg* 1990; **125**: 230–3.
46. Greene FL. Laparoscopy in malignant disease. *Surg Clin N Am* 1992; **72**: 1125–37.
47. Rösch T, Braig C, Gain T *et al.* Staging of pancreatic and ampullary carcinoma by endoscopic ultrasonography. Comparison with conventional sonography, computed tomography and angiography. *Gastroenterology* 1992; **102**: 188–99.
48. Jori GP, Peschle C. Combined peritoneoscopy and liver biopsy in the diagnosis of hepatic neoplasm. *Gastroenterology* 1972; **63**: 1016–19.
49. Bleiberg H, Rozencweig M, Mathieu M, Beyens M, Gompel C, Gerard A. The use of peritoneoscopy in the detection of liver metastases. *Cancer* 1978; **41**: 863–7.
50. Rosen CB, Nagorney DM, Taswell HF *et al.* Perioperative blood transfusion and determinants of survival after liver resection for metastatic colorectal carcinoma. *Ann Surg* 1992; **216**: 493–505.
51. Savage AP, Malt RA. Survival after hepatic resection for malignant tumours. *Br J Surg* 1992; **79**: 1095–101.
52. Lightdale CJ, Winawer SJ, Kurtz RC, Knapper WH. Laparoscopic diagnosis of suspected liver neoplasms: value of prior liver scans. *Dig Dis Sci* 1979; **24**: 588–93.
53. Cosgrove DO, McReady RV. *Ultrasound Imaging: Liver, Spleen, Pancreas*. Chichester, Wiley, 1982.
54. Wernecke K, Henke L, Vassallo P *et al.* Pathological explanation for hypoechoic halo seen on sonograms of malignant liver tumours: an *in vitro* correlative study. *AJR* 1992; **159**: 1011–16.
55. Wernecke K, Vassallo P, Bick U, Diederich S, Peters PE. The distinction between benign and malignant liver tumors on sonography: value of a hypoechoic halo. *AJR* 1992; **159**: 1005–9.
56. Bismuth H, Houssin D, Castaing D. Major and minor segmentectomies "réglées" in liver surgery. *World J Surg* 1982; **6**: 10–24.
57. Yamashita Y, Kurohiji T, Hayashi J, Kimitsuki H, Hiraki M, Kakegawa T. Intraoperative ultrasonography during laparoscopic cholecystectomy. *Surg Laparosc Endosc* 1993; **3**: 167–71.
58. Tio TL, Tytgat GNJ, Cikot RJLM, Houthoff HJ, Sars PRA. Ampullopancreatic carcinoma; preoperative TNM classification with endosonography. *Radiology* 1990; **175**: 455–61.

59. Grimm H, Maydeo A, Soehendra N. Endoluminal ultrasound for the diagnosis and staging of pancreatic cancer. *Baillière's Clin Gastroenterol* 1990; **4**: 869–88.
60. Grimm H, Hamper K, Binmoeller KF, Soehendra N. Enlarged lymph nodes: malignant or not? *Endoscopy* 1992; **24** (suppl. 1): 320–23.
61. Pietrabissa A, Shimi SM, Vander Velpen G, Cuschieri A. Localisation of insulinoma by laparoscopic infragastric inspection of the pancreas and contact ultrasonography. *Surg Oncol* 1993; **2**: 83–6.

Overview

Staging of abdominal malignancy

It may seem curious to most laparoscopic surgeons that before the advent of laparoscopic cholecystectomy they had given little thought to the role of diagnostic laparoscopy in the staging of intra-abdominal malignancy. It may be that, despite the enthusiastic reports by some workers, the majority of surgeons considered the information likely to be obtained from diagnostic laparoscopy was unlikely to change their clinical decision making. Clearly, the value of diagnostic laparoscopy has been augmented with the introduction of laparoscopic ultrasound, and a more complete evaluation of solid organs such as the liver can now be undertaken. Similarly, the improved ability to evaluate retroperitoneal structures such as the pancreas is likely to revolutionize the evaluation of patients with pancreatic malignancy.

16.1

Upper Thoracic Sympathectomy – Open Approaches

M. HASHMONAI and M. SCHEIN

INTRODUCTION

Historical Observations

The knowledge of the anatomy and physiology of the sympathetic nervous system evolved initially with experimental and later with clinical observations made on sympathectomy and its sequelae. In 1852, Claude Bernard[1] remarked that section of the cervical sympathetic trunk resulted in increased skin temperature of the ipsilateral side of the head associated with more active circulation. In the same year, Brown-Séquart[2] reported that stimulation of the sympathetic nerves resulted in vasoconstriction. Gaskell mapped out the anatomy and clarified functional concepts of the autonomous ("involuntary") nervous system.[3]

The initial clinical application of sympathectomy was not devoted to the treatment of vasospastic disorders. The first clinical surgical sympathectomy was performed by Alexander in 1889[4] for the treatment of epilepsy. Jonnesco in 1896[5] and Jaboulay in 1899[6] extended its application to the treatment of exophthalmic goitre, François-Franck in 1899[7] considered its application to the treatment of glaucoma and Jonnesco in 1916[8] treated angina pectoris by sympathectomy. The wider application of sympathectomy to various painful visceral conditions was advocated by Leriche during the early decades of the present century.[9]

The potential value of this operation in the treatment of vasospastic disorders was first realized by Jaboulay in 1899[6] and more widely employed by his pupil Leriche.[10] Brüning[11] by 1922 had used it extensively for the treatment of Raynaud's phenomenon and scleroderma. In 1920, Kotzareff[12] demonstrated its effectiveness in abolishing hyperhidrosis. In 1924 Hunter,[13] Royle[14] and subsequently Brown and Adson[15] extended the use of sympathectomy to the treatment of spastic paralysis, meticulously recording their observations on the effects of the operation on skin microcirculation, its temperature and sweating capacity. Following the first lumbar sympathectomy performed by Diez[16] and the experience accumulated by Adson and Brown,[17] sympathectomy became established as a therapeutic modality for the treatment of vascular disorders of the limbs.

Anatomical and Physiological Considerations in the Development of Surgical Methods

The sympathetic innervation arises from the intermediomedial and intermediolateral columns of the spinal cord. The preganglionic neurons are located in the spinal cord segments C8 to L2. The preganglionic fibres emerge from the cord by way of the ventral roots of the spinal nerves and reach the paravertebral sympathetic ganglionic trunk as the white rami communicantes. The uppermost pathway for the emerging preganglionic fibres is usually T2 and only rarely higher pathways (T1 and C8) exist. Within the trunk, they make synaptic connections with the postganglionic neurons mostly at the level of the same segment or they may pass upwards or downwards to higher or lower segments before doing so. In the upper part of the sympathetic trunk, the C7 and T1 sympathetic ganglia are fused to form the stellate ganglion. Cranially, there are two additional (the middle and upper cervical) sympathetic ganglia, whose preganglionic fibres emerge all from lower segments and ascend through the stellate ganglion.[18,19] The postganglionic fibres emerge from the ganglia as the grey rami communicantes which merge with the peripheral nerves, while some branches join the major arteries. The postganglionic neurons innervate the smooth muscle fibres of blood vessels, the piloerector muscles and the sweat glands. The vasomotor sympathetic postganglionic fibres were considered to be cholinergic, whereas the sudomotor fibres were adrenergic.[19] However, more recent studies have shown dual adrenergic and cholinergic innervation of the sweat glands.[20]

The sympathetic innervation of vasomotor and sudomotor functions is claimed to be dependent upon different pathways, which would explain the occasional recurrence of vasospasm of a hand after an initially successful sympathectomy, although its sudomotor function remains abolished.[21] Anatomical variations exist. It has been demonstrated by anatomical studies that accessory or intermediate sympathetic ganglia may be present outside the sympathetic trunk.[22] Preganglionic fibres make synaptic connections in these ganglia and their postganglionic fibres actually bypass the major sympathetic ganglionic trunk, functioning as independent sympathetic pathways.[18,21,23] Another alternative route is the inconsistent nerve of Kuntz, a branch of the ventral root of the second spinal nerve containing communicating rami, which merges with the first thoracic nerve, bypassing the second thoracic ganglion.[21] The presence of such independent pathways is considered by many authors to be the cause for recurrent sympathetic activity to the upper limb following an initially successful sympathectomy.[21,22,24,25] Presently, there is ample evidence that mainly the second thoracic ganglion is responsible for the sympathetic innervation of the hand,[20,21,24,26–32] whereas T4 supplies the axilla.[28,33,34]

The initial method of sympathectomy was through periarterial dissection. It was developed by Jaboulay[6] and further extended by Leriche.[10] Proximal periarterial sympathectomy, however, was abandoned particularly after Kramer and Todd[35] demonstrated that sympathetic fibres run peripherally with the sensory nerves which they abandon to join the arteries at successive levels. To overcome this anatomical obstacle Brüning[11] performed the first cervicothoracic (stellate) ganglionectomy. The results of this procedure, mostly performed in vasospastic and occlusive vascular conditions, were more disappointing than the results of lumbar sympathectomy and return of sympathetic vasomotor activity to the hand was often observed. This led Telford[32,36] and Smithwick[37] to develop what they considered a preganglionic ramisectomy. Their technique consisted of dividing the rami connecting T2 and T3 ganglia, transecting the chain between T3 and T4, raising the two ganglia and suturing the T3 ganglion outside the chest cavity. This procedure was considered to be a preganglionic ramisectomy. Their belief was based on the assumption that the preganglionic fibres to the upper limbs penetrate the sympathetic chain at a level lower than T1, ascend within the chain and synapse within the stellate ganglion, which remained undisturbed by their technique. That this is not the case was proven by Haxton[38] who also performed a T2–T3 ramisectomy, but unlike Telford and Smithwick transected the chain between T1 (the stellate) and T2 ganglia, rotating the T2–T3 ganglia downwards and into the extrathoracic position. At present, it is almost unanimously accepted that T2–T3 ganglionectomy efficiently achieves sympathetic denervation of the upper limb.[20,21,24,28,29,31] Nevertheless, as stated by Ray,[23] there is no absolute guarantee of achieving complete sympathetic denervation of the upper limb whatever operation is performed.

Pathophysiology of Sympathectomy

Sudomotor Effect

Upper thoracic sympathectomy arrests the secretory activity of eccrine sweat glands in the denervated parts of the upper limb. This effect is total or near total in practically all operated patients and permanent in the vast majority.[28,29,31,39–42]

Circulatory Effect

There are few reports on the vasomotor effect of sympathectomy in subjects with normal circulation. From animal studies it is obvious that sympathectomy substantially increases blood inflow to the limb[43] as well as venous return.[44] Increased limb flow is not accompanied by a significant improvement of oxygen consumption[45] and is attributed to the opening of arteriovenous precapillary

Table 16.1.1 Indications for upper thoracic sympathectomy

1.	Arteriospastic disorders	
	a.	Raynaud's disease
	b.	Acrocyanosis
2.	Occlusive arteriolar disorders	
	a.	Raynaud's phenomenon (associated with underlying diseases): i. Collagen diseases, like scleroderma ii. Haematological disorders, like cryoproteinaemia
	b.	Microembolism, including intra-arterial drug injection
	c.	Thrombangiitis obliterans
	d.	Arteriosclerosis
	e.	Occupational digital thrombosis
	f.	Early stages of cold injury
3.	Neurological disorders	
	a.	Post-traumatic sympathetic dystrophy
	b.	Causalgia
	c.	Vibrating tools syndrome
	d.	Late sequelae of cold injury
4.	Hyperhidrosis	

anastomoses.[45,46] In response to sympathectomy skin capillary flow is increased in humans with occlusive arterial disease of the lower extremity as proven by ^{133}Xe,[47] ^{141}Ce, ^{51}Cr and ^{85}Sr[48] clearance tests. This is accompanied by a marked increase in the skin temperature.[49] Furthermore, there is a shift in distribution of blood flow from muscles to skin as shown in studies of normal humans in whom chemical sympathectomy was performed.[49]

Cardiovascular Effect

The cardiovascular effect of bilateral upper thoracic sympathectomy in healthy subjects treated for hyperhidrosis was studied by Adar's group.[50] They found a significant reduction in mean pulse rate and systolic blood pressure after the operation, both at rest and after effort. These changes persisted for two years after the operation and were considered to be permanent.

INDICATIONS

The initial indications for cervical/upper thoracic sympathectomy, namely epilepsy,[4] exophthalmic goitre,[5,6] glaucoma[7] and angina pectoris,[8] are obsolete today. The modern indications for upper thoracic sympathectomy are listed in Table 16.1.1. Some of the indications are rare conditions. In some others, like the vasospastic disorders, the long term results are rather poor and sympathectomy is reserved only for extreme conditions. As for the occlusive arterial disorders, they affect mainly the lower limb and the development of modern vascular surgery has markedly reduced the role of sympathectomy in their treatment. Thus, hyperhidrosis is by far the most common indication for which upper dorsal sympathectomy is performed today.

TECHNIQUES OF UPPER THORACIC SYMPATHECTOMY

There are three basic approaches to upper thoracic sympathectomy, which by order of invasiveness are:

1. non-surgical;
2. endoscopic;
3. open surgical.

This chapter deals with non surgical and open surgical methods.

Non-Surgical Methods

Percutaneous Phenol Sympathectomy

Neural block by means of paravertebral alcohol injections was first performed by Swetlow in 1926.[51] It was aimed for angina pectoris and the intercostal nerves. The technique was successfully developed by White,[52] who used alcohol to destroy the upper thoracic ganglia. It was commonly followed by a prolonged and painful neuritis.[53] To overcome this problem, Haxton[53] advocated the use of a phenol aqueous solution. All injections were performed by blind percutaneous needle insertion. In experienced hands, this procedure was successful, although relapses have been recorded. It had a certain value in patients whose general condition was too poor to be suitable for general anaesthesia. The advance of radiological methods facilitated the positioning of the needle in the exact required location. Fluoroscopically guided percutaneous sympathetic lysis was reported by Walker *et al.*[54] Later, computed tomographic (CT) guidance was employed[55,56] and Dondelinger and Kurziel[57] were the first to report phenol block of the upper thoracic sympathetic chain by this method.

Percutaneous Radiofrequency Sympathectomy

Wilkinson reported in 1984 a new method of percutaneous sympathectomy of the upper thoracic ganglia.[58] His technique is based on the fluoroscopically guided introduction of a probe to the desired location. Radiofrequency applied through this probe achieves high temperatures which destroy adjacent tissues.

Open Surgical Methods

Supraclavicular Approach

The classical description of this technique was given by Telford[32,36] and subsequently modified to include resection of the upper thoracic ganglia. This is the approach preferred by us and discussed herein in detail.

The operation is undertaken under general anaesthesia. A head light is helpful for illumination. A skin incision, 6–8 cm in length, is made 1 cm above and parallel to the clavicle, beginning from the sternoclavicular junction. The platysma and clavicular head of the sternocleidomastoid muscle are divided. The internal jugular vein is exposed on the medical part of the incision. The prescalene fat pad with crossing veins, arteries and lymphatics is divided or mobilized and retracted aside along with the omohyoid muscle in most instances. On the left side, care must be taken to avoid injury to the thoracic duct. At this stage the phrenic nerve overlying the anterior scalene muscle is exposed. The nerve is mobilized medially and the muscle is divided, exposing the subclavian artery. When crossing the field, the thyrocervical trunk is also divided, which allows gentle retraction of the subclavian artery in a caudal direction. The Sibson's fascia is opened between the brachial nerve plexus on the craniolateral side and the subclavian artery inferiorly. The dome of the pleura is thus exposed and mobilized anterolaterally by blunt dissection.

The sympathetic chain is visualized over the heads of the ribs and is transected between the stellate and second thoracic ganglia. Care must be taken to avoid trauma to the stellate ganglion in order to prevent Horner's syndrome. The second and third ganglia are resected by clipping and dividing all rami. If sympathectomy of the axilla is to be achieved, the fourth ganglion should be excised as well. Whenever in doubt, frozen section of the resected specimen should confirm that sympathetic ganglionectomy has indeed been performed. A thin suction tube is inserted in the extrapleural space. The sternocleidomastoid and platysma muscles are closed, the air is aspirated while the lungs are inflated and the suction tube is removed. The skin is closed.

Bilateral sympathectomy may be performed simultaneously by two experienced surgical teams, thus shortening the length of the operation. A chest radiograph is obtained in the recovery room to exclude a pneumothorax.

Posterior Approach

The classic description of this technique was given by Adson[59] and modifications were suggested by White *et al.*[60] and Smithwick.[37,61] Briefly, the heads of the upper ribs are approached by either a midline incision over the upper thoracic vertebrae with lateral traction of the back muscles which are separated from the vertebrae[17,62] or a vertical[61] or an oblique[60] paravertebral skin incision with muscle splitting. About 3 cm of the heads of the ribs (usually the second and third) must be resected together with the transverse processes of the corresponding vertebrae. This approach allows the resection of the intercostal nerves with their posterior roots and root ganglia[25,61] together with the sympathetic ganglia. Both unilateral and bilateral sympathectomy have been performed in one stage.

Axillary Approach

Devised by Schultze and Goetz,[63] this method was described and published by Atkins.[64] A transverse skin incision is made in the axilla parallel to the ribs, from the pectoralis major anteriorly to the latissimus dorsi posteriorly. When the axillary fat is incised the long thoracic nerve should be safeguarded. Next the intercostal muscles are incised at what is judged to be the second intercostal space[64] or lower down at the third or fourth spaces.[65] At this point the pleura is incised, the lung is retracted and the sympathetic chain approached by an additional longitudinal pleural incision over the heads of the ribs. At completion, a thoracic drain is recommended[65] although omitted by Atkins.[64] An extrapleural transaxillary approach with the resection of the first rib has also been described.[66] Bilateral sympathectomy by the transaxillary approach is usually performed as a staged procedure.

Transthoracic Approach

This approach was first suggested by Goetz and Marr[26] and later supported by Palumbo.[67] An incision is made over the first, the second or the third intercostal space commencing at the sternal margin. The pectoralis major is split and the pleural cavity is opened by incising the intercostal muscles. The lung is retracted downwards and the posterior parietal pleura is incised over the sympathetic chain. This allows a direct approach to the sympathetic ganglia and resection of T2 is possible without any trauma to the stellate ganglion. Originally, Goetz and Marr closed the chest without drainage.[26]

Digital Sympathectomy

The method is based on the anatomic distribution of sympathetic fibres in the hand. For each finger, the neurovascular digital bundles are exposed from the distal palm and interdigital web to the proximal phalanx. The digital nerves are gently separated from the artery and retracted, thus transecting all fibres supplying the artery. Following that, the loose adventitia surrounding the digital artery is dissected in a circumferential fashion over a length of 2 cm and removed. The procedure is repeated with the other digital artery of the same finger.

This method is usually restricted to cases in which the disease is restricted to one digit, although multiple fingers may be operated upon at the same time.[68]

RESULTS

Evaluation of the results of upper thoracic sympathectomy is complex and based mainly on the indication for which the operation has been performed, the approach chosen, the recurrence rate of sympathetic tone and the specific surgical complications.

Evaluation Based on Indications

Arteriospastic Disorders

The results published are variable: Linder *et al.*[69] reported that 80% of their patients with Raynaud's disease were improved on long term follow-up. However, similar results have not been obtained by others[18,25,41,70] and in a large recent series the operation failed within a year in two thirds of the patients[71] or more.[72] Overall, it appears that surgical sympathectomy should be reserved only for cases with imminent tissue loss or established ulcers.

Occlusive Arterial and Arteriolar Disorders

With the development of modern vascular surgical techniques, the role of sympathectomy in atherosclerosis has decreased and in the case of the upper limb it is rarely performed. Only small series appeared recently: Linder *et al.*[69] reported very good results, those of Koikkalainen *et al.*[18] were "fair" in half of the cases and poor in one quarter of them. Thrombangiitis obliterans (Buerger's disease) affects the upper limb only in its advanced stages, but its response to sympathectomy is apparently better.[18] In cases of microembolism, intra-arterial powder drug injections and occupational digital thrombosis, good results have been reported.[41] The response to sympathectomy for digital ischaemia due to collagen disease is of limited benefit[24] and should also be reserved only for cases of imminent tissue loss or established ulcers.

Neurological Disorders

Causalgia is a syndrome of severe burning pain experienced after injury to a main peripheral nerve or nerve trunk. This indication is one of the few for which sympathectomy gives excellent long term results.[41,73] Mimocausalgia (or post-traumatic sympathetic dystrophy, Sudek's atrophy, reflex dystrophy, etc.) is a group of similar pain syndromes, all related to trauma other than that to a major nerve. In a group of 35 patients with this syndrome excellent responses to sympathectomy were obtained in 74% of cases and poor results in only 9%.[74] Frostbite affects both small vessels and nerves. The late sequelae are burning pain and paraesthesia in cold and profusely sweating limbs. Sympathectomy is the most effective measure in the early stages of severe congelation trauma and is also very valuable in the management of late sequelae.[75]

Hyperhidrosis

This is probably the indication for which upper thoracic sympathectomy gives the most rewarding results. Several very large series have been published.[28,29,31,34,40,42,76–82] The short and long term results are excellent and permanent cure may be expected in about 90% of cases or more.[39,42]

Evaluation Based on Surgical Approach and Recurrence Rate

The three basic open surgical approaches to upper thoracic sympathectomy – the supraclavicular, the dorsal and the transaxillary–transthoracic – give approximately the same long term results. Large series of upper thoracic sympathectomy performed for hyperhidrosis by the supraclavicular approach,[40,42,76,77,79] the dorsal approach[29,31,80] and the transaxillary approach[65,69,83,84] show a high long term success rate (more than 90%). The choice of surgical approach should therefore be based on factors other than the rate of success of the operation.

Evaluation Based on Sequelae

Besides the usual local and general complications following surgery, a few specific postoperative sequelae have been reported: Horner's syndrome, phantom sweating, gustatory sweating, compensatory hyperhidrosis, neuralgia and waxy hands.

Horner's Syndrome

This is a distressing but preventable complication consisting of ptosis, miosis and anhydrosis of the face. In the early period of upper thoracic sympathectomy, when the stellate ganglion was routinely resected, it was an obligatory result of the operation. Since it has been established that the second thoracic ganglion is mostly responsible for the sympathetic innervation of the upper limb, the stellate ganglion is no longer resected and Horner's syndrome should not follow this procedure. Nevertheless, the syndrome is reported with an incidence which varies between zero[31,79] and 40%.[78] This wide variation in results implicates not only the surgical approach, but also the technical expertise and experience of the surgeon. It also indicates how meticulously the signs have been looked for on follow-up and the definition given by different authors to these signs. It should be emphasized that in the majority of cases the severity of the syndrome is mild and a slight eyelid drop is the only sign. It results from handling of the sympathetic chain before the trunk between the stellate and second thoracic ganglia is transected. Many patients improve during the postoperative period and the syndrome disappears altogether in the majority of cases. To prevent its occurrence, special attention must be given during sympathectomy and any handling of, or traction on, the stellate ganglion must be avoided.

Phantom Sweating

This is a feeling of sweating in the palms after sympathectomy, without any actual sweating.[85] On specific enquiry it has been reported in 26–59% of patients who underwent upper thoracic sympathectomy for hyperhidrosis.[18,42] However, the number of patients who complained spontaneously of such feeling was much smaller, which may explain why this complication is not mentioned in some large series.[29,31,76,77] In many patients this phenomenon disappears spontaneously.[18]

Gustatory Sweating

This is a bizarre response to upper thoracic sympathectomy. Described in 1931 by Guttmann,[86] it consists mainly of facial sweating triggered by spicy and some other specific foods and has been reported in up to 56% of patients.[42] Vagal reinnervation of denervated sympathetic ganglion cells,[87] proliferation of cut axons of preganglionic sympathetic cells within the spinal cord,[88] aberrant regeneration or collateral sprouting of preganglionic fibres with abnormal synapses in the superior cervical ganglion[89] and the presence of accessory sweat fibres presumably arising in the brainstem[31] are the different suggested mechanisms by which this phenomenon is explained. Kux[90] claimed that resection of the lower third of the stellate ganglion (T1) prevents this phenomenon while Bloor[91] suggested that stellate ganglionectomy was required for that purpose. Shih and Wang,[31] however, stated that gustatory phenomena are not side effects of T2–T3 ganglionectomy via the dorsal approach. They estimated that operative injury of the stellate or other cervical ganglia may be the cause. The aetiology of the phenomenon appears to be still obscure.

Compensatory Sweating

This is another unexplained sequela of upper thoracic sympathectomy, consisting of an increased perspiration in other parts of the body appearing in a large proportion of patients.[39,42,92] It is considered to be a compensatory thermoregulating mechanism,[92,93] namely that the total amount of perspiration is unchanged by sympathectomy while the sweating area is decreased.[94] However, it has been noticed to appear within six months postoperatively,[93] not necessarily at once, and it often abates spontaneously.[29,92] Furthermore, the opposite effect, namely decrease in sweating in other parts of the body following sympathectomy, has also been reported.[29,42] The mechanism of this phenomenon thus appears to be more complex than simple compensation for thermoregulatory purposes.

Neuralgia

This is another sequela of sympathectomy. It consists of pain in the sympathectomized limb, which appears some time after the operation and is reported usually to be temporary.[63,81] It has been postulated that the mechanism may be either that sensory receptors in the periphery are directly activated by a hyperfunctioning of residual postganglionic fibres spared by sympathectomy or that a simple shunting of current occurs at the damaged nerve endings from sympathetic efferent to afferent fibres.[95] Welch and Geary[41] reported the syndrome in 32% of their sympathectomies, half of the cases being permanent. However, this seems to be an exceptional figure. We have not observed it in our series[42] and it has not been reported by others.[29,31,34,40,65,69,76–78,80,83,96] Bogokowsky *et al.*[79] claimed that what is considered to be postoperative neuralgia is in many cases the result of trauma to the brachial plexus. However, it has also been observed in the dorsal approach[81] in which the plexus cannot be damaged either by direct trauma or by stretch due to positioning on the operating table. Greenhalgh *et al.*[28] claimed that in upper limb sympathectomy, neuralgia only occurs when the dorsal or transaxillary approach is used. Further studies are required to elicit the aetiology of this sequela of sympathectomy.

Waxy Hands

The waxy appearance of the hands resulting from upper thoracic sympathectomy is a very rare event. We have observed it only once. The palm of the hand becomes glossy, pink and appears to be wet, yet is completely dry. On palpation, it is very smooth and cool. The mechanism of this phenomenon is unknown.

DISCUSSION

Which approach is preferable for upper thoracic sympathectomy? When advocated by Haxton[53] in 1949, chemical percutaneous block presented a definitive advantage over surgical sympathectomy in patients posing a high anaesthetic risk, although it was recognized that return of sympathetic activity occurred in the majority of cases.[53] Today, when anaesthesia poses incomparably fewer hazards than 50 years ago, the method to be employed should be selected based on its long term success rate and on the amount of postoperative complications it involves. Chemical sympathectomy has certainly a place for indications in which the results of sympathectomy are dubious as a means to ascertain its possible affect, for cases in which only a temporary sympathicolytic effect is required or for the rare poor risk patients. For patients in whom sympathectomy is predicted to be highly effective, the method by which the best results are obtained should be used. Few long term results of CT guided upper dorsal sympathectomy are available. In a series of 63 patients from our institution, on a mean follow-up of 27 ± 14 months, only 63% showed persisting good or satisfactory results, all others representing immediate or late failures.[97] The percutaneous radiofrequency technique, devised a decade ago,[58] has not gained popularity and there are no long term reported results. Surgery is today the best method of achieving upper thoracic sympathectomy with permanent effect.

If open sympathectomy is to be performed, which of the three basic approaches – supraclavicular, dorsal or transaxillary–transthoracic – is the most appropriate? The supraclavicular route has been considered as being technically difficult, jeopardizing several important anatomic structures (the jugular vein, the thoracic duct, the phrenic nerve, the subclavian artery and the brachial plexus). Exposure is relatively difficult. Moreover, the stellate ganglion is exposed and may be damaged. Lastly, the supraclavicular scars have often been regarded as unaesthetical. Without underestimating the potential danger to the abovementioned structures, we consider the procedure to be easy in the hands of any experienced surgeon possessing a good technique. A bilateral operation may not only be performed under one anaesthetic, but even simultaneously by two teams, thus shortening the procedure. Recovery is rapid, the operation is not very painful, the postoperative hospitalization is short and scars in the neck which are parallel to the clavicle, and hence to the skin lines, are usually inconspicuous.

Based on a comparative study, the transaxillary approach was recommended by Little and May.[96] It was felt to offer superior exposure and better cosmetic results than the supraclavicular approach, but postoperative pain was apparently more severe and lung disease presented a contraindication to the transaxillary approach. Although this approach is usually considered unsuitable for a one stage bilateral sympathectomy, it has been so applied in a group of patients without increased morbidity.[70] Unlike these authors, the group of Adar[40] reported six patients who were operated upon by both the supraclavicular approach on one side and the transaxillary route on the other. All patients preferred the former approach. The posterior approach is the most painful, involving a partial resection of one or two ribs and the splitting or retraction of the dorsal muscles. Although bilateral procedures have been routinely performed,[29,31] this method implies a longer operation and more painful postoperative course. Haxton carried out several upper thoracic sympathectomies by the supraclavicular approach on one side and the dorsal route on the other.[39] He concluded that "From the surgeon's point of view the posterior approach was more difficult and time consuming, and from the patient's standpoint it proved much more painful and for a much longer period". The main advantage of the posterior approach is that it allows the resection of the spinal ganglia, anterior roots, intercostal nerves and corresponding fibres besides the sympathetic ganglia, resulting in a more radical sympathectomy of the upper limb.[25]

In conclusion, we consider the supraclavicular approach to be the easiest for the patient, although requiring an excellent surgical technique in order to keep the postoperative complications down to the minimum. The transaxillary–transthoracic approach is easier for the surgeon, but not for the patient. The dorsal approach should be reserved for exceptional cases and we cannot recommend it for routine use.

Is there a place for resympathectomy? Failure to achieve sympathectomy may be due either to inadequate resection or to recurrent sympathetic tone in the limb. For instance, if the second thoracic ganglion has not been resected, relapse of sympathetic tone in the hand is to be expected and properly performed reoperation should achieve effective sympathectomy. If the T2 and T3 ganglia have been removed in the first operation, resympathectomy should be preferably performed by the dorsal approach as suggested by Lemmens.[25] The anterior root, spinal ganglion, intercostal nerve and surrounding tissue should be removed at the level of the T2 and T3 segments. By this approach, satisfactory results have been obtained.[24] It is our personal experience that open resympathectomy after previous failed chemical or surgical procedures involves a more difficult operation due to local fibrosis and distortion of tissue planes. Therefore, reoperation should be reserved for those indications in which sympathectomy is expected to be highly effective. A different route than the first procedure is recommended.

What is the place of the open sympathectomy in the era of endoscopic surgery? The results obtained by the open surgical approaches are the gold standard with which any new method should be compared. Few large series of thoracoscopic sympathectomy have so far been reported. That of Byrne *et al.*[98] showed that on long term follow-up, only 76% were "very much improved" by the operation. Other large series[30,90] do not report long term follow-up. To answer this question a well-planned prospective randomized study is necessary. The decision regarding which method is superior should be based not only on the sympathectomy effect obtained on a long term basis, but also on the amount of immediate and late side effects, as well as the cost effectiveness of the operation. Such a trial is presently under way in our department.

REFERENCES

1. Bernard C. Sur les effets de la section de la portion céphalique du grand sympathique. *Comptes Rend Soc Biol* 1852; **4**: 168–70.
2. Brown-Séquart CE. Experimental researches applied to physiology and pathology. *M Exam* 1852; **8**: 481, 549, 617, 698.
3. Gaskell WH. *The Involuntary Nervous System*. London, Longmans, Green & Co, 1916.

4. Alexander W. *The Treatment of Epilepsy*, p. 228. Edinburgh, YJ. Pentland; 1889.
5. Jonnesco T. Resectia totala si bilaterala a simpaticulu cervical in cazuri di epilepsie si gusa exophtalmica. *Romania Med 1896;* **4**: 479–96.
6. Jaboulay M. *Chirurgie du Grand Sympathique et du Corps Thyroïde (Les Differents Goîtres).* Articles originaux et observations réunis et publiés par le Dr. Etienne Martin. Lyon, A. Storck & Cie, 1900.
7. François-Frank M. Signification physiologique de la résection du sympatique dans la maladie de Basedow, l'épilepsie, l'idiotie et le glaucome. *Bull Acad Med Paris* 1899; **41**: 565–94.
8. Jonnesco T. Angine de poitrine guérie par la résection du sympatique cervicothoracique. *Bull Acad Med Paris* 1920; **84**: 93–102.
9. Leriche R. The surgery of pain. London, Baillière, Tindall & Cox, 1939.
10. Leriche R. De l'élongation et de la section des nerfs périvasculaires dans certains syndromes douloureux d'origine artérielle et dans quelques troubles trophiques. *Lyon Chir* 1913; **10**: 378–82.
11. Brüning F. Zur Tecknik der kombinierten Resektionsmethode samtlicher sympathischen Nervenbahnen am Halse. *Zentralbl Chir* 1923; **5**: 1056–9.
12. Kotzareff A. Résection partielle du tronc sympatique cervical droit pour hyperhidrose unilatérale (régions faciale, cervicale, thoracique et brachiale droites). *Rev Med Suisse Rom* 1920; **40**: 111–13.
13. Hunter JI. The influence of the sympathetic nervous system in the genesis of the rigidity of striated muscle in spastic paralysis. *Surg Gynecol Obstet* 1924; **39**: 721–43.
14. Royle ND. A new operative procedure in the treatment of spastic paralysis and its experimental basis. *Med J Aust* 1924; **1**: 77–86.
15. Brown GE, Adson AW. Calorimetric studies of extremities following lumbar sympathetic ramisection and ganglionectomy. *Am J Med Sci* 1925; **170**: 232–40.
16. Diez J. Un nuevo método de simpatectomia periférica para el tratamiento de las afecciones tróficas y gangrenosas de los miembros. *Bol Soc Cir Buenos Aires* 1924; **8**: 792–806.
17. Adson AW, Brown GE. The treatment of Raynaud's disease by resection of the upper thoracic and lumbar sympathetic ganglia and trunks. *Surg Gynecol Obstet* 1929; **48**:577–603.
18. Koikkalainen K, Luosto R, Keskitalo E, Melartin E. Upper limb sympathectomy. *Ann Chir Gynaecol Fenn* 1974; **63**: 318–25.
19. Baljet B, Groen GJ. Anatomical considerations of the autonomic nervous system. In: Symposium on pathological blushing and sweating (ed. Gelderman PW.). *Acta Neurochir* 1985; **74**: 149–51.
20. Sato K, Kang WH, Saga K, Sato KT. Biology of sweat glands and their disorders. I. Normal sweat gland function. *J Am Acad Dermatol* 1989; **20**: 537–63.
21. Lemmens HAJ. Importance of the second thoracic segment for the sympathetic denervation of the hand. *Vasc Surg* 1982; **16**: 23–6.
22. Ehrlich E, Alexander WF. Surgical implications of upper thoracic independent sympathetic pathways. *Arch Surg* 1951; **62**: 609–14.
23. Ray BS. Sympathectomy of the upper extremity; evaluation of surgical methods. *J Neurosurg* 1953; **10**: 624–33.
24. Van Rhede van der Kloot EJH, Jörning PJG. Resympathectomy of the upper extremity. *Br J Surg* 1990; **77**: 1043–5.
25. Lemmens HAJ. Thoracic resympathectomy. *Int Angiol* 1982; **1**: 147–8.
26. Goetz RH, Marr JAS. The importance of the second thoracic ganglion for the sympathetic supply of the upper extremities – two new approaches for its removal. *Clin Proc* 1944; **3**: 102–14.
27. Hyndman OR, Wolkin J. Sympathectomy of the upper extremity. Evidence that only the second dorsal ganglion need be removed for complete sympathectomy. *Arch Surg* 1942; **45**: 145–55.

28. Greenhalgh RM, Rosengarten DS, Martin P. Role of sympathectomy for hyperhidrosis. *Br Med J* 1971; **1**: 332–4.
29. Cloward RB. Hyperhidrosis. *J Neurosurg* 1969; **30**: 545–51.
30. Edmondson RA, Banerjee AK, Rennie JA. Endoscopic transthoracic sympathectomy in the treatment of hyperhidrosis. *Ann Surg* 1992; **215**: 289–93.
31. Shih CJ, Wang YC. Thoracic sympathectomy for palmar hyperhidrosis. Report of 457 cases. *Surg Neurol* 1978; **10**: 291–6.
32. Telford ED. The technique of sympathectomy. *Br J Surg* 1935; **23**: 448–50.
33. Malone PS, Cameron AEP, Rennie JA. The surgical treatment of upper limb hyperhidrosis. *Br J Dermatol* 1986; **115**: 81–4.
34. Hartfall WG, Jochimsen PR. Hyperhidrosis of the upper extremity and its treatment. *Surg Gynecol Obstet* 1972; **135**: 586–8.
35. Kramer JG, Todd TW. The distribution of nerves to the arteries of the arm, with a discussion on the clinical value of results. *Anat Rec* 1914; **8**: 243–55.
36. Telford ED. Sympathetic denervation of the upper extremity. *Lancet* 1938; **1**: 70–2.
37. Smithwick RH. Modified dorsal sympathectomy for vascular spasm (Raynaud's disease) of the upper extremity; a preliminary report. *Ann Surg* 1936; **104**: 339–50.
38. Haxton H. The technique and results of upper limb sympathectomy. *J Cardiovasc Surg* 1970; **11**: 27–34.
39. Moran KT, Brady MP. Surgical management of primary hyperhidrosis. *Br J Surg* 1991; **78**: 279–83.
40. Kurchin A, Zweig A, Adar R, Mozes M. Upper dorsal sympathectomy for palmar primary hyperhidrosis by the supraclavicular approach. *World J Surg* 1977; **1**: 667–74.
41. Welch E, Geary J. Current status of thoracic dorsal sympathectomy. *J Vasc Surg* 1984; **1**: 202–14.
42. Hashmonai M, Kopelman D, Klein O, Schein M. Upper thoracic sympathectomy for primary palmar hyperhidrosis: long term follow-up. *Br J Surg* 1992; **79**: 268–71.
43. May AG, DeWeese JA, Rob CG. Effect of sympathectomy on blood flow in arterial stenosis. *Ann Surg* 1963; **158**: 182–8.
44. Gaskell WH. Further researches on the vasomotor nerves of ordinary muscles. *J Physiol* 1879; **1**: 262–302.
45. Kreutzer W, Schenk WC Jr. Hemodynamic responses to lumbar sympathectomy. *J Cardiovasc Surg* 1972; **13**: 532–7.
46. Delaney J, Scarpino J. Limb arteriovenous shunting following sympathetic denervation. *Surgery* 1973; **73**: 202–6.
47. Moore WS, Hall AD. Effects of lumbar sympathectomy on skin capillary blood flow in arterial occlusive disease. *J Surg Res* 1973; **14**: 151–7.
48. Rutherford RB, Valenta J. Extremity blood flow and distribution: the effects of arterial occlusion, sympathectomy and exercise. *Surgery* 1971; **69**: 332–44.
49. Wright CJ, Cousins MJ. Blood flow distribution in the human leg following epidural sympathetic blockade. *Arch Surg* 1972; **105**: 334–7.
50. Papa MZ, Schneiderman J, Tuker E, Bass A, Drori Y, Adar R. Cardiovascular changes after bilateral upper dorsal sympathectomy. *Ann Surg* 1986; **204**: 715–18.
51. Swetlow GI. Alcoholic injections into nerve tissues for relief of pain. *Am J Med Sci* 1926; **171**: 397–407.
52. White JC. *The Autonomic Nervous System.* London, H. Kimpton, 1935.
53. Haxton HA. Chemical sympathectomy. *Br Med J* 1949; **1**: 1026–8.
54. Walker PM, Key JA, MacKay IM, Johnston KW. Phenol sympathectomy for vascular occlusive disease. *Surg Gynecol Obstet* 1978; **146**: 741–4.
55. Von Schild H, Günther R, Hoffmann J, Goedecke R. CT-gesteuerte Blockade des Plexus coeliacus mit ventralem Zugang. *Fortschr Röntgenstr* 1983; **139**: 202–5.
56. Rosen RJ, Miller DL, Imparato AM, Riles TS. Percutaneous phenol sympathectomy in advanced vascular disease. *Am J Roentgenol* 1983; **141**: 597–600.

57. Dondelinger RF, Kurziel JC. Percutaneous phenol block of the upper thoracic sympathetic chain with computed tomography guidance. *Acta Radiol* 1987; **28**: 511–15.
58. Wilkinson HA. Percutaneous radiofrequency upper thoracic sympathectomy: a new technique. *Neurosurgery* 1984; **15**: 811–14.
59. Adson AW, Brown GE. Raynaud's disease of the upper extremities; successful treatment by resection of the sympathetic cervicothoracic and second thoracic ganglions and the intervening trunk. *JAMA* 1929: **92**: 444–9.
60. White JC, Smithwick RH, Allen AW, Mixter WJ. A new muscle splitting incision for resection of the upper thoracic sympathetic ganglia. *Surg Gynecol Obstet* 1933; **56**: 651–7.
61. Smithwick RH. The rationale and technic of sympathectomy for the relief of vascular spasm of the extremities. *New Eng J Med* 1940; **222**: 699–703.
62. Cloward RB. Upper thoracic sympathectomy: surgical technique. *Surgery* 1969; **66**: 1120–6.
63. Atkins HJB. Sympathectomy by the axillary approach. *Lancet* 1954; **1**: 538–9.
64. Atkins HJB. Peraxillary approach to the stellate and upper thoracic sympathetic ganglia (letter). *Lancet* 1949; **2**: 1152.
65. Sternberg A, Brickman S, Kott I, Reiss R. Transaxillary thoracic sympathectomy for primary hyperhidrosis of the upper limbs. *World J Surg* 1982; **6**: 458–63.
66. Roos DB. Experience with first rib resection for thoracic outlet syndrome. *Ann Surg* 1971; **173**: 429–42.
67. Palumbo LT. Anterior transthoracic approach for upper thoracic sympathectomy. *Arch Surg* 1956; **72**: 659–66.
68. Shaw Wilgis EF. Digital sympathectomy. In: *Current Therapy in Vascular Surgery*, 2nd edition (eds Ernst CB, Stanley JC.), pp. 208–12. Toronto, B C Decker Inc, 1991.
69. Linder F, Jenal G, Assmus H. Axillary transpleural sympathectomy: indication, technique, results. *World J Surg* 1983; **7**: 437–9.
70. Campbell WB, Cooper MJ, Sponsel WE, Baird RN, Peacock JH. Transaxillary sympathectomy – is a one-stage bilateral procedure safe? *Br J Surg* 1982; **69**(suppl.): S29–S31.
71. De Trafford JC, Lafferty K, Potter CE, Roberts VC, Cotton LT. An epidemiological survey of Raynaud's phenomenon. *Europ J Vasc Surg* 1988; **2**: 167–70.
72. Cotton LT, Khan O. Raynaud's phenomenon: a review. *Int Angiol* 1986; **5**: 215–36.
73. Buker RH, Cox WA, Scully TJ, Seitter G, Pauling FW. Causalgia and transthoracic sympathectomy. *Am J Surg* 1972; **124**: 724–7.
74. Olcott IV C, Eltherington LG, Wilcosky BR, Shoor PM, Zimmerman JJ, Fogarthy TJ. Reflex sympathetic dystrophy – the surgeon's role in management. *J Vasc Surg* 1991; **14**: 488–95.
75. Kyösola K. Clinical experiences in the management of cold injuries: a study of 110 cases. *J Trauma* 1974; **14**: 32–6.
76. Soliman SM. Modified supraclavicular approach for upper thoracic sympathectomy. *J Roy Coll Surg Edinb* 1984; **29**: 162–6.
77. Conlon KC, Keaveny TV. Upper dorsal sympathectomy for palmar hyperhydrosis. *Br J Surg* 1987; **74**: 651.
78. Adar R, Kurchin A, Zweig A, Mozes M. Palmar hyperhidrosis and its surgical treatment: a report of 100 cases. *Ann Surg* 1977; **186**: 34–41.
79. Bogokowsky H, Slutzki S, Bacalu L, Abramsohn R, Negri M. Surgical treatment of primary hyperhidrosis. A report of 42 cases. *Arch Surg* 1983; **118**: 1065–7.
80. Gruszkiewicz J, Doron Y, Guilburd JN, Zaaroor M. Hyperhidrosis and its surgical treatment. *Acta Neurochir* 1986; **81**: 128–31.
81. Golueke PJ, Garrett WV, Thompson JE, Talkington CM, Smith BL. Dorsal sympathectomy for hyperhidrosis – the posterior paravertebral approach. *Surgery* 1988; **103**: 568–72.

82. Law NW, Ellis H. Transthoracic sympathectomy for palmar hyperhidrosis in children under 16 years of age. *Ann Roy Coll Surg Eng* 1989; **71**: 70–1.
83. Jochimsen PR, Hartfall WG. Peraxillary upper extremity sympathectomy: technique reviewed and clinical experience. *Surgery* 1972; **71**: 686–93.
84. Ellis H. Transaxillary sympathectomy in the treatment of hyperhidrosis of the upper limb. *Am Surg* 1979; **45**: 546–51.
85. Kurchin A, Mozes MD, Walden R, Adar R. Phantom sweating. *Angiology* 1977; **28**: 799–802.
86. Guttmann L. Die Schweisssekretion des Menschen in ihren Beziehungen zum Nervensystem. *Z Neurol Psychiat* 1931; **135**: 1–48.
87. Murray JG, Thompson JW. Collateral sprouting in response to injury of the autonomic nervous system, and its consequences. *Br Med Bull* 1957; **13**: 213–19.
88. Bloor K. Gustatory sweating and other responses after cervico-thoracic sympathectomy. *Brain* 1969; **92**: 137–46.
89. Kurchin A, Adar R, Zweig A, Mozes M. Gustatory phenomena after upper dorsal sympathectomy. *Arch Neurol* 1977; **34**: 619–23.
90. Kux M. Thoracic endoscopic sympathectomy in palmar and axillary hyperhidrosis. *Arch Surg* 1978; **113**: 264–6.
91. Bloor K. Regeneration after cervicothoracic sympathectomy producing gustatory responses. *Angiology* 1966; **17**: 143–7.
92. Shelley WB, Florenc R. Compensatory hyperhidrosis after sympathectomy. *New Eng J Med* 1960; **263**: 1056–8.
93. Gjerris F, Olesen HP. Palmar hyperhidrosis. Long-term results following high thoracic sympathectomy. *Acta Neurol Scand* 1975; **51**: 167–72.
94. Shoenfeld Y, Shapiro Y, Machtiger A, Magazanik A. Sweat studies in hyperhidrosis palmaris and plantaris. A survey of 60 patients before and after cervical sympathectomy. *Dermatologica* 1976; **152**: 257–62.
95. Raskin NH, Levinson SA, Hoffman PM, Picket III JBE, Fields HL. Postsympathetic neuralgia. Amelioration with diphenylhydantoin and carbamazepine. *Am J Surg* 1974; **128**: 75–8.
96. Little JM, May J. A comparison of the supraclavicular and axillary approaches to upper thoracic sympathectomy. *Aust NZ J Surg* 1975; **45**: 143–6.
97. Saranga D. Upper thoracic sympathectomy by percutaneous extra-pleural phenol injection under computerized tomography guidance as management of primary palmar hyperhidrosis. MD thesis, University of Tel Aviv, 1992.
98. Byrne J, Walsh TN, Hederman WP. Endoscopic transthoracic electrocautery of the sympathetic chain for palmar and axillary hyperhydrosis. *Br J Surg* 1990; **77**: 1046–9.

16.2

Thoracoscopic Sympathectomy

N. J. STANDFIELD

INTRODUCTION

Upper thoracic sympathectomy is a well-tried and recognized procedure for the treatment of hyperhidrosis, causalgia, hypothermic injury, circulatory disorders and other poorly understood conditions such as erythromelalgia, acrocyanosis and following prolonged disuse of a limb in spastic paralysis or poliomyelitis. Until recently most surgeons have performed this procedure by one of several possible open approaches (see Chapter 16.1) and the use of chemical sympathectomy using phenon[1] has never really become established.[2] Upper thoracic sympathectomy, perhaps more than any other surgical operation, is most suitable to the endoscopic approach as the actual operation is simple, whereas the open surgical approach is difficult and associated with a definite morbidity. Specialist centres have been performing endoscopic sympathectomy for over 15 years now[3] and many large series are now available for comparison with the open procedures.[2,4]

TECHNIQUE OF ENDOSCOPIC UPPER THORACIC SYMPATHECTOMY

Preoperative assessment

Once the decision has been taken to perform upper thoracic sympathectomy a preoperative chest X-ray is performed to exclude any concommitant lung or pleural pathology. Although minor pleural adhesions may be safely divided thoracoscopically, dense adhesions may obscure the sympathetic chain. Bilateral sympathectomies can be performed at the same operation, but if so it is best to commence with the right side as this carries a higher potential morbidity due to the proximity of the azygos vein.

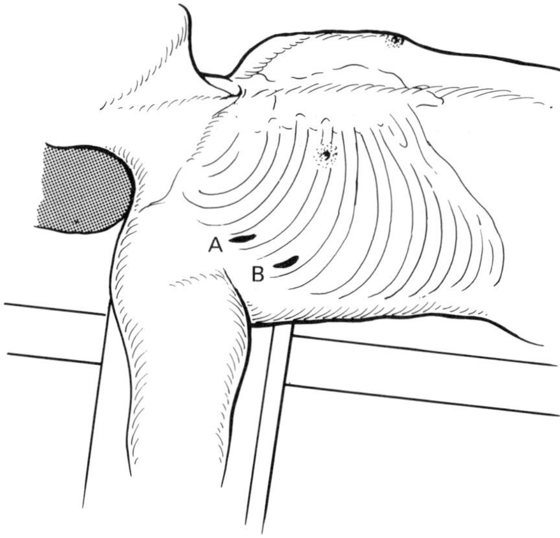

Figure 16.2.1 Position of the patient on the operating table for thoracoscopic sympathectomy. The points for insertion of the laparoscope (A) and electrocoagulation hook (B) are demonstrated.

Procedure

General anaesthesia is instituted and a double lumen endotracheal tube inserted. The patient is placed on the operating table in a reverse Trendelenburg position with both arms abducted to 90° and supported on arm boards (Fig. 16.2.1). Once the anaesthetist has collapsed the appropriate lung a small incision is made over the second or third intercostal space in the anterior axillary line (so as to avoid injury to the long thoracic nerve) and a Veress needle inserted into the pleural cavity. Approximately 500 ml of carbon dioxide is insufflated to ensure complete collapse of the underlying lung before inserting a 10 mm port through which an end-viewing video laparoscope is passed. It is not usually necessary to maintain insufflation of the pleural cavity, but if required a pressure not exceeding 6 mmHg should be used. Excessive insufflation pressure will lead to oxygen desaturation and cardiac arrhythmias. If these occur the carbon dioxide should be released and the lung temporarily re-expanded.

The sympathetic chain is easily visualized as it runs over the necks of the ribs and can usually be followed from the second to fifth ribs. A second 5 mm port is inserted through the fourth intercostal space in the same line as the first port. Some surgeons prefer to place this second port more anteriorly in the midclavicular line[4] but for cosmetic reasons the anterior axillary line is to be preferred if possible. An electrocoagulation probe or hook is inserted through this second port (some surgeons do not use a port and simply insert the hook directly through a small skin incision) and if the sympathetic chain cannot be clearly

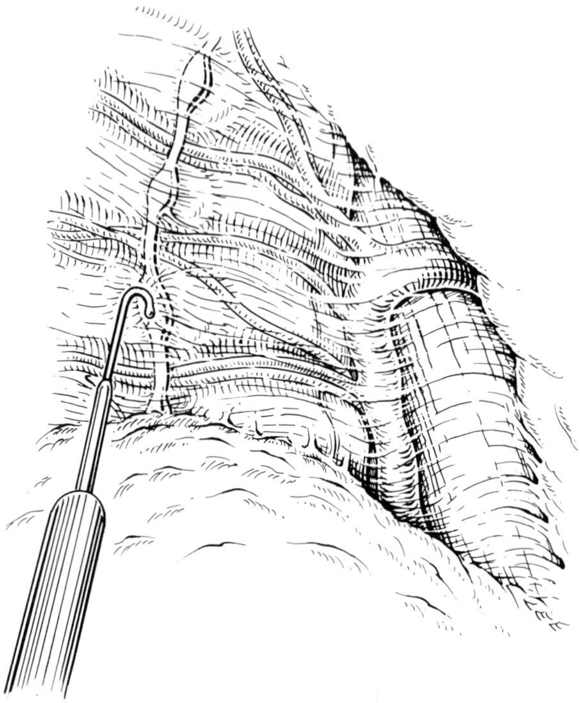

Figure 16.2.2 The view during thoracoscopic sympathectomy on the patient's right side. The collapsed lung is visible inferiorly, the azygos vein medial to the sympathetic chain and the dome of the pleura superiorly.

recognized it can be "palpated" using this hook (Fig. 16.2.2). If identification remains a problem the pleura can be incised with electrocoagulation and the hook used to pick up the sympathetic chain. The second, third and fourth sympathetic ganglia with the intervening chain are then systematically destroyed with electrocoagulation. The fifth ganglion should be included if denervation of the axilla is required although there has been some debate recently as to whether ablation down to the fourth ganglion is adequate. Occasionally access to the fifth ganglion is obscured by the apex of the collapsed lung. Insertion of a third port to retract the lung will solve this problem. Using this approach the stellate ganglion is not visualized as it is obscured by the apical fascia at the dome of the pleural cavity and is therefore protected from injury.

When upper thoracic sympathectomy is performed on the right side, care must be taken to avoid injury to the azygos vein as it ascends medial to the chain (Fig. 16.2.2). When this technique was first introduced many surgeons – making do with gynaecological laparoscopic instruments – performed the procedure using a single port and a laparoscope with an operating channel. However, the improved manipulation which is associated with a second port makes the "two port" technique preferable.

On completion of the procedure a small irrigating catheter is passed down the second port and 5 ml of 0.5% bupivacaine flushed over the area of surgery, following which the lung is re-expanded under endoscopic vision. A small paediatric chest drain connected to an underwater seal can be inserted through one of the port sites to ensure there is no residual pneumothorax. This is then removed in the recovery area after a chest X-ray has confirmed complete re-expansion of the lung. Some surgeons remove this drain on the operating table once the anaesthetist has fully expanded the collapsed lung by manual ventilation, after first observing complete re-expansion endoscopically.

The incisions are closed with interrupted sutures after infiltrating with 0.5% bupivacaine. Peroperative antibiotics are not required. Confirmation of the success of the sympathectomy may be obtained by recording palmar temperature before and after the procedure. This should rise by a mean of 1.6°C after sympathectomy.[5]

Potential complications

Bleeding from adjacent vessels and problems related to raised intrathoracic pressure are the main potential complications although these can be kept to a minimum by careful dissection and insufflating only small volumes of carbon dioxide. Minor complications related to wound pain and paraesthesia in the upper limb should only be transient. If care is taken to ensure complete re-expansion of the lung, clinically significant postoperative pneumothoraces should not occur.

RESULTS

In a series of 41 transthoracic endoscopic sympathectomies performed by the author there have been no complications related to bleeding and no patient has required a postoperative chest drain for pneumothorax. Patients with underlying pulmonary disease, particularly those who smoke, are at risk of postoperative chest infection, but to date only two patients in the author's series have required antibiotics and none have needed hospitalization. Because the stellate ganglion is difficult to identify, postoperative Horner's syndrome is rare and in the author's experience has occurred in one patient, but resolved by six weeks. The majority of patients leave hospital on the first postoperative day, although unilateral procedures could be performed on a day case basis if required.

Since the introduction of endoscopic upper thoracic sympathectomy in 1978[3] large series are now available for long term analysis. One such series from the Mater Hospital in Dublin reviewed 85 patients with palmar/axillary hyperhidrosis who underwent bilateral thoracoscopic sympathectomies since 1980.[4]

Mean hospital stay was three days and immediate postoperative results were assessed by the patients as "very much improved" or "moderately improved" in 92%. This assessment persisted in 85% after a mean follow-up of 43 months. Transient postoperative Horner's syndrome occurred in three patients, surgical emphysema in three and only one patient required a postoperative chest drain for pneumothorax. One patient required a repeat procedure for an inadequate initial operation. Compensatory hyperhidrosis, a recognized complication of thoracic sympathectomy usually affecting the waist, back of the trunk and thighs,[2] was reported in 64% of patients.

DISCUSSION

The problem with upper thoracic sympathectomy in the past has always been the large and often technically demanding surgical access required with its associated morbidity. The ability to achieve similar long term results using thoracoscopy has resulted in the endoscopic approach becoming the operation of choice when upper thoracic sympathectomy is required.[2] In cases of axillary hyperhidrosis, when ablation of the fifth ganglion is required, the endoscopic approach facilitates access with relative ease when compared with the open approaches. Only in occasional cases when dense apical pleural adhesions are encountered might open surgery be required, although this would appear to be rare from current reports.

REFERENCES

1. Reid W, Watt SK, Gray TG. Phenol injection of the sympathetic chain. *Br J Surg* 1970; **57**: 45–50.
2. Hederman WP. Endoscopic sympathectomy. *Br J Surg* 1993; **80**: 687–8.
3. Kux M. Thoracic endoscopic sympathectomy in palmar and axillary hyperhidrosis. *Arch Surg* 1978; **113**: 264–6.
4. Byrne, J, Walsh TN, Hederman WP. Endoscopic transthoracic electrocautery of the sympathetic chain for palmar and axillary hyperhidrosis. *Br J Surg* 1990; **77**: 1046–9.
5. Chester JF, Jeddy TA, Taylor RS, Dormandy JA, Allt-Graham J. Efficacy of endoscopic transthoracic sympathectomy assessed by peroperative palmar temperature measurement. *Br J Surg* 1992; **79**: 752.

Overview

Thoracic sympathectomy

The use of the endoscopic technique for upper thoracic sympathectomy is not new but has recently reached a much wider audience on the back of the laparoscopic revolution. The ability to perform the identical surgical procedure using thoracoscopic techniques, with results equally good (if not better) than those performed using large and painful incisions, even in the hands of experts such as Hashmonai and Schein, has now rendered open thoracic sympathectomy all but obsolete. It would appear that only those patients with severe intrapleural adhesions cannot be offered the endoscopic operation, and palmar hyperhydrosis, an affliction for which surgery is the only chance of cure, can now be treated endoscopically as a day case procedure in the majority of patients.

Index